# THE CAL... W9-APR-095
## Calorie, Fat & Carbohydrate Counter

## Contents

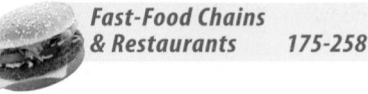

## EXTRA DIET GUIDES & COUNTERS

# Weight Control Tips

## Eat & Drink Sensibly

- Avoid fad diets. Eat 3 sensible portion-controlled meals daily.
- Limit fats, high-fat foods/snacks and sugar. Eat adequate fresh fruit & vegetables.
- Limit soft drinks, energy drinks, fruit juice and alcohol. Quench your thirst on water. (See Sample Meal Plan ~ Page 11)

## Exercise Daily

- Aim for at least 30 minutes daily – even in 5-10 minute lots. For motivation, find an exercise buddy, personal trainer or join a gym. (Extra Notes ~ Page 12)

## Reshape Eating Behaviors

- Be aware of eating and shopping behaviors that lead to overeating.
- Also focus on social and emotional situations that may trigger compulsive eating. (Extra Notes ~ Page 14)

## Keep a Food & Exercise Journal

- A journal helps you see exactly what you eat and drink, and how much you exercise. (Extra Notes ~ Page 15)
- An excellent motivator and proven weight loss aid. Keeps you honest!

## Arrange Moral Support

- Gain the support of family and friends.
- Get extra professional help if required, from your doctor, dietitian, psychologist, exercise trainer, or slimming group.
- Beware of family saboteurs who discourage you from adopting a healthier lifestyle!

### DOCTOR CHECK-UP

*Ask your doctor to check your blood pressure, blood sugar and blood cholesterol levels.*

## HEALTHY WEIGHTS
### ~ MEN & WOMEN ~
#### (Over 18 Years)

Based on weights with least risk of disease or death from heart disease, diabetes, stroke and cancer.

Based on Body Mass Index of 20-25

BMI calculated as: $\dfrac{\text{Weight (kg)}}{\text{Height (m)}^2}$

| Height (No Shoes) Ft Ins | | Healthy Weight Range (Pounds) |
|---|---|---|
| 4'7" | ~ | 86-108 |
| 4'8" | ~ | 88-110 |
| 4'9" | ~ | 92-114 |
| 4'10" | ~ | 97-121 |
| 4'11" | ~ | 99-123 |
| 5'0" | ~ | 101-127 |
| 5'1" | ~ | 105-132 |
| 5'2" | ~ | 110-136 |
| 5'3" | ~ | 112-140 |
| 5'4" | ~ | 114-145 |
| 5'5" | ~ | 119-149 |
| 5'6" | ~ | 123-156 |
| 5'7" | ~ | 127-158 |
| 5'8" | ~ | 129-162 |
| 5'9" | ~ | 134-167 |
| 5'10" | ~ | 138-173 |
| 5'11" | ~ | 143-178 |
| 6'0" | ~ | 145-182 |
| 6'1" | ~ | 149-187 |
| 6'2" | ~ | 156-193 |
| 6'3" | ~ | 158-198 |
| 6'4" | ~ | 162-202 |
| 6'5" | ~ | 170-211 |
| 6'6" | ~ | 172-215 |
| 6'7" | ~ | 175-220 |

## Body Fat Distribution & Health

Moderate amounts of body fat do not compromise health. However, excess fat above the hips carries a far greater health risk than fat on or below the hips - better to be a 'pear-shape' than an 'apple-shape'.

**Abdominal obesity** greatly increases the risk of developing diabetes, heart disease, high blood fats, hypertension, stroke, sleep apnea, arthritis and some cancers. So-called 'cellulite' carries no extra health risk.

**Waist Circumference** directly reflects the increased health risk of abdominal obesity. Waist size associated with a high health risk:

**Men** ~ Over 40 inches    **Women** ~ Over 35 inches

## Body Mass Index (BMI)

BMI is a general (but not specific) indicator of body fatness. Although BMI alone is not diagnostic, the higher the BMI, the greater the health risk of developing diabetes, high blood pressure and heart disease. BMI does not apply to heavily muscled persons. BMI is used in a different way for children.

*Abdominal obesity greatly increases the risk of ill-health and earlier death.*

**Check Your BMI:** Find your height (no shoes) - look across the row to the weight nearest your own. Then track down to BMI.

| Ht | WEIGHT (LBS) ~ ADULTS | | | | | | | | | | | | | |
|-----|-----|-----|-----|-----|-----|-----|-----|-----|-----|-----|-----|-----|-----|-----|
| 5'1" | 100 | 106 | 111 | 116 | 122 | 127 | 132 | 137 | 143 | 148 | 153 | 158 | 185 | 211 |
| 5'2" | 104 | 109 | 115 | 120 | 126 | 131 | 136 | 142 | 147 | 153 | 158 | 164 | 191 | 218 |
| 5'3" | 107 | 113 | 118 | 124 | 130 | 135 | 141 | 146 | 152 | 158 | 163 | 169 | 197 | 225 |
| 5'4" | 110 | 116 | 122 | 128 | 134 | 140 | 145 | 151 | 157 | 163 | 169 | 174 | 204 | 232 |
| 5'5" | 114 | 120 | 126 | 132 | 138 | 144 | 150 | 156 | 162 | 168 | 174 | 180 | 210 | 240 |
| 5'6" | 118 | 124 | 130 | 136 | 142 | 148 | 155 | 161 | 167 | 173 | 179 | 186 | 216 | 247 |
| 5'7" | 121 | 127 | 134 | 140 | 146 | 153 | 159 | 166 | 172 | 178 | 185 | 191 | 223 | 255 |
| 5'8" | 125 | 131 | 138 | 144 | 151 | 158 | 164 | 171 | 177 | 184 | 190 | 197 | 230 | 262 |
| 5'9" | 128 | 135 | 142 | 149 | 155 | 162 | 169 | 176 | 182 | 189 | 196 | 206 | 236 | 270 |
| 5'10" | 132 | 139 | 146 | 153 | 160 | 167 | 174 | 181 | 188 | 195 | 202 | 207 | 243 | 278 |
| 5'11" | 136 | 143 | 150 | 157 | 165 | 172 | 179 | 186 | 193 | 200 | 208 | 215 | 250 | 286 |
| 6'0" | 140 | 147 | 154 | 162 | 169 | 177 | 184 | 191 | 199 | 206 | 213 | 221 | 258 | 294 |
| 6'1" | 144 | 151 | 159 | 166 | 174 | 182 | 189 | 197 | 204 | 212 | 219 | 227 | 265 | 302 |
| 6'2" | 148 | 155 | 163 | 171 | 179 | 186 | 194 | 202 | 210 | 218 | 225 | 233 | 272 | 311 |
| 6'3" | 152 | 160 | 168 | 176 | 184 | 192 | 200 | 208 | 216 | 224 | 232 | 240 | 279 | 319 |
| 6'4" | 156 | 164 | 172 | 180 | 189 | 197 | 205 | 213 | 221 | 230 | 238 | 246 | 287 | 328 |

| BMI | 19 | 20 | 21 | 22 | 23 | 24 | 25 | 26 | 27 | 28 | 29 | 30 | 35 | 40 |

**BMI Classification:**

**BMI Below 19**
Underweight

**BMI 19-24.9**
Healthy Weight
(Low Health Risk)

**BMI 25-29.9**
Overweight
(Moderate Health Risk)

**BMI 30-40**
Obese (High Health Risk)

**BMI Over 40**
Morbid Obesity
(Very High Risk)

Interactive BMI Calculator
www.calorieking.com

# Calories & Weight Loss

## Calories in Food

Calories in food are derived from protein, fat and carbohydrate. Alcohol also provides calories. Vitamins, minerals and water provide no calories.

### Calorie Values Per Gram

| | |
|---|---|
| **Fat/Oil** | ~ 9 Calories |
| Carbohydrate | ~ 4 Calories |
| **Protein** | ~ 4 Calories |
| Alcohol | ~ 7 Calories |

Note that fats have over double the calories of protein and carbohydrate. The higher the fat content of food, the higher the calories.

### Sample Calculation

QUARTER POUNDER®
WITH CHEESE
has 510 calories
derived from:

| | | |
|---|---|---|
| 26g Fat (x 9 cals/gram) | = | 234 |
| 40g Carbohyd.(x 4 cals/gram) | = | 160 |
| 29g Protein (x 4 cals/gram) | = | 116 |
| Total Calories | = | 510 |

## Calorie Levels for Weight Loss

Start with a calorie-controlled diet that allows a moderate weight loss of ½ - 1 pound per week. Weight loss is usually much greater in the first few weeks due to extra fluid losses.

Note: It is better to increase exercise rather than lessen food calories too drastically.

### Suggested Calories for Weight Loss

| | | |
|---|---|---|
| **Women:** | Non-active | 1000 - 1200 |
| | Active | 1200 - 1500 |
| **Men:** | Non-active | 1200 - 1500 |
| | Active | 1500 - 1800 |
| **Teenagers:** | | 1200 - 1800 |

Choose**MyPlate**.gov

The MyPlate symbol **represents the recommended proportion of foods from each food group. It focuses on the importance of making smart food choices in every food group, every day. Daily physical activity is also important.** *(More info: www.ChooseMyPlate.gov)*

## Examples of Single Serving Sizes

**Grains (Eat 6 servings per day):**
- 1 slice wholegrain bread (1 oz)
- ½ bun, small bagel or English muffin
- 4 small crackers or 1 tortilla
- 1 oz ready-to-eat wholegrain cereal
- ½ cup cooked cereal, rice or pasta

**Vegetables (Eat 3-5 servings per day):**
- 1 cup raw leafy vegetables
- 1½ cups raw chopped vegetables
- ½ cup cooked vegetables
- ½ - ¾ cup vegetable juice

**Fruit (Eat 3-5 servings per day):**
- 1 medium apple, orange, banana
- ½ cup canned fruit (in own juice)
- ¼ cup dried fruit
- ½ cup fruit juice (unsweetened)
- ¼ medium avocado

**Protein (2-3 servings per day):**
- 2-3 oz (cooked) lean meat/poultry/fish
- 2 eggs **or** 6 oz tofu **or** ¼ cup nuts
- 1 cup (cooked) dried beans **or** chickpeas

**Dairy (2-3 servings per day):**
- 1 cup (8 fl.oz) milk/soy (enriched)/yogurt
- 1½ oz cheese or ½ cup cottage cheese

## Portion Size Counts!

Food portion size is critical to controlling calorie intake for weight control.

Super-sized food servings have become more common when eating out and in the home. This can mean a day's worth of calories being consumed in one meal; or a snack being equivalent to a full meal.

It is easy to underestimate portion size of foods and drinks, and unwittingly consume excess calories – even if the fat content is low or even zero!

To more accurately estimate portion size of different foods, weigh and measure your food with food scales, measuring spoons and cups. Better control of calories will result.

**For a visual idea of portion sizes, visit www.CalorieKing.com** See examples (fries and cola) on this page.

### Allow for Extra Calories in Packaged Food

The actual weight of packaged foods is usually 5-10% more than the label net weight (the minimum legal weight) – and in some cases up to 50% more. However, manufacturers calculate the calories based on the net weight. For actual calories, weigh the product and calculate the extra calories.

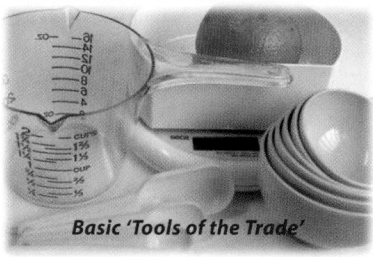

*Basic 'Tools of the Trade'*

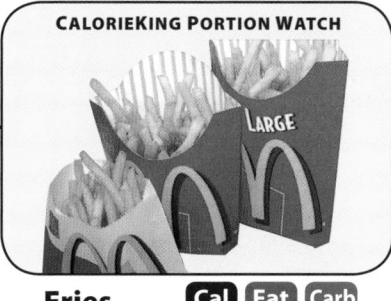

**CALORIEKING PORTION WATCH**

| Fries | Cal | Fat | Carb |
|---|---|---|---|
| Small | 230 | 11 | 29 |
| Medium | 380 | 19 | 48 |
| Large | 500 | 25 | 63 |

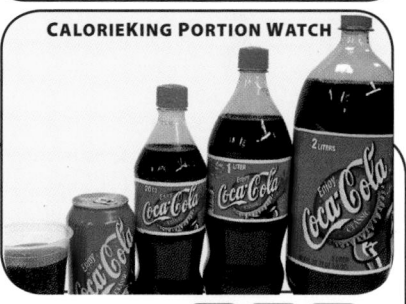

**CALORIEKING PORTION WATCH**

| Cola | Cal | Fat | Carb |
|---|---|---|---|
| 8 fl.oz Cup | 100 | 0 | 25 |
| 12 fl.oz Can | 150 | 0 | 37 |
| 20 fl.oz Bottle | 250 | 0 | 63 |
| 1 Liter Bottle | 400 | 0 | 100 |
| 2 Liter Bottle | 800 | 0 | 200 |

3.75 oz — 4.65 oz

Actual weight of this bun is 24% more than the stated net weight.

## ▶ Fat in the Diet

Fats in the diet are essential for good health. However, too much fat can contribute to obesity and a higher risk of heart disease, high blood pressure, diabetes, gallstone and certain cancers.

Dietary fat and oils have over double the calories of carbohydrates and protein. (Example: Changing from whole-milk to non-fat milk halves the calories.)

### MAXIMUM DESIRABLE FAT INTAKE (DAILY)

| Calories | Fat |
|----------|-----|
| 1200 cals | 30g fat |
| 1500 cals | 40g fat |
| 1800 cals | 50g fat |
| 2000 cals | 60g fat |
| 2200 cals | 70g fat |
| 2500 cals | 80g fat |
| 3000 cals | 110g fat |

### ZERO GRAMS TRANS FAT

*Don't be fooled by **Zero Grams Trans Fat** boldly displayed on some high-fat snacks. They are still high in fat and calories.*

*Examples: Cheetos 99c pkg ~ 24g fat, 380 cals Lay's Chips (2¾ oz pkg) ~ 27g fat, 430 calories*

0 grams
Trans Fat

## ▶ Beware low-fat foods

It is a mistake to think that eating low-fat or fat-free foods allows you to eat double the quantity. You can end up with even more calories than eating smaller amounts of regular-fat products.

Food products which are fat-free but high in calories include soda drinks, fruit juices, beer, alcoholic spirits, sugar and candy. Bread, rice and pasta also have negligible fat but need to be eaten in controlled amounts.

Ultimately, **it is food portion size as well as total calories that count** whether from fat, carbohydrate or protein. Remember, cows get fat on grass!

*Reduced fat and fat-free foods are not necessarily low calorie. Portion size is still important.*

3 Cookies
**140 Calories**

6 oz Fat-Free Muffin:
**450 calories**

### FOOD LABEL MEANINGS

**FDA Nutrition Claim Definitions**
(All are on a Per Serving Basis)

*Low Calorie:* 40 Calories or less

*Light or Lite:* One third fewer calories or, 50% or less fat than regular product

*Fat-Free:* Less than half a gram of fat

*Low-Fat:* 3 grams or less of fat

*Reduced Fat:* 25% less fat than regular product

*Fewer or Less Calories:* At least 25% fewer calories than regular product

# Tips to Reduce Fat

## ► Meats, Poultry, Fish

- **Choose lean cuts** of meat with little marbling. **Trim all visible fat** from meat and remove the skin from poultry. Removal of fat after cooking, is okay (to prevent dryness). Choose 'extra lean' ground beef.
- **Avoid high-fat meat products** such as salami, bacon, sausage and franks.
- **Broil or bake. Avoid frying in oil.** Allow casseroles to cool and skim off surface fat.
- **Avoid fried fish,** frozen fish in batter and canned fish in oil.

## ► Fats & Oils

- **Use minimal amounts** of all types of fat and oil. All are high in calories.
- **Choose** 'light' and 'reduced fat' spreads but still use sparingly.
- Use minimal amounts of oil when stir-frying. Use no-stick sprays like Pam.

## ► Salad Dressings & Sauces

- **Avoid regular mayonnaise and oil dressings.** Choose 'light', 'reduced fat' or 'fat-free' brands.
- **Choose low-fat or fat-free sauces** (mainly tomato-based). Avoid 'pesto', 'alfredo', 'cheese' and 'creamy' sauces.

## ► Milk, Cheese

- **Choose low-fat or nonfat milks and yogurts.** Avoid full-cream milk, cream, Half & Half.
- **Cheese:** Choose fat-free, and low-fat cheese. Part-skim ricotta is still high in fat. Low-fat cottage cheese is a good choice. Cheese substitutes can still be high in fat.

## ► Snacks, Cookies, Candy

- **Avoid** high-fat snacks such as potato chips, corn/tortilla chips, cheese puffs, buttered popcorn, chocolate and carob bars.

## ► Desserts/Sweets

- **Avoid high-fat desserts,** such as cake, pie, pastries, cheesecake, full-fat puddings.
- **Choose** fresh fruits, fresh fruit salad, canned fruit in water pack, low-fat ice cream. Use low-fat yogurt in place of cream.

## ► Fast-Foods & Take-Out

*Check the Fast-Foods Section of this book for actual fat and calorie counts.*

- **Avoid deep-fried foods such as** chicken, french fries and onion rings.
- **Pizzas:** Avoid sausage/pepperoni. Choose vegetarian topping and modest quantity of cheese. Eat a moderate serving. Eat extra salad and fresh fruit.
- **Hamburgers:** Choose medium size, lower fat burgers. Avoid bacon. Have a side salad (with fat-free dressing).
- **Delis:** Choose sandwiches/bread rolls, pitas with low-fat fillings and plain salad. Limit meat/cheese to small portions.
- **Coffees:** Avoid large sizes of latte and frappuccino. Request nonfat milk and no whipped cream. Avoid cookies and pastries.

*Extra Information: www.CalorieKing.com*

### FRYING ADDS FAT!

The greater the surface area of potato exposed to fat or oil, the higher the fat content and calories.

 **Whole Potato (3 oz)** `0g Fat` 65 Cals

 **Roasted Potato (3 oz)** `5g Fat` 155 Cals

 **Fries (Large cut, 3 oz)** `12g Fat` 220 Cals

 **Fries (Small, 3 oz)** `15g Fat` 265 Cals

 **Potato Chips (3 oz)** `30g Fat` 450 Cals

## Naturally-Friendly Carbs

- **Carbohydrate foods in their more natural forms** (not overly processed) are essential to good health. They are the main source of fuel for the body, and also provide important vitamins, minerals, antioxidants and fiber – all of which help protect against heart disease, diabetes, hypertension, constipation-related ailments and many other diseases.

- Carbohydrates even help the body produce serotonin, the 'feel good' brain chemical that helps control appetite and overeating. Too little serotonin can lead to mood swings and depression.

### Carbohydrates are found in different forms in food as:

- Sugars in fruit, sugar cane, milk
- Starches in whole grains, legumes, nuts, seeds and vegetables
- Dietary fiber (See Fiber Guide ~ Page 264)

*Glycemic Index & Diabetes ~ Page 21*

Carbohydrate foods (minimally processed) are essential to good health.

Be sure to eat adequate fruit and vegetables (5 - 7 servings) every day.

| RECOMMENDED CARBOHYDRATE INTAKE | | |
|---|---|---|
| Calories (Daily) | Carbohydrate (Grams) | Percent Carbohydrate Calories |
| 1200 cals | 100-120g | 35-40% |
| 1500 cals | 140-170g | 40-45% |
| 1800 cals | 180-200g | 40-45% |
| 2000 cals | 200-250g | 40-50% |
| 2500 cals | 310-350g | 50-55% |
| 3000 cals | 410-450g | 55-65% |

### How Much Do We Need?

- As shown in the chart, well-balanced diets above 2000 calories contain 50-60% of total calories from carbohydrates.
- At lower calorie levels used for weight control (1200-1500 calories), carbohydrates account for as little as 40% of total calories. This is because protein calories have nutritional priority.
- Carbohydrates & Diabetes ~ *See Page 21*

## Low-Carbohydrate Diets

- Popular low-carbohydrate diets are extreme in their recommendations to initially cut carb intake to as little as 20 grams per day – the amount in 1 thick slice of bread, or 1 medium apple, or 1 small potato.

  This greatly increases the risk of nutritional deficiencies and compromises health, particularly if fat intake is excessive through fatty meats, high-fat dairy products, and fried foods.

- While overweight Americans do need to reduce carbohydrate intake, it should be done **sensibly as part of reducing portion size and total calories.**

- Simply eating 'low-carb' food products without regard to portion size, calories or fats, will do little to promote weight loss or good health.

- **Low-carb diets (and indeed any diet) only work if total calories are reduced.**

- Refined sugars should be one of the first targets in reducing carb intake.

**FAT MATTERS** CARBS COUNT **BUT** CALORIES ARE **KING!**

*Extra Info ~ www.CalorieKing.com*

*Sugar-free & lower carb products may still be high in calories and fat.*

- Many overweight, inactive people consume over 500 calories of refined sugars per day, either self-added or as part of food products. This is equivalent to over 30 level teaspoons – a significant amount in weight control terms. Halving this amount would be reasonable and worthwhile.

**Note:** Naturally occurring sugars in fruits, vegetables and milk are fine when consumed in normal recommended amounts. These foods are also rich in other nutrients.

Refined sugar is referred to as having 'empty calories' because it supplies calories but negligible nutrients and no fiber.

- **Most sugar in our diet is 'hidden'** in processed foods such as soft drinks, fruit drinks, candy, cookies, cake, jam, sauces, ice cream, desserts, canned foods, and breakfast cereals.

Certainly enjoy moderate quantities of these foods, but for serious weight control, look for 'low calorie', 'diet' or 'sugar-free'.

**However, be careful not to substitute sugar-rich foods with high-fat foods which might boost calories even more!**

- Be aware that sugar comes in different forms such as sucrose, glucose, fructose, malt, high-fructose corn syrup, molasses, honey and maple syrup. Check the label.

- **Sugar alcohols such as sorbitol,** mannitol and maltitol are carb-based and have ½ - ¾ the calories of regular sugar. While not counted as sugar on food labels, they do add to the carb count. Excess amounts can cause bloating, gas and diarrhea.

- **Sugar-free sweeteners** such as *Equal, DiabetiSweet, NutraSweet, Splenda, Sweet'n Low* and *Stevia* make it easy to reduce sugar in drinks and recipes. Use only in moderation. Note: Most recipes can be adapted to contain less sugar with little effect on taste or quality.

*Extra Info ~ www.CalorieKing.com*

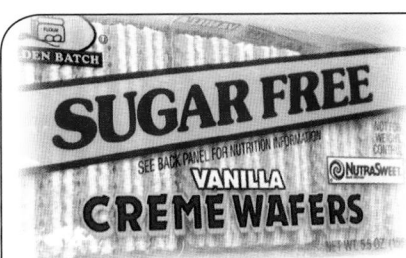

*Sugar-free snacks and foods may be higher in fat and calories than the regular product.*

| Example | ~ Creme Wafers (3): |
|---------|---------------------|
| Regular | ~ 115 cals, 6g fat |
| Sugar-Free | ~ 160 cals, 10g fat |

## SUGAR CONTENT OF SOME COMMON FOODS

### Teaspoons of Sugar

| Food | Teaspoons |
|------|-----------|
| *Coca Cola* or *Pepsi*, 12 fl.oz 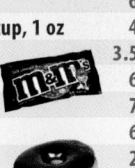 | 10 |
| 20 fl.oz size | 17 |
| Iced Tea, sweetened, 12 fl.oz | 8 |
| Chocolate Milk, 12 fl.oz | 6 |
| *Honey Smacks* Cereal, ¾ cup, 1 oz | 4 |
| Popcorn, caramel, 1 cup | 3.5 |
| Chocolate Bar, 1.5 oz  | 6 |
| *M&M's* 1.7 oz pkg | 7 |
| Muffin, large, 4 oz | 6 |
| Choc Chip Cookie, 1 oz | 2 |
| Donut, iced | 6 |
| Apple Pie, 1 piece | 7 |
| *Jell-O*, ½ cup | 4.5 |
| Jam, 1 Tbsp, ¾ oz | 2.5 |
| Syrup, maple, 1 Tbsp | 3 |

*Reach for fresh fruit when you want to snack instead of candy or snack products rich in sugar and fat.*

### The XL Generation

Some 15% of American kids and adolescents are overweight; and childhood obesity has doubled over the last 20 years. Diabetes, high blood pressure and high cholesterol are major problem areas for overweight children and adolescents, as are depression, low self-esteem, sleep apnea and bone joint problems.

To address this problem, cooperation is required between kids, parents, schools and government. Weight control is a family and community affair.

### *Five Simple Tips To Get Started:*

### ❶ Watch Soda Intake

Limit soda and sugary drinks to one serving on the weekends. Soda should not be an everyday beverage – water should be. When at restaurants or using a soda fountain, choose small servings with ice or choose diet soda instead. Schools should provide water and restrict access to soda as should parents when eating out or in the home!

### ❷ Cut back on Fast-Foods and Eating Out

Many more calories are consumed when you eat out. Healthy meals prepared at home are best for the whole family.

### ❸ Say "No" to Super-Sizing

When meals are upsized, loads more calories are consumed. Choose sensible portion sizes when eating out and at home. Use smaller plates and choose smaller packages.

### ❹ Limit Between-Meal Snacking

Watch out for high-fat and high-calorie snacks – they can have more calories than a meal! Keep your eye on portion sizes and limit salty snack foods and candy to parties and special occasions. Choose fresh fruit, vegetables, nuts and low-fat milk instead.

### ❺ Get Moving ~ Watch Less TV

Kids need at least 60 minutes of physical activity every day. It's critical for their fitness, and greatly lessens the risk of obesity.

Encourage kids to be active out of school hours. Wearing a pedometer can be highly motivational for kids to move more – as can playing dance video games such as *Dance Dance Revolution. Dance Central* (XBox360) and *Wii Fit (Nintendo)* are also excellent fitness motivators.

**Limit TV and non-active computer games** to just one hour per day. Also limit the accompanying snacks! Include exercise in family activities.

*Extra information and tips ~ www.CalorieKing.com*

# Sample Meal Plan - 1400 Calories

**For Healthy, Overweight Persons ~ Not for Persons With Any Medical Condition ~ Please Check With Your Doctor & Dietitian ~**

## Breakfast (approx. 300 cal)

| | |
|---|---|
| | *1 Small Fruit or ½ oz Dried Fruit* |
| *Plus* | *Cereal: 1½ oz Dry (high fiber)* |
| | *or 1 cup cooked Oatmeal* |
| *Plus* | *½ oz Almonds/Seeds* |
| *Plus* | *Milk (from daily allowance) or Yogurt (low-fat)* |

**Daily Milk Allowance (approx. 160 calories)**
*2 cups Non-Fat Milk or 1½ cups Low-fat (1%) Milk or equivalent Soy Drink, Yogurt, Cheese, Tofu*

**Fat Allowance (140 calories; 15g Fat)**
*4 tsp Fat or 6-8 tsp Diet Margarine or 3 tsp Oil or 1½ Tbsp Mayonnaise or ½ medium Avocado or 1½ Tbsp Peanut Butter or 30g Nuts/Seeds*

## Breakfast ~ Choice 2

| | |
|---|---|
| | *1 Small Fruit* |
| *Plus* | *2 Eggs (no added fat)* |
| | *or 2 oz Cheese (low-fat)* |
| | *or 4 oz Cottage Cheese (low-fat)* |
| | *or 2 oz Lean/Canadian Bacon* |
| *Plus* | *1 Tomato* |
| *Plus* | *1 Slice Wholegrain Toast* |

## Between Meals

*Water, Coffee, Tea, Diet drinks, Fruit from main meals; Raw vegetable pieces, Milk from Daily Allowance*

## Lunch (approx. 440 calories)

| | |
|---|---|
| | *2 slices Wholegrain Bread (2 oz)* |
| | *or 4 Crispbreads/Crackers or 6" Pita* |
| *Plus* | *2 oz lean Meat, Chicken or Turkey* |
| | *or 3½oz Tuna (in water) or 2½ oz Salmon* |
| | *or 1 oz Cheese or ½ cup (4 oz) Cottage Cheese* |
| | *or ½ cup (4 oz) Ricotta Cheese (low-fat)* |
| | *or ½ cup (4 oz) Fruit Yogurt (low-fat)* |
| | *or ½ cup (4 oz) Bean Salad* |
| *Plus* | *Large Salad (Oil-free dressing)* |
| *Plus* | *1 small Fruit or ½ oz Dried Fruit* |

## Dinner (approx. 360 calories)

| | |
|---|---|
| | *Soup (fat-free)* |
| *Plus* | *3 oz lean Meat (cooked weight)* |
| | *or 4 oz Chicken Breast (no skin)* |
| | *or 3 oz Chicken Thigh/Leg (no skin)* |
| | *or 5 oz Fish (grilled, no fat)* |
| | *or ¾ cup (6 oz) Beans (Soy, Kidney, Pinto etc)/Lentils* |
| | *or Low-fat Entree (e.g. Lean Cuisine)* |
| *Plus* | *1 small Potato* |
| | *or ½ cup Rice/Pasta/Sweet Corn* |
| | *or 1 slice Wholegrain Bread* |
| *Plus* | *2-3 servings Vegetables/Salad* |
| *Plus* | *1 small Fruit + Diet Gelatin Dessert* |

- **Persons who exercise regularly lose more weight** and keep it off longer than non-exercisers.

- **Exercise also improves general health and well-being.** Mood, confidence and self-esteem are enhanced by a sense of control and accomplishment.

- **Exercise is a good way to 'wake up' a sluggish metabolism** and burn extra fat tissue.

- **Aerobic (huff and puff) exercise most days** is great for burning calories and for cardiovascular fitness. But, it is strength training that mainly builds the muscles that burn calories even while we sleep.

- **Strength training is the key to retaining or rebuilding muscles.** As we age, we lose some 6 pounds of muscle per decade. This results in a lower metabolism and fewer calories being burnt.

  Muscles are the furnaces that burn calories. The more muscle you have, the more calories you will burn.

*Brisk walking each day is a safe and effective way to burn calories and keep fit.*
*Try it – you'll like it!*

- **Regular strength training (2-3 times weekly)** can increase our metabolic rate for several days following exercise – and an extra 100 calories per day being burnt. While 2-3 pounds of muscle may be gained in the first 8-10 weeks, weight from exercised muscles is okay. It is excess fat (particularly abdominal fat) that is a potential health hazard. Gaining muscle and losing fat also helps body reshaping – even if the scales don't show it.

- **Avoid injury** by beginning with walking, low impact aerobics, or weight-supported exercise (e.g. swimming, cycling). Avoid competitive sports. Allow 2-3 days of recovery between strength training sessions. Get professional advice ~ particularly if you have a medical condition.

- **How Much?** Start with 10-20 minutes per day and progress to 30-60 minutes per day.

  Also walk up stairs instead of using elevators. Take a brisk walk at lunch. Use an exercise bike, treadmill or stair machine while watching TV. Walk the dog.

- **How Often?** While aerobic fitness requires only 3-4 sessions weekly, **weight control is a daily event which requires daily exercise to burn calories.** Add in strength training 2-3 times weekly.

- **For motivation,** find an exercise buddy, personal trainer or join a gym.

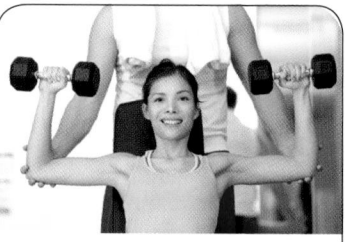

*Strength training is the key to retain or rebuild muscles.*
*Muscles burn extra calories even while you sleep.*

*For extra guidance, seek a qualified trainer or join a gym.*

# Calories Used in Exercise

| LIGHT | MODERATE | HEAVY |
|---|---|---|
| 130 lbs ~ 3 Cals/Min | 130 lbs ~ 5 Cals/Min | 130 lbs ~ 8 Cals/Min |
| 170 lbs ~ 4 Cals/Min | 170 lbs ~ 6 Cals/Min | 220 lbs ~ 12 Cals/Min |
| 220 lbs ~ 5 Cals/Min | 220 lbs ~ 7 Cals/Min | 170 lbs ~ 10 Cals/Min |
| Walking, slow | Walking, brisk | Walking (power), Jogging |
| Cycling, light | Cycling, moderate | Cycling (vigorous), Spinning |
| Frisbee playing | Swimming, crawl | Swimming, strenuous |
| Gardening, light | Weight-training, light | Weight-training, heavy |
| Golf, social | Tennis, moderate | Wrestling/Judo, advanced |
| Tennis, doubles | Racquetball, beginners | Racquetball, advanced |
| Housework, cleaning | Aerobics, light | Tae Bo, Kick Boxing |
| Calisthenics, light | Football, touch | Football, training |
| Bowling | Basketball, Baseball | Basketball (Pro) |
| Ping-pong, social | Walking Downstairs | Climbing Stairs |
| Ice Skating, light | Snow Skiing (downhill) | Skipping Rope |
| Aquarobics, light | Shovelling snow | Skiing (cross country) |
| Skate Boarding | Dancing (ballroom) | Aquarobics, advanced |
| Line/Square Dancing | Rowing, moderate | Dancing (strenuous), Zumba |
| Tai Chi, Yoga | Volleyball, competitive | Rowing, vigorous |
| Volleyball | | Martial Arts |

Note: Only those sports or activities that are sustained over a period of time (e.g running) qualify for heavy exercise. Stop-start sports such as tennis are considered 'moderate'.

## Interactive Calculations ~ www.CalorieKing.com/tools

### WALKING PROGRAM

#### USE DISTANCE, STEPS OR TIME

| Weeks | Distance | Steps Pedometer | Time |
|---|---|---|---|
| 1-2 | 1 mile | 2000 | 20 mins |
| 3-5 | 1.5 miles | 3000 | 28 mins |
| 6-8 | 2 miles | 3500 | 35 mins |
| 9-10 | 2.5 miles | 4500 | 45 mins |
| 11+ | 3.5 miles | 6000 | 60 mins |

### 10,000 STEPS PER DAY

A pedometer can motivate you to be more active. It clips to your belt or waist band and registers each step.

Aim for 8,000 - 10,000 steps per day, instead of an average of only 3,000 - 4,000 steps.

For Extra Information:
www.CalorieKing.com

# Reshaping Eating Behaviors

- Eating is a behavior that is largely controlled by people with whom we live or socialize, places in which we carry out our lives, and our emotions. Become aware of those situations that commonly lead to extra food being eaten.

- We may also be unaware of 'bad' eating habits that can lead to excess calorie intake; e.g. eating quickly, large mouthfuls, eating when tense or bored, finishing a large serving of food when not hungry.

**Tips to help uncover and correct those 'bad' or problem eating habits:**

- **Don't eat while engaged in other activities;** for example, watching TV, reading. Eat only at the table, not at the fridge or while standing.

- **Don't eat quickly.** Chewing slowly allows time to register a feeling of fullness. Don't use fingers, only utensils. Cut food into smaller pieces. Don't load your fork until the previous mouthful is finished.

- **Don't purchase problem high calorie foods.** Shop from a set list to prevent impulse buying. Avoid shopping with children.

- **Buy snack foods** in the smallest package. The larger the serving size or package, the more you are likely to eat or drink.

- **Plan meals in advance. Stick to a set menu.**

- **Plan a strategy to avoid uncontrolled eating** and drinking at social events, or when your emotions urge you to binge.

  Rehearse repeatedly in your mind exactly what you will do in such situations. Remind yourself several times each day that you are in charge of your actions and that you can be strong-willed. Seek counseling or coaching on various strategies.

- **Distract yourself** when you feel the urge to snack impulsively. Engage in some activity that will distract you from thinking about food. Examples: go for a walk, brush your teeth, phone a friend.

  If you eat out of boredom, find some new hobby or interest that gets you out of the house. Even enrol in an adult education class.

*Practice saying 'NO' politely but assertively.*

*Do you use food as an emotional crutch? If so, professional counseling may be helpful.*

**The food journal is the most powerful proven aid for dieters.** Persons who keep a food and exercise journal not only lose more weight, they also keep it off. Here are some of the reasons:

- **Recording your eating and exercise habits** jolts you into realizing just what you do eat and drink each day; and also whether you exercise sufficiently.

- **Helps you identify problem foods** and drinks with excessive calories and fat.

- **Helps identify moods,** situations and events that lead to excessive eating of unwanted calories. You can then plan to overcome or avoid them.

- **Prevents 'calorie amnesia',** the forgetfulness that leads to rebound weight gain after successful weight loss. Recording puts you back on the right track.

- **Helps you develop greater self-discipline.** You will think twice about overindulging if you have to record it - especially if someone checks your journal regularly. It certainly keeps you honest!

- **Motivates you** to carefully plan your meals and to exercise each day.

- **Serves as a check system** for your doctor, dietitian or counselor to assess your progress and make recommendations.

*Write It Down!*

*"Keeping a journal gives me feedback on exactly what I eat and drink each day.*

*It helps prevent 'calorie amnesia' and reminds me to exercise each day.*

*It's a 'must' for successful weight control!"*

## 3 Easy Ways to Track Your Food & Exercise Calories!

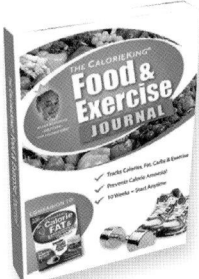

### CalorieKing Online
Part of a comprehensive personalized program that includes tools, reports and a supportive community.

### iPhone
Make smart food choices wherever you are! ControlMyWeight is easy to use & always with you.

### Book
A 10-week journal that fits in your pocket. Includes Weekly Summary page and Progress Checklist

*Extra Information ~ CalorieKing.com*

## What is Diabetes?

**Diabetes occurs when the body has difficulty processing glucose sugar in the blood.**

- **After digestion,** sugar and starches are changed into **glucose** – the simplest form of sugar vital for body energy and growth.
- Insulin is the hormone which acts like a key that opens the door to body cells and allows glucose to enter.
- **Without enough insulin,** glucose builds up in the blood and passes into the urine. High blood glucose levels lead to frequent urination, extreme thirst, and tiredness.
- **Untreated diabetes increases the risk of damage to nerves and blood vessels.** This, in turn, increases the risk of heart disease, stroke, blindness, kidney damage, foot ulcers and gangrene (with amputation), impotence and other complications.

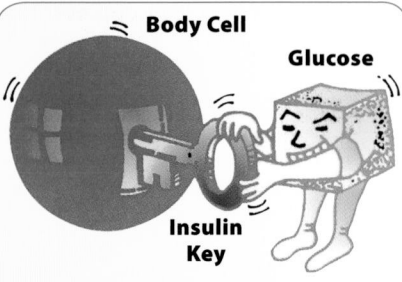

**Body Cell**

**Glucose**

**Insulin Key**

*Insulin acts like a key. It opens the door to body cells and allows glucose to enter.*

**People with type 1 diabetes and some with type 2 have too few or no keys and require insulin injections.**

**Others (primarily type 2) make enough insulin but the body doesn't use it as well as it should – particularly if obese and inactive.**

## SYMPTOMS OF DIABETES

- **Frequent urination**
- **Extreme thirst**
- **Unusual hunger**
- **Rapid weight loss**
- **Extreme fatigue**
- **Blurred vision**
- **Skin infections that are slow to heal**
- **Tingling/numbness in feet**

Note: Diabetes can be present even with no symptoms.

**DON'T IGNORE DIABETES**

*IT'S A SERIOUS DISEASE!*

## TYPE 2 DIABETES

- Occurs in 90% of diabetes cases
- Occurs mainly in adults - particularly in overweight and inactive persons
- Insulin is produced but body cells resist its action and glucose cannot enter cells
- Usually treated with meal planning and physical activity. Sometimes requires medication (pills or insulin)

## TYPE 1 DIABETES

- Occurs in 10% of diabetes cases
- Usually in children and young adults
- Pancreas produces little or no insulin. Daily insulin injections (or use of an insulin pump) are necessary, as well as:
  - matching pre-meal insulin to the amount of carbohydrate eaten
  - weight control and regular physical activity

## GESTATIONAL DIABETES

- Occurs in some women during pregnancy. It usually disappears after the baby's birth.
- Women who have had gestational diabetes still have a high risk of developing type 2 diabetes within 5 to 10 years.
- Requires weight control, a healthy lifestyle and regular medical checks

## Are You At Risk for Diabetes?

### *Pre-Diabetes ~ An Early Warning!*

Pre-diabetes means that your blood glucose levels are higher than normal, but not high enough to be called diabetes.

**If you have pre-diabetes, you have a higher risk for getting diabetes later on.**

The good news is that you can start taking steps to prevent diabetes by making healthy lifestyle changes – such as losing weight if overweight, and being more physically active.

### *WHAT'S YOUR RISK?*

***Find out if you're at risk for diabetes by answering the following questions:***

☐ I have been told I have pre-diabetes

☐ I have a family history of diabetes

☐ I am African American, Latino American, Asian American, Native American or a Pacific Islander

☐ I have had gestational diabetes (diabetes during pregnancy)

☐ I am over age 45

☐ I am overweight

☐ My waist is larger than: 35 inches (for a woman) or 40 inches (for a man)

☐ I get little or no physical activity

☐ My blood pressure is higher than 130 over 85

☐ My HDL (good cholesterol) is too low

☐ My triglycerides (blood fats) are too high

### ✔ CHECK YOUR RESULT

- If you've put a check mark in two or more of the boxes, you may be more likely to develop type 2 diabetes.

- Talk with your healthcare provider to see if you should have a blood test for diabetes.

### BLOOD GLUCOSE CLASSIFICATION OF DIABETES

| | |
|---|---|
| **Normal:** | **Below 100 mg/dl*** |
| **Pre-Diabetes:** | 100-125 mg/dl* |
| **Diabetes:** | **Over 125 mg/dl*** |

(*Fasting Blood Glucose)

### *KNOW YOUR BGL*

*(Blood Glucose Level)*
*Everyone over the age of 45 should have a blood glucose test every three years*

## Importance of Weight Control

- **Type 2 diabetes** is more common in people who are overweight.

- **Being overweight** means that your insulin doesn't work as well to control    blood glucose levels.

- **Losing just 10 to 20 pounds** can help you better manage your diabetes and lower your risk for heart disease.

- **Keys to weight control include:**

- Following a healthy eating plan

- Controlling food portions

- Being physically active most days of the week

- Keeping food records

- Setting realistic goals

- **Work with a registered dietitian** who can help you reach a weight that's ideal for you.

### *KEEP MOVING!*

*Every day, do at least 30 minutes of moderate intensity exercise.*
*(even in 5-minute sets)*

**It's the key to improving insulin action.**
**Add muscle strength training 3-4 times a week to double the benefits.**

## Managing Diabetes

Don't battle diabetes alone. Establish a partnership with your doctor, dietitian, certified diabetes educator, and pharmacist.

**Extra Support:** • *Joslin Diabetes Center*
  • *American Diabetes Association*
  • *American Association of Diabetes Educators*
  • *Juvenile Diabetes Research Foundation*
  • *National Diabetes Education Program*

**Hints to keep blood glucose within safe limits:**

• **Control your food intake.** Know what and when you will eat. Seek referral to a dietitian for expert advice.

• **Exercise regularly.** It assists weight control and can improve sensitivity of body cells to insulin. Plan physical activity into your daily routine.

• **Monitor your blood glucose** at home and work with a blood glucose meter. It will help you become familiar with your blood glucose patterns, and the effects of food, activity and medication.

• **Take insulin or oral medication as prescribed.** If on insulin, know what action to take if hypoglycemia (low blood glucose) occurs. Also educate your family and friends. More Info: www.joslin.org

### Be Heart Smart ~ Know Your ABC's

If you have diabetes, you are at a higher risk for heart attack and stroke than someone without diabetes. But you can fight back!

**Be smart about your heart!**

Take control of the ABC's of diabetes and live a long and healthy life. Talk to your healthcare provider about your ABC targets.

**A is for A1C**
The A1C (A-one-C) test – short for hemoglobin A1C. It reflects your average blood glucose (sugar) over the last 3 months.
**Suggested Target: Below 7%**

**B is for Blood Pressure**
High blood pressure makes your heart work too hard.
**Suggested Target: Below 130/80**

**C is for Cholesterol**
Bad cholesterol, or LDL, can build up and clog your arteries. **Suggested Target: Below 100**

Joslin Diabetes Center, an affiliate of Harvard Medical School, is the world's largest diabetes research center, diabetes clinic and provider of diabetes education.

**MORE INFORMATION**
www.joslin.org or call 800-344-4501

*Be smart about your heart!*

*Take control of the ABC's of diabetes and live a long and healthy life.*

*Talk to your healthcare provider about your ABC targets.*

*Take action now to lower your risk for heart attack, stroke and other diabetes problems.*

\* \* \*

◀ *Note: These targets are suggested by the National Institutes for Health and the American Diabetes Association*

**Guidelines for choosing a healthy diet apply equally to people with or without diabetes.** Eating a wide variety of foods that are mainly low in fat, low in refined sugars, and high in fiber, is recommended.

However, actual food quantities, as well as when you eat, will also influence control of blood glucose. Your dietitian will individualize a meal plan to suit your food preferences, lifestyle and medical status.

### Here are a few tips:

- **Maintain a healthy weight.** If overweight, even a modest weight loss plus daily physical activity can help manage blood glucose in type 2 diabetes.

- **Don't skip meals.** If you take insulin or an oral hypoglycemic agent, regular meals are important.

  **If on insulin,** eat meals at the same time each day. Eat a similar amount of food at each meal. Eating about the same amount of carbohydrate over the day will make best use of insulin and prevent wide variations in blood glucose levels.

- **Know which foods contain carbohydrate;** and learn how to check the *Nutrition Facts Label* on foods. Check the serving size, total fat and total carbohydrate – not just the sugar content. All carbohydrate breaks down to sugars after digestion.

- **Choose wholegrain breads, cereals and pasta.** Eat fresh fruits, vegetables and legumes. These foods contain more fiber and slow the release of glucose into your blood after a meal.

- **Limit foods high in saturated fat, trans fat and cholesterol.** Enjoy fish, soy foods, and other foods rich in omega-3 fats. *(Extra Notes: Page 259)*

- **Limit sugars and foods high in added sugar** particularly if overweight. Small amounts of sugar as part of a meal may occasionally be okay. Check with your dietitian. *(Extra Notes: Page 9)*

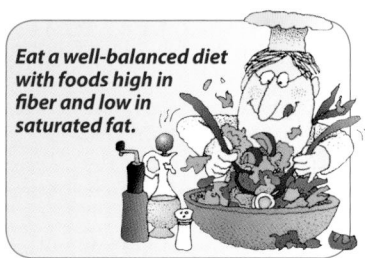

*Eat a well-balanced diet with foods high in fiber and low in saturated fat.*

*The Plate Method is an easy way to eat healthfully. (See next page)*

MAIN MEAL

Vegetables & Salad Greens

Bread • Starch • Grain    Meat • Protein

## ALCOHOL TIPS

- **If you drink alcohol, have only moderate amounts:**
  Men ~ 1-2 drinks/day
  Women ~ 1 drink/day
  For some people, safe drinking will mean no alcoholic drinks at all.

  *(Also see Alcohol Guide ~ Page 23)*

- **Drink along with your food** – especially if you use insulin or diabetes pills.

- **Do not omit any carb food** in exchange for an alcoholic drink. However, non-alcoholic beers (12 fl oz) count as one carb exchange.

- **Alcohol increases the risk of hypoglycemia** (low blood sugar) and drug interactions if you take insulin and certain types of diabetes pills.

- **Check with your doctor and dietitian.**
  *Extra Info: www.joslin.org*

## The Plate Method – An Easy Way to Eat Healthfully

The plate method is a helpful tool to guide your food choices until you see a dietitian for your own meal plan.

**For a healthy meal:**

- Fill half of your plate with non-starchy vegetables (broccoli, green beans, carrots).
- Fill a quarter of your plate with carbohydrate (wholegrain bread, pasta, potato, brown rice).
- Fill the other quarter of your plate with 3-4 ounces of lean meat, poultry, or fish.
- Use 1-2 teaspoons of tub margarine or a heart-healthy vegetable oil.
- Add a small piece of fruit or 8 ounces of skim/low-fat milk or yogurt.

## How Much Carbohydrate Should You Eat?

A dietitian can best determine how much carbohydrate you need at each of your meals, based on your lifestyle, food preferences, and overall diabetes control.

Until you see a dietitian, aim to keep the amount of carbohydrate you eat the same at each of your meals.

**MAIN MEAL**

Vegetables & Salad Greens

Bread • Starch • Grain

Meat • Protein

**PLUS ONE CHOICE**

**Milk, Fruit, Dessert or other Carb Food**

### CARB CHOICES MEAL PLAN
*One Carb Choice = 15 Grams of Carb*

**The amount in:** 1 slice Bread **or** ¾ cup Cereal (unsweetened) **or** 1 small Potato **or** 1 small Fruit

### 🍎 Breakfast
- Eat 2-3 carb choices (30-45 grams)
- Include a low-fat protein source such as egg whites or skim milk.

### 🍎 Lunch and Dinner
- Eat 3-4 carb choices (45-60 grams carb)
- Include fruit and non-starchy vegetables. Choose small portions of low-fat protein foods.

### 🍎 Snacks: If needed, eat 1-2 carb choices (15-30 grams carb).

*Note: Above plan is for adults. Carbohydrate amounts will vary with physical activity level.*

## 🔵 Joslin Diabetes Center

Joslin has books, cookbooks, videos and DVDs to help you manage your diabetes and stay healthy.

*'STAYING HEALTHY WITH DIABETES'*

*BOOK SERIES ($12.⁹⁵ each)*

WEIGHT & WELLNESS
A GUIDE FOR HEALTHY WEIGHT MANAGEMENT

PHYSICAL ACTIVITY & FITNESS

NUTRITION & MEAL PLANNING

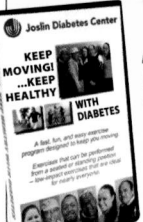

Joslin Diabetes Center

KEEP MOVING! ...KEEP HEALTHY WITH DIABETES

*FUN EXERCISE VIDEO or DVD ($26.⁹⁵)*

**10% DISCOUNT** *for Calorie King Customers!*

*ORDER*
Online: joslin.org/store or Phone 800-344-4501

*DISCOUNT CODE: CALORIEKING*

## Carb Type Affects Blood Glucose

The various forms of carbohydrate affect blood glucose levels in different ways. It is difficult to predict the effect of particular foods, sugars, or meals, simply by their carbohydrate content.

Thus the same amount of carbohydrate from different foods may affect blood sugar levels very differently. Many factors affect the rate of digestion and absorption such as:

- the type of sugar, starch, and fiber
- the degree of processing and cooking (which increases digestion rate)
- the amount of protein and fat (which slow stomach emptying and digestion).

## Glycemic Index (GI)

**The GI is a method of ranking carbohydrate foods on a scale (0-100)** according to how they affect blood glucose levels. (See next column.)

The higher the GI value, the greater the food's ability to rapidly raise blood glucose levels, and the more insulin needed by the body (not desirable).

**Eating low-GI foods may lead to better control of blood glucose and insulin levels** (which in turn lowers the risk of damage to blood vessels and nerves). The slower digestion of low-GI foods may also help to delay hunger pangs and benefit weight control.

## Cautionary Notes on GI

**Choosing low-GI foods is not a license to eat unlimited amounts.** Calorie restriction and portion control for weight control is of prime importance.

**Also remember, Low-GI foods are carbohydrate foods** and must still be counted as part of any dietetic carbohydrate plan.

GI is not meant to be used by itself without regard to portion size, and other dietary recommendations for healthy eating. Foods are not good or bad on the basis of their GI.

While GI may be a helpful tool for some people with diabetes, what is most important is to control the total amount of carbohydrate that you eat.

## LOWER-GLYCEMIC FOODS

### Slower-Acting Carbohydrates

These foods are more slowly digested and absorbed. They help maintain more even blood glucose levels, as long as excessive amounts are not eaten. Use these foods regularly but still limit portion size for weight control.

*Examples:*

- Dried beans, peas, lentils
- Nuts and seeds
- Wholegrain breads
- Bran cereals, oats
- Sweet corn, barley, buckwheat
- Wholegrain pasta, basmati rice
- Fresh fruit: apples, avocados, bananas (firm), cherries, grapefruit, grapes, olives, oranges, peaches, pears, plums. Fresh juices.
- Vegetables: broccoli, yam, sweet potatoes, salad greens
- Milk, yogurt, soy drinks
- Dark chocolate
- Sugar alcohols (sorbitol, maltitol)

## HIGHER-GLYCEMIC FOODS

### Quicker-Acting Carbohydrates

These foods more rapidly raise blood glucose levels. Eat only in moderation.

- White bread, rice cakes, bagels, croissants, doughnuts
- Low-fiber cereals: Cornflakes, *Rice Krispies, Froot Loops*
- White potatoes, white rice
- Watermelon, ripe bananas, cantaloupe, pineapple
- Soda, sugar-sweetened sports and energy drinks
- Sugar, candy, popcorn (plain)
- Ice cream (low-fat), frozen yogurt

*High-GI fruits and potatoes are still healthy choices when eaten in moderate amounts.*

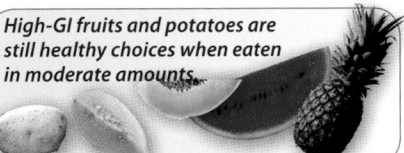

# Notes ◆ Abbreviations ◆ Disclaimer

» Calorie and fat values have been rounded off. **Calories** ~ to the nearest 5 or 10 calories. **Fat** ~ to nearest half gram. **Note:** Trace amounts of fat (less than 0.3 grams) have been treated as zero.

» **Carbohydrate figures** in this book are for total carbohydrate, and not **Net Carbs** (which deducts fiber, polydextrose and sugar alcohols from total carbs).

» Because manufacturers' figures on labels are rounded off, figures in this book may differ slightly from the label. Serving sizes may also vary.

### IMPORTANT DISCLAIMER

* The authors and publishers of this book are not physicians and are not licensed to give medical advice. This book is not a substitute for professional advice. Users should consult their medical professional before making any health, medical or other decisions based on the material contained herein.

* This book is a compilation of original material from other sources intended for educational purposes only. Because food manufacturers constantly change their products, only they are the authoritative source for food's most current nutritional information.

* Persons using the information herein for any medical purposes, such as matching insulin dosage to carbohydrate intake, should not rely solely on the accuracy of figures herein and should independently check food labels or contact the food manufacturer for the latest data.

**Canadian Readers:**

Please note that figures in this book are based on U.S. food products and restaurants. Equivalent Canadian foods may vary and should be checked independently.

### * WARRANTY DISCLAIMER:

THE AUTHOR AND PUBLISHER DISCLAIM ANY LIABILITY ARISING DIRECTLY OR INDIRECTLY FROM THE USE OF THIS BOOK. THE INFORMATION HEREIN IS PROVIDED "AS IS" AND WITHOUT ANY WARRANTY EXPRESSED OR IMPLIED. ALL DIRECT, INDIRECT, SPECIAL, INCIDENTAL, CONSEQUENTIAL OR PUNITIVE DAMAGES ARISING FROM ANY USE OF THIS INFORMATION IS DISCLAIMED AND EXCLUDED.

This information is also provided subject to Family Health Publications' Terms and Conditions found at the website, www.calorieking.com/terms and incorporated herein.

**C** ~ Calories
**F** ~ Fat (grams)
**Cb** ~ Carbohydrate (grams)

### Abbreviations

tsp = teaspoon
Tbsp or T = Tablespoon
oz = ounce(s)
c = cup
fl.oz = fluid ounce(s)
g = gram(s)
avg = average
pkg = package

### Volume Measures

(All measures are level)
3 tsp = 1 Tbsp
2 Tbsp = 1 fl.oz
½ cup = 4 fl.oz
1 cup = 8 fl.oz
2 cups = 1 Pint
2 Pints = 1 Quart

Note: 8 oz weight is not the same as 8 fl oz volume (space occupied). Dense foods weigh more per set volume. Examples:
1 cup popcorn weighs ½ oz
1 cup milk weighs 8½ oz
1 cup pudding weighs 10 oz

### Metric Conversion

½ oz = 14 grams
1 oz = 28.4 grams
2 oz = 57 grams
3½ oz = 100 grams
1 fl.oz = 30 mls
1 cup (8 fl.oz) = 240 mls
33 fl.oz = 1 liter (volume)

## INFORMATION SOURCES

• U.S. Dept. of Agriculture
• U.S. Food Manufacturers
• Food Industry Boards & Councils
• Author extrapolations

## FEEDBACK WELCOME!

Please contact the author with your queries and suggestions.
feedback@calorieking.com

- **Health Hazards: Excessive alcohol intake** contributes to obesity, high blood pressure, stroke, heart and liver disease, some cancers, and even impotence. **Concentration and short-term memory** are reduced as well as athletic performance.

  **Other alcohol hazards include:** Fetal Alcohol Syndrome, stomach upsets, menstrual problems, depression, snoring, sleep problems, work absenteeism, impaired judgement, risky behaviors and social/family problems.

- **Alcohol contributes to obesity** through its high calories and by lessening the body's ability to burn fat. Fat storage is promoted, particularly in the belly — a health danger zone. Alcohol can also stimulate the appetite; and weaken the dieter's resolve!

- **Alcohol is potentially more harmful while dieting:** Blood sugar levels may drop with resultant fatigue and further impairment of concentration, reflexes and driving skills.

*Excess alcohol contributes to obesity, high blood pressure and many other health problems*

### LOWER RISK ALCOHOL LIMITS

 **WOMEN:**
No more than
**1 drink** per day

 **MEN:**
No more than
**2 drinks** per day
(Over 65 y.o. ~ 1 drink)

(At least 2 days a week should be alcohol-free)

**1 DRINK CONTAINS 14 GRAMS ALCOHOL**
➤ 12 fl.oz Regular Beer (5% Alc.)
➤ OR 14 fl.oz Light Beer (4.2% Alc.)
➤ OR 5 fl.oz Wine (12% Alc.)
➤ OR 1½ fl.oz Spirits (80 Proof)

**Note: You cannot save daily drinks for one occasion.**
**Binge drinking is particularly harmful:**
**4 drinks for males or 3 drinks for females (within 2 hours).**

**For some people, safe drinking means no alcohol at all.** Even one drink may impair driving skills, particularly if tired. For women who drink frequently, breast cancer risk is increased by 9% for each drink after the first drink. In men, just 2 drinks a day doubles the risk of cancers of the mouth and throat.

It is advisable not to drink at all if you are:
- pregnant, trying to conceive or breastfeeding
- taking medication or have liver or heart disease (unless approved by your doctor or pharmacist)
- planning to drive, use machinery or play sports
- studying or needing to concentrate
- a child or adolescent

 **Women and adolescents are more prone to alcohol's ill-effects due to their lower body weight, smaller livers and lesser capacity to metabolize alcohol. As we age, our ability to handle alcohol decreases.**

### HOW TO CALCULATE ALCOHOL CONTENT

**Percent alcohol on label refers to alcohol volume (ml alcohol/100ml). Note: 100ml = 3½ fl.oz**

To convert to grams (weight) of alcohol, multiply the alcohol volume by 0.8 — since 1 ml of alcohol weighs only 0.8 grams.

*EXAMPLE:*
*12 fl.oz Can Beer*
*(5% alcohol)*
5% alc. volume
= 5% of 12 fl.oz = 0.6 fl.oz
= 18ml alcohol (Note: 1 fl.oz = 30ml)
Weight (18ml x 0.8) = 14.4g alcohol

### GOVERNMENT WARNINGS!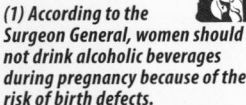

*(1) According to the Surgeon General, women should not drink alcoholic beverages during pregnancy because of the risk of birth defects.*

*(2) Consumption of alcoholic beverages impairs your ability to drive a car or operate machinery, and may cause health problems.*

### EXTRA INFORMATION
*Alcohol & Diabetes ~ See Page 19*
*Alcohol & The Heart ~ See Page 18*
*Tips to Avoid Harmful Drinking ~ Page 19*

## Quick Guide     Alc ~ Alcohol (Grams)     Cb ~ Carbohydrate

### Beer:

| | C | Alc | Cb |
|---|---|---|---|
| **Beer Contains Zero Fat:** | | | |
| **Regular Beer (5% Alc. Vol.):** | | | |
| 7 fl.oz Glass | 80 | 8.5 | 4 |
| 12 fl.oz Bottle/Can/Glass | 140 | 14 | 10 |
| 16 fl.oz Bottle/Can | 185 | 19 | 13 |
| 22 fl.oz Bottle | 260 | 26 | 18 |
| 24 fl.oz Can | 280 | 28 | 20 |
| 32 fl.oz Bottle | 370 | 38 | 28 |
| 40 fl.oz Bottle | 470 | 47 | 35 |
| 50 fl.oz Football | 590 | 59 | 50 |
| **Light Beer (4.2% Alc. Vol.):** | | | |
| 7 fl.oz Glass | 65 | 7 | 4 |
| 12 fl.oz Bottle/Can/Glass | 110 | 12 | 7 |
| 16 fl.oz Bottle/Can | 145 | 16 | 9 |
| 22 fl.oz Bottle | 200 | 22 | 13 |
| 24 fl.oz Can | 220 | 24 | 14 |
| **Non-Alcoholic Brews:** | | | |
| (Less than 0.5% alcohol by volume) | | | |
| Average all Brands, 12 fl.oz | 70 | 1 | 14 |

### Beer ~ Brands

Note: Figure shown are for the United States except for the states of Utah, Colorado, Kansas and Oklahoma who have certain restrictions limiting the alcohol content to not more than 4% by volume (3.2% by weight).

*Percentage alcohol listed is by volume - not by weight.*

*Per 12 fl.oz Serving*

| | C | Alc | Cb |
|---|---|---|---|
| **Amstel,** Light (3.5%) | 95 | 10 | 5 |
| **Anchor:** Porter (5.6%) | 210 | 15 | 23 |
| Steam (4.9%) | 160 | 14 | 14 |
| **Asahi:** Kuronama (5.3%) | 165 | 14 | 14 |
| Select (4.7%) | 140 | 13 | 11 |
| Super Dry (4.9%) | 150 | 14 | 11 |
| **Bass,** Pale Ale (5.1%) | 155 | 14 | 12 |
| **Beck's:** Original (5%) | 145 | 14 | 10 |
| Premier Light (2.3%) | 65 | 7 | 4 |
| Sapphire (6%) | 160 | 17 | 9 |
| **Big Sky:** Original IPA (6.2%) | 195 | 18 | 17 |
| Moose Drool (5.3%) | 175 | 15 | 16 |
| Scape Goat (4.7%) | 155 | 14 | 14 |
| Trout Slayer Ale ( 4.7%) | 145 | 14 | 12 |
| **Blatz:** Original (4.6%) | 145 | 13 | 13 |
| Light (3.9%) | 110 | 11 | 8 |
| **Blue Moon:** Belgian White (5.4%) | 165 | 15 | 13 |
| Grand Cru Ale (8.2%) | 230 | 21 | 14 |
| Harvest Pumpkin Ale (5.7%) | 185 | 16 | 16 |
| Spring Ale (5.4%) | 155 | 16 | 12 |
| Winter Abbey Ale (5.6%) | 180 | 16 | 15 |
| **Bohemia** (4.73%) | 140 | 14 | 12 |

## Brands (Cont)     Alc ~ Alcohol (Grams)

*Per 12 fl.oz Serving*

| | C | Alc | Cb |
|---|---|---|---|
| **Bud,** Ice (5.5%) | 120 | 16 | 4 |
| **Bud Light:** Regular (4.2%) | 110 | 12 | 7 |
| & Clamato Chelada (4.2%) | 150 | 12 | 16 |
| Platinum (6%) | 135 | 17 | 5 |
| Lime (4.2%) | 115 | 12 | 8 |
| Lime-A-Rita (8%), 8 oz | 220 | 15 | 29 |
| Lime Straw-Ber-Rita (8%), 8 oz | 200 | 15 | 24 |
| **Budweiser:** Lager (5%) | 145 | 14 | 11 |
| & Clamato Picante Chelada (5%) | 200 | 14 | 23 |
| Black Crown (6%) | 165 | 17 | 10 |
| Select (4.3%) | 100 | 12 | 3 |
| Select 55 (2.4%) | 55 | 7 | 2 |
| **Busch:** Original (4.3%) | 115 | 12 | 7 |
| Ice (5.9%) | 135 | 17 | 4 |
| Light (4.1%) | 95 | 12 | 3 |
| **Carlsberg,** Pilsner (5%) | 135 | 14 | 10 |
| **Carta Blanca** (4.6%) | 145 | 13 | 11 |
| **Castlemaine XXXX,** | | | |
| Bitter (4.6%) | 140 | 14 | 10 |
| **Cerveza,** Aguila (4%) | 125 | 11 | 11 |
| **Colt 45,** Malt Liquor (5.6%) | 155 | 16 | 11 |
| **Coors:** Banquet (5%) | 145 | 14 | 11 |
| Extra Gold (5%) | 150 | 14 | 12 |
| Light (4.2%) | 100 | 12 | 5 |
| **Corona:** Extra (4.6%) | 150 | 13 | 14 |
| Light (4.1%) | 100 | 12 | 5 |
| **Dos Equis XX:** Ambar (4.7%) | 145 | 14 | 12 |
| Lager (4.5%) | 140 | 13 | 11 |
| **Fosters:** Lager (5%) | 145 | 14 | 11 |
| Premium Ale (5.5%) | 160 | 16 | 13 |
| **Genesee:** Lager (4.5%) | 150 | 13 | 14 |
| Genny Light Lager (4%) | 100 | 10 | 4 |
| **George Killian's,** Irish Red (5.4%) | 170 | 16 | 15 |
| **Grolsch:** Blonde (2.8%) | 120 | 8 | 16 |
| Light (3.6%) | 95 | 11 | 6 |
| Premium (5%) | 145 | 14 | 10 |
| **Guinness:** Draught (4%) | 125 | 12 | 10 |
| Extra Stout (6%) | 175 | 17 | 14 |
| **Hamm's:** Original (4.7%) | 145 | 13 | 12 |
| Special Light (3.9%) | 110 | 12 | 8 |
| **Heineken:** Lager (5%) | 140 | 14 | 10 |
| Special Dark (5%) | 165 | 14 | 15 |
| Premium Light (3.5%) | 100 | 10 | 7 |
| **Henry Weinhard's,** | | | |
| Private Reserve (4.7%) | 150 | 14 | 1 |
| **Hurricane:** Malt Liquor (6%) | 140 | 17 | 4 |
| High Gravity (8.1%) | 185 | 23 | 6 |
| **Icehouse:** Original (5.5%) | 150 | 16 | 10 |
| Light (5%) | 125 | 14 | 7 |
| **Keystone:** Ice (5.9%) | 145 | 17 | 6 |
| Light (4.1%) | 105 | 12 | 5 |
| **Killian's,** Irish Red (5%) | 165 | 14 | 14 |

# Alcohol ~ Beers ◇ Ales (with Alcohol Counts)   A

**Brands (Cont)**   Alc ~ Alcohol (Grams)   Cb ~ Carbohydrate

**Beer Contains Zero Fat:**
*Per 12 fl.oz Serving*

| | C | Alc | Cb |
|---|---|---|---|
| **King Cobra** (6%) | 135 | 17 | 4 |
| **Kirin:** Ichiban (5%) | 145 | 14 | 11 |
| Light (3.2%) | 95 | 9 | 8 |
| **Kokanee Glacier** (5%) | 145 | 14 | 11 |
| **Labatt:** Blue (5%) | 135 | 14 | 10 |
| Blue Light (4%) | 110 | 11 | 8 |
| **Landshark,** Lager (4.6%) | 150 | 13 | 13 |
| **Leinenkugel's:** Original (4.6%) | 150 | 13 | 14 |
| Summer Shandy (4.2%) | 135 | 12 | 12 |
| **Lone Star:** Pale Lager (4.65%) | 135 | 13 | 11 |
| Light (3.85%) | 110 | 11 | 8 |
| **Lowenbrau,** Original (5%) | 140 | 14 | 12 |
| **Magic Hat,** #9 (5.1% alc) | 165 | 15 | 15 |
| **Magnum,** Malt Liquor (5.6%) | 155 | 16 | 11 |
| **Michelob:** Lager (4.8%) | 160 | 14 | 14 |
| Light (4.1%) | 120 | 12 | 9 |
| Amber Bock (5.1%) | 150 | 14 | 12 |
| Golden Draft (4.6%) | 120 | 13 | 7 |
| Golden Draft Light (4.1%) | 110 | 12 | 7 |
| Ultra (4.2%) | 95 | 12 | 2.5 |
| Ultra Amber (3.9%) | 95 | 11 | 3 |
| Ultra Fruit Flavors (4%) | 95 | 11 | 5.5 |
| **Mickey's,** Malt Liquor (5.6%) | 155 | 16 | 11 |
| **Miller:** Chill, 100 Calorie (4.2%) | 100 | 12 | 4 |
| Genuine Draft /High Life (4.6%) | 145 | 13 | 13 |
| High Life Light (4.1%) | 110 | 12 | 7 |
| Lite (4.2%) | 95 | 12 | 3 |
| MGD 64 (2.8%) | 65 | 8 | 2.5 |
| **Milwaukee's Best:** | | | |
| Premium (4.3%) | 130 | 12 | 11 |
| Ice (5.9%) | 145 | 17 | 7 |
| Light (4.1%) | 100 | 12 | 3.5 |
| **Minnesota's Best,** Original (4.9%) | 140 | 14 | 10 |
| **Modelo,** Especial (4.4%) | 145 | 13 | 14 |
| **Molson Canadian:** Lager (5%) | 150 | 14 | 11 |
| Ice (5.6%) | 170 | 16 | 14 |
| Light (3.9%) | 120 | 11 | 10 |
| **Moosehead,** Lager (5%) | 150 | 14 | 11 |
| **Natural:** Ice (5.9%) | 130 | 17 | 4 |
| Light (4.2%) | 95 | 12 | 3 |
| **Negra Modelo** (5.4%) | 175 | 15 | 16 |
| **Newcastle,** Brown Ale (4.7%) | 130 | 13 | 10 |
| **Old English"800",** | | | |
| Malt (5.9%) | 160 | 17 | 11 |
| **Old Milwaukee:** | | | |
| Lager (4.5%) | 150 | 13 | 15 |
| Light (4.3%) | 125 | 12 | 10 |
| Ice (5.5%) | 150 | 16 | 10 |
| **Old Style:** Lager (4.7%) | 145 | 13 | 12 |
| Light (4.2%) | 115 | 12 | 7 |
| **Pabst:** Blue Ribbon (4.7%) | 145 | 13 | 12 |
| Light (3.9%) | 110 | 11 | 8 |

**Cb** ~ Carbohydrate   C   Alc   Cb

*Per 12 fl.oz Serving  Unless Indicated*

| | C | Alc | Cb |
|---|---|---|---|
| **Pacifico,** Clara (4.4%) | 145 | 13 | 13 |
| **Piels,** Lager (4.3%) | 125 | 12 | 9 |
| **Pilsner Urquell,** Lager (4.4%) | 155 | 13 | 16 |
| **Point:** Amber Classic (4.7%) | 160 | 14 | 14 |
| Special Lager (4.7%) | 150 | 14 | 12 |
| **Redbridge,** Lager (4%) | 135 | 10 | 14 |
| **Red Dog,** Lager (5%) | 145 | 14 | 12 |
| **Red Hook:** ESB (5.8%) | 185 | 16 | 16 |
| India Pale Ale (4.7%) | 190 | 13 | 19 |
| **Red Stripe,** Jamaican Ale (5%) | 155 | 14 | 14 |
| **Redd's,** Apple Ale (5%) | 165 | 14 | 17 |
| **Samuel Adams:** | | | |
| Boston Lager (4.9%) | 175 | 14 | 17 |
| **Sam Adams,** Light Lager (4%) | 120 | 13 | 8 |
| **Sapporo,** Prem. Lager (4.9%) | 135 | 14 | 9 |
| **Schaefer:** Lager (4.6%) | 145 | 13 | 12 |
| Light (3.9%) | 110 | 11 | 8 |
| **Schell's:** Deer (4.7%) | 145 | 14 | 13 |
| Light (3.5%) | 100 | 10 | 7 |
| **Schlitz:** Pale Lager (4.6%) | 145 | 13 | 13 |
| Light (3.8%) | 110 | 11 | 8 |
| **Schmidt's:** Pale Lager (4.6%) | 145 | 13 | 13 |
| Light (3.8%) | 110 | 11 | 8 |
| **Sheaf,** Stout (5.7%) | 190 | 16 | 19 |
| **Shock Top:** Belgian White (5.2%) | 165 | 15 | 15 |
| Lemon Shandy (4.2%) | 145 | 12 | 15 |
| **Sierra Nevada:** Bigfoot (9.6%) | 330 | 28 | 32 |
| Draft Pale Ale (5%) | 155 | 14 | 13 |
| Pale Ale (5.6%) | 175 | 16 | 14 |
| Porter (5.6%) | 195 | 16 | 18 |
| **Sol** (4.2%) | 130 | 12 | 11 |
| **Southpaw,** Light (5%) | 125 | 14 | 7 |
| **Sparks,** Lager (6%) | 250 | 17 | 34 |
| **Steel Reserve:** | | | |
| High Gravity Malt Liquor (8.1%) | 220 | 23 | 15 |
| Steel 6 (6%) | 160 | 17 | 11 |
| **Stella Artois,** Pale Lager (5.2%) | 155 | 15 | 12 |
| **Stroh's:** Pale Lager (4.6%) | 145 | 13 | 12 |
| Light (3.9%) | 115 | 11 | 7 |
| **Tecate:** Pale Lager (4.6%) | 140 | 13 | 11 |
| Light (4%) | 110 | 10 | 11 |
| **Third Shift,** Amber Lager (5.3%) | 185 | 15 | 18 |
| **Trader Jose:** | | | |
| Premium Lager (5%), 11.2 fl.oz | 145 | 14 | 14 |
| Light (3.8%), 11.2 fl.oz | 105 | 14 | 8 |
| **Widmer,** Hefeweizen (4.9%) | 155 | 14 | 13 |
| **ZeigenBock,** Amber (4.9%) | 145 | 14 | 11 |

**Alc** ~ Alcohol (Grams)    **Cb** ~ Carbohydrate

## Cider ~ Alcoholic/Hard

*Per 12 fl.oz Unless Indicated*

| | C | Alc | Cb |
|---|---|---|---|
| **Ace:** Cider (5%), average all flavors | 155 | 14 | 12 |
| Joker (6.9%) | 135 | 20 | 12 |
| **Angry Orchard:** Apple Ginger (5%) | 200 | 14 | 26 |
| Crisp Apple (5%) | 220 | 14 | 31 |
| Traditional Dry (5.5%) | 180 | 16 | 20 |
| **Crispin:** Original (5%) | 150 | 14 | 15 |
| Blackberry (5%) | 160 | 14 | 16 |
| Brut (5.5%) | 165 | 16 | 14 |
| Pacific Pear (4.5%) | 160 | 13 | 17 |
| **Hornsby's:** | | | |
| Amber (5.5%), 12 fl.oz | 180 | 16 | 19 |
| Crisp (5.5%), 12 fl.oz | 190 | 16 | 26 |
| **Johnny Appleseed,** (5.5%) | 210 | 16 | 26 |
| **Magners,** (4.5%) | 125 | 13 | 14 |
| **Michelob,** Ultra Light Cider (4%) | 120 | 10 | 10 |
| **Smith & Forge,** (6%) | 220 | 17 | 26 |
| **Stella Artois Cidre,** (4.5%) | 160 | 13 | 17 |
| **Strongbow:** | | | |
| Gold Apple (5%), 11.2 fl.oz | 170 | 13 | 20 |
| Honey & Apple (5%), 11.2 fl.oz | 195 | 13 | 26 |
| **Woodchuck:** Amber (5%) | 200 | 14 | 21 |
| 802 (5%) | 180 | 14 | 16 |
| Granny Smith (5%) | 160 | 14 | 11 |
| Pear (4%) | 150 | 12 | 18 |
| Raspberry (4%) | 170 | 12 | 22 |
| **Wyder's:** Pear (4%) | 140 | 12 | 22 |
| Raspberry (4%) | 120 | 12 | 17 |
| Reposado (6.9%) | 250 | 19 | 30 |

## Quick Guide

**Table Wines:**
*Average all Varieties (11.5% Alc.)*
*(Wine Contains Zero Fat)*

| | C | Alc | Cb |
|---|---|---|---|
| **4 fl.oz,** 1 small wine glass OR ½ large wine glass | 100 | 12 | 3 |
| **6 fl.oz,** (¾ large wine glass) | 145 | 18 | 5 |
| **8 fl.oz,** (1 large wine glass) | 195 | 25 | 7 |
| **½ Carafe/Bottle,** 12 fl.oz | 295 | 37 | 10 |
| **1 Bottle,** 750ml, 25.4 fl.oz | 620 | 78 | 21 |

## Table Wines

| | C | Alc | Cb |
|---|---|---|---|
| **Red:** *Per 4 fl.oz* | | | |
| Burgundy/Cabernet/Merlot, av. | 100 | 11 | 4 |
| **White:** *Per 4 fl.oz* | | | |
| Dry (Chenin; Fume Blanc; Chardonnay) | 95 | 11 | 4 |
| Sparkling, 4 fl.oz | 95 | 11 | 4 |
| Zinfandel Sweet, (Moselle/Sauterne), 4 fl.oz | 85 | 11 | 2 |

## Table Wines (Cont)

| | C | Alc | Cb |
|---|---|---|---|
| **Champagne:** *Per 4 fl.oz* | | | |
| Average all types, 1 glass | 85 | 11 | 2 |
| with Orange Jce (3:1 orange) | 75 | 8 | 4 |
| with Orange Jce (1:1 orange) | 65 | 5 | 7 |
| **Mulled Wine** *(Gluhwein),* 4 fl.oz | 180 | 14 | 20 |
| **Non-Alcoholic Wine:** *Less than 0.5% Alcohol* | | | |
| *Ariel:* White varieties, average, 4 fl.oz | 35 | 0.5 | 8 |
| Red varieties, average, 4 fl.oz | 25 | 0.5 | 5 |
| **Reduced Alcohol Wine:** | | | |
| Average all types, (6%), 4 fl.oz | 80 | 6 | 10 |
| *Skinnygirl,* Red/White, (8.5%), 5 fl.oz | 100 | 10 | 5 |
| **Sake** *(Gekkeikan),* (16%), 4 fl.oz | 120 | 15 | 5 |
| **Sangria** *(Skinnygirl),* (4%), 5 fl.oz | 130 | 5 | 23 |

## Flavored Wines

*Average All Brands (6% alcohol)*
*(Arbor Mist, Wild Vines, Boone's Farm):*

| | C | Alc | Cb |
|---|---|---|---|
| 1 small wine glass, 4 fl.oz | 80 | 6 | 10 |
| 1 large wine glass, 8 fl.oz | 160 | 11 | 20 |
| 1 bottle, 750 ml (25.4 fl.oz) | 510 | 35 | 64 |

## Dessert Wines

| | C | Alc | Cb |
|---|---|---|---|
| **Madeira** (18%), 2 oz | 85 | 9 | 5 |
| **Marsala** (18%), 2 oz | 110 | 9 | 11 |
| **Port,** Muscatel (18%), 2 oz | 85 | 9 | 5 |
| **Sherry** (15%), 2 oz: | | | |
| Dry, 1 Sherry glass | 90 | 7 | 7 |
| Sweet/Cream, average | 90 | 7 | 8 |
| **Vermouth** *(Martini & Rossi):* | | | |
| Extra Dry (18%), 2 oz | 65 | 9 | 2 |
| Martini Rosso (16%), 2 oz | 90 | 8 | 8 |

## Cooking Wines

| | C | Alc | Cb |
|---|---|---|---|
| **Holland House:** | | | |
| **Marsala,** (14%), 2 T., 1 fl.oz | 45 | 4 | 4 |
| **Red/White,** (10%): 2 T., 1 fl.oz | 20 | 2 | 1 |
| 1 cup, 8 fl.oz | 160 | 24 | 8 |
| **Sherry,** (17%), 2 Tbsp, 1 fl.oz | 45 | 5 | 2 |

*Cooking with Wine:*
For alcohol to evaporate, sufficient heat and cooking time (at least 30 minutes) is required.
**Red and white table wines** would then contain negligible residual calories.
**Sweetened wines** (marsala/sherry) would contain 10 calories per 1 fl.oz.
**Flambé Desserts:** Only surface alcohol is burned off, so negligible reduction in alcohol or calories.

## Quick Guide — Alc ~ Alcohol (Grams)

**Spirits/Liquors:**
*Includes Bourbon, Brandy, Gin, Rum, Scotch, Tequila, Vodka, Whiskey.*
Note: All spirits with same alcohol proof have similar calories and zero fat.

| Average All Brands | C | Alc | Cb |
|---|---|---|---|
| **80 Proof (40% Alcohol by Volume):** | | | |
| 1 fl.oz | 65 | 9.5 | 0 |
| 1.5 fl.oz (1 shot) | 100 | 14 | 0 |
| 3 fl.oz (Double shot) | 195 | 28 | 0 |
| ½ Bottle, 350 ml (12 fl.oz) | 770 | 113 | 0 |
| 1 Bottle, 700 ml (24 fl.oz) | 1540 | 227 | 0 |
| **86 Proof (43% Alc):** | | | |
| 1 fl.oz | 70 | 10 | 0 |
| 1.5 fl.oz (1 shot) | 105 | 15 | 0 |
| 1 Bottle (24 fl.oz) | 1670 | 247 | 0 |
| **100 Proof (50% Alc),** | | | |
| 1.5 fl.oz | 125 | 18 | 0 |
| **Shochu (Soju),** | | | |
| average all types (25% alc), 2 fl.oz | 65 | 12 | 0 |

### Flavored Spirits

| Captain Morgan: *Per 1.5 fl.oz* | | | |
|---|---|---|---|
| **Original** (35%) | 85 | 12 | 0.5 |
| **Black Spiced** (47.3%) | 115 | 14 | 1 |
| **Parrot Bay** (21%), average | 90 | 7.5 | 10 |
| **Silver Spiced** (35%) | 95 | 12 | 2 |
| **Malibu Rum,** | | | |
| Original/Fruit Flavors (21%), 1.5 fl.oz | 80 | 8 | 8 |
| **Southern Comfort** (35%), 1.5 fl.oz | 100 | 13 | 3 |

### Hard Lemonade, Sodas & Tea

| Margaritaville: *Per 12 fl.oz* | | | |
|---|---|---|---|
| **Lime Margarita** (8%) | 310 | 23 | 30 |
| **Paradise Punch** (8%) | 340 | 23 | 46 |
| **Mike's:** | | | |
| **Lemonade:** | | | |
| Hard (5%), 11.2 fl.oz | 220 | 13 | 33 |
| Harder (8%) average, 16 fl.oz | 395 | 31 | 44 |
| **Margarita** (5%), 11.2 fl.oz | 220 | 14 | 34 |
| **Punch :** | | | |
| Hard Mango (5.5%), 11.2 fl.oz | 230 | 15 | 33 |
| Harder (8%), 12 fl.oz | 300 | 23 | 36 |
| **Sparks:** *Per 16 fl.oz Can* | | | |
| **Blackberry** (8%) | 385 | 31 | 44 |
| **Iced Tea** (8%) | 375 | 31 | 41 |
| **Lemonade** (8%) | 345 | 31 | 36 |
| **Original** (6%) | 335 | 23 | 45 |
| **Twisted Tea:** Original (5%) | 220 | 14 | 31 |
| Half & Half (5%) | 260 | 14 | 34 |

## Coolers & Premix Cocktails

**Ready-To-Drink:** C Alc Cb
*Zero Fat Unless Indicated*

| Bacardi: *Per 4 fl.oz* | C | Alc | Cb |
|---|---|---|---|
| **Party Drinks (Ready To Pour):** | | | |
| Bahama Mama; Mai Tai (10%) | 130 | 9 | 16 |
| Mojito (15%) | 160 | 14 | 16 |
| Rum Island Ice Tea (12.5%) | 150 | 12 | 16 |
| **Bacardi Silver:** *Per 12 fl.oz* | | | |
| Lemonade/Sangria (6%), av. | 270 | 17 | 41 |
| Raz/Strawberry (5%) | 240 | 14 | 36 |
| Mojito (5%) | 240 | 14 | 36 |
| **Bartles & Jaymes:** *Per 11.2 fl.oz* | | | |
| **Malt Based Coolers** (3.2%): | | | |
| Exotic Berry | 195 | 9 | 31 |
| Margarita | 245 | 9 | 43 |
| Pina Colada | 250 | 9 | 45 |
| Sangria | 240 | 9 | 40 |
| Strawberry Daiquiri | 205 | 9 | 34 |
| **Captain Morgan's,** | | | |
| Parrot Bay (4.1%), all var. av., 11.2 fl.oz | 210 | 10 | 35 |
| **Chi Chi's:** Long Is. Iced Tea, 4 fl.oz | 145 | 12 | 17 |
| Mexican Mudslide, 4 fl.oz (8g fat) | 240 | 1.5 | 42 |
| Mojito, 4 fl.oz | 160 | 11 | 21 |
| Pina Colada, 4 fl.oz (6g fat) | 240 | 4 | 42 |
| White Russian, 4 fl.oz (7g fat) | 245 | 1.5 | 43 |
| **Daily's,** Frozen Pouches (6.9%), | | | |
| average all flavors, 10 fl.oz | 280 | 0 | 46 |
| **Jack Daniels,** Country Cocktails (4.8%), | | | |
| average all varieties, 10 fl.oz | 200 | 9 | 30 |
| **Jose Cuervo:** | | | |
| **Margaritas:** | | | |
| Classic Lime (10%), 6 fl.oz | 210 | 14 | 29 |
| Golden (12.7%), 4.7 fl.oz | 170 | 14 | 19 |
| **Seagram's:** | | | |
| **Escapes Coolers** (3.2%): | | | |
| Bahama Mama, 11.2 fl.oz | 200 | 9 | 36 |
| Strawb. Daiquiri, 11.2 fl.oz | 225 | 9 | 41 |
| **Skinnygirl:** | | | |
| Vodka with flavors (30%), 1.5 fl.oz | 75 | 11 | 0 |
| Cocktails (10%), av., 3 fl.oz | 70 | 8 | 4 |
| **Smirnoff:** | | | |
| **Frozen Lemonades (5%),** av,, 10 oz | 285 | 12 | 53 |
| **Ice,** 4.5%: | | | |
| Cherry Lime, 12 oz | 250 | 13 | 30 |
| Mango/Pineapple, 12 oz | 220 | 13 | 35 |
| Raspberry/Tropical Fruit, 12 oz | 230 | 13 | 38 |
| **TGI Friday's:** | | | |
| **On The Rocks:** *Per 6 fl.oz* | | | |
| Long Island Ice Tea (15%) | 250 | 21 | 28 |
| Margarita (7.5%) | 185 | 11 | 29 |
| Mudslide (10%) | 365 | 14 | 31 |
| **Blenders** (12.5%), | | | |
| Mudslide, 6 fl.oz | 365 | 18 | 31 |

## Coolers & Premix Cocktails (Cont)

**Cocktails**     **Alc** ~ Alcohol (Grams)

| | C | Alc | Cb |
|---|---|---|---|
| **Ready-To-Drink:** | | | |
| **The Club Premix Cocktails:** *Per 3.4 oz Serving (½ can)* | | | |
| Censored on Beach; Margarita (7.5%) | 105 | 6 | 17 |
| Gin/Vodka Martini (21%), average | 155 | 17 | 0.2 |
| Long Island Ice Tea (15%) | 145 | 12 | 17 |
| Manhattan (17%) | 115 | 13 | 5 |
| Mudslide/Pina Colada (10%), average | 200 | 8 | 16 |
| Screwdriver (7.5%) | 95 | 6 | 14 |
| Whiskey Sour (10%) | 95 | 8 | 11 |

### Shooters    **Alc** ~ Alcohol (Grams)

| | | | |
|---|---|---|---|
| Alabama Slammer | 110 | 14 | 2 |
| Amaretto Sour | 120 | 6 | 19 |
| B52 | 145 | 14 | 11 |
| Beam Me Up Scotty | 145 | 13 | 13 |
| Blue Tequila | 160 | 18 | 6 |
| Jager Bomb | 205 | 8 | 30 |
| Jager Bomb, w/ Sugar-Free Red Bull | 155 | 8 | 18 |
| Jell-O Shot: 3 oz, With 1.5 oz Vodka | 180 | 14 | 19 |
| With Diet Jell-O | 110 | 14 | 0 |
| Kamikaze | 75 | 8 | 3 |
| Kool-Aid | 160 | 15 | 14 |
| Orgasm | 100 | 12 | 6 |
| Peppermint Patty | 195 | 8 | 11 |
| Stinger | 170 | 18 | 12 |
| Surfer on Acid | 90 | 7 | 11 |

### Cocktail Mixers ~ Non-Alcoholic

| | | | |
|---|---|---|---|
| **Bacardi:** *Per 8 fl.oz, Prepared from 2 fl.oz Concentrate* | | | |
| Daiquiris; Rum Runner | 120 | 0 | 32 |
| Margarita | 90 | 0 | 25 |
| Mojito | 110 | 0 | 30 |
| Pina Colada | 170 | 0 | 36 |
| **Baja Bob's:** *Per 4 fl.oz* | | | |
| Cranberry Cosmo Martini | 10 | 0 | 2 |
| Pina Colada | 30 | 0 | 4 |
| **Jose Cuervo:** | | | |
| Margaritas: Av. all flav., 4 fl.oz | 85 | 0 | 21 |
| Light (Sugar Free), Lime, 4 fl.oz | 5 | 0 | 1 |
| **Mr & Mrs T:** | | | |
| Bloody Mary: Original, 5 oz | 30 | 0 | 7 |
| Bold & Spicy, 4 oz | 35 | 0 | 7 |
| Mai Tai | 130 | 0 | 32 |
| Margarita | 100 | 0 | 26 |
| Pina Colada | 170 | 0 | 44 |
| Strawberry Daiquiri | 180 | 0 | 46 |
| **TGI Friday's:** | | | |
| Mudslide, 2.3 fl.oz | 110 | 0 | 23 |
| Cosmo; Berrytini, 2 fl.oz | 80 | 0 | 20 |
| Strawb. Daiquiri; Marg., 4 fl.oz | 190 | 0 | 46 |

## Cocktails

**Made to Standard Recipes (Standard Size):**
(Main Reference: The New American Bartender's Guide)
*Zero Fat Unless Indicated*

| | C | Alc | Cb |
|---|---|---|---|
| Adios Mother F. | 260 | 23 | 23 |
| Bacardi & Coke (with 1.5 oz Bacardi) | 160 | 14 | 17 |
| Bellini, 4.5 fl.oz | 95 | 11 | 7 |
| Bloody Mary (with 1.5 oz Vodka) | 125 | 10 | 7 |
| Blushin' Russian (20g fat) | 405 | 14 | 23 |
| Bourbon & Soda (with 2 oz Bourbon) | 130 | 19 | 0 |
| Brandy Alexander (10g fat) | 300 | 20 | 15 |
| Chupa Naranjas (with 1.5 oz Tequila) | 150 | 16 | 8 |
| Cosmopolitan | 215 | 24 | 12 |
| Daiquiri (w/ 2 oz Rum), av. all types | 140 | 19 | 4 |
| Frozen Daiquiri (with 2 oz Rum): | | | |
| Without fruit | 155 | 19 | 6 |
| With fruit (with 1.5 oz Rum) | 145 | 14 | 11 |
| Grasshopper | 260 | 17 | 28 |
| Greyhound (with 1.5 oz Vodka) | 170 | 14 | 17 |
| Harvey Wallbanger (2 oz) | 200 | 19 | 17 |
| Highball (1.5 oz Whiskey) | 100 | 14 | 0 |
| Irish Coffee (10g fat) | 205 | 14 | 2 |
| Kahlua Mudslide: With milk (3g fat) | 145 | 11 | 12 |
| With cream (12g fat) | 230 | 11 | 10 |
| Lemon Drop, 4 fl.oz | 130 | 14 | 10 |
| Long Island Iced Tea (with 3 oz Cola) | 270 | 19 | 32 |
| With 3 oz Diet Cola | 235 | 19 | 22 |
| Mai Tai (with 2 oz Rum) | 290 | 24 | 33 |
| Manhattan | 130 | 17 | 5 |
| Margarita | 160 | 18 | 7 |
| Martini: Dry, with 1.5 oz gin | 100 | 14 | 0 |
| Sour Apple, w/ 2 oz Vodka/1 oz Schnapps | 250 | 31 | 10 |
| Mint Julep (with 2½ oz Bourbon) | 180 | 24 | 4 |
| Mojito (with 2 oz rum) | 170 | 19 | 9 |
| Moscow Mule | 185 | 14 | 24 |
| Pina Colada (10g fat), 6 oz | 250 | 15 | 18 |
| Red Bull & Vodka (with 1.5 oz vodka) | 210 | 14 | 28 |
| With Sugar Free Red Bull | 105 | 14 | 3 |
| Rum & Coke (with 1.5 oz Rum) | 160 | 14 | 17 |
| Sangria: With 1 oz Fruit Juice, 5 oz | 120 | 12 | 9 |
| With 0.5 oz Brandy, 5.5 oz | 150 | 17 | 9 |
| Screwdriver | 160 | 14 | 15 |
| Sex On The Beach | 235 | 19 | 25 |
| Spritzer (with 3 oz Wine) | 65 | 8 | 2 |
| Tequila Sunrise | 200 | 14 | 25 |
| Tom Collins (with 2 oz Gin) | 210 | 19 | 18 |
| Vodka Soda (with 1.5 oz Vodka) | 100 | 14 | 0 |
| Vodka Tonic (with 1.5 oz Vodka) | 165 | 14 | 18 |
| Whiskey Sour (w/ 2 oz Whiskey) | 155 | 19 | 7 |
| White Russian (10g fat) | 240 | 19 | 7 |
| **Non-Alcoholic:** | | | |
| Cinderella | 45 | 0 | 11 |
| Shirley Temple (with 6 oz Ginger Ale) | 140 | 0 | 34 |

## Liqueurs/Cordials  **C** **Alc** **Cb**

*Per 1 fl.oz*

| | C | Alc | Cb |
|---|---|---|---|
| Advocaat (36 Proof; 2g fat) | 85 | 4 | 9 |
| Alizé: Cognac (80 Proof) | 70 | 9 | 2 |
| Gold/Red Passion (32 Proof) | 105 | 4 | 11 |
| Amaretto (56 Proof) | 110 | 7 | 17 |
| Baileys Irish Cream (34 Proof; 4g fat) | 100 | 4 | 8 |
| Benedictine (80 Proof) | 90 | 9 | 5 |
| Chambord (33 Proof) | 105 | 4 | 11 |
| Chartreuse (80 Proof) | 100 | 9 | 9 |
| Cherry Brandy (48 Proof) | 80 | 6 | 9 |
| Coffee Liqueur (53 Proof) | 115 | 7 | 16 |
| Cointreau (80 Proof) | 95 | 9 | 7 |
| Creme de Cacao (54 Proof) | 100 | 6 | 15 |
| Creme de Menthe (72 Proof) | 125 | 9 | 14 |
| Curacao (70 Proof) | 95 | 8 | 6 |
| Drambuie (80 Proof) | 105 | 9 | 9 |
| Frangelico (40 Proof) | 65 | 5 | 12 |
| Galliano (86 Proof) | 100 | 10 | 8 |
| Grand Marnier (80 Proof) | 100 | 9 | 7 |
| Kahlua (40 Proof) | 85 | 5 | 14 |
| Kirsch (68 Proof) | 80 | 8 | 6 |
| Midori (42 Proof) | 80 | 5 | 11 |
| Ouzo (80 Proof) | 105 | 9 | 11 |
| Pernod (80 Proof) | 75 | 9 | 11 |
| Sambuca (84 Proof) | 100 | 10 | 11 |
| Schnapps (100 Proof) | 115 | 12 | 9 |
| Southern Comfort (70 Proof) | 65 | 8 | 3 |

## Liqueur Coffee & Hot Drinks

*Per Standard Drink*

| | C | Alc | Cb |
|---|---|---|---|
| **Liqueur Coffee:** Av. all types | 200 | 10 | 10 |
| Irish, 1.5 oz Whiskey & 1 oz whip | 205 | 9 | 4 |
| **Hot Toddy,** with 1½ oz liquor, av. all | 170 | 9 | 19 |
| **Mulled Wine** (*Glühwein*), 4 fl.oz, av | 195 | 14 | 25 |

*"The doctor told him to cut down to just one glass a day."*

## TEN TIPS TO AVOID HARMFUL DRINKING

1. **Add up the alcohol** you typically drink each day and on social occasions. How does this compare with 'low risk' amounts? (*See page 23*)

2. **Compare the alcohol content** of different drinks and select the lowest. Request half shots of alcohol in cocktails and mixed drinks. Dilute them and keep topping off with non-alcoholic drinks.

3. **Go easy on 'Light' beers.** At 4% alcohol, on average, they are still high in alcohol compared to regular beer (5% alcohol).

4. **Try low alcohol or non-alcohol** alternatives such as fruit juices and mineral water. Take your own to parties.

5. **Before drinking alcohol,** quench your thirst with water and non-alcoholic drinks – particularly after vigorous exercise or sports.

6. **Slow the rate of drinking.** Chugging or drinking fast is the major cause of illness and death from alcohol poisoning.

7. **Avoid drinking in 'rounds'.**

8. **Have a non-alcoholic 'spacer'** between drinks (e.g. mineral water, orange juice).

9. **Don't drink on an empty stomach.** Food slows the rate of alcohol absorption.

10. **Keep track of the number of drinks** and know when to stop. Stick to a set limit.

*Note: Alcohol can be very dangerous when taken with prescription or street drugs, or when you are very tired.*

***Extra Info: www.CalorieKing.com***

## Cocktail Mixers & Extracts

| | C | Alc | Cb |
|---|---|---|---|
| Angostura Bitters, ¼ tsp | 2 | 0 | 0.5 |
| Grenadine, ½ tsp | 6 | 0 | 2 |
| Lime/Lemon Juice, 2 Tbsp, 1 oz | 10 | 0 | 2 |
| Maraschino Cherry, 1 small | 8 | 0 | 2 |
| Simple Syrup, 1 Tbsp, av. | 50 | 0 | 14 |
| Sweet & Sour Mix, 2 Tbsp, 1 oz | 30 | 0 | 7 |
| Tonic Water, 8 fl.oz | 80 | 0 | 22 |
| **Flavor Extracts** (*McCormick*): | | | |
| Pure Lemon (83%), 1 tsp | 0 | 3.5 | 0 |
| Pure Vanilla (35%), 1tsp | 0 | 1.5 | 0 |

| Baking Ingredients | C | F | Cb |
|---|---|---|---|
| **Almond Paste**, (Marzipan), 2 Tbsp | 170 | 7 | 24 |
| **Apple Pie Filling**, Sweetened, 9.4 oz | 290 | 0 | 69 |
| **Baking Powder**: Regular, 1 tsp | 5 | 0 | 1 |
| Cream of Tartar, 1 tsp | 10 | 0 | 2 |
| Baking Mix (*Bisquick*): Original, ⅓ cup, 1.5 oz | 160 | 5 | 26 |
| **Batter Mix (***Golden Dipt***)**, All Purpose, ¼ cup | 100 | 0 | 20 |
| **Butter/Margarine**, ½ cup, 4 oz | 800 | 88 | 1 |
| Stick (*Land O' Lakes*), 0.5 oz | 100 | 11 | 0 |
| **Cacao Butter**, 2 Tbsp, 1 oz | 240 | 28 | 0 |
| **Cacao Nibs**, raw, 3 Tbsp, 1 oz | 180 | 14 | 8 |
| **Cacao Powder**, raw: 1 Tbsp, 0.3 oz | 35 | 2 | 3 |
| ¼ cup, 1 oz | 150 | 9 | 11 |
| **Carob Flour**, ½ cup | 115 | 0.5 | 46 |
| **Chocolate Baking Bars:** *Average all Brands* | | | |
| Sweet (*Baker's*): | | | |
| 1 oz portion | 120 | 7 | 16 |
| 4 oz bar | 470 | 28 | 64 |
| Semi-sweet, 1 oz | 140 | 9 | 16 |
| White Baking, 1 oz | 160 | 9 | 16 |
| Unsweetened: 1 oz | 140 | 14 | 8 |
| Grated, 1 cup, 4.5 oz | 660 | 69 | 39 |
| **Chocolate Baking Chips:** *Average all Brands* | | | |
| Milk Choc./Semi Sweet, 1 oz | 140 | 8 | 18 |
| ½ cup, 3 oz | 420 | 24 | 54 |
| 1 cup, 6 oz | 840 | 48 | 108 |
| Dark, 1 Tbsp, 0.5 oz | 70 | 5 | 3 |
| Mini Kisses (*Hershey*), 1 piece | 5 | 0.5 | 1 |
| **Cocoa Powder**, unsweetened: | | | |
| 1 Tbsp, 0.2 oz | 15 | 0.5 | 3 |
| ⅓ cup, 1 oz | 60 | 4 | 17 |
| **Coconut**, dried: | | | |
| Sweetened/Flaked: | | | |
| 1 oz | 130 | 8 | 15 |
| ½ cup, 1.3 oz | 195 | 12 | 22 |
| Toasted (*Baker's*), 1 oz | 170 | 13 | 13 |
| Unsweetened, 1 oz | 190 | 18 | 7 |
| **Coconut Cream/Milk** ~ *See Page 89* | | | |
| **Coconut Manna** (*Nutiva*), 1 Tbsp | 100 | 9 | 3 |
| **Cornstarch**, 1 Tbsp | 30 | 0 | 7 |
| **Eggs:** Large (1) | 75 | 5 | 0 |
| Jumbo (1) | 90 | 6 | 0.5 |
| **Egg White:** 1 Egg White | 15 | 0 | 0 |
| ½ cup (4 egg whites), 4 oz | 60 | 0 | 1 |
| **Flour:** | | | |
| White: 1 Tbsp, 0.3 oz | 25 | 0 | 5.5 |
| 1 cup, 4.2 oz | 400 | 1 | 88 |
| Whole Wheat, 1 cup, 4.2 oz | 400 | 2 | 84 |

| | C | F | Cb |
|---|---|---|---|
| **Flavor Extracts:** *Av. all Brands* | | | |
| Imitation, 1 tsp | 10 | 0 | 2 |
| Pure Extract, 1 tsp | 10 | 0 | 0.5 |
| Almond; Vanilla, 1 tsp | 10 | 0 | 0.5 |
| **Fruit Pectin:** Swtnd, ¼ tsp | 5 | 0 | 1 |
| Unsweetened, ¼ tsp | 0 | 0 | 0 |
| **Gelatin**, dry, unsweetened, 0.3 oz | 20 | 0 | 0 |
| **Glaze** (*Duncan Hines*): Choc., 2 T. | 150 | 7 | 21 |
| Vanilla, 2 Tbsp | 140 | 6 | 22 |
| *Golden Dipt,* Batter Mix | | | |
| ¼ cup, 1 oz | 100 | 0 | 23 |
| **Honey**, ½ cup, 6 oz | 515 | 0 | 140 |
| **Lemon/Orange Peel**, ¼ cup | 25 | 0 | 6 |
| **Lighter Bake** (*Sunsweet*): | | | |
| (Butter & Oil replacement) | | | |
| 1 Tbsp, ½ oz | 35 | 0 | 9 |
| ¼ cup, 2.7 oz | 140 | 0 | 36 |
| **Milk:** Whole, 1 cup, 8 fl.oz | 150 | 8 | 12 |
| 2%, 1 cup, 8 fl.oz | 120 | 5 | 12 |
| 1%, 1 cup, 8 fl.oz | 100 | 2.5 | 12 |
| Fat-Free, 1 cup, 8 fl.oz | 90 | 0.5 | 13 |
| **Pastry** ~ *See Page 134* | | | |
| **Pie Crusts** ~ *See Page 134* | | | |
| **Pie Fillings, Fruits** ~ *See Page 134* | | | |
| Lemon Creme, ⅓ cup | 130 | 1.5 | 28 |
| Mincemeat, 3.5 oz | 190 | 5 | 45 |
| Pumpkin, 1 cup, 9.3 oz | 270 | 1.5 | 60 |
| **Prune Puree**, ¼ cup, 3 oz | 220 | 0 | 55 |
| **Raisins**, ½ cup, 2.8 oz | 240 | 0.5 | 63 |
| **Rennin**, 0.4 oz pkt | 10 | 0 | 2 |
| **Soy Milk** ~ *See Pages 49-50* | | | |
| **Sprinkles**, all types, 1 tsp | 20 | 1 | 3 |
| **Sugar:** 1 Tbsp, 0.5 oz | 55 | 0 | 14 |
| 1 oz | 110 | 0 | 28 |
| 1 cup, 7 oz | 775 | 0 | 195 |
| 1 lb, 16 oz | 1760 | 0 | 454 |
| **Sweeteners & Sugar Substitutes** ~ *See Page 156* | | | |
| **Vinegar**, average all types, 1 oz | 5 | 0 | 1 |
| **Whey**, sweet, dry, 1 oz | 100 | 0.5 | 21 |
| **Yeast:** | | | |
| Active, dry, 0.3 oz pkg | 25 | 0.5 | 3 |
| Bakers, compressed, 1 oz | 30 | 0.5 | 5 |
| *Fleischmann's*, 0.6 oz pkg | 0 | 0 | 0 |

**For Full Nutritional Data & Product Updates**
~ *See Author's Website*
www.CalorieKing.com

Note: Actual weight of bars is usually 5-10% more than label Net Weight. Weigh bar and allow extra calories.

| **Bars ~ Brands** | **C** | **F** | **Cb** |
|---|---|---|---|

*Per Bar*
AdvantEdge ~ *See EAS*
**Annie's Homegrown:**

**Organic Granola Bars:** *Per 1 oz Bar*

| | C | F | Cb |
|---|---|---|---|
| Berry Berry | 120 | 3.5 | 20 |
| Chocolate Chip | 120 | 4 | 19 |
| PB & J; Peanut Butter | 120 | 4.5 | 18 |

**Atkins:**

**Meal Bars:**

| | C | F | Cb |
|---|---|---|---|
| Blueberry Greek Yogurt Bar, 1.7 oz | 200 | 8 | 22 |
| Chocolate Chip Cookie Dough, 2 oz | 220 | 10 | 32 |
| Chocolate Chip Granola, 1.7 oz | 200 | 9 | 19 |
| Choc. Peanut Butter, 2 oz | 250 | 14 | 23 |
| Choc. Peanut Butter Pretzel, 1.7 oz | 210 | 10 | 19 |
| Cinnamon Bun; Mudslide, 1.7 oz | 210 | 10 | 19 |
| Cookies 'n Crème, 1.7 oz | 200 | 11 | 22 |
| Strawb. Almond, 1.7 oz | 200 | 9 | 20 |

**Snack Bars:** *Per 1.6 oz bar*

| | C | F | Cb |
|---|---|---|---|
| Caramel Chocolate Nut Roll | 190 | 13 | 19 |
| Caramel Chocolate Peanut Nougat | 170 | 11 | 20 |
| Caramel Double Chocolate Crunch | 160 | 9 | 22 |
| Cashew Trail Mix Bar | 170 | 11 | 19 |
| Cranberry Almond Bar | 150 | 6 | 16 |
| Coconut Almond Delight | 200 | 15 | 18 |
| Dark Choc. Almond Coconut Crunch | 190 | 15 | 17 |
| Dark Chocolate Decadence Bar | 160 | 9 | 22 |
| Triple Chocolate | 160 | 9 | 17 |

*Note: Snack Bar Carb figures  includes 4-15g sugar alcohol*

**Attune Bars:**

**Probiotic Bars:** *Per 0.7 oz Bar*

| | C | F | Cb |
|---|---|---|---|
| Dark Chocolate | 80 | 6 | 11 |
| Milk Choc. Crisp | 90 | 6 | 12 |
| Mint Chocolate | 90 | 6 | 12 |

**Balance:**

| | C | F | Cb |
|---|---|---|---|
| Original, average, 1,8 oz | 200 | 7 | 21 |
| Bare, 1.2 oz | 160 | 9 | 17 |
| Dark varieties, 1.6 oz | 180 | 6 | 20 |
| Gold varieties, average, 1.8 oz | 200 | 7 | 23 |

**Cascadian Farms** *(General Mills):*

| | C | F | Cb |
|---|---|---|---|
| Chewy Granola, av. all var., 1.2 oz | 135 | 3 | 26 |
| Crunchy Granola, all var., 2 bars, 1.4 oz | 185 | 8 | 27 |
| Granola Bark, average, 1 oz piece | 140 | 8 | 16 |
| Protein Granola Bars, av. all var., 1.8 oz | 250 | 15 | 21 |

*Per Bar*
**Clif:**

| | C | F | Cb |
|---|---|---|---|
| **Original,** average all varieties., 2.4 oz | 240 | 5 | 45 |
| **Builder's:** Av. all varieties, 2.4 oz | 270 | 8 | 30 |
| Max, average all varieties, 3.4 oz | 385 | 13 | 40 |
| **Kid,** ZBar, av. all varieties, 1.3 oz | 125 | 3.5 | 23 |
| **Mojo,** average, 1.6 oz | 190 | 11 | 21 |

**Corazonas:**

**Oatmeal Squares:** *Per 1.8 oz Bar*

| | C | F | Cb |
|---|---|---|---|
| White Chocolate Macadamia | 200 | 8 | 29 |
| Av. other varieties | 185 | 7 | 28 |

**Detour:**

| | C | F | Cb |
|---|---|---|---|
| **Original,** Caramel Peanut, 3 oz | 350 | 11 | 32 |

**Lean Muscle:**

Peanut Butter Chocolate Crunch:

| | C | F | Cb |
|---|---|---|---|
| 1..6 oz | 190 | 9 | 15 |
| 3.2 oz | 420 | 18 | 33 |
| Other flavors, 3.2 oz | 370 | 12 | 33 |

**Lower Sugar,** average all varieties:

| | C | F | Cb |
|---|---|---|---|
| 1.4 oz Bar | 170 | 5.5 | 16 |
| 2.8 oz Bar | 340 | 11 | 33 |

*Note: Low Sugar Carb figures includes 12-28g sugar alcohol*

| | C | F | Cb |
|---|---|---|---|
| **Oatmeal,** av. all varieties,  4.3 oz | 450 | 11 | 60 |

**dotFIT:**

**dotBAR:**

| | C | F | Cb |
|---|---|---|---|
| Chocolate Mint, 2 oz | 160 | 5 | 15 |
| Choc. Peanut Butter Crunch, 2 oz | 190 | 6 | 23 |
| Peanut Buter Crisp, 1.4 oz | 150 | 5 | 16 |

*Note: dotBAR Carb figures includes 7g sugar alcohol*

| | C | F | Cb |
|---|---|---|---|
| **dotSTICK,** Iced, av. all var., 2 oz | 190 | 6 | 26 |

*Note: dotSTICK Carb figure includess 8g sugar alcohol*

**EAS:**

**AdvantEDGE:**

Carb Control:

| | C | F | Cb |
|---|---|---|---|
| Crisp Bars, 2 oz | 240 | 8 | 27 |
| Other varieties,  2 oz | 230 | 8 | 27 |

*Note: AdvantEDGE Carb figures includes 17-19g sugar alcohol*

| | C | F | Cb |
|---|---|---|---|
| **Myoplex 30,** av. all varieties, 3 oz | 350 | 10 | 36 |

**Extend Bar:**

| | C | F | Cb |
|---|---|---|---|
| Crunch, av., 1.4 oz | 150 | 2.5 | 30 |
| Anytime, av. all varieties, 1.4 oz | 145 | 4 | 22 |

*Note: Extend Bar Carb figures includes 8-9g sugar alcohol*

**Fiber One:**

**Chewy:**

| | C | F | Cb |
|---|---|---|---|
| Protein Caramel Nut, 1.2 oz | 130 | 6 | 16 |
| Other Nut Varieties, 1.2 oz | 140 | 6 | 17 |
| Other Chewy varieties, 1.4 oz | 135 | 5 | 29 |
| **90-Calorie Bar,** av. all var.,  0.8 oz | 90 | 2 | 17 |
| **Meal Bar,** av. all varieties,  1.6 oz | 185 | 8 | 21 |

| Bars ~ Brands (Cont) | C | F | Cb |
|---|---|---|---|
| *Per Bar* | | | |
| **FiberPlus** *(Kellogg's):* | | | |
| **Antioxidants:** Choc. Chip, 1.3 oz | **120** | 4 | 26 |
| Other varieties, 1.3 oz | **130** | 5 | 25 |
| **GeniSoy:** *Per 2 oz Bar* | | | |
| **Protein:** Chunky PB Fudge | **220** | 6 | 30 |
| Chocolate Fudge Brownie | **220** | 6 | 30 |
| Crispy Choc. Mint | **210** | 4.5 | 33 |
| **General Mills:** *Per 1.6 oz Bar* | | | |
| Milk 'n Cereal Bar, | | | |
| Honey Nut Cheerios | **160** | 4 | 28 |
| **Glenny's:** *Per 1 oz Bar* | | | |
| Cashew/Cranberry & Almond, av. | **145** | 7 | 17 |
| Cherry & Almond | **130** | 6 | 18 |
| Classic Fruit & Nut | **140** | 6 | 18 |
| Peanuts & Peanut Butter | **170** | 13 | 10 |
| **Glucerna:** | | | |
| Crispy Delights Nutrition Bars, | | | |
| Peanut/Choc. Chip, av., 1.4 oz | **155** | 6 | 20 |
| *Note: Crispy Bars Carb figure includess 7g sugar alcohol* | | | |
| Mini Snack Bar, average, 0.7 oz | **80** | 3 | 11 |
| *Note: Mini Snack Carb figure includess 2-5 g sugar alcohol* | | | |
| **Health Valley,** | | | |
| **Cobbler Cereal Bars,** 1.3 oz | **130** | 2.5 | 27 |
| **Herbalife,** | | | |
| Protein Deluxe!, average, 1.3 oz | **160** | 6 | 17 |
| **HMR,** Benefit Bars, av. all, 1.4 oz | **155** | 4 | 24 |
| **Jenny Craig:** S'mores, 1.3 oz | **140** | 4 | 22 |
| Yogurt Dream Bar, 1.2 oz | **130** | 4.5 | 20 |
| **Kashi:** | | | |
| Cereal Bars, 1.3 oz | **130** | 3 | 24 |
| Granola & Seed Bars (2), | | | |
| average all flavors, 1.4 oz | **180** | 7 | 27 |
| **Granola Bars:** | | | |
| Chewy, av. all var., 1.3 oz | **135** | 3 | 21 |
| Crunchy, all varieties, | | | |
| 2 bars, 1.4 oz | **170** | 6 | 26 |
| Layered, | | | |
| average all varieties, 1 oz | **125** | 4 | 21 |
| **Go Lean,** Chewy Granola, 1.2 oz | **140** | 5 | 19 |
| **Kellogg's,** | | | |
| Cinnabon Bar, Original, 1.3 oz | **150** | 4.5 | 26 |
| **Fiber Plus** ~ *See page 31* | | | |
| **Nutrigrain** ~ *See page 33* | | | |
| **Special K** ~ *See page 34* | | | |

| *Per Bar* | C | F | Cb |
|---|---|---|---|
| **Kind:** *Per 1.4 oz Bar* | | | |
| **Fruit & Nut:** | | | |
| Almond & Apricot | **180** | 10 | 23 |
| Apple Cinnamon & Pecan | **190** | 12 | 20 |
| Nut Delight | **210** | 16 | 14 |
| Peanut Butter & Strawberry | **190** | 11 | 19 |
| **Nuts & Spices:** | | | |
| Cashew & Ginger Spices | **200** | 14 | 16 |
| Dark Chocolate, all varieties | **200** | 13 | 16 |
| Madagascar Vanilla Almond | **210** | 16 | 14 |
| **Plus,** average all varieties | **185** | 12 | 18 |
| **Kudos,** av. all varieties, 0.9 oz | **100** | 3 | 17 |
| **Labrada:** | | | |
| **Lean Body Protein Bars:** | | | |
| Caramel Peanut; S'mores | **360** | 14 | 33 |
| P'nut Butter & Jelly | **350** | 12 | 36 |
| **Larabar:** | | | |
| Apple Pie, 1.6 oz | **190** | 10 | 24 |
| Cherry Pie, 1.7 oz | **200** | 8 | 30 |
| Chocolate Chip Brownie, 1.6 oz | **200** | 9 | 31 |
| Coconut Pineapple Cake, 1.6 oz | **190** | 8 | 28 |
| Peanut Butter & Jelly, 1.7 oz | **210** | 10 | 27 |
| Strawberry Shortcake, 1.6 oz | **200** | 11 | 24 |
| **Lindora,** av. all varieties, 1.6 oz | **155** | 5 | 17 |
| **Luna:** | | | |
| **Bars For Women,** | | | |
| average all varieties, 1.7 oz | **180** | 4.5 | 27 |
| **Protein,** av. all varieties, 1.6 oz | **180** | 7 | 21 |
| **Marathon** *(Snickers):* | | | |
| **Energy:** Chewy, av. all var., 2 oz | **210** | 8 | 26 |
| Crunchy, Dark Chocolate, 1.6 oz | **150** | 4.5 | 22 |
| **Protein,** average all, 2.8 oz | **285** | 9 | 40 |
| **Market Pantry** *(Target):* | | | |
| **Granola Bars:** | | | |
| Chewy: Choc Chip, 0.8 oz | **100** | 3 | 17 |
| Choc. Chunk; S'Mores, 0.8 oz | **90** | 1.5 | 18 |
| Crunchy, Oats & Honey, 1.5 oz | **180** | 6 | 28 |
| **Mariani:** *Per 1.4 oz Bar* | | | |
| **Honey Bars:** Cranb.; Granola, av. | **170** | 8 | 23 |
| Sesame | **200** | 14 | 16 |
| **Medifast:** Chewy, all var., 1.3 oz | **110** | 3 | 15 |
| Crunch, all varieties, 1.2 oz | **110** | 3 | 13 |
| *Note: Crunch Bar Carb figure includes 2-3g sugar alcohol* | | | |
| Maintenance, Cararmel Nut, 1.5 oz | **170** | 5 | 22 |

| **Bars ~ Brands (Cont)** | **C** | **F** | **Cb** |
|---|---|---|---|

*Per Bar*
**Met-Rx:** *Per 3.5 oz Bar Unless Indicated*

| | **C** | **F** | **Cb** |
|---|---|---|---|
| **Big 100,** average all varieties | 375 | 6 | 49 |
| **Big 100 Colossal:** | | | |
| Crispy Apple Pie | 400 | 10 | 47 |
| Choc. Toasted Almond | 410 | 13 | 46 |
| Peanut Butter Caramel | 410 | 13 | 44 |
| **Protein Plus,** Choc. Choc. Chunk | 310 | 10 | 29 |
| **Mojo Bars ~** *See Clif* | | | |
| **Muscle Milk** *(Cytosport):* | | | |
| **High Protein:** | | | |
| Choc. Peanut Caramel, 2.6 oz | 320 | 11 | 30 |
| Vanilla Toffee Crunch, 2.6 oz | 310 | 11 | 29 |
| **Protein Crunch,** | | | |
| Chocolate PB, 2.9 oz | 360 | 13 | 31 |
| **Nature's Path:** | | | |
| **Granola Bars:** | | | |
| Gluten Free, 5 Bar Box, | | | |
| 1 bar, av., 1.3 oz | 145 | 4 | 22 |
| 10 Bar Box, 2 bars, av. all, 1.4 oz | 195 | 7 | 28 |
| **Nature Valley:** | | | |
| **Crunchy Granola Bars:** | | | |
| Apple Crisp (2), 1.5 oz | 160 | 6 | 26 |
| Average other var. (2), 1.5 oz | 185 | 7 | 28 |
| **Granola Thins,** av. all var., 0.6 oz | 85 | 4.5 | 11 |
| **Protein,** all varieties, 1.4 oz | 190 | 12 | 14 |
| **Trail Mix,** Chewy, av. all, 1.3 oz | 135 | 4 | 25 |
| **Yogurt,** Chewy, all varieties, 1.2 oz | 140 | 4 | 26 |
| **NuGo:** | | | |
| **Dark,** average all varieties | 200 | 5 | 29 |
| **Family:** Choc. Banana | 190 | 2.5 | 25 |
| Av. other varieties | 170 | 3 | 26 |
| **Fiber:** Orange Cranberry | 130 | 3 | 32 |
| Coconut Macaroon; P'nut Choc Chip | 160 | 6 | 28 |
| Average other varieties | 140 | 4 | 30 |
| **Gluten Free,** average all varieties | 180 | 4 | 28 |
| **Organic,** all varieties | 190 | 5 | 26 |
| **Slim:** Espresso | 170 | 5 | 20 |
| Average other varieties | 185 | 5 | 19 |
| **Smarte Carb:** Choc. Black Berry | 150 | 3 | 22 |
| Peanut Butter Crunch | 190 | 4 | 19 |

*Note: Smarte Carb figure includes 12-16 g sugar alcohol*

| | **C** | **F** | **Cb** |
|---|---|---|---|
| **Stronger:** | | | |
| Cookies 'N Crm; Caramel Pretzel, av. | 290 | 7 | 36 |
| Average other varieties | 315 | 12 | 35 |
| **Nutri-Grain** *(Kellogg's):* | | | |
| Fruit Crunch, (2), all varieties, 1.5 oz | 185 | 7 | 29 |
| Harvest, average all varieties, 1.5 oz | 180 | 5 | 34 |

*Per Bar*

| | **C** | **F** | **Cb** |
|---|---|---|---|
| **Nutri-Grain** (Cont): | | | |
| **Soft Baked Breakfast Cereal Bars:** | | | |
| Strawberry Greek Yogurt, 1.3 oz | 130 | 3.5 | 25 |
| Other varieties, 1.3 oz | 120 | 3 | 24 |
| **Nutrilite** *(Amway Global):* | | | |
| **High Protein + Fiber Bars,** | | | |
| average all varieties, 1.5 oz | 140 | 5 | 20 |
| **Meal Bars,** all varieties, 1.8 oz | 200 | 7 | 26 |
| **Wellness Bars,** average all varieties | 195 | 12 | 18 |
| **NutriSystem:** | | | |
| **Granola Breakfast Bars:** | | | |
| Chewy Chocolate Chip | 150 | 2 | 27 |
| Peanut Butter | 160 | 5 | 25 |
| **Snack Bars:** Chewy Peanut | 180 | 9 | 19 |
| Chocolate Caramel | 150 | 3.5 | 23 |
| **Odwalla:** | | | |
| **Chewy,** | | | |
| Choc. Alm. Coconut, 1.6 oz | 200 | 8 | 29 |
| **Nourishing:** *Per 2 oz Bar* | | | |
| Choco-walla | 210 | 5 | 39 |
| Dark Chocolate Chip Walnut | 220 | 7 | 36 |
| White Chocolate Macadamia | 210 | 10 | 27 |
| **Protein,** Choc. Chip Peanut, 2 oz | 230 | 8 | 33 |
| **Superfood:** *Per 2 oz Bar* | | | |
| Original | 200 | 3.5 | 39 |
| Berries GoMega | 210 | 6 | 36 |
| Blueberry Swirl | 200 | 3 | 41 |
| Strawberry Pomegranate | 200 | 2 | 42 |
| **Oh Yeah!** *(ISS),* | | | |
| Orig., Almond Fudge Brownie, 3 oz | 350 | 13 | 27 |
| **Optifast,** 800 Bars, av., 1.6 oz | 165 | 4 | 20 |
| **PowerBar:** | | | |
| **Harvest Energy:** Cranb. Oatmeal | 130 | 2.5 | 23 |
| Fruit & Nut/Nut | 210 | 10 | 21 |
| Roasted P'nut Butter | 140 | 4.5 | 21 |
| Average other varieties | 245 | 5 | 42 |
| **Performance Energy: Bars:** | | | |
| Bars, average all varieties | 240 | 4 | 45 |
| Wafers, average all varieties, 1 pkt | 170 | 4.5 | 30 |
| **Protein & Recovery:** | | | |
| 10G Protein, Triple Threat, av. all | 230 | 9 | 30 |
| 20g Protein Plus, av. all varieties | 210 | 5 | 27 |
| 30g Protein Plus, av. all varieties | 350 | 11 | 26 |
| **Power Crunch** *(BNRG),* | | | |
| Protein Bar, av. all var., 1.4 oz | 205 | 12 | 10 |
| **PR Bar:** Chocolate Peanut. 1.8 oz | 200 | 7 | 22 |
| Yogurt Berry, 1.8 oz | 210 | 7 | 22 |
| Granola, Oatmeal Raisin, 1.8 oz | 210 | 7 | 22 |
| **Premier Nutrition:** | | | |
| **Premier Protein:** | | | |
| Crisp Bars, average all var., 1.8 oz | 190 | 6 | 26 |

*Note: Crisp Bar Carb figure includes 3-8g sugar alcohol*

| | | | |
|---|---|---|---|
| Protein Bars, average all var., 2.5 oz | 280 | 7 | 24 |

Note: Actual weight of bars is usually 5-10% more than label Net Weight. Weigh bar and allow extra calories.

### Bars ~ Brands (Cont)

| Per Bar | C | F | Cb |
|---|---|---|---|
| **Promax:** | | | |
| Gluten-Free, av. all varieties, 2.6 oz | 285 | 8 | 37 |
| Lower Sugar, av all varieties, 2.4 oz | 230 | 7 | 33 |
| Proti Bars (Briatrix), av. all var. | 160 | 5.5 | 16 |
| PureFit, av. all varieties, 2 oz | 220 | 7 | 25 |
| **Pure Protein:** | | | |
| **Hi Protein,** average all varieties: | | | |
| 1.8 oz bar | 190 | 5 | 18 |
| 2.8 oz bar | 305 | 10 | 30 |
| Note: Hi Protein Bar Carb figure includes 5-8g Sugar Alcohol | | | |
| **Quaker:** | | | |
| **Chewy Granola Bars:** | | | |
| 25% Less Sugar, Choc. Chip, 08 oz | 100 | 3.5 | 17 |
| 90 Calories, av. all varieties, 1 oz | 90 | 2 | 19 |
| Big, average all varieties, 1.5 oz | 170 | 6 | 29 |
| Dipps, Caramel Nut | 140 | 6 | 21 |
| School Days, Amazing Apple; Best Berry, 1 oz | 100 | 2 | 20 |
| Yogurt, all varieties, 1.2 oz | 150 | 4.5 | 25 |
| **Oatmeal To Go:** | | | |
| Regular, average all varieties, 2 oz | 220 | 4 | 43 |
| High Fiber, Maple Brown Sugar, 2 oz | 210 | 4 | 43 |
| **Soft Baked,** av. all varieties, 1.5 oz | 140 | 3.5 | 26 |
| **Quest Bar:** | | | |
| **Protein Bar,** average all varieties | 185 | 8 | 22 |
| Note: Protein Bar Carb figure includes 1-6g Sugar Alccohol | | | |
| **Revival Soy** (Direct): | | | |
| Chocolate Temptation | 270 | 7 | 32 |
| Marshmallow Crunch | 220 | 2.5 | 30 |
| Peanut Pal | 240 | 6 | 28 |
| **Low Carb**, average all varieties | 235 | 8 | 31 |
| Note: Low Carb Bar figure includes 20-22g Sugar Alcohol | | | |
| **Slim-Fast:** | | | |
| **Meal Bars:** | | | |
| Chewy Chocolate Crisp, 1.7 oz | 200 | 6 | 25 |
| Chocolate P'nut Caramel, 1.6 oz | 200 | 7 | 21 |
| Sweet & Salty Choc. Almond, 1.6 oz | 200 | 8 | 21 |
| **Snack Bars,** average all flavors | 100 | 3 | 16 |
| SoyJoy Bars, av. all var., 1 oz | 135 | 6 | 16 |
| Solo, GI, av. all, 1.8 oz | 200 | 7 | 26 |

| Per Bar | C | F | Cb |
|---|---|---|---|
| **Special K:** | | | |
| **Cereal Bars,** av. all varieties, 0.8 oz | 90 | 1.5 | 17 |
| **Chewy Snack Bars,** av. all varieties, 0.9 oz | 100 | 2 | 18 |
| **Protein Granola Bars,** 1 bar, 0.9 oz | 110 | 3 | 17 |
| **Protein Meal,** av. all varieties, 1.6 oz | 175 | 5 | 25 |
| Steel Bar (ABB), av. all var., 2.5 oz | 250 | 4 | 36 |
| **Supreme Protein:** | | | |
| High Protein: | | | |
| PB Crunch | 390 | 18 | 26 |
| Average other varieties | 390 | 15 | 36 |
| Note: Carb figure includes 14-20g sugar alcohol | | | |
| **thinkThin:** | | | |
| **High Protein:** | | | |
| Choc. Covered Strawberries, 1.8 oz | 200 | 7 | 23 |
| 2 oz Bars, average all varieties | 235 | 8 | 24 |
| Note: Protein Bar Carb figure includes 10-22g sugar alcohol | | | |
| **Protein Nut,** average all var., 1.4 oz | 190 | 12 | 16 |
| **Tiger's Milk:** | | | |
| Protein Rich, 1.2 oz | 140 | 5 | 18 |
| Peanut Butter Crunch, 1.2 oz | 150 | 6 | 18 |
| King Size, average all varieties, 2 oz | 225 | 9 | 28 |
| **Toaster Strudel** ~ see page 64 | | | |
| **Trader Joe's:** | | | |
| **Chewy Coated Granola Bars, 6-Packs:** | | | |
| Chocolate Chip, 1.3 oz | 150 | 4 | 26 |
| Peanut Butter, 1.3 oz | 170 | 8 | 19 |
| Vanilla Almond, 1.3 oz | 150 | 6 | 22 |
| **Fruit Bars:** Fig 1.5 oz | 120 | 2 | 24 |
| Average other varieties, 1.5 oz | 140 | 2.5 | 27 |
| **Granola Bars, 6-packs:** | | | |
| Fiberful, 1.3 oz | 120 | 3.5 | 22 |
| Trail Mix, 1.3 oz | 150 | 5 | 23 |
| **Tri-O-Plex** (Chef Jay's): | | | |
| **High Protein,** Ban. Walnut, 4.2 oz | 405 | 14 | 40 |
| **Duo,** Bursting Peanut Butter | 395 | 17 | 35 |
| **Usana:** | | | |
| Choco Chip, 1.4 oz | 160 | 5 | 17 |
| Go Nuts 'n' Berries, 1.2 oz | 150 | 7 | 18 |
| Peanutt Bliss, 1.2 oz | 160 | 5 | 17 |
| **Zone Perfect:** | | | |
| Blueb. Pomeg., 1.8 oz | 210 | 6 | 24 |
| Choc, Chip Cookie Dough, 1.5 oz | 180 | 5 | 24 |
| Dark Chocolate, av. all varieties, 1.5 oz | 185 | 6 | 22 |
| Fudge Graham, 1.8 oz | 210 | 7 | 23 |
| Strawberry Yogurt, 1.8 oz | 200 | 6 | 25 |
| Sweet & Salty, Cashew Pretzel, 1.6 oz | 200 | 7 | 23 |

## Cocoa & Hot Chocolate  C  F  Cb

**Cocoa:**

| | C | F | Cb |
|---|---|---|---|
| Small (8 fl.oz): | | | |
| With Whole Milk | 205 | 8.5 | 22 |
| With Nonfat Milk | 145 | 1 | 23 |
| Tall (12 fl.oz): With Whole Milk | 280 | 12 | 26 |
| With Nonfat Milk | 185 | 1 | 28 |

**Hot Chocolate:**

| | C | F | Cb |
|---|---|---|---|
| Small (8 fl.oz): With Whole Milk | 180 | 7 | 26 |
| With Nonfat Milk | 140 | 2 | 27 |
| Tall (12 fl.oz): With Whole Milk | 260 | 10 | 36 |
| With Nonfat Milk | 190 | 2 | 37 |
| Cinnabon, Mochalatta Chill, 16 oz | 420 | 17 | 63 |
| Swiss Miss, Mixes, av., 1 packet | 120 | 2.5 | 22 |

## Cocoa - Chocolate Mixes

*Add extra cals/fat/carbohydrate for milk*
**Carnation Breakfast Drinks** ~ *See Page 38*
**Carnation:** *Per 3 Tbsp*

| | C | F | Cb |
|---|---|---|---|
| Malted Milk: Original | 90 | 2 | 15 |
| Chocolate | 90 | 1 | 18 |

**Ghirardelli:**

| | C | F | Cb |
|---|---|---|---|
| Chocolate Mocha, 3 Tbsp, 1.2 oz | 120 | 1.5 | 29 |
| Double Chocolate, 3 Tbsp, 1.3 oz | 120 | 1.5 | 30 |

**Hershey's,** Cocoa,

| | C | F | Cb |
|---|---|---|---|
| Natural, unsweetened, 1 Tbsp, 0.2 oz | 10 | 0.5 | 3 |

**Land O Lakes:**

| | C | F | Cb |
|---|---|---|---|
| Arctic White Coccoa, 1.3 oz | 160 | 6 | 26 |
| Other varieties, 1.3 oz | 140 | 3.5 | 26 |

**Nestle:** *Per Per Single Serve Envelope*

| | C | F | Cb |
|---|---|---|---|
| Chocolate Caramel | 100 | 3 | 19 |
| Dark Chocolate | 100 | 3 | 19 |
| Rich Milk Chocolate: | | | |
| Regular | 80 | 3 | 14 |
| Fat Free | 25 | 0 | 5 |
| No Sugar Added | 50 | 0 | 9 |

**Nesquik Powder:** *Per 2 Tbsp*

| | C | F | Cb |
|---|---|---|---|
| Chocolate; Strawberry | 60 | 0.5 | 15 |
| Chocolate; Strawb., No Added Sugar | 35 | 1 | 7 |

**Ovaltine,** All Natural Cocoa Mixes,

| | C | F | Cb |
|---|---|---|---|
| average all varieties, 2 Tbsp | 40 | 0 | 10 |

**Swiss Miss:** *Per Single Serve Envelope*
**Breakfast Blends:** Great Start

| | C | F | Cb |
|---|---|---|---|
| Breakfast Blends: Great Start | 60 | 1 | 11 |
| Pick Me Up | 110 | 2 | 23 |

**Classics, Milk Chocolate:**

| | C | F | Cb |
|---|---|---|---|
| Hot Cocoa Mix | 90 | 2 | 16 |
| No Added Sugar | 60 | 1 | 10 |
| With Marshmallow | 90 | 2 | 16 |
| Rich Chocolate | 120 | 2 | 23 |

## Instant Coffee  C  F  Cb

**Powder/Granules:** *Regular or Decaffeinated,*

| | C | F | Cb |
|---|---|---|---|
| 1 level tsp | 2 | 0 | 0.5 |
| 1 rounded tsp | 4 | 0 | 1 |
| **Ground,** 3 tsp | 7 | 0 | 2 |
| **Brewed/Percolated,** 1 cup, 8 fl.oz | 4 | 0 | 1 |

**Coffee With Milk/Cream/Creamers:** *Per 8 oz Cup*

| | C | F | Cb |
|---|---|---|---|
| **Black:** | 4 | 0 | 1 |
| With Whole Milk: Dash, 1 Tbsp | 15 | 0.5 | 2 |
| 2 Tbsp, 1 fl.oz | 25 | 1 | 2.5 |
| With 2% Milk, 2 Tbsp | 20 | 0.5 | 2.5 |
| With 1% Milk, 2 Tbsp | 20 | 0.5 | 2.5 |
| With Fat Free Milk, 2 Tbsp | 15 | 0 | 2.5 |
| With Soy Milk: 1 Tbsp | 10 | 0 | 1.5 |
| 2 Tbsp, 1 oz | 15 | 0.5 | 2 |
| With Half & Half: 2 Tbsp | 50 | 3 | 3 |
| ¼ cup, 2 fl.oz | 90 | 6 | 4 |
| With Cream (light coffee), 2 Tbsp | 65 | 6 | 2 |
| With Coffee Mate: Liquid, reg., 1 T. | 20 | 1 | 3 |
| Liquid Fat Free, 1 Tbsp | 25 | 0 | 2 |
| Powder, 1 heaping tsp | 15 | 1 | 2 |
| **Sugar ~ Add Extra:** 1 heaping tsp | 25 | 0 | 6 |
| Single portion, 1 package | 25 | 0 | 6 |
| **Sweeteners,** *(Equal/Splenda/Sweet N Low),* | | | |
| Powder, 1 package | 0 | 0 | 0 |

## Flavored Coffee Mixes

**Chicory:**

| | C | F | Cb |
|---|---|---|---|
| Instant Coffee, 1 tsp | 5 | 0 | 1 |
| Coffee Essence, 1 tsp | 15 | 0 | 4 |

**Caffé D'Vita:**

| | C | F | Cb |
|---|---|---|---|
| Mixes, average all varieties, 3 tsp, | 60 | 1.5 | 11 |
| Sugar Free Mixes, 2 tsp | 35 | 2 | 3 |

**General Foods International:**

| | C | F | Cb |
|---|---|---|---|
| Average all varieties, 0.5 oz | 60 | 3 | 10 |
| Sugar-free, av. all varieties, 1 tsp | 30 | 2.5 | 2 |
| Cappuccino Coolers, all varieties, 0.5 oz | 60 | 0 | 15 |

**Hills Bros:** *Per 3 Tbsp, 1 oz*

| | C | F | Cb |
|---|---|---|---|
| Cappuccino: French Vanilla | 120 | 4.5 | 19 |
| Chocolate Hazelnut | 110 | 3.5 | 19 |
| Classic Cappuccino | 120 | 5 | 17 |
| Dark Chocolate | 110 | 4 | 19 |
| Mocha Mint | 120 | 4 | 20 |

**Nescafe,** Memento, 1 stick,

| | C | F | Cb |
|---|---|---|---|
| average all varieties | 100 | 2.5 | 19 |

**Starbucks,** VIA, Iced Coffee,

| | C | F | Cb |
|---|---|---|---|
| all varieties, 1 stick/packet | 100 | 0 | 24 |

### Coffee Shops/Restaurants

*Per 8 fl.oz Cup (Unless Indicated)*

| | C | F | Cb |
|---|---|---|---|
| **Coffee,** Regular/Percolated/Filtered | 5 | 0 | 0 |
| **Americano Drip Coffee,** 1 cup | 7.5 | 0 | 1 |
| **Cafe Au Lait:** 1 cup, 8 fl.oz | 60 | 3.5 | 5 |
| Nonfat Milk, 1 cup, 8 fl.oz | 35 | 0 | 5 |
| **Caffe Latté:** | | | |
| 8 fl.oz cup: With Whole Milk | 110 | 6 | 9 |
| With 2% Milk | 100 | 3.5 | 9 |
| With Nonfat Milk | 70 | 0 | 10 |
| 12 fl.oz: With Whole Milk | 180 | 9 | 14 |
| With Nonfat Milk | 100 | 0 | 15 |
| 16 fl.oz: With Whole Milk | 220 | 11 | 18 |
| With Nonfat Milk | 130 | 0 | 19 |
| **Cafe Mocha (Mochaccino):** 8 fl.oz | 150 | 6 | 20 |
| 12 fl.oz | 230 | 9 | 31 |
| 16 fl.oz | 290 | 12 | 41 |
| **Cappuccino:** | | | |
| 8 fl.oz cup: With Whole Milk | 90 | 3.5 | 7 |
| With 2% Milk | 80 | 3 | 8 |
| With Nonfat Milk | 50 | 0 | 8 |
| 12 fl.oz: With Whole Milk | 110 | 6 | 9 |
| With 2% Milk | 90 | 3.5 | 9 |
| With Nonfat Milk | 60 | 0 | 9 |
| 16 fl.oz: With Whole Milk | 140 | 7 | 11 |
| With 2% Milk | 120 | 3.5 | 11 |
| With Nonfat Milk | 80 | 0 | 12 |
| **Mocha:** *With Cream* | | | |
| 8 fl.oz: With Whole Milk | 200 | 11 | 22 |
| With Nonfat Milk | 160 | 6 | 22 |
| 12 fl.oz: Whole Milk | 290 | 15 | 33 |
| With Nonfat Milk | 230 | 8 | 34 |
| **Iced Mocha:** *Without Cream* | | | |
| 12 fl.oz: With Whole Milk | 170 | 6 | 26 |
| With Nonfat Milk | 130 | 2 | 27 |
| **Espresso:** Single (Solo), 1 fl.oz | 5 | 0 | 1 |
| Double (Doppio), 2 fl.oz | 10 | 0 | 2 |
| **Espresso con Panna,** | | | |
| (w/ dollop wh. cream), solo, 1 fl.oz | 30 | 2.5 | 2 |
| **Espresso Macchiato,** solo, 1 fl.oz | 5 | 0 | 1 |
| **Frappuccino:** Tall, 12 fl.oz | 180 | 2.5 | 37 |
| Grande, 16 fl.oz | 240 | 3 | 48 |
| **Frappuccino Mocha:** | | | |
| (With Cream): Tall, 12 fl.oz | 280 | 11 | 43 |
| Grande, 16 fl.oz | 380 | 15 | 57 |
| **Iced Latte,** Similar to Caffe Latte | | | |

McCafe (McDonald's) ~ See Fast Food, Page 216
Starbucks ~ See Fast-Foods Section , Page 243

### Coffee Substitute Mixes

| | C | F | Cb |
|---|---|---|---|
| **Roasted Cereal Beverages ~** *(No Caffeine)* | | | |
| Cafix, Instant Beverage, 1 tsp | 5 | 0 | 1 |
| Kaffree Roma, Instant Beverage, 1 tsp | 10 | 0 | 2 |
| Teeccino, Herbal Coffees, 1 tsp | 10 | 0 | 2 |

### Irish & Liqueur Coffees

| | C | F | Cb |
|---|---|---|---|
| **Irish Coffee,** without sugar | 175 | 10 | 0 |
| **Liqueur Coffee,** with cream, | | | |
| all varieties, av., 1 fl.oz | 100 | 5 | 7 |

### Coffee Extras

| | C | F | Cb |
|---|---|---|---|
| Chocolate (Cocoa) Topping, ½ tsp | 5 | 0 | 1 |
| Flavored Syrups: Regular, 2 Tbsp | 80 | 0 | 20 |
| Sugar-free, 2 Tbsp | 0 | 0 | 0 |
| Half & Half Cream: 2 Tbsp | 40 | 3.5 | 1 |
| Single serve pkg, ⅜ fl.oz | 15 | 1.5 | 0.5 |
| Light whipped cream, 2 Tbsp | 15 | 1.5 | 1 |
| Marshmallows, miniature (2) | 5 | 0 | 1 |
| **Sugar:** | | | |
| 1 single portion package | 20 | 0 | 5 |
| 1 level tsp | 15 | 0 | 4 |
| 1 heaping tsp | 25 | 0 | 6 |
| *Equal/Splenda/Sweet 'N Low* | 0 | 0 | 0 |

### Coffee Shop ~ Cakes, Cookies

| | C | F | Cb |
|---|---|---|---|
| **Cookies:** | | | |
| Biscotti, 1 oz | 140 | 6.5 | 18 |
| Chocolate Chip, 3 oz | 350 | 15 | 54 |
| Oatmeal Raisin, 3 oz | 350 | 12 | 56 |
| Peanut Butter, 3 oz | 410 | 25 | 39 |
| White Chocolate Macadamia, 3.33 oz | 420 | 20 | 55 |
| **Cakes/Pastries:** | | | |
| Almond Croissant, 5 oz | 620 | 35 | 67 |
| Apple Danish, 5 oz | 450 | 18 | 67 |
| Banana Walnut, 4.5 oz | 410 | 17 | 60 |
| Brownie, 3 oz | 390 | 24 | 42 |
| Bundt, Chocolate, 4 oz | 440 | 21 | 61 |
| Carrot Cake, 4 oz | 400 | 22 | 45 |
| Chocolate Cake, 5 oz | 530 | 28 | 65 |
| Crumble Coffee Cake, 4.5 oz | 500 | 25 | 65 |
| Cupcake, 3 oz | 330 | 16 | 43 |
| Pound Cake, av., 3 oz | 330 | 17 | 40 |
| **Cinnamon Roll,** 6 oz | 500 | 15 | 83 |
| **Donuts:** | | | |
| Sugared, 1.8 oz | 220 | 11 | 27 |
| Glazed, 2 oz | 250 | 12 | 34 |
| **Pretzel,** large, 4 oz | 290 | 5 | 52 |

Starbucks Bakery Items ~ See Page 244

### Ready To Drink Coffee C F Cb

#### Chilled:
**Full Throttle Coffee & Energy** ~ *See Page 38*
**International Delight,**
   Iced, all varieties, 8 fl.oz | **150** | 2.5 | 29
**Java Monster Energy** ~ *See Page 39*
**Kahlua,** Cappuccino Shake, 10.5 fl.oz | **130** | 2 | 24
**Shock Coffee:**
Triple Latte, 8 fl.oz can | **150** | 3.5 | 27
Triple Mocha, 8 fl.oz can | **150** | 3.5 | 28
**Skinny Cow,** all flavors, 8 fl.oz | **120** | 2.5 | 20
**Starbucks:**
**Doubleshot Energy Drink:** *Per 15 fl.oz*
   Coffee with Millk | **210** | 2.5 | 36
   Hazelnut | **210** | 3 | 31
   Mocha | **200** | 2.5 | 33
   Vanilla | **210** | 2.5 | 34
   Light Vanilla | **130** | 2.5 | 20
   White Chocolate | **210** | 3 | 31
**Frappuccino Coffee Drink:** *Per 9.5 fl.oz*
   Caramel; Vanilla | **200** | 3 | 37
   Light Mocha | **100** | 3 | 12
**Iced Coffee:** Unsweetened, 8 fl.oz | **10** | 0 | 0
   Caramel, 11 fl.oz | **110** | 0.5 | 21
**Iced Espresso Classics:** *Per 8 fl.oz*
   Caffe Mocha | **140** | 2.5 | 23
   Caramel; Vanilla Latte | **130** | 2.5 | 21
   Light Espresso Drink, 6.5 fl.oz | **70** | 4 | 5
**Starbucks Refreshers** ~ *See Page 40*
**TruMoo,** Protein Plus,
   Chocolate; Vanilla, average, 8 fl.oz | **230** | 2.5 | 37

## CALORIE KING TIP!

### Reduce the Calories in Your Coffee Drinks:

- Request non-fat milk in place of whole or 2% milk
- Downsize to 8 fl.oz or 12 fl.oz
- Avoid cream on frappuccinos
- Replace sugar with *Equal, Splenda Stevia* or *Sweet 'N Low*
- Avoid syrup add-ons

### Caffeine Counter

Moderate caffeine intake is not harmful to healthy adults. However, frequent large amounts (over 350mg/day) may cause dependency ('caffeinism') and adversely affect health. To be safe, limit caffeine to 200mg/day. Avoid if pregnant, breast feeding, a child under 8, have sleep problems, an overactive bladder or heart arrhythmia.

**Caffeine** (mg)

**Coffee:** Instant, weak, 1 level teaspoon | 30
   Medium, 1 rounded teaspoon | 60
   Strong, 1 heaping teaspoon | 100
   **Decaffeinated**, 1 round teaspoon | 2
   **Bags (Folgers)**, 1 bag (6-8 fl.oz) | 115
   **Ground**, 1 Tbsp, 0.2 oz | 60
   **Bottled (Ready-To-Drink)**, 9.5 fl.oz | 70
**Coffee Shop:** Brewed, 8 fl.oz | 110-150
   **Cappuccino:** 1 cup, 8 fl.oz | 75
   Tall, 12 fl.oz | 110
   Large, 16 fl.oz | 150
   **Decappuccino**, decaffeinated | 5
   **Espresso**: Regular/Solo | 75
   Double, (Doppio) | 150
   Iced Coffee, 12 fl.oz | 140
   Latte, 1 cup, 8 fl.oz | 75
   Mocha, 1 cup, 8 fl.oz | 90
   Hot Chocolate, 8 fl.oz | 15
**Tea (Black/Green):** Weak, 1 cup | 20
   Medium Strength, 1 cup | 40
   Strong, 1 cup | 70
   Decaffeinated Tea, 1 cup | 0-5
   Herbal Tea, 1 cup | 0
   **Iced Tea**, tall glass/can, 12 fl.oz | 25-30
**Soft Drinks:** *Per 12 fl.oz Can*
   Coca-Cola; Pepsi (Regular/Diet) | 35
   Diet Coke; TAB; RC Cola (Regular) | 45
   Dr. Pepper; Sunkist Orange | 40
   Pepsi One; Mountain Dew; Mellow Yellow; Surge | 55
   Pepsi Max (Regular/Diet) Sun Drop (Reg/Diet) | 70
   7-Up, Fanta, Sprite, Fresca, Diet Rite Cola | 0
**Energy Drinks (with added caffeine):**
   (AMP, Adrenaline Rush, Full Throttle Monster, No Fear, Red Bull, Rockstar)
   **Average all brands:** 8 fl.oz | 80
   16 fl.oz | 160
   **NOS Energy**, 16 fl.oz | 260
**Chocolate Bars:** Milk Chocolate, 2 oz | 20
   Dark Chocolate, 2 oz | 30
**Choc Chip Cookies**, 2 medium, 2 oz | 6
**Chocolate Syrup**, 2 Tbsp, 1.4 oz | 5
**Medicinals:** Excedrin, Extra Strength (2) | 130
   NoDoz Maximum, 1 tablet | 200

| Energy/Protein Drinks | C | F | Cb |
|---|---|---|---|
| 5-hour Energy, 2 fl.oz | 4 | 0 | 1 |
| **ABB:** | | | |
| **Energy:** Speed Shot, 8.5 fl.oz | 0 | 0 | 0 |
| Ripped Force, 18 fl.oz | 90 | 0 | 23 |
| **Hi-Pro:** | | | |
| Pure Pro 35 Shake, all flav., 12 fl.oz | 160 | 0.5 | 5 |
| Pure Pro 50, all flavors, 14.5 fl.oz | 240 | 1.5 | 7 |
| **Recovery,** | | | |
| Maxx Recovery, all flavors, 18 fl.oz | 400 | 0.5 | 60 |
| AdvantEDGE *(EAS)*, | | | |
| Carb Control, av. all flavors, 11 fl.oz | 105 | 2.5 | 3 |
| **AllSport,** | | | |
| Hydration, all flavors, 20 fl.oz | 150 | 0 | 40 |
| AMP: *Per 16 fl.oz Can* | | | |
| **Active:** Lemonade | 130 | 0 | 31 |
| Lemonade, Sugar Free | 15 | 0 | 0.5 |
| **Boost:** Original | 220 | 0 | 58 |
| Original, Sugar Free | 10 | 0 | 0.5 |
| Cherry; Grape | 130 | 0 | 31 |
| **Focus,** Mixed Berry | 130 | 0 | 31 |
| **Arizona,** | | | |
| Caution Extr. Performance, 11 fl.oz | 160 | 0 | 40 |
| Atkins, Advantage Shakes, 11 fl.oz | 155 | 9 | 4 |
| Bariatrix, Proti-Max, | | | |
| Anytime Shakes, av., 8 fl.oz | 100 | 4 | 4 |
| **Bawls:** | | | |
| **Guarana:** Original, 10 fl.oz | 120 | 0 | 32 |
| Cherry, 10 fl.oz | 90 | 0 | 32 |
| Blue Sky, Blue Energy, 8 fl.oz | 120 | 0 | 29 |
| Bolthouse: *Per 8 fl.oz* | | | |
| **Breakfast Smoothies,** | | | |
| Peach/Strawberry Parfait, 8 fl.oz | 190 | 2.5 | 35 |
| **Protein Plus,** | | | |
| Blended Coffee | 190 | 2.5 | 26 |
| Choc.; Mango; Vanilla, av. | 200 | 2 | 30 |
| Boost: *Per 8 fl.oz* | | | |
| Original, all flavors | 240 | 4 | 41 |
| Glucose Control, all flavors | 190 | 7 | 16 |
| High Protein, all flavors | 240 | 6 | 33 |
| Plus, all flavors | 360 | 14 | 45 |
| **Carnation:** | | | |
| **Breakfast Essentials :** | | | |
| Powder Only: | | | |
| Average all flav., 1 env., 1.3 oz | 130 | 1 | 27 |
| No Sug. Added, av. all flav., 0.7 oz | 60 | 1 | 12 |
| **Ready To Drink,** all flavors, 8 fl.oz | 240 | 4 | 41 |
| Celestial Seasoning, Shots, | | | |
| Kombucha, all flavors, 2 oz | 30 | 0 | 8 |
| CeraSport, EX1, Lime Flavor, 8.5 fl.oz | 20 | 0 | 1 |
| Champion Lyte, Sports Drink | 0 | 0 | 0 |

| Champion Nutrition: | C | F | Cb |
|---|---|---|---|
| Heavywt Gainer 900, av., 4 scps, 5.4 oz | 600 | 7 | 102 |
| Ultramet, Original, 1 packet, 2.7 oz | 280 | 2 | 24 |
| **Clif Shot,** | | | |
| Energy Gel, av. all flavors, 1.2 oz pkt | 105 | 1 | 21 |
| Cocaine, Energy, 8.4 fl.oz can | 70 | 0 | 18 |
| Core Power: *20g, av. all,* 11.5 fl.oz | 150 | 3.5 | 16 |
| 26g, average all flavors, 11.5 fl.oz | 240 | 3.5 | 27 |
| Curves, Protein Drink, | | | |
| Choc.; Vanilla, 2 scps, 1 oz | 120 | 1 | 12 |
| **CytoSport:** | | | |
| **Muscle Milk:** | | | |
| Powder, all flavors, av., 2 scoops | 310 | 12 | 18 |
| Ready To Drink: Chocolate, 10 fl.oz | 170 | 7 | 8 |
| 17 fl.oz | 340 | 16 | 16 |
| Drank, Anti Energy, 16 fl.oz bottle | 220 | 0 | 54 |
| EAS ~ *See AdvantEdge & Myoplex* | | | |
| Ensure: *Per Bottle* | | | |
| Original, 8 fl.oz | 220 | 6 | 33 |
| Active: Clear, 10 fl.oz | 180 | 0 | 37 |
| Muscle Health, 8 fl.oz | 250 | 8 | 31 |
| High Protein Shake, 14 fl.oz | 210 | 2.5 | 23 |
| Plus, 8 fl.oz bottle | 350 | 11 | 50 |
| Enterex, Diabetic, all flavors, 8 fl.oz | 240 | 9 | 27 |
| FRS, Energy, Wild Berry; Cherry Limeade | | | |
| average, 12 fl.oz | 90 | 0 | 22 |
| Fruit$_2$O *(Veryfine):* Classic 20 fl.oz | 0 | 0 | 0 |
| Sparkling, 20 fl.oz | 0 | 0 | 1 |
| Full Throttle: *Per 16 fl.oz* | | | |
| **Energy:** Citrus | 220 | 0 | 58 |
| Blue Agave; Red Berry | 230 | 0 | 58 |
| **Fuze:** | | | |
| Blends average, 16.9 fl.oz | 185 | 0.5 | 43 |
| **Juice:** Berry Punch, 8 fl.oz | 80 | 0 | 20 |
| Strawb. Lemonade, 8 fl.oz | 100 | 0 | 25 |
| **Gatorade:** | | | |
| G Series: *Ready To Drink* | | | |
| Endurance, Thirst Quencher: 12 fl oz | 80 | 0 | 21 |
| 32 fl oz bottle | 215 | 0 | 56 |
| G2 Low Calorie Thirst Quencher: | | | |
| 12 fl oz | 30 | 0 | 7 |
| 32 fl oz | 80 | 0 | 19 |
| Prime, Sports Fuel, | | | |
| 4 fl oz pouch | 100 | 0 | 25 |
| Recover: | | | |
| Post-Game Prot. Drink, 16.9 oz | 230 | 0 | 41 |
| Protein Shake, 330 ml carton | 270 | 1 | 46 |
| **Genisoy,** | | | |
| **Protein Powder,** Chocolate; Vanilla, | | | |
| average, 1.3 oz scoop | 125 | 0 | 18 |
| **Glaceau:** | | | |
| Smartwater, 8 fl.oz | 0 | 0 | 0 |
| Vitaminwater, all flav., 20 fl.oz | 120 | 0 | 32 |
| **Glucerna,** | | | |
| **Shakes,** all flavors, 8 fl.oz | 190 | 7 | 23 |

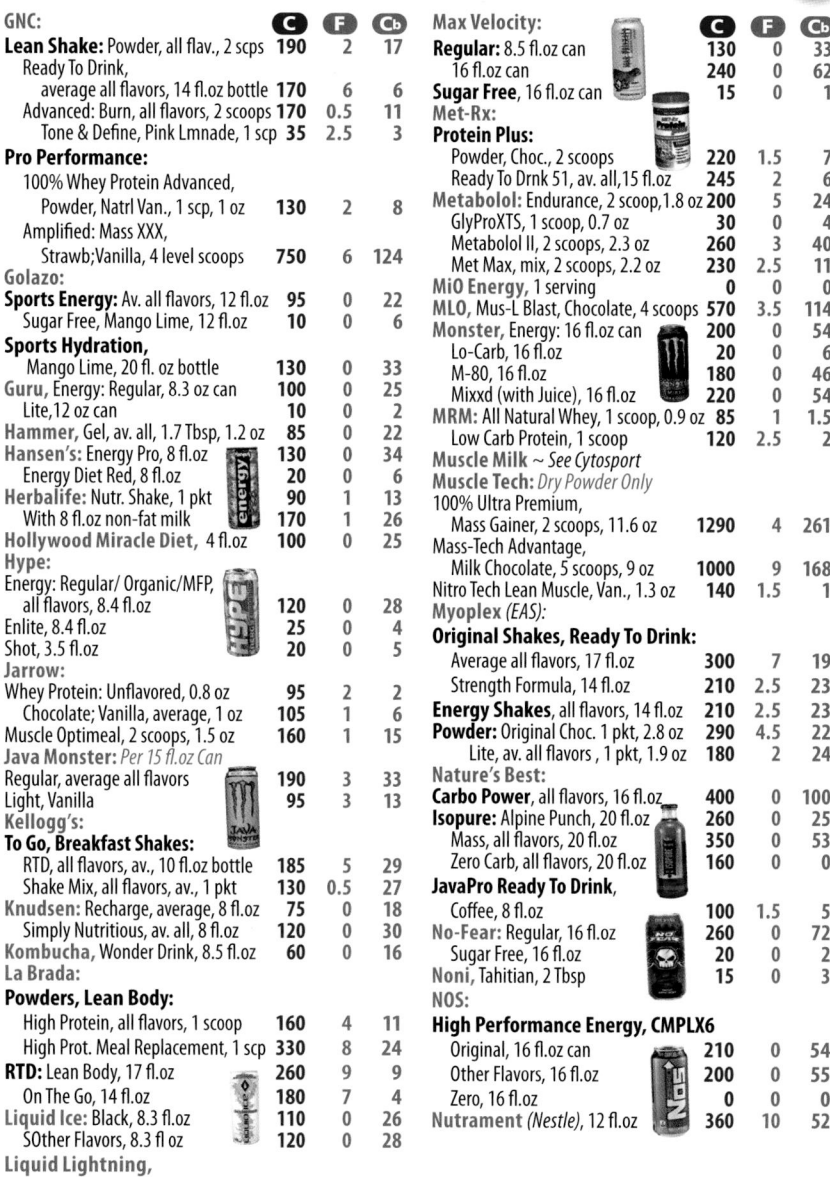

| GNC: | C | F | Cb |
|---|---|---|---|
| **Lean Shake:** Powder, all flav., 2 scps | 190 | 2 | 17 |
| Ready To Drink, | | | |
| average all flavors, 14 fl.oz bottle | 170 | 6 | 6 |
| Advanced: Burn, all flavors, 2 scoops | 170 | 0.5 | 11 |
| Tone & Define, Pink Lmnade, 1 scp | 35 | 2.5 | 3 |
| **Pro Performance** | | | |
| 100% Whey Protein Advanced, | | | |
| Powder, Natrl Van., 1 scp, 1 oz | 130 | 2 | 8 |
| Amplified: Mass XXX, | | | |
| Strawb;Vanilla, 4 level scoops | 750 | 6 | 124 |
| Golazo: | | | |
| **Sports Energy:** Av. all flavors, 12 fl.oz | 95 | 0 | 22 |
| Sugar Free, Mango Lime, 12 fl.oz | 10 | 0 | 6 |
| **Sports Hydration,** | | | |
| Mango Lime, 20 fl. oz bottle | 130 | 0 | 33 |
| **Guru,** Energy: Regular, 8.3 oz can | 100 | 0 | 25 |
| Lite,12 oz can | 10 | 0 | 2 |
| **Hammer:** Gel, av. all, 1.7 Tbsp, 1.2 oz | 85 | 0 | 22 |
| **Hansen's:** Energy Pro, 8 fl.oz | 130 | 0 | 34 |
| Energy Diet Red, 8 fl.oz | 20 | 0 | 6 |
| **Herbalife:** Nutr. Shake, 1 pkt | 90 | 1 | 13 |
| With 8 fl.oz non-fat milk | 170 | 1 | 26 |
| **Hollywood Miracle Diet,** 4 fl.oz | 100 | 0 | 25 |
| **Hype:** | | | |
| Energy: Regular/ Organic/MFP, | | | |
| all flavors, 8.4 fl.oz | 120 | 0 | 28 |
| Enlite, 8.4 fl.oz | 25 | 0 | 4 |
| Shot, 3.5 fl.oz | 20 | 0 | 5 |
| **Jarrow:** | | | |
| Whey Protein: Unflavored, 0.8 oz | 95 | 2 | 2 |
| Chocolate; Vanilla, average, 1 oz | 105 | 1 | 6 |
| Muscle Optimeal, 2 scoops, 1.5 oz | 160 | 1 | 15 |
| *Java Monster: Per 15 fl.oz Can* | | | |
| Regular, average all flavors | 190 | 3 | 33 |
| Light, Vanilla | 95 | 3 | 13 |
| **Kellogg's:** | | | |
| **To Go, Breakfast Shakes:** | | | |
| RTD, all flavors, av., 10 fl.oz bottle | 185 | 5 | 29 |
| Shake Mix, all flavors, av., 1 pkt | 130 | 0.5 | 27 |
| **Knudsen:** Recharge, average, 8 fl.oz | 75 | 0 | 18 |
| Simply Nutritious, av. all, 8 fl.oz | 120 | 0 | 30 |
| **Kombucha,** Wonder Drink, 8.5 fl.oz | 60 | 0 | 16 |
| **La Brada:** | | | |
| **Powders, Lean Body:** | | | |
| High Protein, all flavors, 1 scoop | 160 | 4 | 11 |
| High Prot. Meal Replacement, 1 scp | 330 | 8 | 24 |
| **RTD:** Lean Body, 17 fl.oz | 260 | 9 | 9 |
| On The Go, 14 fl.oz | 180 | 7 | 4 |
| **Liquid Ice:** Black, 8.3 fl.oz | 110 | 0 | 26 |
| SOther Flavors, 8.3 fl oz | 120 | 0 | 28 |
| **Liquid Lightning,** | | | |
| Regular, 8.5 fl.oz | 90 | 0 | 22 |

| Max Velocity: | C | F | Cb |
|---|---|---|---|
| **Regular:** 8.5 fl.oz can | 130 | 0 | 33 |
| 16 fl.oz can | 240 | 0 | 62 |
| **Sugar Free,** 16 fl.oz can | 15 | 0 | 1 |
| **Met-Rx:** | | | |
| **Protein Plus:** | | | |
| Powder, Choc., 2 scoops | 220 | 1.5 | 7 |
| Ready To Drnk 51, av. all,15 fl.oz | 245 | 2 | 6 |
| **Metabolol:** Endurance, 2 scoop,1.8 oz | 200 | 5 | 24 |
| GlyProXTS, 1 scoop, 0.7 oz | 30 | 0 | 4 |
| Metabolol II, 2 scoops, 2.3 oz | 260 | 3 | 40 |
| Met Max, mix, 2 scoops, 2.2 oz | 230 | 2.5 | 11 |
| **MiO Energy,** 1 serving | 0 | 0 | 0 |
| **MLO,** Mus-L Blast, Chocolate, 4 scoops | 570 | 3.5 | 114 |
| **Monster:** Energy: 16 fl.oz can | 200 | 0 | 54 |
| Lo-Carb, 16 fl.oz | 20 | 0 | 6 |
| M-80, 16 fl.oz | 180 | 0 | 46 |
| Mixxd (with Juice), 16 fl.oz | 220 | 0 | 54 |
| **MRM:** All Natural Whey, 1 scoop, 0.9 oz | 85 | 1 | 1.5 |
| Low Carb Protein, 1 scoop | 120 | 2.5 | 2 |
| **Muscle Milk** ~ *See Cytosport* | | | |
| **Muscle Tech:** *Dry Powder Only* | | | |
| 100% Ultra Premium, | | | |
| Mass Gainer, 2 scoops, 11.6 oz | 1290 | 4 | 261 |
| Mass-Tech Advantage, | | | |
| Milk Chocolate, 5 scoops, 9 oz | 1000 | 9 | 168 |
| Nitro Tech Lean Muscle, Van., 1.3 oz | 140 | 1.5 | 1 |
| **Myoplex** *(EAS):* | | | |
| **Original Shakes, Ready To Drink:** | | | |
| Average all flavors, 17 fl.oz | 300 | 7 | 19 |
| Strength Formula, 14 fl.oz | 210 | 2.5 | 23 |
| **Energy Shakes,** all flavors, 14 fl.oz | 210 | 2.5 | 23 |
| **Powder:** Original Choc. 1 pkt, 2.8 oz | 290 | 4.5 | 22 |
| Lite, av. all flavors , 1 pkt, 1.9 oz | 180 | 2 | 24 |
| **Nature's Best:** | | | |
| **Carbo Power,** all flavors, 16 fl.oz | 400 | 0 | 100 |
| **Isopure:** Alpine Punch, 20 fl.oz | 260 | 0 | 25 |
| Mass, all flavors, 20 fl.oz | 350 | 0 | 53 |
| Zero Carb all flavors, 20 fl.oz | 160 | 0 | 0 |
| **JavaPro Ready To Drink,** | | | |
| Coffee, 8 fl.oz | 100 | 1.5 | 5 |
| **No-Fear:** Regular, 16 fl.oz | 260 | 0 | 72 |
| Sugar Free, 16 fl.oz | 20 | 0 | 2 |
| **Noni,** Tahitian, 2 Tbsp | 15 | 0 | 3 |
| **NOS:** | | | |
| **High Performance Energy, CMPLX6** | | | |
| Original, 16 fl.oz can | 210 | 0 | 54 |
| Other Flavors, 16 fl.oz | 200 | 0 | 55 |
| Zero, 16 fl.oz | 0 | 0 | 0 |
| **Nutrament** *(Nestle)* 12 fl.oz | 360 | 10 | 52 |

## Energy/Protein Drinks (Cont)

| | C | F | Cb |
|---|---|---|---|
| **Nutrilite** *(Amway)*: | | | |
| **Meal Replacement Shakes:** | | | |
| Powder, av. all flavors, 1.2 oz scoop | 110 | 3 | 8 |
| Ready To Drink, all flavors, 11 fl.oz | 140 | 3 | 15 |
| **Protein Shake**, Vanilla, 11.5 oz | 190 | 6 | 7 |
| **Optifast:** *(Nestle):* | | | |
| **800:** Shake Mix, 1 pkg | 160 | 3 | 20 |
| Ready To Drink Shakes, 8 fl.oz | 160 | 3 | 20 |
| **HP Shake Mix**, 1 pkg | 200 | 6 | 10 |
| **Optimum Nutrition:** | | | |
| **100%:** Whey, Gold Standard, 1 oz scp | 120 | 1 | 3 |
| Oats & Whey, 1.9 oz scoop | 200 | 1.5 | 22 |
| Soy Protein, 1 oz scoop | 120 | 1.5 | 2 |
| **Optisource** *(Nestle)*, | | | |
| Very High Protein Drink, 8 fl.oz | 200 | 6 | 12 |
| **Powerade:** | | | |
| **Sports Drink:** | | | |
| Regular, av. all flav.,12 fl.oz | 80 | 0 | 22 |
| Zero, 12 fl.oz | 0 | 0 | 0 |
| **PowerBar:** | | | |
| Performance Energy Blends, | | | |
| average, 1 pouch | 80 | 0 | 21 |
| Power Gel, av. all flavors, 1.5 oz pkg | 110 | 0 | 27 |
| **Propel**, Workout Water, | | | |
| all flavors, 12 fl.oz | 0 | 0 | 0 |
| **Radioactive:** | | | |
| Regular: 10.5 oz | 150 | 0 | 37 |
| 16 oz | 220 | 0 | 56 |
| Sugar Free, all sizes | 0 | 0 | 0 |
| **Red Bull:** | | | |
| Energy Drink, all flavors: | | | |
| 8.4 fl.oz | 110 | 0 | 28 |
| 12 fl.oz can | 160 | 0 | 40 |
| Simply Cola, 12 fl.oz | 130 | 0 | 31 |
| Sugar-Free, 8.4 fl.oz | 10 | 0 | 3 |
| Zero Calories, 8.4 fl.oz | 0 | 0 | 0 |
| **Resource** *(Nestle):* | | | |
| Breeze, 8 fl.oz | 250 | 0 | 54 |
| Diabetishield, 8 fl.oz | 150 | 0 | 30 |
| Health Shake: 4 fl.oz | 200 | 4 | 35 |
| No Added Sugar, 4 fl.oz | 200 | 9 | 22 |
| Shake Plus, 8 fl.oz | 480 | 16 | 69 |
| **Revival**, Soy Mix, unsweetened: | | | |
| Plain, 2 scoops, 0.95 oz | 105 | 1 | 4 |
| Chocolate Day Dream, 1 package | 120 | 2.5 | 7 |
| **Rhino's**, Energy Drink, | | | |
| all flavors, 100ml | 50 | 0 | 11 |
| **Rip It**, Energy Fuel, Citrus X, 16 fl.oz | 260 | 0 | 66 |
| **Rockstar:** *Per 16 fl.oz Can* | | | |
| Energy Drink: Punched, av. | 270 | 0 | 62 |
| Sugar Free | 20 | 0 | 0 |
| **Rush:** *Per 8 fl.oz* | C | F | Cb |
| Energy Drink: Regular | 140 | 0 | 31 |
| Lite | 0 | 0 | 0 |
| **SK Energy**, Energy Shot, all flavors, 2 oz | 0 | 0 | 0 |
| **Slim-Fast:** | | | |
| **Protein Meal Shakes,** | | | |
| Ready to Drink, | | | |
| av. all flavors, 10 fl.oz | 190 | 6 | 25 |
| **Protein Shake Mixes,** | | | |
| French Vanilla, 0.9 oz scoop | 200 | 4 | 28 |
| **SoBe:** *Per 20 fl.oz Can/Bottle* | | | |
| **Elixir**, Citrus Energy | 250 | 0 | 64 |
| **Lifewater:** Average all flavors | 100 | 0 | 25 |
| 0-Cal, average all flavors | 0 | 0 | 9 |
| *Note: Carb figures inlude 7-10g sugar alcohol* | | | |
| **Solixir**, Energy Drink, av. all, 12 fl.oz | 55 | 0 | 13 |
| **Special K,** | | | |
| **Protein Shakes,** av. all flavors, | | | |
| 11 fl.oz | 185 | 5 | 28 |
| **Spiru-Tein:** *Per 1.2 oz* | | | |
| **Energy Meal:** | | | |
| Chocolate | 95 | 0 | 10 |
| Vanilla | 100 | 0 | 10 |
| **Starbucks:** | | | |
| Refreshers, av. all flav.,12 fl.oz | 60 | 0 | 19 |
| Doubleshot Energy ~ See page 37 | | | |
| **Steaz:** Energy, all flav., 12 fl.oz | 135 | 0 | 35 |
| Zero Calorie, Berry, 12 fl.oz | 0 | 0 | 0 |
| **The Sports Club/LA:** | | | |
| Beachbody Whey Prot. Powder, | | | |
| Chocolate; Vanilla, 2 scoops, 1.4 oz | 130 | 4 | 7 |
| **Twin Lab**, MVP Fuel, all flavors, | | | |
| 1 scoop, 0.5 oz | 25 | 0 | 6 |
| **Venom:** Mojave Rattler, 16 fl.oz | 50 | 0 | 8 |
| Average other varieties, 16 fl.oz | 235 | 0 | 57 |
| **Verve:** Energy, 8.3 fl.oz can | 70 | 0 | 18 |
| Sugar Free | 5 | 0 | 1 |
| **Weider:** | | | |
| **100% Whey**, 1 scoop, 1.4 oz | 160 | 3 | 12 |
| **Creatine ATP**, ½ cup, 1.7 oz | 210 | 0 | 37 |
| **Dynamic Wght Gainer**, av., 4.5 oz | 450 | 2 | 96 |
| **Mega Mass 2000**, av., 3.5 oz | 400 | 7 | 62 |
| **Pro Carb**, Ultimate Mass Gainer, | | | |
| 6 scoops, average, 7 oz | 770 | 6 | 161 |
| **Worldwide:** | | | |
| Carbo Rush, average, 20 fl.oz | 270 | 0 | 68 |
| Pure Protein Shakes, | | | |
| 35g Protein, 11 fl.oz | 160 | 1 | 2 |
| **Worx**, Energy, | | | |
| Original; Extra Strength, 2 fl.oz | 0 | 0 | 0 |
| **XS** *(Quixtar)*, Energy Drink, 8.4 oz | 10 | 0 | 0 |
| **Zola**, Acai, Original Juice, 8 fl.oz | 125 | 2 | 25 |

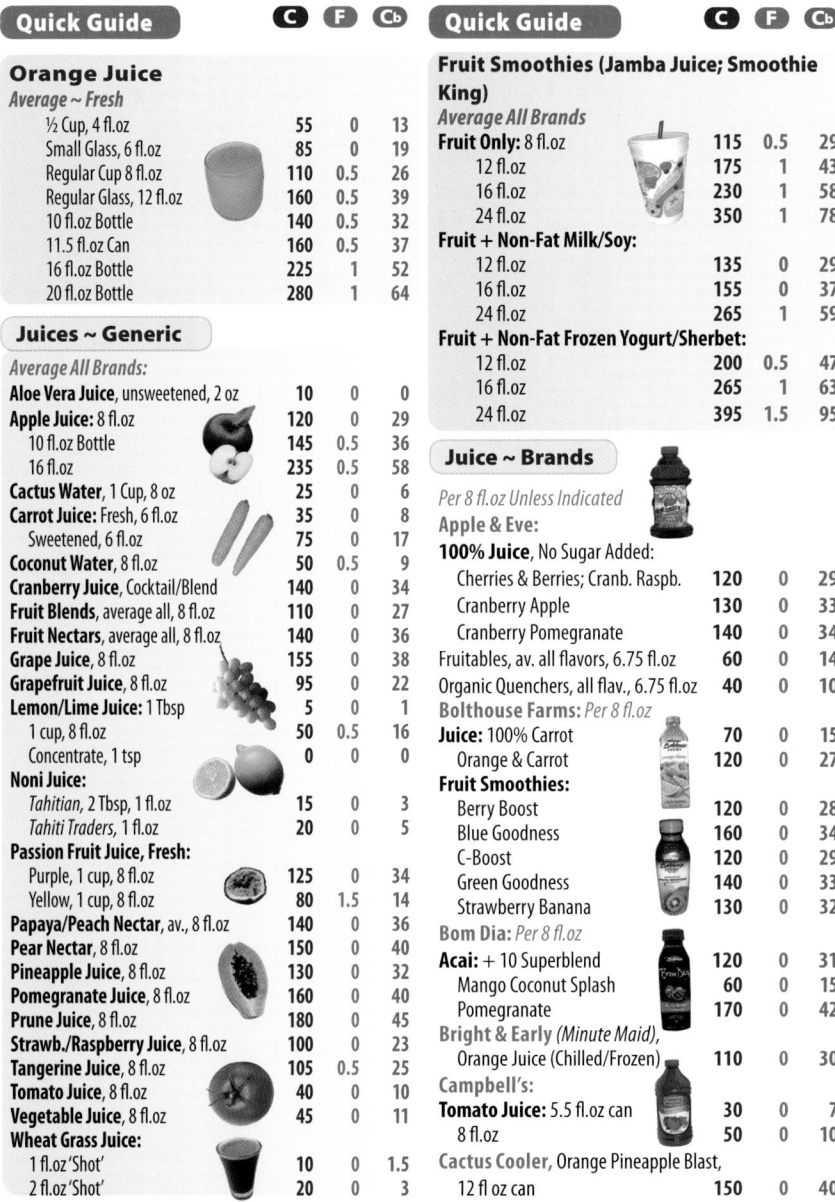

## Quick Guide  C F Cb

### Orange Juice
*Average ~ Fresh*

| | C | F | Cb |
|---|---|---|---|
| ½ Cup, 4 fl.oz | 55 | 0 | 13 |
| Small Glass, 6 fl.oz | 85 | 0 | 19 |
| Regular Cup 8 fl.oz | 110 | 0.5 | 26 |
| Regular Glass, 12 fl.oz | 160 | 0.5 | 39 |
| 10 fl.oz Bottle | 140 | 0.5 | 32 |
| 11.5 fl.oz Can | 160 | 0.5 | 37 |
| 16 fl.oz Bottle | 225 | 1 | 52 |
| 20 fl.oz Bottle | 280 | 1 | 64 |

### Juices ~ Generic
*Average All Brands:*

| | C | F | Cb |
|---|---|---|---|
| Aloe Vera Juice, unsweetened, 2 oz | 10 | 0 | 0 |
| Apple Juice: 8 fl.oz | 120 | 0 | 29 |
| 10 fl.oz Bottle | 145 | 0.5 | 36 |
| 16 fl.oz | 235 | 0.5 | 58 |
| Cactus Water, 1 Cup, 8 oz | 25 | 0 | 6 |
| Carrot Juice: Fresh, 6 fl.oz | 35 | 0 | 8 |
| Sweetened, 6 fl.oz | 75 | 0 | 17 |
| Coconut Water, 8 fl.oz | 50 | 0.5 | 9 |
| Cranberry Juice, Cocktail/Blend | 140 | 0 | 34 |
| Fruit Blends, average all, 8 fl.oz | 110 | 0 | 27 |
| Fruit Nectars, average all, 8 fl.oz | 140 | 0 | 36 |
| Grape Juice, 8 fl.oz | 155 | 0 | 38 |
| Grapefruit Juice, 8 fl.oz | 95 | 0 | 22 |
| Lemon/Lime Juice: 1 Tbsp | 5 | 0 | 1 |
| 1 cup, 8 fl.oz | 50 | 0.5 | 16 |
| Concentrate, 1 tsp | 0 | 0 | 0 |
| Noni Juice: | | | |
| Tahitian, 2 Tbsp, 1 fl.oz | 15 | 0 | 3 |
| Tahiti Traders, 1 fl.oz | 20 | 0 | 5 |
| Passion Fruit Juice, Fresh: | | | |
| Purple, 1 cup, 8 fl.oz | 125 | 0 | 34 |
| Yellow, 1 cup, 8 fl.oz | 80 | 1.5 | 14 |
| Papaya/Peach Nectar, av., 8 fl.oz | 140 | 0 | 36 |
| Pear Nectar, 8 fl.oz | 150 | 0 | 40 |
| Pineapple Juice, 8 fl.oz | 130 | 0 | 32 |
| Pomegranate Juice, 8 fl.oz | 160 | 0 | 40 |
| Prune Juice, 8 fl.oz | 180 | 0 | 45 |
| Strawb./Raspberry Juice, 8 fl.oz | 100 | 0 | 23 |
| Tangerine Juice, 8 fl.oz | 105 | 0.5 | 25 |
| Tomato Juice, 8 fl.oz | 40 | 0 | 10 |
| Vegetable Juice, 8 fl.oz | 45 | 0 | 11 |
| Wheat Grass Juice: | | | |
| 1 fl.oz 'Shot' | 10 | 0 | 1.5 |
| 2 fl.oz 'Shot' | 20 | 0 | 3 |

## Quick Guide  C F Cb

### Fruit Smoothies (Jamba Juice; Smoothie King)
*Average All Brands*

| | C | F | Cb |
|---|---|---|---|
| **Fruit Only:** 8 fl.oz | 115 | 0.5 | 29 |
| 12 fl.oz | 175 | 1 | 43 |
| 16 fl.oz | 230 | 1 | 58 |
| 24 fl.oz | 350 | 1 | 78 |
| **Fruit + Non-Fat Milk/Soy:** | | | |
| 12 fl.oz | 135 | 0 | 29 |
| 16 fl.oz | 155 | 0 | 37 |
| 24 fl.oz | 265 | 1 | 59 |
| **Fruit + Non-Fat Frozen Yogurt/Sherbet:** | | | |
| 12 fl.oz | 200 | 0.5 | 47 |
| 16 fl.oz | 265 | 1 | 63 |
| 24 fl.oz | 395 | 1.5 | 95 |

### Juice ~ Brands
*Per 8 fl.oz Unless Indicated*

**Apple & Eve:**

| | C | F | Cb |
|---|---|---|---|
| **100% Juice,** No Sugar Added: | | | |
| Cherries & Berries; Cranb. Raspb. | 120 | 0 | 29 |
| Cranberry Apple | 130 | 0 | 33 |
| Cranberry Pomegranate | 140 | 0 | 34 |
| Fruitables, av. all flavors, 6.75 fl.oz | 60 | 0 | 14 |
| Organic Quenchers, all flav., 6.75 fl.oz | 40 | 0 | 10 |
| **Bolthouse Farms:** *Per 8 fl.oz* | | | |
| **Juice:** 100% Carrot | 70 | 0 | 15 |
| Orange & Carrot | 120 | 0 | 27 |
| **Fruit Smoothies:** | | | |
| Berry Boost | 120 | 0 | 28 |
| Blue Goodness | 160 | 0 | 34 |
| C-Boost | 120 | 0 | 29 |
| Green Goodness | 140 | 0 | 33 |
| Strawberry Banana | 130 | 0 | 32 |
| **Bom Dia:** *Per 8 fl.oz* | | | |
| **Acai:** + 10 Superblend | 120 | 0 | 31 |
| Mango Coconut Splash | 60 | 0 | 15 |
| Pomegranate | 170 | 0 | 42 |
| **Bright & Early** *(Minute Maid)*, | | | |
| Orange Juice (Chilled/Frozen) | 110 | 0 | 30 |
| **Campbell's:** | | | |
| **Tomato Juice:** 5.5 fl.oz can | 30 | 0 | 7 |
| 8 fl.oz | 50 | 0 | 10 |
| **Cactus Cooler,** Orange Pineapple Blast, | | | |
| 12 fl oz can | 150 | 0 | 40 |

## Juice Brands (Cont)

*Per 8 fl.oz Unless Indicated*

| | C | F | Cb |
|---|---|---|---|
| **Capri Sun:** *Per 6 fl.oz* | | | |
| **100% Juice,** av. all flavors | 85 | 0 | 21 |
| **Juice Drinks,** (25% Less Sugar), | | | |
| all flavors | 60 | 0 | 17 |
| **Roarin' Waters,** all flavors, 6 fl.oz | 30 | 0 | 8 |
| **Clamato:** | | | |
| Original Tomato Cocktail | 60 | 0 | 12 |
| Picante | 60 | 0 | 13 |
| **Crystal Geyser:** | | | |
| **Juice Squeeze:** *Per 12 fl.oz Bottle* | | | |
| Blackberry Pomegranate | 170 | 0 | 43 |
| Ruby Grapefruit | 150 | 0 | 36 |
| Average other flavors | 135 | 0 | 32 |
| **Dole:** *Per 8 fl.oz* | | | |
| **Aguas Frescas,** average all flavors | 110 | 0 | 26 |
| **100% Pure,** Chilled or Frozen, | | | |
| average all flavors | 120 | 0 | 28 |
| **Blended Juices,** average all flavors: | 120 | 0 | 30 |
| **Florida's Natural:** *Per 8 fl.oz* | | | |
| Apple Juice | 120 | 0 | 29 |
| Cranberry Ruby Red Cocktail | 130 | 0 | 32 |
| Lemonade, Premium | 110 | 0 | 28 |
| Orange, No Pulp | 110 | 0 | 26 |
| 100% Juice: Orange Mango | 110 | 0 | 27 |
| Orange Pineapple | 130 | 0 | 31 |
| Orange Strawberry | 110 | 0 | 26 |
| Ruby Red Grapefruit, Original | 90 | 0 | 22 |
| **Fuze:** *Per 16.9 fl.oz Bottle* | | | |
| Banana Colada | 180 | 0.5 | 43 |
| Other Fruit Flavors | 180 | 0 | 45 |
| **Goya:** *Per 12 fl.oz Can* | | | |
| Nectar: Guava; Tamarind | 240 | 0 | 59 |
| Mango | 230 | 0 | 56 |
| Papaya | 220 | 0 | 56 |
| Peach | 220 | 0 | 54 |
| Pear & Passion Fruit | 230 | 0 | 57 |
| Pineapple & Passion Fruit | 220 | 0 | 55 |

*Per 8 fl.oz Unless Indicated*

| | C | F | Cb |
|---|---|---|---|
| **Hansen's:** | | | |
| **Juice Box:** *Per 6.75 fl.oz Box* | | | |
| Awesome Apple; Loud Lemonade, av. | 90 | 0 | 23 |
| Burstin Berry; Totally Tropical | 100 | 0 | 24 |
| Strawberry Banana | 110 | 0 | 27 |
| **Junior Juice,** | | | |
| 100% Juice, av. of flavors, 4.23 oz box | 60 | 0 | 16 |
| **Natural,** (64 fl.oz Bottles): *Per 8 fl.oz* | | | |
| Apple | 120 | 0 | 28 |
| Apple Strawberry | 110 | 0 | 27 |
| Cranberry Apple | 110 | 0 | 27 |
| Cranberry Grape | 140 | 0 | 35 |
| Grape | 120 | 0 | 33 |
| White Grape | 140 | 0 | 36 |
| **Hawaii's Own,** Frozen Concentrate, | | | |
| 10% Juice, average all flavors, | | | |
| 8 fl.oz prepared | 110 | 0 | 27 |
| **Hi-C Juice Drinks:** *Per 6.75 fl.oz Box* | | | |
| Flashin' Fruit Punch | 90 | 0 | 26 |
| Orange Lavaburst | 90 | 0 | 26 |
| Poppin' Lemonade | 100 | 0 | 27 |
| **Hood:** *Per 8 fl.oz* | | | |
| Apple | 120 | 0 | 31 |
| Lemonade | 110 | 0 | 29 |
| Orange | 120 | 0 | 30 |
| **Jamba Juice ~** *See Fast-Foods Section* | | | |
| **Juicy Juice** *(Nestle):* | | | |
| Average all flavors: | | | |
| 4.23 fl.oz box | 60 | 0 | 15 |
| 6.75 fl.oz box | 100 | 0 | 24 |
| **Kerns:** | | | |
| **Nectars:** *Per 11.5 fl.oz Can* | | | |
| Guava | 210 | 0 | 53 |
| Pear; Strawb. Banana, av. | 220 | 0 | 53 |
| Pineapple Coconut | 280 | 8 | 53 |
| Strawberry | 210 | 0 | 52 |
| **Kool Aid:** *Per 6 fl.oz Containers* | | | |
| **Jammers,** | | | |
| Scary Blackberry; Tropical Punch | 70 | 0 | 19 |
| **L & A:** *Per 8 fl.oz* | | | |
| All Cherry | 180 | 0 | 45 |
| All Cranberry | 60 | 0 | 14 |
| Papaya Delight | 130 | 0 | 32 |
| Pineapple Coconut | 140 | 3 | 28 |

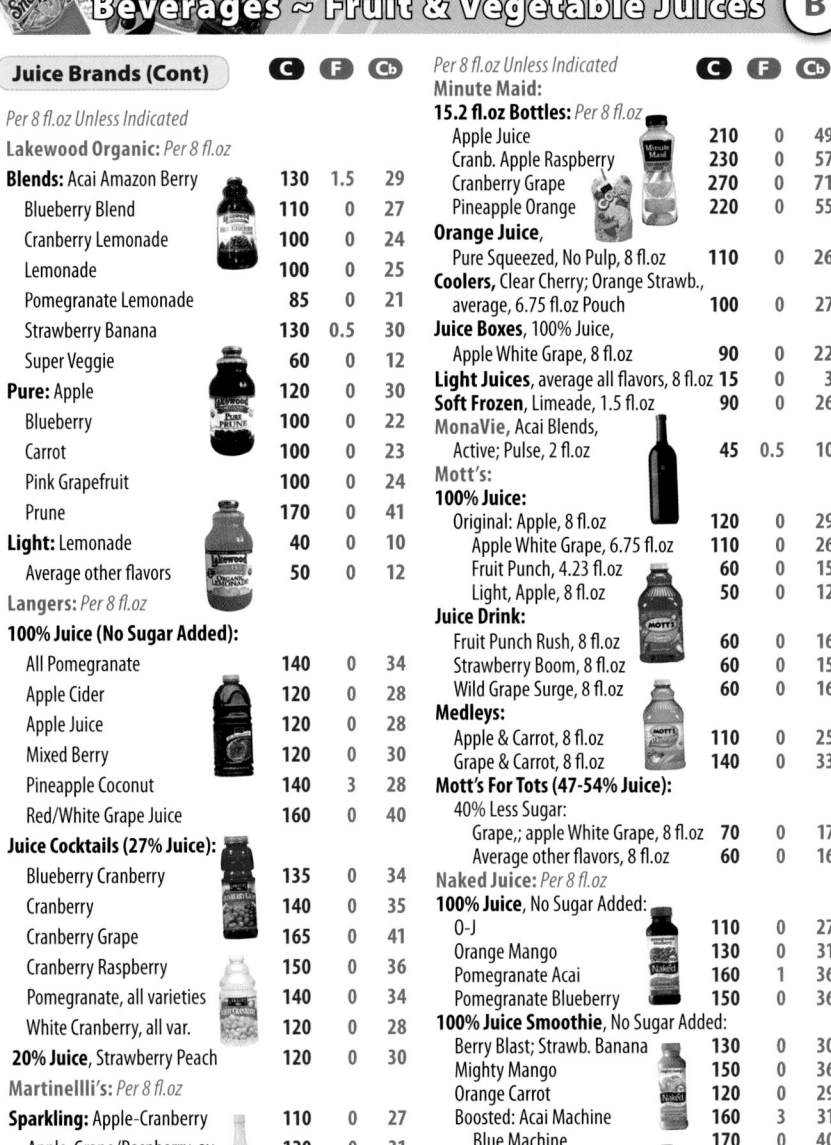

## Juice Brands (Cont) ⓒ ⓕ ⓒb

*Per 8 fl.oz Unless Indicated*

**Lakewood Organic:** *Per 8 fl.oz*

| | C | F | Cb |
|---|---|---|---|
| **Blends:** Acai Amazon Berry | 130 | 1.5 | 29 |
| Blueberry Blend | 110 | 0 | 27 |
| Cranberry Lemonade | 100 | 0 | 24 |
| Lemonade | 100 | 0 | 25 |
| Pomegranate Lemonade | 85 | 0 | 21 |
| Strawberry Banana | 130 | 0.5 | 30 |
| Super Veggie | 60 | 0 | 12 |
| **Pure:** Apple | 120 | 0 | 30 |
| Blueberry | 100 | 0 | 22 |
| Carrot | 100 | 0 | 23 |
| Pink Grapefruit | 100 | 0 | 24 |
| Prune | 170 | 0 | 41 |
| **Light:** Lemonade | 40 | 0 | 10 |
| Average other flavors | 50 | 0 | 12 |

**Langers:** *Per 8 fl.oz*

| | C | F | Cb |
|---|---|---|---|
| **100% Juice (No Sugar Added):** | | | |
| All Pomegranate | 140 | 0 | 34 |
| Apple Cider | 120 | 0 | 28 |
| Apple Juice | 120 | 0 | 28 |
| Mixed Berry | 120 | 0 | 30 |
| Pineapple Coconut | 140 | 3 | 28 |
| Red/White Grape Juice | 160 | 0 | 40 |
| **Juice Cocktails (27% Juice):** | | | |
| Blueberry Cranberry | 135 | 0 | 34 |
| Cranberry | 140 | 0 | 35 |
| Cranberry Grape | 165 | 0 | 41 |
| Cranberry Raspberry | 150 | 0 | 36 |
| Pomegranate, all varieties | 140 | 0 | 34 |
| White Cranberry, all var. | 120 | 0 | 28 |
| **20% Juice**, Strawberry Peach | 120 | 0 | 30 |

**Martinellli's:** *Per 8 fl.oz*

| | C | F | Cb |
|---|---|---|---|
| **Sparkling:** Apple-Cranberry | 110 | 0 | 27 |
| Apple-Grape/Raspberry, av. | 120 | 0 | 31 |
| Apple-Mango/Pomegranate | 150 | 0 | 38 |
| Apple-Pear/Marionberry, av. | 130 | 0 | 32 |
| Apple-Wild Berry | 150 | 0 | 36 |

*Per 8 fl.oz Unless Indicated*

**Minute Maid:**

| | C | F | Cb |
|---|---|---|---|
| **15.2 fl.oz Bottles:** *Per 8 fl.oz* | | | |
| Apple Juice | 210 | 0 | 49 |
| Cranb. Apple Raspberry | 230 | 0 | 57 |
| Cranberry Grape | 270 | 0 | 71 |
| Pineapple Orange | 220 | 0 | 55 |
| **Orange Juice**, | | | |
| Pure Squeezed, No Pulp, 8 fl.oz | 110 | 0 | 26 |
| **Coolers,** Clear Cherry; Orange Strawb., | | | |
| average, 6.75 fl.oz Pouch | 100 | 0 | 27 |
| **Juice Boxes,** 100% Juice, | | | |
| Apple White Grape, 8 fl.oz | 90 | 0 | 22 |
| **Light Juices,** average all flavors, 8 fl.oz | 15 | 0 | 3 |
| **Soft Frozen,** Limeade, 1.5 fl.oz | 90 | 0 | 26 |
| **MonaVie,** Acai Blends, | | | |
| Active; Pulse, 2 fl.oz | 45 | 0.5 | 10 |
| **Mott's:** | | | |
| **100% Juice:** | | | |
| Original: Apple, 8 fl.oz | 120 | 0 | 29 |
| Apple White Grape, 6.75 fl.oz | 110 | 0 | 26 |
| Fruit Punch, 4.23 fl.oz | 60 | 0 | 15 |
| Light, Apple, 8 fl.oz | 50 | 0 | 12 |
| **Juice Drink:** | | | |
| Fruit Punch Rush, 8 fl.oz | 60 | 0 | 16 |
| Strawberry Boom, 8 fl.oz | 60 | 0 | 15 |
| Wild Grape Surge, 8 fl.oz | 60 | 0 | 16 |
| **Medleys:** | | | |
| Apple & Carrot, 8 fl.oz | 110 | 0 | 25 |
| Grape & Carrot, 8 fl.oz | 140 | 0 | 33 |
| **Mott's For Tots (47-54% Juice):** | | | |
| 40% Less Sugar: | | | |
| Grape,; apple White Grape, 8 fl.oz | 70 | 0 | 17 |
| Average other flavors, 8 fl.oz | 60 | 0 | 16 |
| **Naked Juice:** *Per 8 fl.oz* | | | |
| **100% Juice,** No Sugar Added: | | | |
| O-J | 110 | 0 | 27 |
| Orange Mango | 130 | 0 | 31 |
| Pomegranate Acai | 160 | 1 | 36 |
| Pomegranate Blueberry | 150 | 0 | 36 |
| **100% Juice Smoothie,** No Sugar Added: | | | |
| Berry Blast; Strawb. Banana | 130 | 0 | 30 |
| Mighty Mango | 150 | 0 | 36 |
| Orange Carrot | 120 | 0 | 29 |
| Boosted: Acai Machine | 160 | 3 | 31 |
| Blue Machine | 170 | 0 | 40 |
| Green Machine | 140 | 0 | 33 |
| Power-C Machine | 120 | 0 | 29 |
| Red Machine | 170 | 4.5 | 31 |
| **Coconut Water,** Pure, 11.2 fl.oz | 60 | 0 | 14 |

### Juice Brands (Cont)

| | C | F | Cb |
|---|---|---|---|

*Per 8 fl.oz Unless Indicated*

**Nantucket Nectars:**

**100% Juice:** *Per 8 fl.oz*

| | C | F | Cb |
|---|---|---|---|
| Peach Orange | 130 | 0 | 32 |
| Pineapple Orange Banana | 140 | 0 | 34 |
| Pomegranate Cherry | 120 | 0 | 29 |
| Premium Orange Juice | 110 | 0 | 26 |
| Pressed Apple | 120 | 0 | 30 |
| **Juice Cocktail**, Cranberry | 130 | 0 | 33 |

**Juice Drinks:** *Per 8 fl.oz*

| | C | F | Cb |
|---|---|---|---|
| Orange Mango | 120 | 0 | 31 |
| Pineapple Orange Guava | 120 | 0 | 29 |
| Pomegranate Pear | 110 | 0 | 28 |
| Red Plum Juice | 130 | 0 | 31 |
| Watermelon Strawberry | 110 | 0 | 28 |
| **Lemonade**, Squeezed | 110 | 0 | 28 |

**Newman's Own:** *Per 8 fl.oz*

| | C | F | Cb |
|---|---|---|---|
| Lemonade, Regular; Pink | 110 | 0 | 27 |
| Limeade | 140 | 0 | 34 |

**Fruit Juice Cocktail:**

| | C | F | Cb |
|---|---|---|---|
| Gorilla Grape | 140 | 0 | 34 |
| Orange Mango Tango | 130 | 0 | 33 |

**Northland,**

**100% Juice,**

| | C | F | Cb |
|---|---|---|---|
| Cranb. Blackberry/Raspberry/Grape, average | 135 | 0 | 34 |

**Ocean Spray:** *Per 8 fl.oz*

**Juice Cocktails:**

| | C | F | Cb |
|---|---|---|---|
| Blueberry | 110 | 0 | 28 |
| Cranberry | 120 | 0 | 30 |
| With Calcium | 120 | 0 | 30 |

**00% Juice Blends:**

| | C | F | Cb |
|---|---|---|---|
| Citrus Tangerine Orange | 110 | 0 | 28 |
| Cranberry Concord Grape | 130 | 0 | 33 |
| Cranberry Raspberry | 120 | 0 | 30 |
| White Grapefruit | 90 | 0 | 21 |

**Juice Drinks:**

| | C | F | Cb |
|---|---|---|---|
| Cran-Apple | 120 | 0 | 31 |
| Cran-Grape | 120 | 0 | 31 |
| Cran-Raspberry/Strawberry, av. | 105 | 0 | 27 |
| **Diet Juice Drinks**, all flavors | 5 | 0 | 2 |
| **Energy**, average all flavors, 10 fl.oz | 40 | 0 | 10 |
| **Light Juice Drinks**, av. all flavors | 50 | 0 | 13 |
| **Sparkling**, av. all flavors, 8.4 fl.oz | 85 | 0 | 21 |
| **Wave**, average all flavors, 8 fl.oz | 80 | 0 | 20 |

*Per 8 fl.oz Unless Indicated*

**Odwalla:**

| | C | F | Cb |
|---|---|---|---|

**100% Juice:** *Per 15.2 fl.oz Bottle*

| | C | F | Cb |
|---|---|---|---|
| Carrot | 120 | 0 | 26 |
| Orange | 210 | 0 | 47 |

**Smoothies:** *Per 15.2 fl.oz Bottle*

| | C | F | Cb |
|---|---|---|---|
| Blueberry B | 260 | 0 | 65 |
| Mango Tango | 280 | 1.5 | 64 |
| Mo'Beta | 220 | 0 | 51 |
| Original Super Food | 240 | 1 | 56 |
| Red Rhapsody | 200 | 0 | 48 |
| Strawberry C Monster | 300 | 0 | 71 |

**Orange Julius:**

**Originals:** *Per Medium*

| | C | F | Cb |
|---|---|---|---|
| Mango P'apple, 21.5 fl.oz | 450 | 0 | 114 |
| Orange, 17.5 fl.oz | 270 | 0 | 68 |
| Pina Colada, 21 fl.oz | 470 | 7 | 99 |
| Strawberry Banana, 20 fl.oz | 530 | 8 | 114 |

**Smoothies ~** *See Fast-Foods Section*

| | C | F | Cb |
|---|---|---|---|
| **Orangina**, 10 fl.oz bottle | 130 | 0 | 32 |

**Pom Wonderful:** *Per 8 fl.oz*

**100% Juice,**

| | C | F | Cb |
|---|---|---|---|
| Blueberry; Cherry; Pomegranate | 150 | 0 | 36 |

**Juice Blends:** Coconut

| | C | F | Cb |
|---|---|---|---|
| | 95 | 0 | 22 |
| Hula | 140 | 0 | 35 |
| Mango | 140 | 0 | 34 |

**R.W. Knudsen:** *Per 8 fl.oz*

**Organic, 100% Juice:** Apple

| | C | F | Cb |
|---|---|---|---|
| | 120 | 0 | 30 |
| Concord Grape | 150 | 0 | 39 |
| Cranberry Blueberry | 120 | 0 | 31 |

**Natural, 100% Juice:**

| | C | F | Cb |
|---|---|---|---|
| Mango Peach | 120 | 0 | 30 |
| Cranberry Raspberry | 130 | 0 | 32 |
| Kiwi Strawberry | 120 | 0 | 30 |
| Razzleberry | 120 | 0 | 30 |
| Rio Red Grapefruit | 140 | 0 | 34 |

**Just Juice:**

| | C | F | Cb |
|---|---|---|---|
| Just Blueberry | 100 | 0 | 24 |
| Just Black Cherry | 160 | 0 | 37 |
| Just Black Currant | 110 | 0 | 25 |
| **Simply Nutritious:** Mega C | 120 | 0 | 30 |
| Average other flavors | 125 | 0 | 31 |
| **Sparkling:** Blueberry; Cranberry, av. | 110 | 0 | 29 |
| Cherry; Pomegranate | 130 | 0 | 32 |
| Organic Pear | 120 | 0 | 31 |

## Juice Brands (Cont)

**C F Cb**

*Per 8 fl.oz Unless Indicated*
**R.W. Knudsen (Cont):**
**Spritzers:** *Per 10.5 fl.oz Cans*

| | C | F | Cb |
|---|---|---|---|
| Black Cherry; Strawb; Tangerine | 120 | 0 | 29 |
| Mango Fandango; Red Raspb., av. | 110 | 0 | 28 |
| **Very Veggie**, Original, 8 fl.oz | 60 | 0 | 12 |

**ReaLemon – ReaLime:**
Lemon/Lime Juice (from concentrate):

| | C | F | Cb |
|---|---|---|---|
| 1 teaspoon | 0 | 0 | 0 |
| 2Tbsp, 1 fl.oz | 10 | 0 | 2.5 |

**Santa Cruz:** *Per 8 fl.oz*
**Organic, 100% Juice:**

| | C | F | Cb |
|---|---|---|---|
| Apple Juice; Red Tart Cherry | 120 | 0 | 30 |
| Concord/White Grape | 160 | 0 | 39 |
| Hibiscus Cooler | 100 | 0 | 25 |
| Orange Mango | 130 | 0 | 32 |

**Carbonated Beverages:** *Per 10.5 fl.oz Can*

| | C | F | Cb |
|---|---|---|---|
| Lemon Lime | 130 | 0 | 32 |
| Average other flavors | 115 | 0 | 28 |

**Nectars:** Apricot; Berry; Cranberry

| | C | F | Cb |
|---|---|---|---|
| Apricot; Berry; Cranberry | 120 | 0 | 29 |
| Pear | 130 | 0 | 33 |

**Seismic** *(Amway):*
**Super Juices:** *Per 10 fl.oz*

| | C | F | Cb |
|---|---|---|---|
| Citrus; Berry | 180 | 0 | 44 |
| Low Sugar Cherry | 100 | 0 | 26 |

**Simply Orange Juice Company:**

| | C | F | Cb |
|---|---|---|---|
| Lemonade; Limeade | 120 | 0 | 30 |
| Orange Juice, with or without pulp | 110 | 0 | 26 |

**Snap•E• Tom,**

| | C | F | Cb |
|---|---|---|---|
| Tomato & Chili Cocktail, 11.5 fl.oz can | 70 | 0 | 15 |

**Snapple:** *Per 16 fl.oz Bottle*
**Juice Drink Blends:**

| | C | F | Cb |
|---|---|---|---|
| Go Bananas; Rasp. Peach, average | 225 | 0 | 55 |
| Grapeade; Lemonade; Orangeade | 190 | 0 | 46 |
| Fruit Punch | 200 | 0 | 48 |
| **Diet**, Cranberry Raspberry | 20 | 0 | 4 |

**Ssips,** Juice Boxes,

| | C | F | Cb |
|---|---|---|---|
| av. all flavors, 6 fl.oz box | 80 | 0 | 21 |

**Stonyfield Farm:** *Per 10 fl.oz Bottle*
**Smoothies:** Strawberry; Wild Berry

| | C | F | Cb |
|---|---|---|---|
| Strawberry; Wild Berry | 230 | 3 | 39 |
| Peach | 230 | 3 | 41 |
| **6 oz Bottle,** Strawberry Banana | 140 | 2 | 24 |

*Per 8 fl.oz Unless Indicated*
**SunnyD:**
**Original:** *Per 64 fl.oz Ctn*

| | C | F | Cb |
|---|---|---|---|
| Orange, all var., 8 fl.oz | 50 | 0 | 12 |

**Blends,** 64 fl.oz Containers,

| | C | F | Cb |
|---|---|---|---|
| average all flavors, 8 fl.oz | 60 | 0 | 15 |

**Baja Juice:** *Per 12 fl.oz Bottles*

| | C | F | Cb |
|---|---|---|---|
| Red Punch | 170 | 0 | 43 |
| Other flavors | 190 | 0 | 46 |

**Sunsweet:** *Per 8 fl.oz*
**Plum Smart:** Original

| | C | F | Cb |
|---|---|---|---|
| Original | 160 | 0 | 36 |
| Light | 60 | 0 | 15 |

**Prune Juice:** Original

| | C | F | Cb |
|---|---|---|---|
| Original | 180 | 0 | 42 |
| Light | 100 | 0 | 26 |

**Trader Joe's:**
**All Natural Pasteurized,** 32/64 fl.oz Bottle: *Per 8 fl.oz*

| | C | F | Cb |
|---|---|---|---|
| 100% Cranberry | 70 | 0 | 16 |
| Blueberry Pomegranate | 140 | 0 | 34 |
| Just Blueberry | 100 | 0 | 24 |
| Just Pomegranate | 150 | 0 | 37 |
| Mango PassionFruit | 130 | 0 | 32 |
| Omega Orange Carrot | 110 | 0 | 26 |

**Organic,** 32/64 fl.oz Bottle: *Per 8 fl.oz*

| | C | F | Cb |
|---|---|---|---|
| 100% Pomegranate | 140 | 0 | 35 |
| Apple Juice | 120 | 0 | 30 |
| Concord Grape Juice | 160 | 0 | 39 |
| Cranberry | 70 | 0 | 18 |
| Grapefruit Sunset; Lemonade | 120 | 0 | 30 |
| Mango Nectar | 130 | 0 | 32 |
| Pink Lemonade | 130 | 0 | 32 |
| Strawberry Lemonade | 120 | 0 | 29 |
| White Grape Juice | 160 | 0 | 40 |

**Joe's Kids:** *Per 6.75 oz Box*

| | C | F | Cb |
|---|---|---|---|
| From Concentrate: Apple | 90 | 0 | 23 |
| Apple Grape | 100 | 0 | 24 |
| White Grape | 120 | 0 | 30 |
| 10% Juice, Lemonade | 90 | 0 | 22 |

**Sparkling Juices,** 25.4 fl.oz Botle:

| | C | F | Cb |
|---|---|---|---|
| Blueberry, 8 fl.oz | 120 | 0 | 30 |
| Cranberry, 8 fl.oz | 140 | 0 | 35 |
| Pomegranate, 8 fl.oz | 130 | 0 | 31 |

## Juice Brands (Cont)    C   F   Cb

*Per 8 fl.oz Unless Indicated*

**Tree Top:**
**100% Juice Concentrates:**
**64 fl.oz Bottle:** *Per 8 fl.oz*

| | C | F | Cb |
|---|---|---|---|
| Apple Berry/Grape, average | 125 | 0 | 32 |
| Apple Cranb.; Blue Pomegranate | 120 | 0 | 30 |

**11.5 fl.oz Can:** *Per Can*

| | C | F | Cb |
|---|---|---|---|
| Apple Berry/Grape, av. | 180 | 0 | 46 |
| Fruit Punch | 170 | 0 | 42 |

**6.75 fl.oz Box:** *Per Box*

| | C | F | Cb |
|---|---|---|---|
| Apple Pear | 100 | 0 | 25 |
| Fruit Punch | 110 | 0 | 26 |
| Grape Juice | 110 | 0 | 27 |

**Tropicana:** *Per 8 fl.oz*
**Chilled:**

| | C | F | Cb |
|---|---|---|---|
| Orangeade | 130 | 0 | 33 |
| Punch, average all flavors | 125 | 0 | 31 |

**Non-Refrigerated:**

| | C | F | Cb |
|---|---|---|---|
| 100% juice, 10 fl.oz bottles: Apple | 170 | 0 | 40 |
| Fruit Medley | 170 | 0 | 40 |
| **20% Juice**, 15.2 fl.oz Bottle, Cranberry | 270 | 0 | 67 |
| **Farmstand**, 46 fl.oz bottle, average all flavors, 8 fl.oz | 120 | 0 | 30 |
| **Trop50**, 50% less sugar, 59 fl.oz bottle, average all flavors, 8 fl.oz | 50 | 0 | 13 |
| **Trop Twisters**, 20 fl.oz bottle, average all flavors | 300 | 0 | 74 |
| **Tropics**, 59 fl.oz container, average all flavors, 8 fl.oz | 120 | 0 | 30 |

**Tru Nopal:**
**Cactus Water:**

| | C | F | Cb |
|---|---|---|---|
| 1 Cup, 8 fl.oz | 25 | 0 | 6 |
| 16.9 fl.oz carton | 50 | 0 | 12 |

**V8 Juices & Drinks:**
**Original/Spicy 100% Vegetable Juice:**

| | C | F | Cb |
|---|---|---|---|
| 5.5 fl.oz can | 35 | 0 | 7 |
| 8 fl.oz cup | 50 | 0 | 10 |
| 11.5 fl.oz can | 70 | 0 | 14 |
| 12 fl.oz bottle | 75 | 0 | 15 |
| **Splash:** Average all flavors | 75 | 0 | 19 |
| Diet Splash, all flavors | 10 | 0 | 3 |
| **Smoothies:** Strawberry Banana | 80 | 0 | 18 |
| Tropical Colada | 80 | 0 | 18 |
| **V-Fusion:** Grape Raspberry | 120 | 0 | 30 |
| Average other flavors | 110 | 0 | 27 |
| Light Varieties, av. all flavors | 50 | 0 | 13 |
| Refreshers, average all flavors | 100 | 0 | 25 |

*Per 8 fl.oz Unless Indicated*    C   F   Cb

**Veryfine:**

| | C | F | Cb |
|---|---|---|---|
| **100%:** Apple; Orange, 8 fl.oz | 120 | 0 | 29 |
| Apple Strawb., 11.5 fl.oz can | 170 | 0 | 43 |

**Walnut Acres:** *Per 8 fl.oz*
**Organic:** Apple

| | C | F | Cb |
|---|---|---|---|
| Apple | 110 | 0 | 29 |
| Apricot; Raspberry | 130 | 0 | 32 |
| Cherry | 140 | 0 | 34 |
| Cranberry | 110 | 0 | 26 |
| Incredible Vegetable | 50 | 0 | 12 |
| Mango Nectar | 120 | 0 | 29 |

**Welch's:** *Per 8 fl.oz*

| | C | F | Cb |
|---|---|---|---|
| 100% Juice: Concord Grape | 140 | 0 | 36 |
| Red Grape juice | 160 | 0 | 41 |
| White Grape | 140 | 0 | 38 |
| White Grape Cherry/Peach | 140 | 0 | 34 |

**Cocktails**, Refrigerated, 64 fl.oz Ctn:

| | C | F | Cb |
|---|---|---|---|
| Dragon Fruit Mango, 8 fl.oz | 140 | 0 | 35 |
| Passion Fruit, 8 fl.oz | 140 | 0 | 36 |
| Strawberry Breeze, 8 fl.oz | 130 | 0 | 33 |
| **Concentrates,** 100% Juice, Grape; White Grape, 2 fl.oz | 140 | 0 | 39 |
| **Light Juice**, 52 fl.oz Bottle Concord/White Grape, 8 fl.oz | 45 | 0 | 12 |

**Sparkling Juice Cocktail:**

| | C | F | Cb |
|---|---|---|---|
| Blueberry, 8 fl.oz | 150 | 0 | 38 |
| Other flavors, 8 fl.oz | 160 | 0 | 40 |

**Zola:** *Per 12 fl.oz Bottle*
**Acai:**

| | C | F | Cb |
|---|---|---|---|
| Original | 185 | 3 | 39 |
| With Blueberry Juice | 180 | 3 | 38 |

### CALORIEKING PORTION WATCH

| ORANGE JUICE | C | Cb |
|---|---|---|
| 8 fl.oz | 110 | 26 |
| 16 fl.oz | 220 | 52 |
| 24 fl.oz | 330 | 78 |
| 32 fl.oz | 440 | 104 |

### Quick Guide ⒸⒻⒸᵇ

#### Cow's Milk ~ Average All Brands

**Whole (3.25% fat):**

| | C | F | Cb |
|---|---|---|---|
| 2 Tbsp, 1 fl.oz | 20 | 1 | 1.5 |
| 1 Cup, 8 fl.oz | 150 | 8 | 12 |
| 1 Large Glass, 12 fl.oz | 220 | 12 | 17 |
| 1 Pint, 16 fl.oz | 295 | 16 | 22 |
| 1 Quart, 946 ml | 590 | 32 | 44 |

**Reduced-Fat (2% fat):**

| | C | F | Cb |
|---|---|---|---|
| 2 Tbsp, 1 fl.oz | 15 | 0.5 | 1.5 |
| 1 Cup, 8 fl.oz | 120 | 5 | 12 |
| 1 Large Glass, 12 fl.oz | 180 | 7.5 | 18 |
| 1 Pint, 16 fl.oz | 245 | 10 | 23 |
| 1 Quart, 946 ml | 490 | 20 | 46 |

**Light/Low-Fat (1% fat):**

| | C | F | Cb |
|---|---|---|---|
| 2 Tbsp, 1 fl.oz | 15 | 0.3 | 1.5 |
| 1 Cup, 8 fl.oz | 100 | 2.5 | 12 |
| 1 Large Glass, 12 fl.oz | 150 | 4 | 18 |
| 1 Pint, 16 fl.oz | 205 | 5 | 25 |
| 1 Quart, 946 ml | 410 | 10 | 49 |

**Fat Free/Skim:**

| | C | F | Cb |
|---|---|---|---|
| 2 Tbsp, 1 fl.oz | 10 | 0 | 1.5 |
| 1 Cup, 8 fl.oz | 90 | 0.5 | 13 |
| 1 Pint, 16 fl.oz | 180 | 1 | 26 |

**Protein Fortified,**

| | C | F | Cb |
|---|---|---|---|
| 1 cup | 100 | 0.5 | 14 |

**Buttermilk:** *Average All Brands*

| | C | F | Cb |
|---|---|---|---|
| Reduced-Fat (2%), 1 cup, 8 fl.oz | 120 | 5 | 10 |
| Low-Fat (1%), 1 cup, 8 fl.oz | 100 | 2.5 | 12 |

**Lactose-Free:** *Per 8 fl.oz*

| | C | F | Cb |
|---|---|---|---|
| *Dairy Ease:* Whole | 160 | 9 | 11 |
| 2% Reduced-Fat | 130 | 5 | 12 |
| Fat-Free | 90 | 0 | 12 |
| *Lactaid 100:* Whole | 150 | 8 | 12 |
| 2% Reduced-Fat | 130 | 5 | 12 |
| 1% Low-Fat | 110 | 2.5 | 13 |
| Fat-Free; Calcium Fort. | 80 | 0 | 13 |
| *Real Goodness,* 2% Fat | 120 | 5 | 7 |
| *Smart Balance,* | | | |
| FF + Omega-3s & Vit. E | 110 | 1 | 14 |

**Lower Calorie Dairy Drinks:** *Per 8 fl.oz Cup*

Calorie Countdown (*Hood*):

| | C | F | Cb |
|---|---|---|---|
| 2% Reduced-Fat | 90 | 5 | 3 |
| 2% Reduced-Fat, Chocolate | 90 | 5 | 5 |
| Fat-Free | 45 | 0 | 3 |

### Goat/Sheep Milk, Kefir ⒸⒻⒸᵇ

**Goat's Milk** (*Meyenberg*):

| | C | F | Cb |
|---|---|---|---|
| Whole, 1 cup, 8 fl.oz | 140 | 7 | 11 |
| Light/Low-Fat (1%), 8 fl.oz | 100 | 2.5 | 11 |
| Evaporated, reconst., 8 fl.oz | 150 | 8 | 11 |

**Kefir:** *Per 8 fl.oz*

| | C | F | Cb |
|---|---|---|---|
| *Lifeway:* Original | 150 | 8 | 12 |
| Greek Style | 210 | 14 | 12 |
| Green | 170 | 2 | 25 |
| Lowfat, average all flavors | 140 | 1.5 | 20 |
| *Nancy's:* Plain | 110 | 3 | 14 |
| Fruit flavors, average | 180 | 2.5 | 34 |
| *Trader Joe's:* Plain, 1% | 110 | 2.5 | 8 |
| Strawberry | 160 | 2 | 21 |
| **Sheep's Milk,** Whole, 1 cup | 265 | 17 | 13 |

### Canned & Dried Milk

**Condensed:** Sweetened, 2 T., 1 fl.oz

| | C | F | Cb |
|---|---|---|---|
| Condensed: Sweetened, 2 T., 1 fl.oz | 130 | 3 | 23 |
| Low Fat, 2 Tbsp | 120 | 1.5 | 23 |
| Fat-Free, 2 Tbsp | 110 | 0 | 24 |
| **Evaporated:** Whole, 2 Tbsp | 40 | 3 | 3 |
| Whole, ½ cup, 4 fl.oz | 170 | 10 | 13 |
| *Carnation:* Low Fat, 2 Tbsp, 1 oz | 25 | 0.5 | 3 |
| ½ cup, 4 fl.oz | 115 | 2.5 | 14 |
| Fat-Free, 2 Tbsp, 1 oz | 25 | 0 | 4 |
| **Dried:** Whole, ¼ cup, 1 oz | 160 | 9 | 12 |
| Skim/Non-Fat, ⅓ cup | 80 | 0 | 12 |
| Made-up, 1 cup, 8 fl.oz | 80 | 0 | 12 |
| Buttermilk (sweet cream): 1 oz | 110 | 2 | 14 |
| Non-Fat, 1 Tbsp | 25 | 0 | 3 |
| *Carnation,* Malted, dry, 1 Tbsp | 30 | 0.5 | 6 |
| *Horlick's,* Malt Powder, dry, 1 oz | 180 | 4 | 27 |

### Soy/Non-Dairy Drinks ~ See Page 49

*'Whatever happened to sensible portion size?!'*

### Quick Guide    C   F   Cb

**Chocolate Milk:**
*Average All Brands:*

| | C | F | Cb |
|---|---|---|---|
| **Whole Milk,** (3.3%): | | | |
| 8 fl.oz cup | 220 | 8 | 29 |
| 1 Pint, 16 fl.oz | 440 | 16 | 58 |
| **Reduced-Fat,** (2%): | | | |
| 8 fl.oz cup | 190 | 5 | 30 |
| 1 Pint, 16 fl.oz | 380 | 10 | 60 |
| **Low-Fat,** (1%): | | | |
| 8 fl.oz cup | 160 | 3 | 26 |
| 1 Pint, 16 fl.oz | 315 | 5 | 52 |

### Flavored Milk ~ Brands

**Ready-To-Drink:** *Per 8 fl.oz Cup Unless Indicated*

| | | | |
|---|---|---|---|
| **Albertson's,** Choc Milk | 180 | 2.5 | 29 |
| **Hood:** Chocolate | 220 | 8 | 30 |
| Low-Fat (1%), Chocolate | 160 | 2.5 | 28 |
| **Horizon Organic:** | | | |
| Low-Fat: Chocolate with Omega 3 | 150 | 2.5 | 23 |
| Vanilla with Omega 3 | 150 | 2.5 | 23 |
| **Kellogg's:** | | | |
| **To Go, Breakfast Shakes:** *Per 10 fl.oz* | | | |
| Milk Chocolate | 190 | 5 | 29 |
| Strawberry; Vanilla | 180 | 5 | 29 |
| **Mixes,** average all flavors, | | | |
| 1 packet | 130 | 0 | 26 |
| **Kroger,** Simple Truth, | | | |
| Choc Milk, Low-Fat, 1% | 150 | 2.5 | 22 |
| **Land O Lakes:** *Per 8 fl.oz* | | | |
| **Grip 'n Go:** | | | |
| Swiss Chocolate (2% red-fat) | 190 | 5 | 26 |
| Strawberry (whole milk) | 190 | 8 | 22 |
| **Muscle Milk** ~ *See Energy Protein Drinks* | | | |
| **Nesquik:** *Per 8 fl.oz* | | | |
| **Chocolate:** Low Fat | 150 | 2.5 | 24 |
| Average other flavors | 150 | 2.5 | 24 |
| **Chocolate,** No Sugar Added | 100 | 2 | 13 |
| **Prairie Farms:** *Per 8 fl.oz* | | | |
| Chocolate, 2% Reduced Fat | 180 | 5 | 26 |
| Strawberry, 1% Low Fat | 160 | 2.5 | 28 |

### Flavored Milk ~ Brands (Cont)

    C   F   Cb

**Ready-To-Drink:** *Per 8 fl.oz Cup Unless Indicated*

| | | | |
|---|---|---|---|
| **Ralphs,** Chocolate, Low-Fat, 8 fl.oz | 210 | 2.5 | 36 |
| **TruMoo,** Choc.; Strawb., av., 8 fl.oz | 135 | 2.5 | 20 |
| **Yoo-Hoo,** Chocolate,15.5 fl.oz bottle | 230 | 2 | 51 |
| **Bottled Coffee Drinks** ~ *See Page 37* | | | |

### Shakes

**Arby's:** *Per Medium Size*

| | | | |
|---|---|---|---|
| Chocolate; Jamocha, 16 oz | 565 | 15 | 99 |
| Vanilla, 16 oz | 470 | 15 | 75 |
| **Burger King:** | | | |
| Chocolate: | | | |
| Small, 12 fl.oz | 580 | 17 | 97 |
| Medium, 16 fl.oz | 760 | 21 | 131 |
| Large, 20 fl.oz | 980 | 24 | 174 |
| **Other flavors** ~ *See Fast Food Section* | | | |
| **Denny's:** *Per 14 oz* | | | |
| Chocolate | 680 | 31 | 90 |
| Strawberry | 580 | 25 | 78 |
| Vanilla | 640 | 31 | 80 |
| **Hardees,** all varieties, av., 16 fl.oz | 710 | 33 | 87 |
| **McDonalds,** McCafe Shakes: | | | |
| Chocolate & Strawberry: | | | |
| 12 fl.oz cup | 555 | 16 | 91 |
| 16 fl.oz cup | 695 | 20 | 114 |
| 22 fl.oz cup | 850 | 24 | 141 |
| **Other Restaurants** ~ *See Fast-Foods Section* | | | |

### Smoothies

*Made Up Ready-To-Drink:*
**8 fl. oz Milk/Soy + Fruit:** *Per 12 fl.oz*
*Average all flavors:*

| | | | |
|---|---|---|---|
| With Whole Milk | 300 | 8 | 50 |
| + Ice Cream, 1 scoop | 400 | 13 | 62 |
| With Non-Fat Milk | 240 | 0 | 50 |
| **Kroger/Ralph's Smoothies:** *Per 8 fl.oz* | | | |
| Mixed Berry | 210 | 2.5 | 40 |
| Strawberry Banana | 200 | 2.5 | 37 |
| **LALA:** *Per 7 fl.oz Bottle* | | | |
| Frusion C-Charged Smoothie, | | | |
| average all flavors | 180 | 2.5 | 35 |
| **Freshens; Jamba Juice; TCBY** ~ *See Fast-Foods* | | | |

## Nut, Rice & Cereal Drinks

*Per 8 fl.oz Cup Unless Indicated*   **C**  **F**  **Cb**

**Almond Breeze** *(Blue Diamond):*
**Refrigerated/Shelf Stable,** average:

| | C | F | Cb |
|---|---|---|---|
| Original | 60 | 2.5 | 8 |
| Chocolate | 120 | 3 | 22 |
| Vanilla | 80 | 2.5 | 14 |
| Unsweetened, Orig.; Van. | 30 | 2.5 | 1 |

**Almond Dream:**
**Shelf Stable,** Enriched:

| | C | F | Cb |
|---|---|---|---|
| Original | 70 | 3 | 12 |
| Unsweetened | 50 | 3.5 | 3 |

**Alpina:**
**Oat Based Smoothies,**

| | C | F | Cb |
|---|---|---|---|
| all flavors, 8.4 fl.oz | 180 | 4 | 29 |

**Amazake,** Oh So Original,

| | C | F | Cb |
|---|---|---|---|
| Rice Shake | 150 | 0 | 34 |

**Better Than Milk:**
**Rice Vegan Powder Mix,**

| | C | F | Cb |
|---|---|---|---|
| Original; Vanilla, 2 Tbsp, 0.7 oz | 70 | 0 | 17 |

**Cacique,**

| | C | F | Cb |
|---|---|---|---|
| Horchata Rice Drink | 160 | 3.5 | 31 |

**Don Jose:**

| | C | F | Cb |
|---|---|---|---|
| Cereal Match | 100 | 3 | 17 |
| Horchata Rice Drink | 140 | 4 | 25 |

**Pacific:**

| | C | F | Cb |
|---|---|---|---|
| **Rice Drinks,** Plain; Vanilla | 130 | 2 | 27 |
| **Organic Oat,** Original/Vanilla, av. | 130 | 2.5 | 25 |
| **Nut Drinks:** | | | |
| Hazelnut, Original | 110 | 3.5 | 19 |
| Chocolate | 120 | 5 | 19 |
| **Organic Almond:** | | | |
| Original; Vanilla, av. | 65 | 2.5 | 10 |
| Chocolate, single serve container | 100 | 3 | 19 |

**Rice Dream:**
**Refrigerated,** Enriched, Original

| | C | F | Cb |
|---|---|---|---|
| | 120 | 2.5 | 23 |

**Shelf Stable:**

| | C | F | Cb |
|---|---|---|---|
| Classic Carob | 150 | 2.5 | 30 |
| Classic/Enriched Van., av. | 130 | 2.5 | 27 |
| Horchata | 160 | 2.5 | 32 |

**Silk:**

| | C | F | Cb |
|---|---|---|---|
| **Almond:** Original | 60 | 2.5 | 8 |
| Dark Chocolate | 100 | 2.5 | 19 |
| Unswt'nd, Orig.; Vanilla | 30 | 2.5 | 1 |

Note: Rice/Oat/Nut drinks are very low in protein. Unless enriched with protein (and calcium), they are not suitable for infants as a substitute for milk or calcium-enriched soy drinks.

## Soy Milk ~ Ready-To-Drink

*Per 8 fl.oz Cup Unless Indicated*   **C**  **F**  **Cb**

**Trader Joe's:**
**Rice Drinks:**
Unsweetened:

| | C | F | Cb |
|---|---|---|---|
| Original, Organic | 120 | 2.5 | 23 |
| Vanilla | 130 | 2.5 | 26 |
| **WestSoy,** Rice, Plain; Vanilla | 110 | 2.5 | 20 |

**365 Organic** *(Whole Foods):*

| | C | F | Cb |
|---|---|---|---|
| Original, unsweetened | 70 | 4 | 4 |
| Chocolate | 140 | 3.5 | 22 |
| Vanilla | 90 | 3.5 | 10 |
| **Light:** Original | 70 | 1.5 | 9 |
| Vanilla | 70 | 1.5 | 10 |

**8th Continent:**

| | C | F | Cb |
|---|---|---|---|
| Original | 80 | 2.5 | 7 |
| Complete Vanilla | 80 | 2.5 | 8 |
| Vanilla | 100 | 2.5 | 11 |
| Light: Original | 50 | 2 | 2 |
| Chocolate | 90 | 1.5 | 12 |
| Vanilla | 60 | 2 | 5 |
| **Better Than Milk,** Original | 90 | 1.5 | 17 |

**Bolthouse Farms:**
**Perfectly Protein Cafe Drink,**

| | C | F | Cb |
|---|---|---|---|
| Vanilla Chai Tea | 170 | 3.5 | 28 |

**Edensoy:** *Per 32 fl.oz Container*

| | C | F | Cb |
|---|---|---|---|
| **Organic:** Original | 140 | 5 | 14 |
| Unswseetened | 120 | 6 | 5 |
| Carob; Chocolate, av. | 175 | 4 | 28 |
| Vanilla | 150 | 3 | 24 |
| **Extra:** Original | 130 | 4 | 13 |
| Vanilla | 150 | 3 | 23 |

**Kidz Dream:**

| | C | F | Cb |
|---|---|---|---|
| **Smoothies:** Berry Blast | 100 | 2 | 17 |
| Orange Cream | 120 | 2 | 21 |

**Odwalla:** *Per 15.2 fl.oz Bottle*
**Protein Shakes:**

| | C | F | Cb |
|---|---|---|---|
| Strawberry | 300 | 6 | 36 |
| Vanilla | 370 | 6 | 46 |

**Pacific:**

| | C | F | Cb |
|---|---|---|---|
| **Organic,** Original, Unsweetened | 90 | 4.5 | 4 |
| **Select Soy:** Original | 70 | 2.5 | 9 |
| Vanilla | 80 | 2.5 | 11 |
| **Ultra:** Original | 140 | 5 | 12 |
| Vanilla | 140 | 5 | 14 |

## Soy Milk ~ Ready-To-Drink (Cont)

*Per 8 fl.oz Unless Indicated*

| | **C** | **F** | **Cb** |
|---|---|---|---|
| **Silk:** | | | |
| Original | 110 | 4.5 | 9 |
| Chocolate | 120 | 3 | 19 |
| Vanilla | 100 | 3.5 | 10 |
| Very Vanilla | 130 | 3.5 | 18 |
| Light: Original | 60 | 1.5 | 5 |
| Chocolate | 90 | 1.5 | 16 |
| Vanilla | 70 | 1.5 | 7 |
| **Organic:** Original | 100 | 4 | 8 |
| Unsweetened | 80 | 4 | 3 |
| **Slim-Fast ~ See Page 40** | | | |
| **Soy Dream:** | | | |
| **Enriched:** Original | 100 | 3.5 | 9 |
| Vanilla | 120 | 3.5 | 14 |
| **Shelf Stable:** | | | |
| Classic Vanilla | 140 | 4 | 18 |
| Enriched: Original | 100 | 4 | 8 |
| Chocolate | 150 | 4 | 21 |
| Vanilla | 120 | 4 | 14 |
| **Soy Slender,** | | | |
| average all varieties | 70 | 3 | 4 |
| **Trader Joe's:** | | | |
| **Soy Milk:** Original | 110 | 2 | 13 |
| Chocolate | 130 | 2.5 | 23 |
| Vanilla | 100 | 2 | 16 |
| **Organic:** Original | 130 | 3 | 17 |
| Chocolate | 120 | 3 | 17 |
| Vanilla | 130 | 3 | 19 |
| **WestSoy:** | | | |
| **Organic Plus,** (25% Less Sugar): | | | |
| Plain | 110 | 4.5 | 11 |
| Vanilla | 110 | 4.5 | 11 |
| **Low-Fat:** Plain | 90 | 2 | 15 |
| Vanilla | 120 | 2 | 23 |
| **Non-Fat:** Plain | 70 | 0 | 10 |
| Vanilla | 80 | 0 | 12 |
| **Unsweetened:** Plain | 90 | 4.5 | 5 |
| Chocolate; Vanilla, average | 100 | 4.5 | 6 |

## Soy Powder Mix

| | **C** | **F** | **Cb** |
|---|---|---|---|

*1 oz (¼ cup) mix makes 8 fl.oz Cup*

| | **C** | **F** | **Cb** |
|---|---|---|---|
| **Soy Protein Isolate,** dry, 1 oz | 95 | 1 | 2 |
| **Better Than Milk:** | | | |
| Original, 2 Tbsp | 90 | 1.5 | 18 |
| Vanilla, 2 Tbsp | 90 | 1.5 | 18 |
| **Genisoy:** *Per Scoop* | | | |
| **Protein Shake Powder:** | | | |
| Natural, 1 oz | 100 | 0 | 0 |
| Chocolate, 1.2 oz | 120 | 0 | 17 |
| Vanilla, 1.2 oz | 130 | 0 | 18 |
| **Now:** | | | |
| **Soy Protein Isolate:** | | | |
| Plain, ⅓ cup, 0.8 oz | 90 | 0.5 | 0.5 |
| Natural: | | | |
| Chocolate, 1 level scoop, 1.6 oz | 160 | 1.5 | 9 |
| Vanilla, 1 level scoop, 1.6 oz | 180 | 2.5 | 13 |
| **Revival:** *Per Packet* | | | |
| **Unsweetened Shakes:** Plain | 105 | 1 | 4 |
| Cappuccino; Strawberry Smile | 115 | 2 | 4 |
| Chocolate | 120 | 2.5 | 7 |
| Vanilla Pleasure | 120 | 2 | 6 |
| Average other flavors | 115 | 2 | 4 |
| **Whole Foods:** | | | |
| Chocolate, with Spirulina, 1 oz | 100 | 1 | 10 |
| Vanilla, with Spirulina, 1 oz | 100 | 0 | 11 |

## Coconut Milk Drink

| | **C** | **F** | **Cb** |
|---|---|---|---|
| **So Delicious:** *Per 8 fl.oz cup* | | | |
| Original | 70 | 4.5 | 8 |
| Vanilla | 80 | 4.5 | 10 |
| Unsweetened, Original | 45 | 4.5 | 2 |
| **Trader Joes:** *Per 8 fl.oz cup* | | | |
| Unsweetened | 60 | 5 | 1 |
| Vanilla | 90 | 5 | 9 |

(Enriched with calcium + vitamins D & B12)

*Confucious say:*
**"Man who eat with one chopstick never have problem with obesity"**

## Quick Guide | C | F | Cb

**Cola:**

**Drinks:** *Average all Brands*

| | C | F | Cb |
|---|---|---|---|
| 8 fl.oz Cup/Can | 100 | 0 | 26 |
| 12 fl.oz Can | 150 | 0 | 39 |
| 16 fl.oz Bottle | 200 | 0 | 52 |
| 20 fl.oz Bottle | 250 | 0 | 65 |
| 24 fl.oz (Pepsi) | 300 | 0 | 84 |
| 1-Liter Bottle (34 fl.oz) | 400 | 0 | 100 |
| 2-Liter Bottle (68 fl.oz) | 800 | 0 | 200 |

**Other Soda Drinks:** *Per 12 fl.oz, average all brands*

| | C | F | Cb |
|---|---|---|---|
| **Club Soda** | 0 | 0 | 0 |
| **Cream Soda** | 190 | 0 | 48 |
| **Ginger Ale** | 125 | 0 | 31 |
| **Lemonade,** Regular/Pink | 180 | 0 | 45 |
| **Orange** | 180 | 0 | 45 |
| **Root Beer** | 150 | 0 | 39 |
| **Tonic Water** | 125 | 0 | 32 |
| **Mineral Water:** Plain | 0 | 0 | 0 |
| Sweetened/flavored | 150 | 0 | 37 |
| With Fruit Juice | 120 | 0 | 30 |
| **Soda Water/Seltzer:** Plain/Diet | 0 | 0 | 0 |
| Sweetened/flavored | 155 | 0 | 39 |
| With Fruit Juice | 160 | 0 | 40 |

## Fountain, Movie Theater & Take-Out

*Average All Flavors*

| | C | F | Cb |
|---|---|---|---|
| **Small Cup,** 12 fl.oz: No Ice | 160 | 0 | 40 |
| With ⅓ Ice | 120 | 0 | 30 |
| **Regular,** 16 fl.oz: No Ice | 215 | 0 | 53 |
| With ⅓ Ice | 160 | 0 | 40 |
| **Medium,** 22 fl.oz: No Ice | 295 | 0 | 73 |
| With ⅓ Ice | 220 | 0 | 55 |
| **Large,** 32 fl.oz: No Ice | 430 | 0 | 105 |
| With ⅓ Ice | 320 | 0 | 80 |

*Note: ⅓ Cup of Ice = ¼ Cup Liquid*

## Soft Drink ~ Brands

*Per 12 fl.oz Unless Indicated*

| | C | F | Cb |
|---|---|---|---|
| **365 Organic** *(Whole Foods),* Spritzers, all flavors | 110 | 0 | 28 |
| **A&W:** Root Beer | 170 | 0 | 47 |
| Ten | 10 | 0 | 3 |
| **Albertson's:** | | | |
| Super Chill: Cola | 160 | 0 | 43 |
| Root Beer | 180 | 0 | 48 |
| **Barq's,** Root Beer | 160 | 0 | 45 |
| **Big Red,** Soda, 20 fl.oz | 250 | 0 | 63 |
| **Blue Sky,** Natural Soda, Cola | 160 | 0 | 42 |

## Soft Drink Brands (Cont)

*Per 12 fl.oz Unless Indicated*

| | C | F | Cb |
|---|---|---|---|
| **Bubble Up,** Lemon-Lime Soda, 8 fl.oz | 110 | 0 | 28 |
| **Cactus Cooler** | 150 | 0 | 40 |
| **Canada Dry:** *Per 8 fl.oz* | | | |
| Club Soda; Diet Ginger Ale | 0 | 0 | 0 |
| Ginger Ale; Tonic Water, average | 90 | 0 | 25 |
| **Cheerwine** | 150 | 0 | 42 |
| **Coca-Cola:** | | | |
| Classic; Caffeine Free | 140 | 0 | 39 |
| Diet Coke, all varieties | 0 | 0 | 0 |
| Cherry Coke; Vanilla Coke | 150 | 0 | 42 |
| Life | 90 | 0 | 24 |
| **Country Time** *(Dr Pepper/Snapple),* Lemonade, all varieties, 20 fl.oz | 230 | 0 | 58 |
| **Crush:** *Per 20 fl.oz Bottle* | | | |
| Grape; Orange | 270 | 0 | 72 |
| Peach; Pineapple, average | 315 | 0 | 85 |
| Strawberry | 290 | 0 | 77 |
| **Dad's:** Orange Cream Soda | 180 | 0 | 46 |
| Root Beer | 165 | 0 | 41 |
| **Diet Rite,** Pure Zero | 0 | 0 | 0 |
| **Dr Pepper:** *Per 12 fl.oz Can* | | | |
| Regular | 150 | 0 | 40 |
| Cherry | 160 | 0 | 43 |
| Ten | 10 | 0 | 3 |
| **Fanta:** Orange | 160 | 0 | 45 |
| Other flavors | 180 | 0 | 48 |
| **Fresca,** all flavors | 0 | 0 | 0 |
| **GuS,** average all flavors | 95 | 0 | 23 |
| **Hansen's:** | | | |
| Natural Cane Sugar: | | | |
| Creamy Root Beer | 160 | 0 | 43 |
| Original Cola | 160 | 0 | 41 |
| Pomegranate | 130 | 0 | 35 |
| Diet, all flavors | 0 | 0 | 0 |
| **Hawaiian Punch:** *Per 12 fl.oz Can* | | | |
| Aloha Morning, 40% less sugar, all flavors | 90 | 0 | 20 |
| Maizin Melon Mix; Wild Purple Splash | 165 | 0 | 44 |
| Average other flavors | 100 | 0 | 27 |
| **Henry Weinhard's:** Root Beer | 170 | 0 | 43 |
| Orange/Vanilla Cream, av. | 180 | 0 | 44 |
| **Hires,** Root Beer | 170 | 0 | 46 |
| **IBC:** Root Beer | 160 | 0 | 44 |
| Cream Soda; Black Cherry | 180 | 0 | 48 |
| **Icee:** Coca-Cola; Orange Fanta | 100 | 0 | 27 |
| Lemon Lime Fanta | 90 | 0 | 24 |
| Minute Maid, Raspberry Lemonade | 100 | 0 | 27 |
| **Jarritos,** all flavors, 8 fl.oz | 110 | 0 | 28 |
| **Jelly Belly,** all flavors | 180 | 0 | 42 |
| **Jolt,** Cola | 150 | 0 | 41 |

## Soft Drink Brands (Cont)

*Per 12 fl.oz Unless Indicated*

| | C | F | Cb |
|---|---|---|---|
| Jones Soda: Cola | 170 | 0 | 43 |
| Whoopass, 16 fl.oz | 200 | 0 | 52 |
| Average other flavors | 185 | 0 | 46 |
| Kool Aid, Bursts, av., 6.75 fl.oz | 35 | 0 | 9 |
| Mello Yello, Regular | 170 | 0 | 47 |
| Mountain Dew: All flavors | 170 | 0 | 46 |
| Diet varieties | 0 | 0 | 0 |
| Dewshine | 160 | 0 | 42 |
| Mug, Root Beer | 160 | 0 | 43 |
| Natural Brew: Chai Cola | 170 | 0 | 41 |
| Draft Root Beer | 170 | 0 | 43 |
| Outrageous Ginger Ale | 180 | 0 | 44 |
| Vanilla Cream Soda | 160 | 0 | 39 |
| Nehi, Peach | 190 | 0 | 51 |
| Pepsi: | | | |
| Regular; Caffeine Free | 150 | 0 | 41 |
| Diet Pepsi; Jazz; Pepsi One | 0 | 0 | 0 |
| Pepsi Next | 60 | 0 | 16 |
| Pepsi True: 7.5 fl.oz can | 60 | 0 | 17 |
| 12 fl.oz can | 100 | 0 | 27 |
| Perrier, Carbonated Water | 0 | 0 | 0 |
| Pibb, Xtra | 140 | 0 | 39 |
| RC Cola: Regular | 160 | 0 | 43 |
| Ten | 10 | 0 | 3 |
| Reed's, Ginger Brew, | | | |
| all varieties | 145 | 0 | 38 |
| 7•UP: Lemon Lime; Cherry | 140 | 0 | 39 |
| Diet flavors | 0 | 0 | 0 |
| Ten, Lemon Lime | 10 | 0 | 3 |
| Safeway: *Per 8 fl.oz* | | | |
| Refreshe: Cola | 110 | 0 | 29 |
| Grape | 140 | 0 | 36 |
| Lemon Lime | 110 | 0 | 27 |
| Mtn Breeze; Strawberry | 120 | 0 | 30 |
| Santa Cruz: Or. Mango, 10.5 fl.oz | 120 | 0 | 29 |
| Raspberry Lemonade, 10.5 fl.oz | 100 | 0 | 26 |
| Average other varieties, 10.5 fl.oz | 135 | 0 | 33 |
| Schweppes: Ginger Ale | 120 | 0 | 33 |
| Tonic Water | 130 | 0 | 33 |
| Shasta: Cream Soda | 190 | 0 | 47 |
| Cherry Cola | 180 | 0 | 45 |
| Club Soda; Diet, all flavors | 0 | 0 | 0 |
| Dr. Shasta | 150 | 0 | 38 |
| Ginger Ale | 130 | 0 | 33 |
| Tiki Punch; Pineapple; Orange | 200 | 0 | 50 |
| Average other flavors | 170 | 0 | 41 |
| Sierra Mist, Lemon Lime | 140 | 0 | 37 |
| Sprite: Regular | 140 | 0 | 38 |
| Zero | 0 | 0 | 0 |

*Per 12 fl.oz Unless Indicated*

| | C | F | Cb |
|---|---|---|---|
| Squirt, Ruby Red | 170 | 0 | 45 |
| Stewarts: Root Beer | 160 | 0 | 41 |
| Grape; Orange 'n Cream | 190 | 0 | 48 |
| Sun Drop: Citrus Soda, 20 fl.oz | 290 | 0 | 76 |
| Diet Citrus Soda | 10 | 0 | 1 |
| Sunkist: Orange | 170 | 0 | 44 |
| Ten, Orange | 10 | 0 | 2 |
| Surge, 16 fl.oz | 230 | 0 | 62 |
| TAB | 0 | 0 | 0 |
| Tampico: | | | |
| **64 fl.oz Container:** | | | |
| Blue Raspberry Punch | 45 | 0 | 21 |
| Pineapple Coconut | 105 | 0 | 25 |
| Average other flavors | 90 | 0 | 21 |
| Thomas Kemper: | | | |
| Black Cherry | 170 | 0 | 44 |
| Ginger Ale; Vanilla Cream | 150 | 0 | 36 |
| Root Beer | 160 | 0 | 41 |
| Trader Joe's: | | | |
| **Sparkling:** | | | |
| French Berry Lemonade: | | | |
| 1 cup, 8 fl.oz | 130 | 0 | 31 |
| 1 bottle, 33.8 fl.oz | 520 | 0 | 124 |
| Lime Ade: 1 cup, 8 fl.oz | 110 | 0 | 28 |
| 1 bottle, 33.8 fl.oz | 440 | 0 | 108 |
| Pink Lemonade: 1 cup, 8 fl.oz | 130 | 0 | 31 |
| 1 Bottle, 33.8 fl.oz | 520 | 0 | 124 |
| Vernors, Ginger Soda, 20 fl.oz | 240 | 0 | 65 |
| Virgil's, Root Beer | 160 | 0 | 42 |
| Walgreens: *Per 20 fl.oz* | | | |
| Orchard Grape Soda | 300 | 0 | 84 |
| Cola; Zesty Lemon Lime, av. | 225 | 0 | 65 |
| Root Beer | 225 | 0 | 75 |
| Zevia, all flavors | 0 | 0 | 4 |
| (Contains between 4-7g Erythritol) | | | |

## Powdered Soft Drink Mixes

*Per 8 fl.oz Prepared, Unless Indicated*

| | C | F | Cb |
|---|---|---|---|
| Country Time: | | | |
| Lemonade; Pink Lemonade | 60 | 0 | 16 |
| Strawberry Lemonade | 80 | 0 | 19 |
| Crystal Light *(Kraft):* | | | |
| Fruit Drinks, all flavors, ½ tsp | 5 | 0 | 0 |
| Pure Fitness, average all flavors, 1 pkt | 15 | 0 | 4 |
| Flavor Aid, ⅛ package | 0 | 0 | 0 |
| Kool-Aid, sweetened, 0.6 oz | 60 | 0 | 16 |
| Tang, Regular, 2 Tbsp, 1 oz | 90 | 0 | 24 |

### Quick Guide | C | F | Cb

**Teas**

**Regular:** Bag, Loose or Instant

| | C | F | Cb |
|---|---|---|---|
| Brewed, 1 cup, 8 fl.oz | 2 | 0 | 0.5 |
| (Add extra for sugar/milk) | | | |

**Herbal:** All flavors, average, 1 cup | 2 | 0 | 0.5
*Bigelow,* all flavors | 0 | 0 | 0
*Celestial Seasonings,* all flavors | 0 | 0 | 0
**Bubble Milk Tea,** w/ Pearls, 8 fl.oz | 175 | 0 | 41
**Chai Tea,** 2 Tbsp | 120 | 3.5 | 21
**Starbucks ~ See Fast-Foods Section**

**Iced Tea**

*Average All Brands*

| | C | F | Cb |
|---|---|---|---|
| **Sweetened:** 8 fl.oz cup | 90 | 0 | 22 |
| 12 fl.oz glass/can | 140 | 0 | 35 |
| 16 fl.oz bottle | 180 | 0 | 45 |
| 20 fl.oz bottle | 225 | 0 | 55 |
| **Unsweetened,** 8 fl.oz | 0 | 0 | 0 |

### Iced Tea Mixes

*Per 8 fl.oz Made-Up*

**4C Iced Tea:**

| | C | F | Cb |
|---|---|---|---|
| Average all flavors, 0.67 oz | 70 | 0 | 18 |
| Totally Light, all flavors | 0 | 0 | 0 |
| **Crystal Light,** sugar free | 5 | 0 | 0 |

**Lipton:**

| | | | |
|---|---|---|---|
| **Sweetened:** Lemon | 70 | 0 | 18 |
| Mango; Peach | 80 | 0 | 19 |
| Unsweetened | 0 | 0 | 0 |
| Diet, all varieties | 5 | 0 | 1 |

### Bottled & Canned Teas

**Arizona:** *Per 8 fl.oz*

| | | | |
|---|---|---|---|
| **Black:** Cranberry | 80 | 0 | 22 |
| Sweet | 90 | 0 | 23 |
| With Ginseng | 60 | 0 | 15 |
| **Green Tea,** average all flavors | 70 | 0 | 18 |
| **Fuze,** Iced Lemon | 70 | 0 | 19 |
| **Gold Peak,** Lemon, 12 fl.oz | 120 | 0 | 30 |

**Honest Tea:** *Per 16 fl.oz Bottle*

| | | | |
|---|---|---|---|
| Just Black/Green | 0 | 0 | 0 |
| Assam Black | 35 | 0 | 9 |
| Community/Jasmin | | | |

### Bottled & Canned Teas (Cont)

**Lipton:**
**Iced Tea:** *Per 20 fl.oz Unless Indicated* | C | F | Cb

| | C | F | Cb |
|---|---|---|---|
| Citrus Green Tea | 120 | 0 | 33 |
| Diet, all flavors | 0 | 0 | 0 |
| Half & Half | 120 | 0 | 31 |
| Lemon | 120 | 0 | 32 |
| Peach | 120 | 0 | 30 |
| Sparkling: Peach | 70 | 0 | 18 |
| Diet | 0 | 0 | 0 |
| Sweet Iced Tea, 8 fl.oz | 80 | 0 | 23 |
| White Tea, with Raspberry, 16.9 fl.oz | 110 | 0 | 29 |

**Nestea:**
**Iced Tea,** with Lemon:

| | | | |
|---|---|---|---|
| 8 fl.oz | 50 | 0 | 12 |
| 20 fl.oz bottle | 125 | 0 | 30 |
| **Diet,** Green/Lemon | 0 | 0 | 0 |

**POM:**
**Antioxidant Super Tea:** *Per 12 fl.oz*
Pomegranate:

| | | | |
|---|---|---|---|
| Lemonade Tea | 140 | 0 | 35 |
| Peach Passion White Tea | 130 | 0 | 11 |
| Sweet Tea | 120 | 0 | 30 |
| Honey Green Tea | 130 | 0 | 35 |

**Snapple:** *Per 16 fl.oz*

| | | | |
|---|---|---|---|
| Green Tea | 120 | 0 | 31 |
| Diet Green Tea | 0 | 0 | 0 |
| Lemon/ Raspberry Tea | 150 | 0 | 37 |
| Diet Lemon/Raspberry Tea | 10 | 0 | 0 |
| **SnapTea:** Lemon | 120 | 0 | 31 |
| Peach Green Tea | 160 | 0 | 42 |
| Sweet Tea | 170 | 0 | 46 |
| **SoBe,** Infusion, Green Tea, 20 fl.oz | 200 | 0 | 52 |
| **Ssips,** Lemon Iced, 6.fl.oz | 70 | 0 | 18 |
| **Steaz,** Green Tea, average all flavors, 16 fl.oz | 80 | 0 | 20 |
| **Tazo,** Org. Iced Black Tea, 13.8 fl oz | 60 | 0 | 15 |
| **TeaZazz:** Original; Peach, 20 fl.oz | 50 | 0 | 12 |
| Green Tea Lemon, 20 fl.oz | 60 | 0 | 17 |

**Trader Joe's:** *Per 8 fl.oz*

| | | | |
|---|---|---|---|
| Organic Tea & Lemonade | 100 | 0 | 25 |
| Pomegranate Green Tea | 60 | 0 | 15 |
| Unsweetened *(Kettle/Green)* | 0 | 0 | 0 |
| **Turkey Hill:** Iced Tea, 16 fl.oz | 180 | 0 | 42 |
| Peach Tea, 16 fl.oz | 200 | 0 | 46 |
| Green Tea, Mango | 180 | 0 | 42 |

**365 Organic** *(Whole Foods):*

| | | | |
|---|---|---|---|
| Unsweetened: Black Tea | 0 | 0 | 0 |
| Green Tea | 0 | 0 | 0 |

Note: Most breads have similar calories on a weight basis. However, volume may vary.

For example, 1 oz of bread may equal 1 slice regular bread or 2 slices of a lighter bread. It is best to weigh bread used and calculate using: 1 oz bread = 70 calories, 14g carb.

### Quick Guide

| | C | F | Cb |
|---|---|---|---|
| **Bread** | | | |
| **White or Wheat:** *Average Per Slice* | | | |
| **Thin or Light,** 0.75 oz | 50 | 0.5 | 9 |
| **Sandwich slice,** 1 oz | 70 | 1 | 12 |
| **Thick or Large,** 1.5 oz | 105 | 1.5 | 18 |
| **Thick,** 2 oz | 140 | 2 | 23 |
| **Extra Thick,** 3 oz | 210 | 3 | 35 |
| **Whole Loaf:** 16 oz | 1120 | 15 | 185 |
| 24 oz Loaf | 1680 | 24 | 280 |
| **Multi Grain/Whole Grain:** *Per Slice* | | | |
| **Sandwich Slice,** 1 oz | 75 | 1.5 | 12 |
| **Thick Slice,** 2 oz | 150 | 2.5 | 25 |
| **Toast:** *Based on same counts as White/Wheat as above* | | | |
| **1 Slice (1 oz fresh):** | | | |
| With 1 tsp butter/margarine | 105 | 5 | 12 |
| With 1 tsp "light" butter/marg. | 90 | 3.5 | 12 |
| With 2 tsp butter/margarine | 140 | 9 | 12 |
| With 2 tsp "light" butter/marg. | 110 | 6 | 12 |

### Breads

*Per Slice Unless Indicated*

| | C | F | Cb |
|---|---|---|---|
| **12-Grain,** 1.5 oz | 110 | 1.5 | 22 |
| **Bran style/Dark,** 1 oz | 70 | 1 | 14 |
| **Buttermilk,** average, 1.5 oz | 110 | 1 | 22 |
| **Challah,** 0.75 oz | 85 | 1.5 | 17 |
| **Chapati,** 1 oz | 110 | 3 | 18 |
| **Ciabatta,** 2 oz | 130 | 1 | 26 |
| **Cornbread,** average, 3 oz | 220 | 6 | 37 |
| **Cracked Wheat Sourdough,** 1.5 oz | 130 | 0.5 | 27 |
| **Croissants** ~ *See Page 134* | | | |
| **Crustless Bread,** regular, slice, 0.75 oz | 40 | 0.5 | 8.5 |
| **Crusts Only,** regular slice, 0.25 oz | 30 | 0 | 7 |
| **English Toasting,** 2 oz | 140 | 1.5 | 27 |
| **Flax & Grain,** 1.5 oz | 120 | 3 | 19 |
| **Foccacia:** Plain, 2 oz serve | 150 | 2.5 | 28 |
| Cheese & Garlic; Pesto, 2 oz serve | 160 | 6 | 21 |
| Tomato & Olive, 2 oz serve | 150 | 5 | 21 |

### Breads (Cont)

| | C | F | Cb |
|---|---|---|---|
| *Per Slice Unless Indicated* | | | |
| **French Stick/Baguette,** 1 oz | 70 | 1 | 15 |
| **French Toast:** Slices, 1.5 oz | 140 | 2 | 26 |
| *Aunt Jemima,* Sticks, av., 2 oz | 110 | 2 | 18 |
| **Garlic Bread/Toast:** | | | |
| Small slice + 1 tsp spread, 0.75 oz | 80 | 5 | 7 |
| Medium slice + 2 tsp spread, 1.5 oz | 160 | 10 | 14 |
| Thick slice + 3 tsp spread, 1.8 oz | 220 | 14 | 20 |
| *Pepperidge Farm,* 1 slice, 1.4 oz | 160 | 10 | 15 |
| **Hawaiian Sweet Bread,** 1.5 oz | 110 | 2 | 19 |
| **Hemp Bread,** 1.2 oz | 95 | 2 | 12 |
| **Italian Bread,** 2 oz | 140 | 1 | 28 |
| **Lower Carb,** (higher protein/fiber), average all brands, 1 oz | 60 | 1.5 | 9 |
| **MultiGrain,** 1.5 oz | 100 | 2 | 21 |
| **Naan Flatbread,** 2 oz | 160 | 3.5 | 29 |
| **Nut/Health Nut,** 1.35 oz | 90 | 1.5 | 18 |
| **Oatmeal/Oatbran Bread,** 1.5 oz | 90 | 0.5 | 19 |
| **Pita,** average all types: | | | |
| Small (4" diam), 1 oz | 90 | 0 | 18 |
| Large (6½" diam), 2 oz | 140 | 1.5 | 27 |
| Extra Large (9" diam), 4 oz | 300 | 1.5 | 60 |
| **Popovers,** (1), without butter | 130 | 2 | 18 |
| **Pumpernickel:** | | | |
| Cocktail/Party size | 30 | 0.5 | 6 |
| Large slice, 1.35 oz | 80 | 0 | 15 |
| **Raisin Bread,** 1 oz | 80 | 1 | 15 |
| **Rye:** 1 thin slice, av., 1 oz | 80 | 1 | 14 |
| 1 thick slice, 2 oz | 150 | 2 | 25 |
| Cocktail size, 0.4 oz | 25 | 0.5 | 4 |
| **Sandwich Pockets,** 2 oz | 140 | 1.5 | 27 |
| **Sourdough:** Regular, 1.5 oz | 120 | 1 | 25 |
| French Style, 1 oz | 75 | 0 | 14 |
| **Spelt,** 1.6 oz | 130 | 1 | 26 |
| **Sprouted 7-Grain,** 1.5 oz | 110 | 0.5 | 18 |
| **Squaw,** 1.1 oz | 85 | 0.5 | 13 |
| **Tacos/Tortillas** ~ *See Page 172* | | | |
| **Turkish/Middle Eastern,** 1 oz | 80 | 1.5 | 16 |
| **Wheat-Free Breads:** Spelt, 1.6 oz | 130 | 1 | 26 |
| Rice, with Fruit Juice, 1.5 oz | 110 | 2 | 21 |
| Healthseed Rye, 1.6 oz | 90 | 1 | 20 |
| Millet, 1.5 oz | 100 | 1 | 20 |

## Bread ~ Brands

*Per Slice Unless Indicated*

| | **C** | **F** | **Cb** |
|---|---|---|---|
| **Ener-G,** Gluten-Free Breads: | | | |
| Brown Rice Loaf, | | | |
| Regular, 1.3 oz | 100 | 3 | 16 |
| High Fiber Loaf, 1.4oz | 90 | 4.5 | 16 |
| Tapioca, regular, sliced, 1 oz | 80 | 3 | 11 |
| **Ezekiel:** | | | |
| Sprouted: | | | |
| 7 Sprouted Grains, 1.2 oz | 80 | 0.5 | 15 |
| Sesame, 1.2 oz | 80 | 0.5 | 14 |
| Whole Grain, 1.3 oz | 80 | 0.5 | 15 |
| **French Meadow:** *Per Slice* | | | |
| Flax & Sunflower, 1.2 oz | 90 | 1.5 | 15 |
| Hemp, 1.2 oz | 100 | 2.5 | 12 |
| Spelt, 1.2 oz | 85 | 0.5 | 17 |
| **Francisco International:** | | | |
| Extra Sourdough Loaf, | | | |
| 1 slice, 1.7 oz | 130 | 1 | 24 |
| French, 2 slices, 1.6 oz | 120 | 1 | 22 |
| **Oroweat:** | | | |
| 3 Seed Oatnut, 1.35 oz | 110 | 2.5 | 18 |
| 100% Whole Wheat, 1.3 oz | 100 | 1.5 | 18 |
| Country Buttermilk, 1.3 oz | 100 | 1 | 19 |
| Honey Wheat Berry, 1.2 oz | 80 | 1 | 17 |
| **Pepperidge Farm:** *Per Slice Unless Indicated* | | | |
| 100% Whole Wheat, Very Thin, 3 slices | 110 | 2 | 20 |
| 15 Grain | 110 | 2 | 20 |
| Farmhouse, Hearty White | 110 | 1.5 | 22 |
| Italian, with Sesame Seeds | 90 | 1 | 15 |
| Light Style, average all varieties | 130 | 1 | 26 |
| **Frozen Breads:** | | | |
| Garlic Bread: | | | |
| Original | 180 | 8 | 21 |
| Five Cheese | 200 | 10 | 20 |
| Texas Toast: Cheddar | 160 | 9 | 16 |
| Garlic | 150 | 8 | 15 |
| **Roman Meal:** Orig. Multigr., 2 slices | 110 | 1.5 | 21 |
| Honey Oat Bran, 1.5 oz | 110 | 1.5 | 20 |
| **Sara Lee:** Honey Wheat, 1 oz | 75 | 1 | 15 |
| 100% Whole Wheat, 1 oz | 70 | 1 | 13 |
| 45 Cals & Delightful Wheat | 45 | 0.5 | 9 |
| **Schwan's,** Frozen: | | | |
| Cheese Stuffed Breadsticks, 1.7 oz | 130 | 5 | 15 |
| French Baguette, ¼ loaf, 1.7 oz | 130 | 0.5 | 26 |
| **Trader Joe's:** Gourmet White, 1.5 oz | 120 | 3.5 | 19 |
| Soft 10 Grain, 1.5 oz | 90 | 1.5 | 16 |
| Sprouted Rye, 1.2 oz | 90 | 1 | 15 |

## Biscuits, Bread Rolls & Buns

**Biscuits:** *Average, 2½" diameter*

| | **C** | **F** | **Cb** |
|---|---|---|---|
| Plain/Butter Milk: | | | |
| Prepared from Recipe | 210 | 10 | 27 |
| Refrig. Dough, Baked | 95 | 4 | 13 |
| Brown 'n Serve, av., 1 oz | 70 | 1 | 13 |
| Refrigerated Dough: | | | |
| *Pillsbury,* Buttermilk Biscuit, | | | |
| (3), 2.25 oz | 150 | 2 | 30 |
| **Buns:** | | | |
| Frankfurter/Hot Dog: 1.25 oz | 110 | 1.5 | 21 |
| 1.5 oz | 130 | 2 | 25 |
| Hamburger: Regular, 1.5 oz | 110 | 1.5 | 22 |
| Large, 3 oz | 210 | 3 | 40 |
| Hoagie/Submarine, Plain, 2.3 oz | 200 | 1 | 38 |
| **Rolls:** | | | |
| Ciabatta Roll, 3.5 oz | 230 | 4 | 41 |
| Crescent Roll, Original, 1 oz | 100 | 6 | 11 |
| Dinner: | | | |
| 1 small, 1 oz | 90 | 1.5 | 17 |
| 1 medium (3" diam),1.5 oz | 110 | 1 | 23 |
| French: 1 med, 1.3 oz | 110 | 1.5 | 22 |
| 1 large, 3 oz | 230 | 2.5 | 42 |
| Kaiser: | | | |
| Small, 2 oz | 200 | 2.5 | 35 |
| Large, 3.5 oz | 350 | 4 | 61 |
| Plain, 6", average all, 2.5 oz | 200 | 1 | 38 |
| Sourdough, 1.3 oz | 110 | 1 | 21 |
| Wheat Rolls: Small, 1.2 oz | 100 | 1 | 17 |
| Medium, 1.8 oz | 130 | 1.5 | 23 |
| Large, 3.5 oz | 260 | 3 | 46 |

## Breadsticks, Croutons

**Breadsticks:**

| | **C** | **F** | **Cb** |
|---|---|---|---|
| Salt Sticks, plain, 1 oz | 110 | 1 | 20 |
| Fresh baked (1), 2 oz | 180 | 2.5 | 34 |
| *Stella D'oro:* Original (1) | 45 | 1 | 7 |
| Sesame (1) | 50 | 2 | 7 |
| **Croutons:** Seasoned, 2 Tbsp, 0.3 oz | 35 | 1.5 | 4 |
| *Pepp. Farm,* Zesty Italian, 6 croutons | 30 | 1 | 5 |

## Bread Products

| | | | |
|---|---|---|---|
| **Bread Crumbs,** dry: | | | |
| Plain or seasoned: 1 oz | 110 | 1.5 | 20 |
| 1 cup, 3.5 oz | 385 | 5 | 70 |
| **Corn Flake Crumbs,** 1 oz | 120 | 0 | 29 |
| **Graham Cracker Crumbs** *(Keebler),*1 oz | 110 | 2.5 | 20 |
| **Bread Dough,** average: | | | |
| Frozen, 1 slice, 2 oz | 140 | 2 | 26 |
| Refrigerated: French, 1" sl. | 60 | 1 | 13 |
| Wheat; White, 1" slice | 80 | 2 | 14 |
| **Coating Mixes,** av., 2 Tbsp., 1 oz | 100 | 0.5 | 20 |
| **Stuffing:** Dry mix, average all,1 oz | 110 | 1 | 10 |
| Prepared, ½ cup, 4 oz | 180 | 9 | 22 |

## Quick Guide    C F Cb

### Bagels
*Average All Brands*

| **Plain/Onion:** | C | F | Cb |
|---|---|---|---|
| 1 mini/bagelette, 1 oz | 65 | 0.5 | 13 |
| 1 small bagel, 2 oz | 145 | 1 | 29 |
| 1 medium bagel, 3 oz | 220 | 1.5 | 43 |
| 1 large bagel, 4 oz | 290 | 2 | 57 |
| **Bagel Chips,** 1 oz | 130 | 4.5 | 19 |
| **Pizza Bagel Bites** (Bagel Bites), | | | |
| average all varieties., 4 pieces, 3 oz | 190 | 5.5 | 27 |
| **Bagel Crisps** (New York Style), | | | |
| average all varieties, 6 crisps, 1 oz | 130 | 5 | 17 |
| **Bagel Thins** (Thomas'), 1, 1.5 oz | 110 | 1 | 25 |

## Bagel ~ Brands

*Per Bagel*

| | C | F | Cb |
|---|---|---|---|
| **Bubba's:** Plain; Onion, average | 240 | 2 | 48 |
| Blueberry | 150 | 0.5 | 32 |
| Cinnamon Raisin | 250 | 1.5 | 51 |
| **Costco Bakery:** Plain | 330 | 1.5 | 70 |
| Cinnamon Raisin | 340 | 1.5 | 73 |
| Whole Grain | 300 | 5 | 56 |
| **Lender's,** Fresh, NY Style: | | | |
| Plain, 3.3 oz | 240 | 2 | 46 |
| Blueberry, 2 oz | 150 | 0.5 | 32 |
| Whole Grain, 3.3 oz | 250 | 1.5 | 49 |
| Whole Wheat, 3.3 oz | 210 | 1.5 | 41 |
| **Panera Bread:** Plain | 290 | 1.5 | 59 |
| Cinnamon & Raisin Swirl, 3.8 oz | 320 | 2 | 65 |
| Everything, 4 oz | 300 | 2.5 | 59 |
| Whole Grain, 4.3 oz | 340 | 2.5 | 67 |
| **Sara Lee:** Mini, average, 1.3 oz | 100 | 0.5 | 20 |
| Plain, 3.4 oz | 260 | 1 | 50 |
| Blueberry, 3.7 oz | 280 | 1 | 54 |
| Cinnamon Raisin, 3.7 oz | 270 | 1 | 54 |
| Everything, 3.7 oz | 280 | 3.5 | 50 |
| Onion, 3 oz | 270 | 1 | 52 |
| **Western,** The Alternatives, av., 2 oz | 120 | 0.5 | 29 |

## Bagel Spreads

| **Cream Cheese:** | C | F | Cb |
|---|---|---|---|
| Plain: 2 Tbsp, 1 oz | 100 | 9 | 1 |
| 2 oz mini-tub | 200 | 18 | 2 |
| Reduced Fat: 2 Tbsp, 1 oz | 60 | 5 | 2 |
| 2 oz mini-tub | 120 | 10 | 4 |
| **Flavors:** Lox, 1 oz | 90 | 8 | 2 |
| Honey Nut, 1 oz | 80 | 7 | 4 |
| Strawberry, 1 oz | 90 | 7 | 5 |
| Sundried Tomato, 1 oz | 80 | 7 | 2 |
| Vegetable, 1 oz | 90 | 8 | 2 |

## English Muffins    C F Cb

*Average All Brands*

| **Plain/Whole Wheat:** | C | F | Cb |
|---|---|---|---|
| Regular, 2 oz | 135 | 1.5 | 26 |
| Heavier, 2.5 oz | 155 | 2 | 31 |
| Super Size, 3.2 oz | 190 | 2 | 38 |
| **Raisin-Cinnamon,** 2.2 oz | 150 | 1 | 30 |

Note: Actual weight of packaged muffins can be 10-15% heavier than stated net weight.

## Rice Cakes

| | C | F | Cb |
|---|---|---|---|
| Regular size (1), average, 0.3 oz | 35 | 0.5 | 7.5 |
| **Hain,** Mini, Mild Cheddar (10) | 70 | 2.5 | 11 |
| **Lundberg,** | | | |
| all varieties, 0.4 oz | 70 | 0.5 | 14 |
| **Quaker,** Apple Cinn., 0.5 oz | 50 | 0 | 11 |

## Tortillas & Shells

**Tortillas:** *Per Tortilla*

| Corn Flour: | C | F | Cb |
|---|---|---|---|
| White/Yellow: 6", 1 oz | 55 | 1 | 11 |
| 7", 1.2 oz | 75 | 1 | 14 |
| Wheat Flour: | | | |
| 6", 1.2 oz | 100 | 3 | 16 |
| 8", 1.4 oz | 130 | 4 | 20 |
| 10", 2.3 oz | 200 | 6 | 31 |

**Shells:** *Per Shell, Without Fillings*

| Corn Taco Shells: | C | F | Cb |
|---|---|---|---|
| Mini, 3", 0.2 oz | 25 | 1 | 3 |
| Medium, 5", 0.5 oz | 60 | 2.5 | 8 |
| Large, 6½", 0.7 oz | 100 | 4.5 | 13 |
| Salad Shell, 10" | 310 | 17 | 34 |
| **Tostada Shells,** fried: | | | |
| White Corn, 5½" diam., 0.4 oz | 55 | 2.5 | 8 |
| Yellow Corn, 5½" diam., 0.5 oz | 80 | 3.5 | 11 |
| **Sopes,** 1 shell, 4" 2 oz | 110 | 1.5 | 23 |
| **La Tortilla Factory:** | | | |
| **100 Calorie,** Whole Wheat, 2 oz | 100 | 1.5 | 24 |
| **Hand Made Style:** | | | |
| Flour, 1.7 oz | 150 | 5 | 21 |
| Green Chile, 2.5 oz | 90 | 1 | 14 |
| **Traditional,** White/Yellow Corn, | | | |
| 2 Tortillas, 2.3 oz | 130 | 1.5 | 27 |
| **Whole Wheat,** Low Carb High Fiber, | | | |
| Original; Garlic & Herb, 1.3 oz | 50 | 2 | 10 |
| **Mission Foods:** | | | |
| **Corn,** Yellow/White, Super Soft: | | | |
| Regular size, 2 Tortillas, 1.7 oz | 100 | 1.5 | 20 |
| Super size (1), 1.2 oz | 70 | 1 | 13 |
| **Flour:** Estilo Casero, 1 Tortilla, 1.8 oz | 170 | 6 | 24 |
| Homestyle, 1 Tortilla, 2.2 oz | 190 | 4.5 | 32 |

## Quick Guide    **C** **F** **Cb**

### Cooked Cereals

| | C | F | Cb |
|---|---|---|---|
| **Barley,** pearled, cooked, 1 cup | 195 | 0.5 | 44 |
| **Buckwheat Groats,** roasted: | | | |
|   Dry, ½ cup, 3 oz | 285 | 2 | 61 |
|   Cooked, 1 cup, 6 oz | 155 | 1 | 34 |
| **Bulgur:** Dry, ½ cup, 2.5 oz | 240 | 1 | 53 |
|   Cooked, 1 cup, 6.5 oz | 150 | 0.5 | 34 |
| **Corn/Hominy Grits:** | | | |
|   Dry: Regular, ¼ cup, 1.4 oz | 140 | 0.5 | 32 |
|   Instant: 0.8 oz packet | 75 | 0 | 18 |
|     W/ Imitation Bacon Bits, 1 oz | 100 | 0.5 | 22 |
|   Cooked, ¾ cup, 6.5 oz | 110 | 0.5 | 23 |
| **Cream of Rice,** cooked, ¾ cup, 6.5 oz | 95 | 0 | 21 |
| **Cream of Wheat:** | | | |
|   Cooked: Regular, ¾ cup, 6.5 oz | 95 | 0.5 | 20 |
|   Instant, ¾ cup, 6.5 oz | 105 | 0.5 | 21 |
|   Quick, ¾ cup, 6.5 oz | 100 | 0.5 | 22 |
| **Farina,** cooked, ¾ cup, 6 oz | 95 | 0.5 | 19 |
| **Millet,** dry, ¼ cup, 1.8 oz | 190 | 2 | 36 |
| **Oat Bran:** Raw, ⅓ cup, 1 oz | 70 | 2 | 19 |
|   Cooked, ½ cup, 3.8 oz | 45 | 1 | 13 |
| **Oatmeal:** | | | |
|   Dry: Regular, ⅓ cup, 1 oz | 100 | 1.5 | 18 |
|   Instant: Regular, average, 1 oz | 105 | 1.5 | 18 |
|     Flavored, average, 1.5 oz | 165 | 2 | 34 |
|   Cooked: Regular, ¾ cup, 6 oz | 125 | 2.5 | 21 |
|     1 cup, 8 oz | 165 | 3.5 | 28 |
| **Whole Wheat,** cooked, ¾ cup, 6.5 oz | 115 | 0.5 | 25 |

### Brans, Wheat Germ, Add-Ons

| | C | F | Cb |
|---|---|---|---|
| **Bee Pollen Granules,** 1 Tbsp, 0.3 oz | 25 | 1 | 2 |
| **Bran:** | | | |
|   **Oat Bran:** Raw, 1 Tbsp, 0.2 oz | 20 | 0.5 | 3 |
|     ⅓ cup, 1 oz | 100 | 2 | 17 |
|   **Rice Bran:** Raw, 1 Tbsp, 0.2 oz | 15 | 1 | 2.5 |
|     ¼ cup, 1 oz | 95 | 6 | 15 |
| **Fruit:** Dried, average, 1 oz | 70 | 0 | 18 |
|   Banana, ½ medium | 55 | 0 | 14 |
|   Prunes in Syrup (5), 3 oz | 90 | 0 | 23 |
| **Honey,** 1 Tbsp, 0.75 oz | 65 | 0 | 17 |
| **Lecithin Granules,** 1 Tbsp, 0.4 oz | 55 | 4 | 0.5 |
| **Nuts,** Almonds (6), 0.3 oz | 40 | 4 | 1.5 |
| **Psyllium Husks,** 1 Tbsp, 0.2 oz | 10 | 0 | 4 |
| **Wheat,** unprocessed, 1 Tbsp | 5 | 0 | 2 |
| **Wheat Germ:** Raw, 1 Tbsp, 0.3 oz | 25 | 0.5 | 4 |
|   ¼ cup, 1 oz | 105 | 3 | 15 |

### Hot/Cooked Cereals ~ Brands

*Per Serving, Dry Mix only*    **C** **F** **Cb**

| | C | F | Cb |
|---|---|---|---|
| **Albers,** | | | |
|   Quick Grits, ¼ cup, 1.4 oz | 140 | 0.5 | 31 |
| **B&G:** | | | |
| **Cream of Wheat Instant:** | | | |
|   Original, 1 oz | 100 | 0 | 19 |
|   Cinn. Swirl, Maple Br. Sugar, 1.3 oz | 130 | 0 | 29 |
| **Bobs Red Mill,** | | | |
|   10 Grain, ¼ cup, 1.5 oz | 130 | 1 | 26 |
| **Country Choice:** | | | |
|   Multigrain Hot Cereal, ½ cup | 130 | 1 | 29 |
|   Oat varieties, ½ cup | 150 | 3 | 27 |
| **Dr. McDougall's:** *With Brown Sugar* | | | |
|   Apple Flax, 2.3 oz | 250 | 3.5 | 48 |
|   Cranberry Almond & Grains, 3 oz | 330 | 4 | 64 |
|   Hemp Peach, 3 oz | 330 | 5 | 63 |
|   Maple, 2.5 oz | 270 | 3.5 | 55 |
| **Great Value** *(Walmart):* | | | |
|   **Instant Oatmeal:** | | | |
|     Maple & Brown Sugar, 1.5 oz pkg | 160 | 2 | 33 |
|     Strawberries & Cream, 1.2 oz pkg | 130 | 2 | 27 |
| **McCann's:** | | | |
|   **Instant Irish Oatmeal:** | | | |
|     Regular, 1 oz package | 100 | 2 | 19 |
|     Apple & Cinn., 1.3 oz | 130 | 1.5 | 27 |
|     Maple & Brown Sugar, 1.5 oz | 160 | 2 | 32 |
| **Malt-O-Meal:** Original; Choc., 1.2 oz | 130 | 0.5 | 27 |
|   Maple Brown Sugar, ¼ cup | 170 | 0 | 37 |
| **Natures Path:** | | | |
|   **Oatmeal:** Flax Plus, 1.8 oz | 210 | 3 | 38 |
|     Apple Cinnamon, 1.7 oz | 210 | 2.5 | 40 |
|     Maple Nut, 1.7 oz | 210 | 4 | 38 |
| **NutriSystem:** | | | |
|   Oatmeal, Apple Cinnamon, 1 pkt | 130 | 1.5 | 26 |
| **Quaker:** | | | |
|   **Grits:** | | | |
|     Instant, average all flavors, 1 oz | 100 | 1 | 22 |
|     Quick, Original, ¼ cup, 1.3 oz | 130 | 0.5 | 29 |
|   **Instant Oatmeal:** | | | |
|     Original, Organic 1 oz | 100 | 2 | 19 |
|     Peaches & Cream, 1.3 oz | 130 | 2 | 27 |
|     Other varieties, 1.5 oz | 160 | 2 | 32 |
|   **Old Fash'nd/Quick Oats,** ½ c., 1.4 oz | 150 | 3 | 27 |
|   **Real Medleys:** | | | |
|     Blueb. Hazelnut, 2.5 oz | 270 | 7 | 49 |
|     Summer Berry, 2.5 oz | 250 | 3 | 51 |
|     Av. other varieties, 2.6 oz | 290 | 8 | 49 |
| **Wegmans:** | | | |
|   **Food You Feel Good About:** | | | |
|     Instant Oatmeal: Original, 1oz pkt | 100 | 2 | 19 |
|     Maple & Brown Sugar, 1.5 oz pkt | 160 | 2 | 32 |

# B. Breakfast Cereals

## Quick Guide    C   F   Cb

### Cold Cereals
*Average All Brands*

| | C | F | Cb |
|---|---|---|---|
| Bran Flakes, ¾ cup, 1 oz | 95 | 0.5 | 24 |
| Corn Flakes, 1 cup, 1 oz | 100 | 0 | 22 |
| Frosted Flakes, ¾ cup, 1 oz | 110 | 0 | 27 |
| Granola, 100% Nat., ½ cup, 1.7 oz | 205 | 6 | 35 |
| Oat Bran Cereal, ½ cup, 1.5 oz | 145 | 3 | 25 |
| Puffed Rice, 1 cup. 0.5 oz | 55 | 0 | 13 |
| Puffed Wheat, 1 cup, 0.5 oz | 45 | 0 | 10 |
| Raisin Bran, ½ cup, 1 oz | 90 | 0.5 | 22 |
| Rice Crisps, 1 cup, 1 oz | 105 | 0.5 | 24 |
| Shredded Wheat, 1 biscuit, 1 oz | 85 | 0.5 | 20 |
| Wheat Flakes, ¾ cup, 1 oz | 105 | 1 | 24 |

**Breakfast/Cereal Bars ~** *See Page 31*

## Ready-To-Eat Cereal ~ Brands

**Arrowhead Mills:**

| | C | F | Cb |
|---|---|---|---|
| **Flakes:** Amaranth, 1.2 oz | 140 | 2 | 26 |
| Kamut, 1 oz | 120 | 1 | 25 |
| Oat Bran, 1.2 oz | 140 | 2.5 | 24 |
| Spelt, 1 oz | 120 | 1 | 24 |
| Sprouted Wheat Berry & Quinoa, 1.5 oz | 100 | 1 | 22 |
| **Breadshop Granola,** | | | |
| Blueberry 'n Cream, ½ cup, 1.8 oz | 210 | 6 | 36 |
| **Puffed:** Corn, 0.5 oz | 60 | 1 | 12 |
| Kamut, 0.5 oz | 50 | 0 | 11 |
| Millet, 0.5 oz | 60 | 0.5 | 11 |
| Rice, 0.5 oz | 60 | 0 | 14 |
| Wheat, 0.5 oz | 60 | 0 | 12 |
| **Shredded Wheat:** | | | |
| Bite Size: | | | |
| Regular, 1.7 oz | 190 | 1 | 38 |
| Sweetened, 1.8 oz | 200 | 1 | 42 |

**Back to Nature:** *Per ½ Cup, Unless Indicated*

| | C | F | Cb |
|---|---|---|---|
| **Granola:** Apple Blueberry, 1.8 oz | 200 | 2.5 | 39 |
| Banana Walnut, 1.8 oz | 200 | 5 | 36 |
| Chocolate Delight, 1.8 oz | 220 | 6 | 37 |
| Classic, 1.8 oz | 200 | 3 | 39 |
| Cranberry Pecan, 1.6 oz | 200 | 5 | 35 |
| Orange Crunch, 1.8 oz | 200 | 4 | 37 |
| Sunflower & Pumpkin Seed, 1.8 oz | 210 | 7 | 31 |
| Vanilla Almond Agave, 1.8 oz | 200 | 5 | 37 |

**Barbara's Bakery:**

**Classics, Organic & Sweetened:**

| | C | F | Cb |
|---|---|---|---|
| Brown Rice Crisps, 1 oz | 120 | 1 | 25 |
| Corn Flakes, 1 cup, 1 oz | 110 | 1 | 25 |
| Honest O's, Original, 1 oz | 120 | 2 | 24 |
| **High Fiber:** | | | |
| Original, 12 oz | 180 | 1.5 | 42 |
| Cranberry, 2 oz | 190 | 1.5 | 42 |
| **Morning Oat Crunch:** | | | |
| Original, 2 oz | 210 | 2 | 44 |
| Cinnamon, 2 oz | 230 | 3 | 43 |
| Vanilla Almond, 2 oz | 220 | 3 | 42 |
| **Puffins:** | | | |
| Original, ¾ cup, 1 oz | 90 | 1 | 23 |
| Cinnamon, ⅔ cup, 1 oz | 90 | 1 | 26 |
| Multigrain, ¾ cup, 1 oz | 110 | 0 | 25 |
| PB/PB & Choc., av., ¾ cup, 1 oz | 110 | 2 | 24 |
| **Snackanimals,** av. all varieties, 1 oz | 110 | 0.5 | 26 |
| **Shredded Wheat,** 2 biscuits, 1.4 oz | 140 | 1 | 31 |
| **Spoonfuls,** Multigrain, ¾ cup, 1 oz | 120 | 1.5 | 24 |
| **Squarefuls,** Multigrain, 1 cup, 1.9 oz | 200 | 1 | 47 |

**Cascadian Farm:**

| | C | F | Cb |
|---|---|---|---|
| Buzz Crunch, 1 cup, 2.1 oz | 230 | 2.5 | 47 |
| Cinn. Crunch, 1 cup, 1 oz | 110 | 2.5 | 22 |
| Graham Crunch, ¾ cup, 1 oz | 110 | 2 | 23 |
| Granola: Ancient Grains, ⅔ cup, 2 oz | 230 | 5 | 43 |
| French Vanilla Almond, ⅔ cup, 2 oz | 240 | 6 | 43 |
| Oats & Honey, ⅔ cup, 2 oz | 230 | 6 | 42 |
| Av. other varieties, ¾ cup, 1.8 oz | 210 | 5 | 39 |
| Honey Nut O's, 1 cup, 1 oz | 110 | 1 | 25 |
| Multi Grain Squares, 1 cup, 1.9 oz | 210 | 1 | 44 |
| Raisin Bran, 1 cup, 1.8 oz | 180 | 1 | 41 |

**EnviroKidz:** *Per 1 oz*

| | C | F | Cb |
|---|---|---|---|
| Amazon Frosted Flakes, ⅔ cup | 120 | 0 | 26 |
| Gorilla Munch, ¾ cup | 120 | 1 | 26 |
| Koala Crisp, ¾ cup | 110 | 1 | 25 |
| Leapin' Lemurs, ¾ cup | 120 | 1.5 | 25 |
| Panda Puffs, ¾ cup | 130 | 3.5 | 23 |

**Erewhon:**

| | C | F | Cb |
|---|---|---|---|
| Corn Flakes, 1 cup, 1.2 oz | 130 | 0 | 30 |
| Crispy Brown Rice: Original, 1 oz | 110 | 0.5 | 25 |
| W/ Mixed Berries, 1 cup, 1 oz | 120 | 0.5 | 27 |
| Raisin Bran, 1 cup, 1.8 oz | 180 | 1 | 40 |
| Rice Twice, ¾ cup, 1 oz | 120 | 0 | 26 |
| Strawb. Crisps, ¾ cup, 1 oz | 120 | 0.5 | 28 |

## Ready-To-Eat Cereal (Cont)

| | **C** | **F** | **Cb** |
|---|---|---|---|
| **Ezekiel 4.9:** | | | |
| **Sprouted Whole Grain Cereals:** | | | |
| Original, ½ cup, 2 oz | 190 | 1 | 40 |
| Almond, ½ cup, 2 oz | 200 | 3 | 38 |
| Cinnamon Raisin, 2 oz | 190 | 1 | 41 |
| Golden Flax, ½ cup, 2 oz | 180 | 2.5 | 37 |
| **General Mills:** | | | |
| **Cheerios:** *Per ¾ Cup Unless Indicated* | | | |
| Original, 1 cup, 1 oz | 100 | 2 | 20 |
| Apple Cinn., ¾ cup, 1 oz | 120 | 1.5 | 24 |
| Banana Nut, ¾ cup, 1 oz | 100 | 1 | 24 |
| Cinnamon Burst, 1 c., 1.2 oz | 120 | 2 | 27 |
| Chocolate; Fruity, ¾ cup, 1 oz | 100 | 1.5 | 22 |
| Dulce de Leche; Frosted, ¾ cup, 1 oz | 100 | 1.5 | 22 |
| Honey Nut, ¾ cup, 1 oz | 110 | 1.5 | 22 |
| **Multigrain:** | | | |
| Regular, 1 cup, 1oz | 110 | 1 | 24 |
| Dark Choc. Crunch, ¾ cup, 1 oz | 110 | 1.5 | 23 |
| Peanut Butter, ¾ cup, 1 oz | 110 | 1.5 | 23 |
| **Protein:** Cinnamon Almond, 1¼ c. | 220 | 4.5 | 40 |
| Oats & Honey, 1¼ cups, 2 oz | 210 | 3 | 42 |
| **Chex:** Corn, 1 cup, 1 oz | 120 | 0.5 | 26 |
| Apple Cinn; Choc., average, 1 oz | 130 | 2.5 | 26 |
| Honey Nut, ¾ cup, 1 oz | 120 | 0.5 | 28 |
| Rice, 1 cup, 1 oz | 100 | 0.5 | 23 |
| Vanilla, ¾ cup, 1 oz | 120 | 2 | 25 |
| Wheat, ¾ cup, 1.7 oz | 160 | 1 | 39 |
| **Cinnamon Toast Crunch,** ¾ cup, 1.1 oz | 130 | 3 | 25 |
| **Fiber One:** Original, ½ cup, 1 oz | 60 | 1 | 25 |
| Honey Clusters, 1 cup, 1.8 oz | 170 | 1.5 | 44 |
| Nutty Clusters & Almonds, 1.9 oz | 190 | 4 | 44 |
| Protein, av. all flavors, 1 cup, 2 oz | 220 | 5 | 41 |
| **Kix:** Original, 1¼ cups, 1 oz | 110 | 1 | 25 |
| Berry Berry; Honey, 1¼ cup, 1.2 oz | 120 | 1.5 | 28 |
| **Lucky Charms,** all varieties, average, ¾ cup, 1 oz | 110 | 1.5 | 23 |
| **Monsters,** Count Chocula, ¾ cup, 1 oz | 100 | 1.5 | 23 |
| **Total:** Original, ¾ cup, 1 oz | 100 | 0.5 | 22 |
| Raisin Bran, 1 cup, 2 oz | 160 | 1 | 40 |
| **Trix,** 1 cup, 1 oz | 120 | 1.5 | 27 |
| **Wheaties,** | | | |
| Original, ¾ cup, 1 oz | 100 | 0.5 | 22 |

| | **C** | **F** | **Cb** |
|---|---|---|---|
| **Great Value** *(Walmart):* | | | |
| Apple Blasts, 1 cup, 1.2 oz | 120 | 0 | 29 |
| Crunch Honey Oats, with Almonds, ¾ cup, 1 oz | 130 | 2 | 26 |
| Extra Raisin Bran, 1 cup, 2 oz | 200 | 1 | 43 |
| Frosted Shredded Wheat, 1.9 oz | 180 | 1 | 42 |
| Fruit Spins, 1 cup, 1 oz | 110 | 1 | 25 |
| **Health Valley:** | | | |
| **Crunch-Ems!:** Corn, 1 cup, 1 oz | 110 | 0 | 27 |
| Rice, 1¼ cups, 1 oz | 110 | 0 | 26 |
| **Organic Flakes:** | | | |
| Amaranth, 1¼ cups, 2 oz | 210 | 2 | 43 |
| Fiber 7, Multigrain , 1 cup, 1.8 oz | 160 | 1 | 37 |
| Oat Bran: 1 cup, 1.8 oz | 190 | 1.5 | 39 |
| With Raisins, 1 cup, 1.9 oz | 200 | 1.5 | 43 |
| **Heartland:** | | | |
| **Granola:** | | | |
| Original, ½ cup, 2.3 oz | 240 | 6 | 40 |
| Harvest Spice, ½ cup, 1.8 oz | 210 | 5 | 37 |
| Low-Fat with Raisin, ½ cup, 2 oz | 200 | 3 | 40 |
| **Hershey's,** Cookies 'n' Creme, 1 oz | 110 | 3 | 21 |
| **Kashi** | | | |
| **7 Whole Grain:** Flakes, 1 c., 1.8 oz | 170 | 0.5 | 41 |
| Honey Puffs, 1 cup, 1 oz | 120 | 1 | 25 |
| Nuggets, ½ cup, 2 oz | 210 | 1.5 | 47 |
| Puffs, 1 cup, 0.7 oz | 70 | 0.5 | 15 |
| **GoLEAN:** Original, 1¼ cups, 2 oz | 180 | 2 | 40 |
| Crunch!: Original, ¾ cup, 2 oz | 190 | 3 | 38 |
| Honey Almond Flax, ⅔ cup, 2 oz | 200 | 5 | 35 |
| Van. Graham Clusters, 1 c., 1.8 oz | 170 | 1.5 | 36 |
| **Good Friends,** Orig., 1 cup, 2 oz | 160 | 1.5 | 42 |
| **Heart to Heart:** | | | |
| Honey Toasted Oat, ¾ cup, 1.2 oz | 120 | 1.5 | 26 |
| Oat Flakes & Blueb. Clusters, 1 c., 2 oz | 210 | 2 | 44 |
| **Organic Promise:** | | | |
| Berry Fruitful, 29 bisc., 1.8 oz | 170 | 0.5 | 42 |
| Indigo Morning, ¾ cup | 100 | 1 | 22 |
| Raisin Vineyard, ¾ c., 1.8 oz | 170 | 0.5 | 40 |
| Simply Maize, ¾ cup, 1 oz | 100 | 1 | 23 |
| **Kellogg's:** | | | |
| **All-Bran:** | | | |
| Original, ½ cup, 1 oz | 80 | 1 | 23 |
| Bran Buds, ⅓ cup, 1 oz | 80 | 1 | 24 |
| Compl. Wheat Flakes, 1 oz | 90 | 0.5 | 24 |
| **Apple Jacks,** 1 cup, 1 oz | 110 | 1 | 25 |
| **Cinnabon,** 1 cup, 1 oz | 120 | 2 | 25 |

*continued next page...*

## Ready-To-Eat Cereal (Cont)

| Kellogg's (Cont): | C | F | Cb |
|---|---|---|---|
| **Cinnabon,** 1 cup, 1 oz | 120 | 2 | 25 |
| **Corn Flakes,** Original, 1 cup, 1 oz | 100 | 0 | 24 |
| **Corn Pops,** 1 cup, 1 oz | 120 | 0 | 27 |
| **Cracklin' Oat Bran,** ¾ cup, 1.8 oz | 200 | 7 | 34 |
| **Crispix,** Original, 1 cup, 1 oz | 110 | 0 | 25 |
| **Crunchy Nut,** Golden Nut Flakes, ¾ cup, 1 oz | 120 | 1 | 26 |
| **Froot Loops:** Original, 1 cup, 1 oz | 110 | 1 | 26 |
| Marshmallow, 1 cup, 1 oz | 110 | 1 | 26 |
| **Frosted Flakes:** | | | |
| Original, ¾ cup, 1 oz | 110 | 0 | 27 |
| Reduced Sugar with Fiber, 1 cup, 1 oz | 110 | 0 | 26 |
| **Honey Smacks,** ¾ cup, 1 oz | 100 | 0.5 | 24 |
| **Krave:** | | | |
| Chocolate, ¾ cup, 1.1 oz | 120 | 3.5 | 24 |
| Double Choc., ¾ c., 1.1 oz | 120 | 3.5 | 23 |
| **Mini-Wheats, Frosted:** | | | |
| Big Bites (7), 2 oz | 200 | 1 | 49 |
| Bite Size, Orig. (21), 2 oz | 190 | 1 | 46 |
| Little Bites: | | | |
| Original, 1 cup, 2 oz | 200 | 1 | 47 |
| Chocolate, 1 cup, 2 oz | 200 | 2 | 46 |
| Touch of Fruit In Middle, Raspberry (24), 2 oz | 190 | 1 | 45 |
| **Mini Wheats,** unfrosted, Bite Size (30), 2 oz | 190 | 1 | 45 |
| **Mueslix,** ⅔ cup, 2 oz | 200 | 3 | 41 |
| **Product 19,** 1 cup, 1 oz | 110 | 0 | 25 |
| **Raisin Bran:** | | | |
| Regular, 1 cup, 2 oz | 190 | 1 | 46 |
| Crunch, 1 cup, 2 oz | 190 | 1 | 45 |
| **Rice Krispies:** | | | |
| Original, 1¼ cups, 1.2 oz | 130 | 0 | 29 |
| Frosted, ¾ cup, 1 oz | 120 | 0 | 27 |
| Treats, ¾ cup, 1 oz | 120 | 1 | 26 |
| **Scooby-Doo,** 1 cup, 1.1 oz | 120 | 1.5 | 27 |
| **Smart Start,** | | | |
| Original Antioxidants, 1 cup, 1.8 oz | 190 | 1 | 44 |

| Kellogg's (Cont): | C | F | Cb |
|---|---|---|---|
| **Special K:** | | | |
| Chocolate Almond, ⅔ cup, 1 oz | 110 | 1.5 | 23 |
| Cinnamon Pecan, ¾ cup, 1.1 oz | 110 | 2 | 24 |
| Granola, Touch of Honey, low fat, ½ cup, 1.8 oz | 190 | 3 | 39 |
| Oats & Honey, ¾ cup, 1 oz | 100 | 0.5 | 25 |
| Protein, average, ¾ cup, 1.1 oz | 115 | 1 | 21 |
| Vanilla Almond, ¾ cup | 110 | 1.5 | 25 |
| **Malt-O-Meal:** | | | |
| Apple Zings, 1 cup, 1.2 oz | 130 | 1 | 30 |
| Cocoa Dyno-Bites, ¾ cup | 120 | 1 | 26 |
| Coco Roos, ¾ cup, 1 oz | 120 | 1.5 | 26 |
| Colossal/Berry Crunch, ¾ cup, 1 oz | 120 | 1.5 | 26 |
| Frosted Flakes, ¾ cup, 1 oz | 120 | 0 | 28 |
| Frosted Mini Spooners, 1 cup | 190 | 1 | 45 |
| Golden Puffs, ¾ cup, 1 oz | 100 | 0 | 24 |
| Honey Nut Scooters, 1 cup, 1 oz | 120 | 1.5 | 24 |
| Raisin Bran, 1 cup, 2 oz | 220 | 1.5 | 45 |
| **Nature's Path:** | | | |
| **Flax Plus:** Flakes, ¾ c. 1 oz | 110 | 1.5 | 23 |
| Maple Pecan Crunch, ¾ cup | 220 | 7 | 38 |
| Pumpkin Raisin Crunch, ¾ c. | 210 | 4.5 | 40 |
| Raisin Bran Flakes, ¾ c., 2 oz | 190 | 2.5 | 41 |
| Heritage Flakes, ¾ cup, 1 oz | 120 | 1 | 24 |
| Honey'd Cornflakes, ¾ cup, 1 oz | 120 | 0 | 27 |
| Kamut Puffs, 1 cup, 0.5 oz | 50 | 0 | 11 |
| Multigrain Oatbran Flakes, ¾ cup, 1 oz | 110 | 1 | 24 |
| Qi'a, all varieties, av., 2Tbsp, 1 oz | 135 | 6.5 | 14 |
| Optimum Power, Blueb. Cinn. Flax, 2 oz | 200 | 3 | 38 |
| **New England Natural Bakers:** | | | |
| **Granola Pouches:** | | | |
| All Natural: | | | |
| Banana Walnut, ½ cup, 2 oz | 260 | 12 | 34 |
| Honey Nut Cinn., ½ cup, 2 oz | 270 | 12 | 35 |
| Probiotic Raspb., ½ cup, 1.7 oz | 200 | 3 | 37 |
| **Organic:** | | | |
| High Protein Clusters: | | | |
| Blueb. Harvest, ⅔ cup, 2 oz | 260 | 10 | 35 |
| Five Seed Granola, unsweetened, ½ cup, 2 oz | 270 | 14 | 28 |
| Muesli, Cinn. Raisin, ⅔ cup, 1.9 oz | 200 | 3.5 | 38 |

## Ready-To-Eat Cereal ~ Brands (Cont)

| | C | F | Cb |
|---|---|---|---|
| **NutriSystem:** *Per Packet* | | | |
| Granola, Low-Fat | 160 | 2.5 | 31 |
| NutriFlakes | 110 | 1 | 23 |
| Sweetened O's | 110 | 0 | 22 |
| **Peace:** | | | |
| **Clusters & Flakes:** | | | |
| Cherry Almond, 2 oz | 240 | 6 | 42 |
| Av,.other varieties, 2 oz | 235 | 5 | 43 |
| Low Fat, Hearty Raisin Bran, 2 oz | 190 | 2 | 44 |
| Crispy Rice & Flakes, | | | |
| Blueberry Pomegranate, 2 oz | 240 | 6 | 41 |
| Granola, average all varieties, ⅔ cup | 240 | 6 | 41 |
| **Post:** | | | |
| Alpha Bits, 1 cup, 1 oz | 120 | 1.5 | 24 |
| Bran Flakes, ¾ cup, 1 oz | 100 | 0.5 | 24 |
| Good Mornings, average, 1 oz | 120 | 1.5 | 25 |
| **Grape-Nuts:** Original, 2 oz | 210 | 1 | 47 |
| Fit, ⅔ cup, 2 oz | 220 | 3 | 44 |
| Flakes, ¾ cup, 1 oz | 110 | 1 | 24 |
| **Great Grains:** | | | |
| Banana Nut Crunch, 1 cup, 2 oz | 230 | 5 | 42 |
| Cranb. Alm. Crunch, 1cup, 2 oz | 210 | 3.5 | 41 |
| Protein Blend, av. all varieties, 2oz | 230 | 5 | 38 |
| **Honey Bunches of Oats:** | | | |
| With Almonds, ¾ cup, 1 oz | 130 | 2.5 | 26 |
| Wholemeal, with Van. Bunches, 2 oz | 220 | 3 | 46 |
| Honeycomb, Original, 1½ cups, 1 oz | 130 | 1 | 28 |
| Mini Cinnamon Churros, 1 cup, 1.2 oz | 130 | 3 | 26 |
| Pebbles, average all varieties, ¾ cup, 1 oz | 120 | 1 | 24 |
| Raisin Bran, 1 cup, 2 oz | 190 | 1 | 47 |
| **Selects**, Blueberry Morning, 1¼ cups, 2 oz | 220 | 3 | 45 |
| **Shredded Wheat**, Spoon Size: | | | |
| Original, 1.7 oz | 170 | 1 | 40 |
| Honey Nut, 2.1 oz | 220 | 2 | 49 |
| Waffle Crisp, 1 cup, 1 oz | 120 | 1.5 | 25 |
| **Quaker:** | | | |
| King Vitaman, 1½ cups, 1 oz | 120 | 1 | 26 |
| Life, all types, ¾ cup, 1 oz | 120 | 1.5 | 25 |
| **Natural Granola:** | | | |
| Apple Cranberry Almond, 1.7 oz | 200 | 5 | 37 |
| Oats, Honey, & Alm., ½ cup, 1.7 oz | 200 | 6 | 35 |
| Oatmeal Squares, Honey Nut, 1 cup, 2 oz | 210 | 2.5 | 44 |
| Quisps, 1 cup 1 oz | 100 | 1.5 | 23 |

| | C | F | Cb |
|---|---|---|---|
| **Stop & Shop:** | | | |
| Oats & O's, ½ cup, 1.8 oz | 110 | 1.5 | 22 |
| Raisin Bran, 1 cup, 2 oz | 190 | 1 | 46 |
| **Sweet Home Farm:** | | | |
| Honey Nut Granola, 1.9 oz | 250 | 10 | 37 |
| Other varieties, 2 oz | 250 | 8 | 40 |
| Low-Fat Granola, | | | |
| ½ cup, 1.9 oz | 210 | 3 | 44 |
| **Trader Joe's:** | | | |
| **Clusters:** Raisin Bran, 1 cup, 2 oz | 190 | 3 | 41 |
| Super Nutty Toffee, ¾ cup, 2 oz | 250 | 9 | 38 |
| Average other varieties, | | | |
| ⅔ cup, 1.3 oz | 145 | 3.5 | 26 |
| Corn Flakes, 1 cup, 1 oz | 110 | 0 | 26 |
| Golden Flax Cereal, 1.7 oz | 200 | 3.5 | 37 |
| **Granola:** Mango Passion, 2 oz | 240 | 7 | 38 |
| Pecan Praline, ½ cup, 1.6 oz | 210 | 7 | 31 |
| Trek Mix, ⅔ cup, 2 oz | 240 | 8 | 37 |
| High Fiber, ⅔ cup, 1 oz | 80 | 0.5 | 23 |
| Honey Nut O's, ¾ cup, 1 oz | 120 | 1.5 | 24 |
| Joe's O's, 1 cup, 1 oz | 110 | 1.5 | 22 |
| Shredded Wheats, Bite Size, 1 cup, 1.7 oz | 180 | 1 | 38 |
| Triple Berry O's, ¾ cup, 1 oz | 110 | 1 | 25 |
| Toasted Oatmeal Flakes, ¾ cup, 1 oz | 110 | 1 | 23 |
| Wheats, average all var., 1 cup, 2 oz | 200 | 1 | 42 |
| **Uncle Sam:** | | | |
| Original, ¾ cup, 2 oz | 210 | 6 | 37 |
| Raisin Bran, 1 cup, 2 oz | 190 | 1 | 42 |
| **Weetabix,** | | | |
| 2 biscuits, 1.3 oz | 130 | 1 | 29 |
| **Wegmans:** | | | |
| Cinnamon Muffin Squares, ¾ cup, 1 oz | 130 | 3.5 | 24 |
| Cinnamon Oat Crisps, ¾ cup, 1 oz | 120 | 1 | 26 |
| Chocolaty Rice Crisps, 1 oz | 120 | 1 | 26 |
| Corn Flakes, 1 cup, 1 oz | 100 | 0 | 24 |
| Frosted Flakes, 1 oz | 120 | 0 | 28 |
| Granola, Vanilla, ⅔ cup | 240 | 6 | 41 |
| Raisin Bran, 1 cup, 2 oz | 190 | 1 | 46 |
| **Whole Foods** *(365):* | | | |
| Corn Flakes, 1 cup, 1 oz | 110 | 0 | 26 |
| Frosted Flakes, ¾ cup, 1 oz | 110 | 0 | 27 |
| Hon. Flakes & Oat Clusters, | | | |
| ¾ cup, 1 oz | 120 | 1 | 25 |
| Protein & Fiber Crunch, 1 cup, 1.8 oz | 190 | 1 | 33 |
| Raisin Bran, 1 cup, 2 oz | 180 | 1 | 44 |
| **Wheat Squares:** | | | |
| Bite Sized, 1.7 oz | 180 | 1 | 38 |
| Frosted, 1 cup, 1.9 oz | 210 | 1 | 45 |

| Ready-to-Eat | C | F | Cb |
|---|---|---|---|
| *Per Piece/Slice* | | | |
| **Angel Food**, Plain: Without oil, 2 oz | 145 | 0 | 33 |
| With oil, 2 oz | 145 | 1 | 27 |
| With Cream Frosting | 255 | 7 | 45 |
| **Almond Croissant**, 5 oz | 620 | 35 | 67 |
| **Apple Danish**, 5 oz | 450 | 18 | 67 |
| **Apple Pie** ~ *See Pies/Tarts Page 134* | | | |
| **Baklava**, 1½" square, 1.75 oz | 200 | 10 | 27 |
| **Banana Cake**, with Butter Cream, 2 oz | 230 | 9 | 37 |
| **Banana Walnut Cake**, 3 oz | 270 | 11 | 40 |
| **Bear Claw**, 4.5 oz | 540 | 24 | 71 |
| **Black Forest**, 3 oz | 345 | 11 | 59 |
| **Brownie:** Small, 2" Square, 1 oz | 130 | 8 | 14 |
| Large, 3 oz | 390 | 24 | 42 |
| **Bundt Cakes**, average all types: | | | |
| 3 oz slice | 300 | 13 | 42 |
| Mini-Bundt, 5 oz | 500 | 22 | 70 |
| **Cannoli's:** Mini, 1 oz | 85 | 3 | 11 |
| Regular, 2.5 oz | 215 | 8 | 28 |
| **Carrot Cake:** Plain, 3 oz | 300 | 16 | 37 |
| With Cream Cheese Frosting | 400 | 22 | 48 |
| **Cheesecake:** | | | |
| Small serving, 3 oz | 240 | 13 | 26 |
| Large serving, 5 oz | 400 | 21 | 44 |
| With Low-Fat Cheese/Fruit, 3 oz | 170 | 4 | 28 |
| *Denny's*, NY Style, 5oz | 510 | 34 | 43 |
| **Chocolate Cake:** | | | |
| With Chocolate Frosting, 4 oz | 415 | 18 | 62 |
| Without Frosting, ¹⁄₁₂ of 9", 3.5 oz | 340 | 14 | 51 |
| **Chocolate Croissant**, 4.25 oz | 470 | 26 | 54 |
| **Chocolate Eclair**, w/ custard, 3.5 oz | 260 | 16 | 24 |
| **Chocolate Fudge Cake**, 3 oz | 270 | 12 | 40 |
| **Chocolate Meringue**, 2.5 oz | 320 | 13 | 48 |
| **Churros**, 1 stick, 1.5 oz | 165 | 8 | 21 |
| **Cinnamon Crumb Cake**, 2.5 oz | 260 | 9 | 40 |
| **Cinnamon Rolls:** Small, 2 oz | 220 | 8 | 34 |
| Regular, 4 oz | 440 | 16 | 68 |
| Large, 6 oz | 660 | 24 | 102 |
| **Brands** ~ *See Page 67* | | | |
| **Coffee Cake**, 2 oz | 180 | 6 | 30 |
| **Concha:** Small, 2 oz | 240 | 9 | 33 |
| Large (5" diameter), 5.5 oz | 615 | 23 | 85 |
| **Cream Puff**, custard filled, 4.6 oz | 335 | 20 | 30 |
| **Cream Horn**, 3 oz | 210 | 5 | 36 |
| **Crumble Coffee Cake**, 4.5 oz | 500 | 25 | 65 |
| **Danish Pastries:** | | | |
| Small, 2.5 oz | 250 | 14 | 25 |
| Large, 5 oz | 500 | 28 | 50 |
| **Donuts** ~ *See Page 66* | | | |
| **Eclair**, Chocolate, custard filled, 3.5 oz | 260 | 16 | 24 |
| **Fig Bars**, average | 160 | 3 | 31 |

| Ready-to-Eat (Cont) | C | F | Cb |
|---|---|---|---|
| *Per Piece/Slice* | | | |
| **Fruit Cake**, Dark/Light, 2 oz | 185 | 5 | 34 |
| **Fudge Nut Brownie**, 3.5 oz | 380 | 18 | 54 |
| **Gingerbread**, from mix, 3" square | 210 | 4 | 41 |
| **Honey Bun**, 2.7 oz | 310 | 15 | 39 |
| **Jelly Roll**, ½ roll, 1.8 oz | 150 | 2 | 32 |
| **Key Lime Pie**, 4.3 oz | 400 | 25 | 41 |
| **Kringles:** Almond; Pecan, average | 205 | 12 | 24 |
| Blueberry: Cherry; Raspberry, av. | 165 | 8 | 24 |
| **Lady Finger**, 3 oz | 310 | 4.5 | 59 |
| **Lemon Cake**, 4 oz | 440 | 24 | 49 |
| **Lemon Poppy Seed Creme**, 1.6 oz | 180 | 9 | 23 |
| **Marble Cake**, 4 oz | 430 | 23 | 50 |
| **Mississippi Mud Pie**, 4 oz | 480 | 22 | 67 |
| **Mud Cake**, 4.5 oz | 380 | 20 | 44 |
| **Muffins** ~ *See Page 67* | | | |
| **Palmier Cookie**, large, 4.5 oz | 490 | 25 | 62 |
| **Pineapple Upside Down Cake**, | | | |
| 2.5 oz | 230 | 9 | 36 |
| **Peach Melba**, 3.5 oz | 300 | 8 | 52 |
| **Pecan Sticky Roll**, 6.5 oz | 690 | 22 | 91 |
| **Pecan Twirls**, 1.3 oz | 170 | 7 | 26 |
| **Pies & Tarts** ~ *See Page 134* | | | |
| **Pound Cakes:** Iced Lemon, 3.5 oz | 360 | 17 | 50 |
| Marble, 3.75 oz | 350 | 13 | 53 |
| **Raspberry Rugulah**, | | | |
| 1.2 oz | 110 | 9 | 7 |
| **Scone**, fruit, 2 oz | 200 | 9 | 30 |
| **Sponge Cake:** Plain, 2.5 oz | 220 | 10 | 33 |
| With Chocolate Frosting | 290 | 12 | 45 |
| With Cream & Strawberry Jam | 390 | 12 | 69 |
| **Starbucks Cakes** ~ *Page 244* | | | |
| **Strawberry Creme Cake**, 4.7 oz | 400 | 27 | 33 |
| **Strudel Bites**, 0.75 oz | 60 | 2.5 | 9 |
| **Strudel**, fruit, av., 4.5 oz | 300 | 17 | 32 |
| **Swiss Rolls**, 1 oz | 135 | 6 | 19 |
| **Tiramisu**, 4.5 oz | 440 | 22 | 34 |
| **Turnovers**, fruit, average, 3 oz | 290 | 15 | 35 |

| Cupcakes | | | |
|---|---|---|---|
| *Average all Varieties* | | | |
| **Regular:** | | | |
| Cake only, 1.5 oz | 140 | 5.5 | 20 |
| Cake + Icing, 2.5 oz | 260 | 13 | 34 |
| **Large**, (Muffin Size): | | | |
| Cake only, 2.5 oz | 235 | 9 | 34 |
| Cake + Icing, 5 oz | 520 | 27 | 67 |
| **Mini**, (2-Bite): | | | |
| Cake only, 0.4 oz | 40 | 1.5 | 5.5 |
| Cake + Icing, 1 oz | 110 | 5.5 | 13 |
| **Icing Only:** Per 1 oz | 115 | 7 | 13 |
| Thick/Tall amount, 2.5 oz | 290 | 17 | 32 |

## Cakes ~ Brands  **C** **F** **Cb**

**Albertson's Bakery:**
**Ring Cakes:** *Per ⅛ Cake*

| | C | F | Cb |
|---|---|---|---|
| Angel Food, 2 oz | 160 | 0 | 36 |
| Butter; Chocolate, av., 3 oz | 305 | 15 | 39 |

**Cake Slices:** *Per Slice Unless Indicated*

| | | | |
|---|---|---|---|
| Banana Nut Loaf | 330 | 17 | 39 |
| Butter Creme | 110 | 6 | 20 |
| Creme Cake (2), 3.2 oz | 300 | 12 | 43 |
| Cinnamon Streusel (2), 3.2 oz | 350 | 18 | 43 |

**Bimbo Bakery:**

| | | | |
|---|---|---|---|
| Concha, Vanilla, 2 oz | 260 | 11 | 35 |

**Pound Cakes:** *Per Slice*

| | | | |
|---|---|---|---|
| Panquecitos, 1.8 oz | 170 | 4.5 | 29 |
| Pecan, 2.3 oz | 260 | 11 | 36 |
| Raisin, 2.3 oz | 240 | 9 | 38 |

**Bon Appetit Bakery:**

| | | | |
|---|---|---|---|
| Banana Bread, 4 oz | 440 | 25 | 49 |
| Cream Cheese Cake, 4 oz slice | 430 | 24 | 49 |

**Danish:**

| | | | |
|---|---|---|---|
| Apple (1), 5 oz | 210 | 11 | 25 |
| Bear Claw (1), 5 oz | 240 | 13 | 27 |
| Cheese & Berries (1), 5 oz | 250 | 14 | 26 |
| Vienna Cream (1), 5 oz | 240 | 14 | 27 |

**Slices:**

| | | | |
|---|---|---|---|
| Cheesecake, 4 oz | 430 | 24 | 49 |
| Lemon Cake, 4 oz | 430 | 24 | 49 |
| Marble Cake, 4 oz | 430 | 24 | 50 |
| Walnut Brownie, 3.5 oz | 380 | 18 | 54 |

**Cheesecake Factory** ~ *See Fast-Foods Section*
**Entenmann's:** *Per Slice*

**Crumb Cakes:**

| | | | |
|---|---|---|---|
| All Butter French, 1.8 oz | 210 | 10 | 29 |
| Chocolate, ⅛ cake | 270 | 12 | 39 |

**Danish:**

| | | | |
|---|---|---|---|
| Pecan Danish Twist, ⅙ cake | 260 | 16 | 27 |
| Cheese-Filled Crumb Coffee, 2 oz | 200 | 10 | 25 |
| Raspberry Danish Twist, 2 oz | 220 | 11 | 29 |

**Dessert Cakes:**

| | | | |
|---|---|---|---|
| Banana, 2.3 oz | 270 | 14 | 36 |
| Carrot, Iced, 2.4 oz | 260 | 12 | 37 |
| Chocolate Fudge, 2.3 oz | 240 | 10 | 37 |
| Red Velvet, Iced, ⅛ cake | 270 | 14 | 36 |

**Loaf Cakes:**

| | | | |
|---|---|---|---|
| Chocolate, ⅙ loaf | 190 | 8 | 29 |
| Cinnamon Crunch, ⅙ loaf | 270 | 14 | 33 |

**Glenny's:**
**100 Calorie:**

| | | | |
|---|---|---|---|
| Blondie, Choc. Chip, 1.5 oz | 100 | 4 | 15 |
| Brownies: Chocolate Chip, 1.5 oz | 100 | 4 | 12 |
| Peanut Butter, 1.5 oz | 100 | 4 | 15 |

**Muffins/Sweet Rolls** ~ *See Page 67*

**Great American Cookies:**  **C** **F** **Cb**
**Cookie Cakes:** *Per Slice*

| | | | |
|---|---|---|---|
| By the Slice, 4.5 oz | 580 | 27 | 83 |
| Heart Shaped, 3.5 oz | 440 | 21 | 64 |
| M&M, 4 oz | 500 | 24 | 73 |

**Great Value** *(Walmart):*

| | | | |
|---|---|---|---|
| Chocolate Cup Cakes (1), 1.8 oz | 170 | 5 | 31 |
| Devil's Food Cake (1), 1.4 oz | 160 | 7 | 23 |
| Swiss Roll Snack Cakes (2), 2.2 oz | 240 | 10 | 35 |

**Hostess:**

| | | | |
|---|---|---|---|
| Twinkies, (1) | 135 | 4.5 | 23 |

**Cup Cakes:**

| | | | |
|---|---|---|---|
| 100 Calorie, Lemon Golden (1) | 100 | 2.5 | 21 |
| Chocolate, 8-pack, 1 cupcake, 1.5 oz | 160 | 6 | 26 |

**Donettes** ~ *See Page 66*
**Little Debbie,** Snack Cakes:

| | | | |
|---|---|---|---|
| Brownie: Choc Chip (1), 2.2 oz | 270 | 11 | 41 |
| Fudge (1), 2.2 oz | 300 | 13 | 43 |
| Choc. Chip Cake, 2 oz | 300 | 14 | 42 |
| Chocolate Cup Cake, Creme Filled (1) | 430 | 17 | 65 |
| Cocoa Cremes (1), 1.5 oz | 170 | 8 | 24 |
| Devil Cremes (1), 1.7 oz | 260 | 11 | 38 |
| Devil Squares (2), 2.2 oz | 260 | 11 | 38 |
| Fancy Cakes (2) | 310 | 15 | 43 |
| Frosted Fudge Cake, 1.5 oz | 190 | 9 | 27 |
| Rolls: Blueberry Creme, 2.2 oz | 240 | 8 | 40 |
| Boston Creme, 2.2 oz | 270 | 12 | 40 |
| Star Crunch Cosmic Snacks, 2.2 oz | 290 | 12 | 43 |
| S'mores (1) | 190 | 7 | 30 |
| Zebra Cake (2), 2.5 oz | 320 | 14 | 48 |

**Nemo's:**

| | | | |
|---|---|---|---|
| Brookie (1), 1.5 oz | 160 | 7 | 26 |

**Cake Squares:**

| | | | |
|---|---|---|---|
| Banana, 3 oz | 300 | 12 | 45 |
| Carrot, 3.6 oz | 390 | 21 | 47 |
| Chocolate, 3 oz | 300 | 12 | 44 |

**Crumble Cake:**

| | | | |
|---|---|---|---|
| Blueberry (1), 4 oz | 390 | 17 | 54 |
| Cinnamon Streusel (1), 4 oz | 420 | 18 | 59 |
| Lemon Rasp. (1), 4 oz | 400 | 19 | 55 |

**Oreo:**
**Soft Cakesters:**

| | | | |
|---|---|---|---|
| Chocolate (2), 2 oz | 250 | 12 | 36 |
| Double Stuf (2), 2.6 oz pkg | 350 | 18 | 48 |

## Cakes ~ Brands (Cont)

**Pepperidge Farm:**
**3-Layer Cakes:** *Per ⅛ Cake*

| | | | |
|---|---|---|---|
| Chocolate Fudge | 240 | 13 | 32 |
| Coconut | 250 | 12 | 34 |
| Key Lime | 240 | 12 | 34 |
| Orange Cream | 210 | 9 | 32 |
| Average other varieties | 240 | 11 | 33 |

**Turnovers (Frozen):**

| | | | |
|---|---|---|---|
| Apple; Cherry (1) | 260 | 13 | 31 |
| Chocolate (1) | 350 | 22 | 35 |
| Peach; Raspberry (1) | 270 | 13 | 34 |

**Pop Tarts** *(Kellogg's):*

| | | | |
|---|---|---|---|
| Fruit/Frosted/Unfrosted, av. | 200 | 5 | 36 |
| Gone Nutty, | | | |
| average all varieties, 1.8 oz | 195 | 5 | 35 |
| Mini Crisps, all flavors, 1 pouch, 0.5 oz | 60 | 1.5 | 11 |

**Safeway Select,**

| | | | |
|---|---|---|---|
| Molten Chocolate Lava Cake, 4.5 oz | 440 | 26 | 50 |

**Sara Lee:**
**Carrot Cake**, ⅙ cake  340  18  41
**Cheesecakes:**

| | | | |
|---|---|---|---|
| Classic: French, 4.7 oz slice | 410 | 26 | 38 |
| Strawberry, 4.3 oz slice | 320 | 18 | 37 |
| New York Style, 5 oz slice | 480 | 29 | 48 |
| Limited Edition, | | | |
| NY Style, Chocolate, 5 oz slice | 500 | 29 | 55 |
| Original Cream: | | | |
| Cherry, 4.8 oz slice | 320 | 11 | 50 |
| Classic, 4.3 oz slice | 340 | 18 | 38 |
| Strawberry, 4.7 oz slice | 330 | 12 | 51 |

**Coffee Cake**, Butter Streusel, ⅙ cake  190  9  24
**Pound Cakes:**

| | | | |
|---|---|---|---|
| All Butter, 1.9 oz slice | 260 | 9 | 42 |
| Lemon, 2.7 oz slice | 270 | 9 | 42 |
| Individual Slices: | | | |
| All Butter, 1 oz | 100 | 3 | 15 |
| Double Choc., 1.8 oz | 180 | 7 | 28 |
| Lemon, 1 oz | 100 | 3.5 | 15 |
| Original, 1.6 oz | 160 | 5 | 25 |

**Smart Ones** *(Weight Watchers):*
**Smart Delights:** *Per Sundae*

| | | | |
|---|---|---|---|
| Chocolate Chip Cookie Dough | 140 | 3 | 26 |
| Peanut Butter Cup | 130 | 3 | 23 |
| Strawberry Shortcake | 120 | 4 | 19 |

| | C | F | Cb |
|---|---|---|---|
| **Special K,** | | | |
| Pastry Crisps, all varieties, (2), 1 oz | 100 | 2 | 20 |
| **Tastykake:** | | | |
| **Chocolate Creme Cups**, (2), 1.9 oz | 210 | 8 | 32 |
| **Kandy Kake**, Peanut Butter, 1.7 oz | 230 | 13 | 25 |
| **Krimpets**, Butterscotch, | | | |
| Creme Filled (2), 2.4 oz | 220 | 6 | 39 |
| **Toaster Strudel** *(Pillsbury): Per 2 oz* | | | |
| Boston Cream Pie | 180 | 7 | 25 |
| Cream Cheese, | | | |
| average all varieties | 185 | 9 | 24 |
| Fruit flavors, all varieties | 180 | 7 | 27 |

**Trader Joe's:**
**Bakery Fresh:**

| | | | |
|---|---|---|---|
| Apricot Almond Tart, | | | |
| 4 oz slice | 450 | 24 | 56 |
| Cheesecake Brownie Bites (1) | 110 | 7 | 9 |
| Chocolate Ganache Cake, 3 oz slice | 390 | 22 | 44 |
| Flourless Chocolate Cake, | | | |
| 1 slice, 2 oz | 260 | 17 | 23 |
| Lemon Cake, 3.3oz slice | 350 | 19 | 43 |
| Mini Bundt, Triple Choc., ½ cake | 340 | 21 | 41 |
| Mini Carrot Cake, 5 oz | 450 | 19 | 68 |
| Whoopie Pie (1), 2.5 oz | 350 | 14 | 54 |

**Bread Cake:**

| | | | |
|---|---|---|---|
| Banana Bonanza, 2.6 oz slice | 250 | 9 | 39 |
| Pumpkin Nut, 2.6 oz slice | 270 | 10 | 43 |
| Walnut Streusel Coffee, 2 oz slice | 180 | 8 | 25 |
| Zucchini Carrot, 2 oz slice | 200 | 7 | 32 |

**Loaf Cake:**

| | | | |
|---|---|---|---|
| Cranberry Pumpkin, 2 oz slice | 140 | 2 | 30 |
| Pumpkin Nut, 2.6 oz slice | 270 | 10 | 43 |

**Frozen:**

| | | | |
|---|---|---|---|
| Apple Raspberry Turnover, 3.2 oz | 280 | 14 | 34 |
| Chocolate Dilemma Cheesecake: | | | |
| Plain, 3.5 oz | 320 | 19 | 30 |
| Choc. Chip; Triple Choc, av., 3.5 oz | 345 | 20 | 35 |
| Tuxedo, 3.5 oz | 320 | 17 | 34 |
| Choc Lava Cake (1), 4 oz | 360 | 23 | 40 |
| Karat Cake, 3 oz slice | 320 | 19 | 37 |
| N.Y. Style Cheesecake, 4.5 oz slice | 400 | 28 | 32 |
| Tiramisu Torte, 3.2 oz slice | 230 | 12 | 24 |

**Tarts:**

| | | | |
|---|---|---|---|
| Pear, 3.5 oz slice | 250 | 9 | 39 |
| Raspberry, 5 oz slice | 290 | 10 | 51 |
| Wild Blueberry, 3.5 oz slice | 260 | 6 | 52 |

## Cakes ~ Mixes

| | C | F | Cb |
|---|---|---|---|

*Prepared as Directed*

**Arrowhead Mills:**
**Brownie Mix:**

| | C | F | Cb |
|---|---|---|---|
| Regular, ½o package, 1 oz | 150 | 7 | 21 |
| Gluten Free, Fudge Brownie | | | |
| ½o package, 1 oz | 160 | 8 | 21 |

**Cake Mix:**

| | C | F | Cb |
|---|---|---|---|
| Chocolate, organic, ¹⁄₁₂ pkg., 1.5 oz | 260 | 11 | 39 |
| Vanilla, ¹⁄₁₂ package, 1.8 oz | 260 | 10 | 39 |

**Betty Crocker:**
**Bars:**

| | C | F | Cb |
|---|---|---|---|
| Reese's, ¹⁄₁₅ package | 180 | 13 | 20 |
| Sunkist Lemon, ¹⁄₁₆ pkg | 140 | 4 | 24 |

**Brownie Mix:**

| | C | F | Cb |
|---|---|---|---|
| Dark Chocolate Fudge, ½o package | 160 | 7 | 24 |
| Fudge, ½o package | 170 | 8 | 23 |
| Low-Fat Fudge, ¹⁄₁₈ pkg | 140 | 3 | 28 |
| Premium: | | | |
| Choc. Chunk, ¹⁄₁₆ pkg | 170 | 7 | 26 |
| Original Supreme, ¹⁄₁₆ package | 190 | 8 | 27 |
| P'nut Butter/Walnut, av., ¹⁄₁₆ pkg | 170 | 7 | 24 |
| Triple Chunk, ¹⁄₁₆ package | 180 | 7 | 28 |
| Ultimate Fudge, ¹⁄₁₆ package | 170 | 6.5 | 26 |

**Cake Mixes:** *Per ¹⁄₁₀ Package*

| | C | F | Cb |
|---|---|---|---|
| SuperMoist: | | | |
| Butter Recipe Yellow | 240 | 9 | 36 |
| Carrot | 310 | 18 | 35 |
| Cherry Chip | 280 | 14 | 36 |
| Devil's Food | 280 | 14 | 35 |
| French Vanilla | 280 | 14 | 35 |
| Milk Chocolate | 250 | 10 | 35 |
| Average other Chocolate varieties | 280 | 14 | 35 |

If using No-Cholesterol Recipe, deduct 40 cals and 4g fat.

**Cupcakes:** *Per 0.8 oz Mix & 0.4 oz Filling*

| | C | F | Cb |
|---|---|---|---|
| FUN da-middles: | | | |
| Chocolate Cake, Vanilla Filling | 200 | 9 | 27 |
| Yellow Cake, Chocolate Filling | 190 | 9 | 25 |

**Duncan Hines:**
**Brownie Mix:** *Per ¹⁄₂₀ Pkg Unless Indicated*

| | C | F | Cb |
|---|---|---|---|
| Decadent, Caramel Turtle, ¹⁄₁₆ pkg | 150 | 7 | 23 |
| Premium: Chewy Fudge | 180 | 8 | 24 |
| Snack Size, ¹⁄₁₂ pkg | 140 | 7 | 20 |
| Milk Chocolate | 160 | 8 | 21 |

**Cake Mix**,

| | C | F | Cb |
|---|---|---|---|
| Classic, Dark Choc. Fudge, ½o pkg | 220 | 11 | 28 |

*Prepared as Directed*

**Duncan Hines (Cont):**

| | C | F | Cb |
|---|---|---|---|

**Decadent:** *Per ¹⁄₁₂ Package*

| | C | F | Cb |
|---|---|---|---|
| Classic Carrot | 260 | 10 | 39 |
| Devil's Food | 230 | 11 | 30 |

**Signature:**

| | C | F | Cb |
|---|---|---|---|
| Banana Supreme | 270 | 12 | 36 |
| Coconut Supreme; Red Velvet, av. | 250 | 12 | 34 |
| French Vanilla; German Choc., av. | 270 | 12 | 34 |

**Jell-O:**
**No Bake Cheesecake:**

| | C | F | Cb |
|---|---|---|---|
| Cherry, ¹⁄₉ pkg, 2.4 oz | 290 | 11 | 48 |
| Real Cheesecake, ¹⁄₈ pkg, 2.1 oz | 360 | 21 | 42 |

| | C | F | Cb |
|---|---|---|---|
| **Krusteaz:** Cinn. Swirl Crumb Cake, 2" | 210 | 5 | 39 |
| Lemon; Key Lime Bar, 2½x2" bar | 160 | 4.5 | 29 |

**Pillsbury:**
**Brownies, Premium Mix:** *Dry Mix Only*

| | C | F | Cb |
|---|---|---|---|
| Caramel Swirl, ¹⁄₁₂ pkg, 1.2 oz | 120 | 1 | 28 |
| Cheesecake Swirl, ¹⁄₁₅ pkg, 1 oz | 110 | 1.5 | 25 |
| Chocolate Extreme, ¹⁄₁₅ pkg, 1 oz | 120 | 2 | 24 |
| Double Chocolate, ¹⁄₁₆ pkg, 1 oz | 100 | 0.5 | 24 |

**Cakes:**

| | C | F | Cb |
|---|---|---|---|
| Funfetti: Bold Purple ⅙ pkg, 1.4 oz | 140 | 1.5 | 32 |
| Neon Yellow, ⅙ pkg, 1.4 oz | 140 | 1.5 | 21 |
| Moist Supreme: Per ¹⁄₁₀ Pkg, Dry Mix Only | | | |
| Classic White/Yellow, 1.5 oz | 160 | 1.5 | 35 |
| Devils Food, Regular, 1.5 oz | 150 | 2 | 34 |

## Cake Frostings

**Betty Crocker:**
Rich & Creamy,

| | C | F | Cb |
|---|---|---|---|
| average all flavors, 2 Tbsp, 1.2 oz | 140 | 6 | 23 |
| Whipped, av. all flavors., 2 T., 0.9 oz | 100 | 4.5 | 15 |
| **Cool Whip**, Original, 2 Tbsp, 0.3 oz | 25 | 1.5 | 2 |

**Duncan Hines:**

| | C | F | Cb |
|---|---|---|---|
| Creamy Homestyle, av. all flav., 2T. | 140 | 6 | 23 |
| Whipped, av. all flavors, 3 Tbsp | 150 | 7 | 21 |

**Pillsbury:** *Per 2 Tbsp*
**Creamy Supreme:**

| | C | F | Cb |
|---|---|---|---|
| Choc Fudge; Milk Choc., | | | |
| 1.2 oz | 130 | 6 | 20 |
| Classic White; Vanilla, 1.2 oz | 140 | 5 | 22 |
| **Fluffy**, av. all flavors, 2 Tbsp, 0.8 oz | 100 | 5 | 14 |
| **Funfetti**, av. all flavors, 2 Tbsp,1.2 oz | 140 | 5 | 23 |
| **Sugar Free**, Chocolate Fudge | 100 | 6 | 16 |

## Quick Guide | C | F | Cb

### Donuts
*Average All Brands*

| | | C | F | Cb |
|---|---|---|---|---|
| **Cake:** Plain, 1.8 oz | | 205 | 12 | 23 |
| Chocolate Iced, 2 oz | | 255 | 14 | 29 |
| Sugared, 0.8 oz | | 205 | 10 | 29 |
| **Non-Cake,** Glazed, 2 oz | | 225 | 11 | 29 |

### Croissant-Donuts
**(Includes Cronuts/Frissants)**
*Average all Brands*

| | C | F | Cb |
|---|---|---|---|
| Cream-filled, 3.5 oz | 430 | 26 | 45 |
| Custard-filled, 3.5 oz | 360 | 19 | 45 |

**Extra Listings** ~ *See CalorieKing.com*

*(Cronut is a trademark of Dominique Ansel Bakery, New York)*

## Donuts ~ Brands

**Albertson's:**
**Donut Holes:**

| | C | F | Cb |
|---|---|---|---|
| Glazed Old Fashioned (4) | 240 | 12 | 31 |
| Powdered Sugar (4) | 210 | 12 | 24 |
| **Gem Donuts:** Plain Cake (3) | 190 | 12 | 20 |
| Cinnamon Sugar (3) | 240 | 15 | 23 |
| Glazed (1) | 140 | 6 | 21 |

**Bon Appetit:**
**Mini Donuts:**

| | C | F | Cb |
|---|---|---|---|
| Chocolate (4) | 270 | 16 | 29 |
| Crumb (4) | 240 | 12 | 32 |
| Powdered (4) | 250 | 12 | 34 |

**Dunkin' Donuts:**

| | C | F | Cb |
|---|---|---|---|
| Apple Crumb | 490 | 18 | 80 |
| Apple N' Spice | 270 | 14 | 32 |
| Barvarian Kreme | 270 | 15 | 31 |
| Blueberry Cake | 340 | 17 | 44 |
| Blueberry Crumb | 500 | 18 | 84 |
| Boston Scream | 310 | 16 | 39 |
| Chocolate Frosted Cake | 370 | 23 | 45 |
| Chocolate Glazed Cake | 370 | 24 | 35 |
| Chocolate Peanut Butter Kreme | 360 | 19 | 43 |
| Glazed Cake | 360 | 22 | 44 |
| Jelly Filled | 270 | 14 | 32 |
| Powdered Cake | 340 | 22 | 38 |
| Vanilla Kreme Filled | 380 | 23 | 42 |

**Extra Listings** ~ *See Fast Food Section*

## Donuts ~ Brands (Cont) | C | F | Cb

**Entenmann's:**
**8 Pack:** *Per Donut*

| | C | F | Cb |
|---|---|---|---|
| Chocolate Lovers, 2 oz | 300 | 20 | 31 |
| Crumb, 2 oz | 250 | 12 | 36 |
| Frosted Devil's, 2.4 oz | 310 | 18 | 36 |
| Rich Frosted, 2 oz | 300 | 20 | 30 |
| Strawberry Crumb Topped | 220 | 10 | 33 |

**Pop'ems:**

| | C | F | Cb |
|---|---|---|---|
| Frosted (4), 2 oz | 320 | 23 | 28 |
| Powdered (4), 2 oz | 270 | 16 | 30 |

**Great Value** *(Walmart):*

| | C | F | Cb |
|---|---|---|---|
| **Minis:** Chocolate Frosted (4) | 280 | 16 | 32 |
| Powdered (4) | 210 | 10 | 30 |

**Hostess:**

| | C | F | Cb |
|---|---|---|---|
| **Mini Donettes:** Crumb, 6-pack, 4 oz | 430 | 18 | 63 |
| Frosted, 6-pack, 3 oz | 360 | 22 | 38 |
| Powdered, 6-pack, 3 oz | 340 | 17 | 43 |

**Krispy Kreme:**

| | C | F | Cb |
|---|---|---|---|
| Apple Fritter, 3.5 oz | 390 | 20 | 50 |
| Baseball Donut, 2.2 oz | 280 | 15 | 34 |
| Chocolate: Iced Cake, 2.2 oz | 240 | 12 | 32 |
| Iced Custard Filled, 3.5 oz | 350 | 22 | 35 |
| Iced Glazed Cruller, 2.5 oz | 300 | 18 | 34 |
| Iced Glazed, 2.3 | 240 | 12 | 32 |
| Iced Kreme Filled, 3 oz | 340 | 17 | 42 |
| Iced Glazed w/ Sprinkles, 2.3 oz | 250 | 12 | 34 |
| Cinnamon Twist, 2 oz | 230 | 2 | 30 |
| Glazed Cruller, 2 oz | 250 | 17 | 23 |
| Glazed Doughnut Holes: | | | |
| Original (4) | 200 | 9 | 27 |
| Blueberry (4) | 180 | 10 | 22 |
| Chocolate Cake (4) | 180 | 10 | 21 |
| Glazed Kreme Filled, 3 oz | 370 | 23 | 38 |
| Maple Iced Glazed, 2.3 oz | 230 | 11 | 31 |
| New York Cheesecake, 3.3 oz | 400 | 26 | 37 |
| Original Glazed, 1.7 oz | 190 | 11 | 21 |
| Powdered Cake, 2.3 oz | 260 | 16 | 26 |
| Traditional Cake, 2 oz | 230 | 15 | 20 |

**Little Debbie,**

| | C | F | Cb |
|---|---|---|---|
| Donut Sticks (2), 2.8 oz | 360 | 20 | 43 |

**Tastykake:**

| | C | F | Cb |
|---|---|---|---|
| Cinnamon, 1.8 oz | 210 | 11 | 26 |
| Mini: Coated, 3 oz | 380 | 22 | 42 |
| Powdered Sugar (6), 2.5 oz | 280 | 13 | 37 |

## Quick Guide    **C**   **F**   **Cb**

### Muffins: Ready-To-Eat
*Average All Brands*

| | C | F | Cb |
|---|---|---|---|
| Small, 1 oz | 90 | 3.5 | 14 |
| Medium, 2 oz | 185 | 6.5 | 28 |
| Large, 3 oz | 275 | 10 | 42 |
| Extra Large, 4 oz | 365 | 13 | 57 |
| Giant, 6 oz | 550 | 20 | 84 |
| Super Size, 8 oz | 730 | 27 | 112 |

## Muffins Ready-To-Eat ~ Brands

| | C | F | Cb |
|---|---|---|---|
| **Albertsons:** | | | |
| **Minis:** Banana Nut (2) | 200 | 12 | 20 |
| Blueberry (2) | 180 | 10 | 21 |
| Honey Raisin Bran (2) | 170 | 7 | 24 |
| **Entenmann's,** | | | |
| Blueberry; Choc. Chip; Corn (1) | 190 | 9 | 26 |
| **Great Value** *(Walmart):* | | | |
| Double Banana (1), 4 oz | 360 | 16 | 52 |
| Double Blueberry (1), 4 oz | 430 | 16 | 65 |
| Triple Chocolate (1), 4 oz | 420 | 18 | 61 |
| **Little Debbie:** Banana Nut (1), 1.9 oz | 210 | 9 | 30 |
| Blueberry (1), 1.9 oz | 190 | 8 | 27 |
| Chocolate Chip (1), 1.9 oz | 210 | 9 | 28 |
| **My Favorite Muffin:** *Per 6 oz Muffin* | | | |
| Banana Nut | 585 | 33 | 63 |
| Blueberry | 505 | 24 | 66 |
| Boston Cream Pie | 530 | 21 | 78 |
| Chocolate Chip | 635 | 33 | 81 |
| Lemon Poppyseed | 605 | 30 | 75 |
| **Otis Spunkmeyer:** | | | |
| Banana Nut, 4oz | 440 | 22 | 58 |
| Chocolate Chip, 4 oz | 460 | 24 | 58 |
| Wild Blueberry, 4 oz | 400 | 16 | 58 |
| **Starbucks** ~ *See Fast-Foods Section* | | | |
| **Trader Joe's:** *Per Muffin* | | | |
| Apple Cranberry, 4.8 oz | 220 | 5 | 38 |
| Banana Chocolate Chip, 4 oz | 400 | 18 | 57 |
| Carrot, 4 oz | 320 | 11 | 52 |
| Triple Berry, 4 oz | 310 | 11 | 49 |
| **Vitalicious:** | | | |
| **VitaMuffins:** Average all, 2 oz | 100 | 1 | 24 |
| Large, average all varieties., 4 oz | 200 | 2 | 50 |
| Sugar-Free, Banana Nut, 2 oz | 90 | 2.5 | 21 |
| **VitaTops:** Average all varieties, 2 oz | 100 | 1.5 | 25 |
| Sugar free, av. all varieties, 2 oz | 90 | 2.5 | 22 |
| **Weight Watchers,** | | | |
| Blueb.; Double Choc, av., 2.5 oz | 185 | 2.5 | 42 |

## Muffin Mixes    **C**   **F**   **Cb**
*Per Muffin, Prepared*

| | C | F | Cb |
|---|---|---|---|
| **Betty Crocker:** Banana Nut | 170 | 8 | 22 |
| Cinnamon Streusel | 180 | 8 | 26 |
| Wild Blueberry | 160 | 6.5 | 24 |
| Pouch Mix: | | | |
| Banana Nut | 120 | 3 | 22 |
| Blueberry; Triple Berry | 120 | 2.5 | 23 |
| Chocolate Chip | 130 | 3.5 | 22 |
| **Fiber One,** | | | |
| Apple Cinnamon; Blueberry, av. | 160 | 6 | 29 |
| **Krusteaz:** | | | |
| Choc Chunk | 260 | 13 | 33 |
| Lemon Poppyseed | 170 | 4 | 31 |
| Oat Bran | 180 | 4.5 | 32 |
| **Trader Joe's,** Triple Berry | 150 | 2 | 28 |

## Sweet Rolls & Buns

Note: It is best to weigh for accuracy as actual weight can be 10-50% higher than label weight·
*Per Sweet Roll or Bun Unless Indicated*

| | C | F | Cb |
|---|---|---|---|
| **Bimbo,** Bimbolete, 2.2 oz | 250 | 10 | 36 |
| **Bon Appetit,** | | | |
| Cinnamon Roll, 2.5 oz | 230 | 8 | 34 |
| **Cinnabon:** Classic | 880 | 36 | 127 |
| Caramel Pecanbon | 1080 | 51 | 146 |
| **Cloverhill Bakery,** | | | |
| Jumbo Honey Bun, 4.8 oz | 600 | 35 | 64 |
| **Entenmann's,** Cinn. Swirl Bun, 3 oz | 320 | 14 | 44 |
| **Little Debbie:** | | | |
| Honey Bun: 2.3 oz | 280 | 16 | 32 |
| 4 oz | 480 | 26 | 56 |
| With Chocolate Icing, 2 oz | 310 | 20 | 29 |
| With White Icing, 4 oz | 490 | 25 | 60 |
| Pecan Spinwheels, 1 oz | 100 | 3.5 | 17 |
| **McDonald's,** Cinnamon Melts, 4 oz | 460 | 19 | 66 |
| **Pillsbury:** | | | |
| **Sweet Rolls,** Refrigerated: *Per Roll Unless Indicated* | | | |
| Cinnamon, w/ Icing, all varieties | 140 | 5 | 23 |
| Reduced Fat | 130 | 3.5 | 24 |
| Orange Flavored, with Icing, 1.7 oz | 160 | 6 | 26 |
| Twists, Flaky Cinnamon, with Icing | 160 | 7 | 23 |
| **Grands,** Refrigerated: *Per Roll* | | | |
| Cinnabon: Cinnamon Roll, with Cream Cheese Icing | 360 | 17 | 48 |
| Caramel Rolls, with Icing, 3.5 oz | 310 | 9 | 53 |
| Flaky Supreme Cinnamon Roll, with Icing, 3.5 oz | 360 | 17 | 48 |
| Flaky Caramel Roll, w/ Icing, 1.6 oz | 170 | 8 | 22 |
| **7-Eleven:** Iced Honey Bun, 6 oz | 820 | 58 | 68 |
| Glazed Honey Bun, 5 oz | 620 | 35 | 70 |
| **Sara Lee,** Cinnamon Roll, 2.4 oz | 260 | 12 | 33 |

## Quick Guide

| | C | F | Cb |
|---|---|---|---|
| **Chocolate:** | | | |
| *Average All Brands* | | | |
| **Milk Chocolate**, regular: | | | |
| **Plain/Nuts/Fruit,** average, 1 oz | 150 | 9 | 17 |
| 1.5oz Bar | 230 | 13 | 25 |
| 2 oz Bar | 305 | 17 | 34 |
| 4 oz Block | 610 | 34 | 68 |
| 8 oz Block | 1220 | 68 | 136 |
| 1 Pound, 16 oz | 2440 | 136 | 272 |
| **Dark/White Chocolate:** 1 oz | 155 | 9 | 17 |
| *Hershey's,* Sugar Free, 5 pieces | 110 | 13 | 24 |
| **Milk Chocolate-Coated:** | | | |
| Almonds, 5-6, 1 oz | 150 | 10 | 15 |
| Cherry Cordial Centers, 2 pcs, 1 oz | 145 | 6 | 21 |
| Clusters, Nut, 3 pieces, 1.2 oz | 210 | 14 | 20 |
| Coffee Beans, 1.4 oz | 220 | 13 | 22 |
| Macadamias, 10 pieces, 1.4 oz | 220 | 16 | 21 |
| Mints, 1 medium, 0.5 oz | 55 | 1 | 11 |
| Nougat & Caramel, 1 oz | 150 | 9 | 15 |
| Peanuts, 12 medium, 1 oz | 145 | 10 | 14 |
| Raisins, 28 medium, 1 oz | 110 | 4 | 19 |
| **Baking Chocolate:** | | | |
| *Baker's:* Bittersweet, 1 oz | 140 | 12 | 14 |
| Semi-sweet, 1 oz | 140 | 9 | 16 |
| *Nestle,* Chips: Dark, 1 Tbsp. 0.5 oz | 70 | 5 | 3 |
| Semi-Sweet, 1 Tbsp. 0.5oz | 70 | 4 | 9 |
| Unsweetened, 1 oz | 140 | 14 | 8 |
| **Carob**, Plain, 1 oz | 155 | 9 | 16 |

## Candy ~ Brands & Generic

*Per Piece/Serving*

| | C | F | Cb |
|---|---|---|---|
| **3 Musketeers:** Orig., 1 bar, 1.9 oz | 240 | 7 | 42 |
| 2 To Go, 1.7 oz Bar | 200 | 6 | 36 |
| Fun Size, 3 bars, 1.6 oz | 190 | 6 | 34 |
| Minis, 7 pieces, 1.4 oz | 170 | 5 | 32 |
| **100 Grand:** 1.5 oz bar | 190 | 8 | 30 |
| Snack Size (1), 0.8 oz | 95 | 4 | 15 |
| Super Size, 2.8 oz | 360 | 14 | 58 |
| **Abba Zabba,** 2 oz bar | 250 | 5 | 48 |
| **After Dinner Mints,** 1 small | 25 | 1.5 | 3 |
| **After Eight Mint,** each | 35 | 1.5 | 4 |
| **Airhead,** 1 bar, 0.5 oz | 60 | 1 | 14 |
| **Almond Joy:** 2 bars, 1.6 oz | 220 | 13 | 26 |
| King Size, 4 bars, 3.2 oz | 440 | 26 | 53 |
| Snack Size, 0.6 oz bar | 80 | 4.5 | 10 |
| Pieces (46), 1.4 oz | 200 | 10 | 27 |

*Per Piece/Serving*

| | C | F | Cb |
|---|---|---|---|
| **Almond Roca,** 3 pieces, 1.3 oz | 200 | 15 | 17 |
| **Almond:** Sugar-coated (15), 1.4 oz | 190 | 7 | 27 |
| *Jordan,* 15 pieces, 1.4 oz | 180 | 8 | 28 |
| **Almond Clusters:** | | | |
| *True North,* 1 oz | 170 | 12 | 9 |
| *Trader Joe's,* 1.2 oz | 190 | 14 | 13 |
| **Altoids,** 3 pieces | 10 | 0 | 2 |
| **Andes,** Thins (8), av. all var., 1.4 oz | 205 | 13 | 22 |
| **Anthon Berg:** | | | |
| Creamy Mint (4), 1.4 oz | 180 | 6 | 31 |
| Marzipan with Plum, in Madeira | 120 | 6 | 14 |
| **Atomic Fireball,** 1 piece, 0.3 oz | 35 | 0 | 9 |
| **Baby Ruth:** King Size, 3.5 oz bar | 500 | 24 | 66 |
| 2 oz bar | 280 | 14 | 39 |
| Fun size, 2 bars | 170 | 8 | 24 |
| Minis, 4 bars | 210 | 11 | 28 |
| **Baci** (Perugina), | | | |
| 1 piece, 0.5 oz | 75 | 6 | 7 |
| **Baskin-Robbins:** Sugar Candy, 3 pcs | 60 | 1 | 12 |
| Sugar Free, 4 pieces, average, 0.6 oz | 40 | 1 | 16 |
| *Carbs include 16g sugar alcohol* | | | |
| **Big Hunk,** 2 oz Bar | 230 | 3 | 47 |
| **Bit-O-Honey:** | | | |
| 1.7 oz bar | 180 | 3.5 | 39 |
| Chews, 6 pieces, 1.4 oz | 150 | 3 | 32 |
| **Bliss** (Hershey's): | | | |
| Milk/Dark Choc./Caramel, 6 pieces | 120 | 14 | 25 |
| Meltaway Centers: | | | |
| Milk Chocolate, 6 pieces | 220 | 15 | 24 |
| Raspberry, 6 pieces | 220 | 14 | 24 |
| **Blow Pops,** each, 0.6 oz | 60 | 0 | 17 |
| **Bon Bons,** 3 pieces | 65 | 0 | 15 |
| **Boston Baked Beans,** (11), 0.5 oz | 70 | 2 | 11 |
| **Brach's:** | | | |
| Almond Supremes (10) | 200 | 14 | 20 |
| Bridge Mix (15), 1.4 oz | 190 | 10 | 26 |
| Double Dippers (15), 1.4 oz | 210 | 14 | 22 |
| Gummi Bears (14), 1.4 oz | 130 | 0 | 30 |
| Lemon Drops, Sugar Free, 4 pieces | 35 | 0 | 17 |
| *Carbs include 17g Sugar Alcohol* | | | |
| Mandarin/Orange Slices (3), 1.6 oz | 150 | 0 | 37 |
| Maple Nut Goodies (8), 1.5 oz | 190 | 9 | 27 |
| Milk Maid Crmls (4), 1.3 oz | 150 | 4 | 25 |
| Peanut Cluster (3), 1.4 oz | 210 | 15 | 20 |
| **Breath Savers,** all varieties, each | 5 | 0 | 2 |
| **Bubble Gum** ~ *See Page 75* | | | |
| **Bulls Eyes,** 3 pieces, 1.2 oz | 130 | 3 | 23 |
| **Buncha Crunch:** ⅓ cup, 1.4 oz | 180 | 9 | 25 |
| Movie Box, 3.2 oz | 450 | 20 | 65 |
| **Burnt Peanuts**, (31), 1.4 oz | 170 | 6 | 29 |

## Candy ~ Brands & Generic (Cont)

*Per Piece/Serving*

| | C | F | Cb |
|---|---|---|---|
| **Butterfinger:** 2 oz bar | 270 | 11 | 43 |
| King Size (3 bars), 3.5 oz | 480 | 18 | 75 |
| Fun Size, (1), 0.8 oz | 100 | 4 | 15 |
| Giant, (Pieces in Chocolate), | | | |
| ¼ bar, 1 oz | 150 | 8 | 21 |
| Miniatures: | | | |
| 1 piece, 0.4 oz | 45 | 2 | 8 |
| 4 pieces, 1.4 oz | 180 | 8 | 32 |
| Snack Pack, 4 pcs, 1.4 oz | 180 | 7 | 29 |
| Crisp Bar: Original, 2 oz bar | 270 | 11 | 43 |
| King Size, 3 pieces, 2 oz | 310 | 17 | 38 |
| Minis, 2 bars, 1.4 oz | 210 | 11 | 25 |
| Snackerz: | | | |
| Single, 1.3 oz | 170 | 8 | 23 |
| Fun Size, 2 pcs, 1.2 oz | 150 | 7 | 21 |
| King Size, 10 pcs, 1.4 oz | 190 | 8 | 25 |
| **Butter Mints,** 7 pieces, 0.5 oz | 50 | 0 | 12 |
| **Butterscotch:** 3 pieces | 60 | 0 | 15 |
| Discs (*Walgreens*), 3 pieces, 0.6 oz | 70 | 0 | 17 |
| **Cadbury:** Caramello Bar, 1.6 oz | 220 | 10 | 29 |
| Caramel Egg, 1.2 oz | 170 | 8 | 22 |
| Dairy Milk Bar, 7 pieces, 1.4 oz | 200 | 11 | 23 |
| Mini Eggs (Candy), 12 pcs, 1.4 oz | 190 | 8 | 28 |
| **Candy Apple,** medium, 6.5 oz | 280 | 0 | 60 |
| **Candy Cane,** medium, 5", 0.5 oz | 40 | 0 | 14 |
| **Candy Corn,** 20 pieces, 1.4 oz | 150 | 0 | 38 |
| **Candy Jar Mix** (*Jewel*), 3 pcs, 0.6 oz | 60 | 0 | 14 |
| **Candy Necklace** (*Smarties*), (1), 0.8 oz | 90 | 0.5 | 20 |
| **Caramels:** Each, 0.4 oz | 40 | 1 | 8 |
| Chocolate, each, 0.3 oz | 25 | 0.3 | 6 |
| Creams (3), 1.3 oz | 130 | 3 | 23 |
| **Caramel Popcorn,** ⅔ cup | 150 | 6 | 23 |
| **Cella's,** | | | |
| Milk Choc. Cherries, 3 pieces, 1.5 oz | 160 | 6 | 27 |
| **Certs,** Breath Mints, 1 piece | 5 | 0 | 2 |
| **Charleston Chew:** | | | |
| Chocolate Bar (1), 1.4 oz | 160 | 4.5 | 30 |
| Mini Bars, 13 pieces | 190 | 6 | 34 |
| **Charms:** Blow Pop | 60 | 0 | 17 |
| Flat Pop, 0.5 oz | 50 | 0 | 14 |
| **Chew-ets,** Peanut Chews, | | | |
| Original (4), 1.6 oz | 230 | 12 | 29 |
| **Chewz,** 1 roll, 1 oz | 120 | 1 | 28 |
| **Chick O Stick,** 2 oz | 240 | 9 | 42 |

*Per Piece/Serving*

| | C | F | Cb |
|---|---|---|---|
| **Chunky Bar** (*Nestlé*), | | | |
| King Size, 2.5 oz | 340 | 19 | 44 |
| **Chupa Chups,** 1 Pop | 50 | 0 | 12 |
| **Cinn. Buttons** (*Walgreens*), 3 pieces | 60 | 0 | 16 |
| **Cinnamon Disks** (*Walmart*), 3 pieces | 70 | 0 | 18 |
| **Circus Peanuts** (*Spangler*), | | | |
| 6 pieces, 1.3 oz | 165 | 0 | 41 |
| **CocoaVia,** Orig., 0.8 oz | 100 | 6 | 12 |
| **Coconut Stacks,** (8) | 320 | 16 | 46 |
| **Coffee Go,** Candy, (4) | 60 | 1 | 12 |
| **Conversation Hearts** (*Necco*): | | | |
| Small (40), 1.4 oz | 160 | 0 | 39 |
| 1 large | 10 | 0 | 3 |
| **Cookie Dough Bites,** 1.4 oz | 200 | 10 | 27 |
| **Cote d'Or:** Dark 86% Coca, 4 pcs | 270 | 22 | 14 |
| Dark, 70%, Orange, 3.5 oz | 575 | 46 | 34 |
| Dark, Raspberry, 3.5 oz | 580 | 46 | 34 |
| Milk, Intense, 3.5 oz | 575 | 40 | 45 |
| **Cotton Candy,** 1 oz | 110 | 0 | 28 |
| **Cough Drops ~** *See Page 75* | | | |
| **Cracker Jack,** ½ cup, 1 oz | 120 | 2 | 23 |
| **Creme Savers:** 3 pieces, 0.5 oz | 60 | 1 | 11 |
| Sugar-Free, 3 pieces | 30 | 1 | 8 |
| **Crisped Rice,** Choc Chip, 1 bar, 1 oz | 115 | 4 | 20 |
| **Crows,** 11 pieces, 1.4 oz | 130 | 0 | 33 |
| **Crunch Bar ~** *See Nestle* | | | |
| **Dots,** 11 dots, 1.4 oz | 130 | 0 | 33 |
| **Double Dip Stick,** 1 stick | 15 | 0.5 | 3 |
| **Dove:** | | | |
| Milk Choc: Singles Bar, 1.4 oz | 220 | 13 | 24 |
| Large Tablet Bar, 9 pieces, 1.5 oz | 230 | 13 | 25 |
| Choc. Covered Almonds, 13 pcs, 1.4 oz | 220 | 15 | 19 |
| Promises: Milk Choc., 1 piece, 0.3 oz | 45 | 2.5 | 5 |
| With Caramel, 1 piece, 0.3 oz | 40 | 2 | 5 |
| With Peanut Butter, 1 piece, 0.3 oz | 45 | 3 | 4 |
| Swirls, all varieties, 9 pieces 1.5 oz | 230 | 14 | 25 |
| Dark Choc: Singles Bar, 1.3 oz | 220 | 13 | 24 |
| Large Tablet Bar, 9 pieces, 1.5 oz | 220 | 14 | 25 |
| Choc. Covered. Almds, 13 pcs, 1.4 oz | 210 | 15 | 19 |
| Promises, Almond, 1 piece, 0.3 oz | 40 | 3 | 4 |
| Swirls, Raspberry, 9 pieces, 1.4 oz | 220 | 14 | 24 |
| Sugar Free, all varieties, 5 pcs, 1.4 oz | 195 | 15 | 21 |
| **Dum Dum Pops** (*Spangler*), 1 pop | 25 | 0 | 7 |
| **Drops** (*Hershey's*): | | | |
| Cookies 'n' Creme, 14 pieces, 1.5 oz | 210 | 11 | 26 |
| Milk Chocolate, 15 pieces, 1.4 oz | 200 | 12 | 25 |

## Candy ~ Brands & Generic (Cont)

| Per Piece/Serving | **C** | **F** | **Cb** |
|---|---|---|---|
| **English Toffee**, 1 piece, 0.4 oz | 70 | 4 | 6 |
| **5th Avenue:** 2 oz bar | 260 | 12 | 38 |
| King Size, 3.5 oz | 440 | 20 | 64 |
| **Fannie May:** | | | |
| Mint Meltaway (1) | 230 | 15 | 24 |
| Pixie (1), 1.5 oz | 210 | 12 | 24 |
| Trinidad (1), 1.5 oz | 200 | 12 | 23 |
| **Fast Break** (Reese's): 2 oz bar | 260 | 12 | 35 |
| 3.5 oz bar | 460 | 22 | 62 |
| **Ferrero Rocher:** 1 piece | 75 | 5 | 5 |
| 3 pieces, 1.3 oz | 220 | 16 | 16 |
| Rondnoir, 3 pieces, 1 oz | 180 | 13 | 14 |
| **Fifty 50 Snack Bars:** | | | |
| Milk Chocolate: 5 pieces, 1 oz | 135 | 11 | 14 |
| Almond, 5 pieces, 1 oz | 135 | 12 | 14 |
| Crunch Bar, 7 pcs, 1 oz | 140 | 12 | 16 |
| Dark Chocolate, 5 pieces, 1 oz | 120 | 11 | 15 |
| *Carb figures include 9-12g Sugar Alcohol* | | | |
| **Fluffy Stuff** (Charms), | | | |
| Cotton Candy, 1.4 oz | 150 | 0 | 40 |
| **Fondant:** Choc-coated, 1.2 oz | 125 | 3 | 27 |
| Mint, 1 oz | 105 | 0 | 25 |
| **Fran's:** | | | |
| Gold Bar, Almond (1) | 250 | 14 | 27 |
| GoldBite, Almond (1) | 120 | 7 | 13 |
| **Fruit Drops**, (1), ¼ oz | 20 | 0 | 4 |
| **Fruit Gems** (Sunkist), (4), 1.4 oz | 130 | 0 | 33 |
| **Fruit Leathers**, average, 0.5 oz | 50 | 0.5 | 12 |
| **Fruit Pastilles** (Rowntree), 1 roll | 185 | 0 | 45 |
| **Fruit Roll-Ups** (Betty Crocker/Sunkist), | | | |
| 1 roll, 0.5 oz | 50 | 1 | 12 |
| **Fruit Runts** (Walgreens), | | | |
| 12 pieces | 60 | 0 | 14 |
| **Fruit Flavored Shapes** (Betty Crocker), | | | |
| all varieties, 0.8 oz | 80 | 0 | 19 |
| **Fudge:** | | | |
| Chocolate; Mint, 1 oz | 130 | 8 | 14 |
| Peanut Butter & Choc., 1 oz | 130 | 8 | 13 |
| *Brevin's:* Cashew, 1 oz | 195 | 9 | 28 |
| Triple Decker, 1 oz | 165 | 7 | 25 |
| **Ghirardelli:** | | | |
| 3 oz Bars: Dark Chocolate, 4 squares | 220 | 17 | 23 |
| Filled, Peanut Butter, 4 squares | 250 | 17 | 22 |
| Intense Dark Bars, Ev'ng Dream, 3 pcs | 190 | 15 | 20 |
| Squares: | | | |
| Dark Chocolate (4), 1.5 oz | 210 | 16 | 23 |
| Milk & Caramel (3), 1.5 oz | 220 | 12 | 27 |
| Sea Salt Escape (4), 1.5 oz | 210 | 15 | 24 |

| Per Piece/Serving | **C** | **F** | **Cb** |
|---|---|---|---|
| **Godiva:** | | | |
| Bars: Milk/Dark, av., 1.5 oz | 230 | 14 | 26 |
| Extra Dark: 75%, 1.5 oz | 230 | 17 | 18 |
| 85%, 1.4 oz | 260 | 21 | 14 |
| Chocoiste: | | | |
| Dark Chocolate Cherries (12) | 190 | 7 | 30 |
| Milk Chocolate Cashews (14) | 230 | 15 | 19 |
| Hearts: Dark Ganache (4) | 200 | 12 | 23 |
| Milk Praline (4) | 220 | 13 | 23 |
| **Go Lightly:** | | | |
| Assorted Toffee, 5 pieces, 1 oz | 85 | 2 | 24 |
| Fruit Chews, 5 pieces, 1 oz | 95 | 2 | 26 |
| Hard Candy, Assorted (4), 0.5 oz | 45 | 0 | 15 |
| *Carb figures include 15-25g sugar alcohol* | | | |
| **Goobers Peanuts,** 1 package, 1.4 oz | 200 | 13 | 21 |
| **Good & Plenty** (Hershey's), (33), 1.4 oz | 140 | 0 | 35 |
| **GooGoo Clusters,** 1 piece, 1.8 oz | 240 | 12 | 30 |
| **Gum** ~ See Page 75 | | | |
| **Gum Drops:** 1 small, 0.1 oz | 15 | 0 | 3 |
| 5 pieces, 0.5 oz | 75 | 0 | 15 |
| **Gummi** (Shur Fine): | | | |
| Bears (15 ), 1.4 oz | 130 | 0 | 29 |
| Chewy Sweet Tarts (4) | 160 | 0 | 36 |
| Worms (9), 1.5 oz | 140 | 0 | 31 |
| **Guylian:** | | | |
| Bars: Dark Chocolate (3), 1 oz | 150 | 12 | 11 |
| Milk Choc. with Hazelnuts (3),1 oz | 170 | 11 | 15 |
| No Sugar Added Bars: | | | |
| Milk Chocolate, 3 squares | 150 | 11 | 16 |
| 54% Cocoa, Dark Choc., 3 squares | 140 | 11 | 16 |
| Seashells: | | | |
| Bar, 1.4 oz | 210 | 13 | 21 |
| Boxed, Originals (1), 0.4 oz | 60 | 4 | 6 |
| Truffles (1), 0.4 oz | 70 | 5.5 | 5 |
| **Heath:** Original (1), 1.4 oz | 210 | 13 | 24 |
| King Size, 2.8 oz | 410 | 22 | 49 |
| Snack Size, 3 pieces, 1.5 oz | 230 | 14 | 27 |
| **Hershey's:** | | | |
| **Cookies 'n' Creme**, 1.6 oz Bar | 220 | 12 | 26 |
| **Milk Chocolate:** | | | |
| Bars: 1.6 oz | 210 | 13 | 26 |
| With Almonds, 1 bar, 1.4 oz | 210 | 14 | 21 |
| King Size, 1 Bar, 2.5 oz | 370 | 22 | 44 |
| Kisses, 9 pieces, av., 1.4 oz | 200 | 12 | 25 |
| Nuggets: 4 pieces, 1.4 oz | 200 | 13 | 20 |
| W/ Toffee & Alm., 4 pcs, 1.3 oz | 200 | 13 | 21 |
| Sugar Free Choc., 5 pieces, 1.4 oz | 160 | 13 | 24 |
| **Extra Dark Choc.**, 4 pieces, 1.4 oz | 180 | 14 | 21 |
| **Simple Pleasures**, 6 pieces, av. | 180 | 8 | 29 |
| **Special Dark Choc.**, 1.5 oz bar | 190 | 12 | 25 |

## Candy ~ Brands & Generic (Cont)

*Per Piece/Serving*   **C** **F** **Cb**

**Hershey's,** (Cont):

**Pot of Gold Chocolate Asstd:**

| | C | F | Cb |
|---|---|---|---|
| Carmel, 4 pieces, 1.4 oz | 190 | 10 | 26 |
| Average other var., 4 pieces, 1.4 oz | 210 | 12 | 24 |

**Candy-Coated Eggs:**

| | C | F | Cb |
|---|---|---|---|
| Milk Chocolate: (8) 1.2 oz | 170 | 8 | 27 |
| With Almonds (8) 1.2 oz | 200 | 12 | 18 |
| **Honeycomb:** Plain, 1 oz | 115 | 0 | 27 |
| Choc-coated, 2 pieces | 180 | 7 | 31 |

**Hot Tamales,**

| | C | F | Cb |
|---|---|---|---|
| 20 pieces, 1.4 oz | 150 | 0 | 36 |

**Hugs** ~ *See Kisses*

| | C | F | Cb |
|---|---|---|---|
| **Jawbreakers** *(Sathers)*, (15), 0.6 oz | 60 | 0 | 16 |
| **Jells** *(Joyva)*, Raspb., 3 pieces, 1.6 oz | 160 | 0 | 38 |

**Jelly Beans,** average all brands

| | C | F | Cb |
|---|---|---|---|
| Small Size *(Jelly Belly)*: 1 bean | 5 | 0 | 1 |
| 12 beans, 0.5 oz | 50 | 0 | 13 |
| Regular Size: 1 bean | 10 | 0 | 2 |
| 10 beans, 1 oz | 105 | 0 | 26 |
| Large Size: 1 bean | 15 | 0 | 38 |
| 10 beans, 1.5 oz | 150 | 0 | 38 |

**Sugar Free,**

| | C | F | Cb |
|---|---|---|---|
| average all brands, 25 beans, 1 oz | 60 | 0 | 26 |

*Carb figures include 26g sugar alcohol*

**Jelly Belly:** 

| | C | F | Cb |
|---|---|---|---|
| 25 beans, 1 oz | 105 | 0 | 26 |
| 3.5 oz package | 360 | 0 | 90 |

Sugar Free,

| | C | F | Cb |
|---|---|---|---|
| 25 beans, 1 oz | 60 | 0 | 26 |

*Carb figures include 26 sugar alcohol*

Chocolate Dips:

| | C | F | Cb |
|---|---|---|---|
| All flavors: 1 bean | 4 | 0 | 1 |
| 10 beans | 40 | 1 | 8 |
| 2.8 oz bag | 300 | 8 | 62 |
| **Jelly Rings** *(Jewel)*, 5 pieces, 1.4 oz | 110 | 0 | 26 |

**Jolly Rancher:**

| | C | F | Cb |
|---|---|---|---|
| Bites: Soft, 15 pieces | 150 | 1.5 | 32 |
| Sours, 16 pieces | 130 | 0 | 34 |
| Crunch 'N Chew, 1 oz pkg | 160 | 0.5 | 40 |
| Filled Fruity Bites, 22 pieces | 140 | 1 | 31 |
| Gummies, 9 pieces | 120 | 0 | 28 |
| Hard Candy, 3 pieces | 70 | 0 | 17 |
| Jelly Beans/Sours, 1.4 oz | 140 | 0 | 36 |
| Lollipops (1), 0.55 oz | 60 | 0 | 15 |
| **Jujubes,** all varieties (52), 1.4 oz | 110 | 0 | 28 |
| **Juju Bears,** 5 pieces | 130 | 0 | 34 |
| **Juju Mix** *(Sathers)*, 11 pieces, 1.5 oz | 150 | 0 | 36 |
| **Jujyfruits,** 16 pieces, 1.4 oz | 120 | 0 | 32 |
| **Junior Caramels:** 13 pieces, 1.5 oz | 190 | 6 | 33 |
| Mini, 2 boxes, 1 oz | 130 | 4 | 23 |

*Per Piece/Serving*   **C** **F** **Cb**

| | C | F | Cb |
|---|---|---|---|
| **Junior Mints:** 1.8 oz | 220 | 4 | 45 |
| 16 pieces, 1.4 oz | 170 | 3 | 35 |

**Justin's,** Peanut Butter Cups,

| | C | F | Cb |
|---|---|---|---|
| Milk Choc, 2 cups, 1.4 oz pkg | 200 | 14 | 18 |

**Kisses** *(Hershey's)*:

| | C | F | Cb |
|---|---|---|---|
| Air Delights (11), 1.4 oz | 200 | 12 | 24 |
| Cookies 'n' Creme (9), 1.5 oz | 220 | 12 | 26 |
| Hugs (9), 1.4 oz | 210 | 12 | 24 |
| Milk Chocolate: (1), 0.16 oz | 25 | 1.5 | 3 |
| (9), 1.4oz | 200 | 12 | 25 |
| With Almonds (9), 1.4 oz | 200 | 13 | 22 |
| Caramel Filled (9), 1.5 oz | 190 | 9 | 27 |
| Special Dark (9), 1.4 oz | 180 | 12 | 25 |

**Kit Kat** *(Nestle)*:

**Milk Chocolate:**

| | C | F | Cb |
|---|---|---|---|
| 4 piece bar, 1.5 oz | 210 | 11 | 28 |
| Extra Crispy, 1.6 oz bar | 220 | 12 | 29 |
| King Size, 8 pcs, 3 oz bar | 420 | 22 | 56 |
| Minis, 5 pieces | 210 | 11 | 28 |
| Snack Size, 6 pcs, 1.5 oz | 210 | 11 | 27 |
| **White Chocolate**, 4 pieces, 1.5 oz | 220 | 12 | 26 |
| **Peanut Bar** *(Lance)*, 2.2 oz package | 340 | 19 | 29 |
| **Lemon Drops:** (4), 0.6 oz | 60 | 0 | 16 |
| *Walgreens*, Sugar Free (3), 0.6 oz | 50 | 0 | 17 |
| **Lemonhead,** (26), 1.4 oz | 140 | 0 | 36 |

**Licorice:**

| | C | F | Cb |
|---|---|---|---|
| Avaerage all varieties, 1oz | 100 | 0 | 25 |
| Chews *(Panda)*, (1) | 10 | 0 | 3 |
| Tid Bits (1) | 10 | 0 | 2 |
| Twists: Black/Red, av., 1 pc | 35 | 0 | 8 |
| Sugar Free, 1 piece | 15 | 0 | 2.5 |

**American Licorice Co.:**

| | C | F | Cb |
|---|---|---|---|
| Natural Vines: Black (9), 1.4 oz | 140 | 1 | 33 |
| Strawberry (9), 1.4 oz | 150 | 1 | 34 |
| Red Vines (4), 1.4 oz | 140 | 0 | 34 |
| Sip-n-Chew, 1 oz package | 100 | 1 | 23 |
| Snaps (31), 1.4 oz | 140 | 0.5 | 33 |
| Sour Punch (6), 1.4 oz | 150 | 0.5 | 34 |
| Super Ropes (1), 2 oz | 200 | 0 | 46 |
| **Lifesavers:** Large size, 1 candy | 15 | 0 | 3 |
| Regular: All flavors, 1 candy | 10 | 0 | 3 |
| 1 Roll (14 candies), 1.2 oz | 140 | 0 | 35 |
| Creme Savers: 3 pieces, 0.5 oz | 60 | 1 | 11 |
| Sugar Free (4) | 45 | 1.5 | 13 |
| Pep-o-mint (3), 0.2 oz | 20 | 0 | 5 |
| Fruit Splosion (10), 1.4 oz | 130 | 0 | 31 |

Sugar-Free Delites,

| | C | F | Cb |
|---|---|---|---|
| Orchard Fruits; Summer Blend (1) | 5 | 0 | 2 |
| Butter Toffee; European Collection | 10 | 1 | 3 |

## Candy ~ Brands & Generic (Cont)

| Per Piece/Serving | C | F | Cb |
|---|---|---|---|
| **Lik-m-aid** (Nestle), Fun Dip, 1 package | 50 | 0 | 13 |
| **Lindt:** Lindor Truffles (1), average | 75 | 6 | 5 |
| Swiss Milk Chocolate Bars: | | | |
| 70% Cocoa, 4 pieces | 220 | 17 | 13 |
| Classic, with Hazelnuts, 10 pieces | 230 | 16 | 20 |
| Raspberry filled, 7 pieces | 200 | 10 | 25 |
| Dark Choc. Truffles, | | | |
| with filling, 7 pieces | 240 | 18 | 18 |
| **Lollipops:** Mini, 0.3 oz | 25 | 0 | 6 |
| Small, 0.5 oz | 50 | 0 | 12 |
| Medium, 1 oz | 100 | 0 | 25 |
| Giant (4" diam), 7 oz | 790 | 0 | 198 |
| **M & M's:** | | | |
| Dark Chocolate: 1.5 oz package | 210 | 10 | 29 |
| Peanuts, 1.5 oz | 220 | 12 | 25 |
| Milk Chocolate: 28 piece, 1 oz | 145 | 6.5 | 21 |
| 1.5 oz package | 210 | 9 | 30 |
| 1.7 oz package | 240 | 10 | 34 |
| Almond Choc., 1.5 oz | 220 | 12 | 25 |
| Minis, 1 tube, 1 oz | 150 | 7 | 21 |
| Peanut: 28 pieces, 1 oz | 155 | 8 | 17 |
| 1.75 oz pkg | 250 | 13 | 30 |
| Peanut Butter, 1.6 oz package | 240 | 14 | 26 |
| Premiums: Chocolate Trio, 1.5 oz | 230 | 14 | 25 |
| Mint Thrills, 1.5 oz | 240 | 14 | 25 |
| Pretzels, ½ pkg, 1.4 oz | 180 | 6 | 29 |
| Snack Mix, av. all var., ⅓ cup, 1.5 oz | 200 | 9 | 25 |
| **Mamba Sours,** Fruit Chews, | | | |
| 6 pieces, 1 oz | 100 | 1 | 22 |
| **Marshmallow Egg**, 1 egg, 1 oz | 120 | 3 | 22 |
| **Mary Jane** (Necco), 5 pieces, 1.4 oz | 160 | 3.5 | 32 |
| **Marshmallows:** Firm/Soft, 1 oz | 90 | 0 | 23 |
| Regular size, 4 pieces, 1 oz | 100 | 0 | 24 |
| Mini-Marshmallow, ⅔ cup, 1 oz | 95 | 0 | 24 |
| Joyva, Choc-coated Twists | 95 | 2 | 10 |
| Fluff, 2 Tbsp, 0.6 oz | 60 | 0 | 15 |
| Kraft: Creme, 0.5 oz | 45 | 0 | 11 |
| Funmallows, ⅔ cup, 1 oz | 100 | 0 | 24 |
| Jet-Puffed, 5 pieces, 1 oz | 100 | 0 | 24 |
| Mini, 1 oz | 90 | 0 | 23 |
| **Marzipan**, 2 Tbsp, 1.4 oz | 160 | 4 | 29 |
| **Mauna Loa,** Mountains, 4 pcs | 230 | 17 | 21 |
| **Mexican Hats**, (7), 1.4 oz | 120 | 0 | 30 |
| **Mentos:** Regular | 10 | 0 | 3 |
| Sugar Free | 5 | 0 | 2 |
| **Mike & Ike:** | | | |
| Original: 2.1 oz package | 220 | 0 | 55 |
| 23 pieces, 1.4 oz | 140 | 0 | 36 |
| **Milk Duds,** 1 box, 1.8 oz | 230 | 8 | 38 |

| Per Piece/Serving | C | F | Cb |
|---|---|---|---|
| **Milky Way** (Mars): | | | |
| Bars: Single, 2 oz | 240 | 9 | 37 |
| Fun Size, 2 bars, 1.2 oz | 160 | 6 | 24 |
| To Go, 1.8 oz | 230 | 9 | 36 |
| Minis, 5 pieces, 1.5 oz | 190 | 7 | 30 |
| Midnight Bars: 1.8 oz | 230 | 8 | 36 |
| Minis, 5 pieces, 1.4 oz | 190 | 7 | 30 |
| Simply Caramel, 1.9 oz | 250 | 11 | 37 |
| **Mints:** Uncoated, 3 pieces | 70 | 0 | 17 |
| 1 mint , medium | 7 | 0 | 1 |
| 1 large mint | 15 | 0 | 3 |
| **Mon Cheri** (Ferrero), 4 pieces, 2 oz | 260 | 18 | 20 |
| **Mounds:** 1.75 oz bar | 240 | 13 | 28 |
| King Size, 4 pieces, 3.5 oz | 480 | 26 | 56 |
| Snack Size, 1 piece, 0.6 oz | 80 | 4.5 | 10 |
| **Mr Goodbar:** 1.8 oz bar | 250 | 17 | 26 |
| King Size, 2.6 oz bar | 380 | 26 | 38 |
| **Munch Bar,** 1.4 oz | 220 | 15 | 18 |
| **Necco,** Candy Wafers (40), 2 oz | 220 | 0 | 56 |
| **Nestle Crunch:** Orig.,1.6 oz bar | 220 | 11 | 30 |
| Fun Size, 3 bars, 1.4 oz | 180 | 9 | 26 |
| Miniatures, 4 bars, 1.4 oz | 200 | 10 | 27 |
| Buncha Crunch, ⅓ cup, 1.2 oz | 180 | 9 | 25 |
| Crunch Crisp, 1.8 oz | 240 | 13 | 32 |
| **Newman's Own:** | | | |
| Milk Chocolate: Caramel Cups (3) | 160 | 8 | 21 |
| Peanut Butter Cups (3) | 180 | 12 | 17 |
| Dark Chocolate: Caramel Cups (3) | 160 | 9 | 20 |
| Peanut Butter Cups (3) | 180 | 13 | 16 |
| **Nips,** all varieties, 2 pieces, 0.5 oz | 60 | 2 | 11 |
| **Nougat:** 3 pieces, 1.5 oz | 170 | 1 | 39 |
| Chocolate Covered, 1 oz | 125 | 4 | 22 |
| **Nuggets** ~ See Hershey's | | | |
| **Nutrageous Bar** (Reese's), 1.8 oz | 260 | 16 | 28 |
| **Oh Henry!:** Fun Size, 0.9 oz | 120 | 5 | 16 |
| 1.8 oz bar | 230 | 11 | 33 |
| **Orange Slices:** | | | |
| Jewel, 3 pieces, 1.5 oz | 140 | 0 | 35 |
| Walgreens, 4 pieces, 1.6 oz | 160 | 0 | 39 |
| **Pastel Mints** (Walgreens), 20 pieces | 60 | 0 | 14 |
| **PayDay Bar:** 1.8 oz bar | 240 | 13 | 27 |
| King Size, 3.5 oz bar | 440 | 24 | 50 |
| Snack Size, 0.7 oz | 90 | 5 | 10 |
| Avalanche, 1.8 oz bar | 250 | 13 | 29 |
| **Peanut Bar** (Planter's), 1.6 oz | 240 | 14 | 21 |
| **Peanut Butter Cups** ~ See Reese's; Newman's Own | | | |
| **Peanut Brittle:** 1 piece, 1.5 oz | 190 | 5 | 32 |
| Sugar Free (Russell Stover), | | | |
| 4 pieces, 1.3 oz | 140 | 10 | 24 |

## Candy ~ Brands & Generic (Cont)

*Per Piece/Serving*

| | **C** | **F** | **Cb** |
|---|---|---|---|
| **Peanuts**, choc-covered, 14 pieces | 230 | 14 | 23 |
| *Pearson's,* Mint Patties, (5), 1.3 oz | 150 | 2.5 | 31 |
| **Peppermints:** 7 small, 0.5 oz | 60 | 0 | 15 |
| Brach's, Star Brites (3) | 60 | 0 | 16 |
| *Pez,* 1 roll | 35 | 0 | 9 |
| *Planters,* | | | |
| Double Peanut Bar, 1.6 oz | 240 | 14 | 21 |
| *Pop Rocks,* 0.4 oz package | 35 | 0 | 9 |
| *Pot of Gold* (Hershey's): | | | |
| Assortment: Caramel, 4 pieces | 190 | 10 | 25 |
| Nut, 4 pieces | 210 | 13 | 23 |
| **Pretzels:** Choc-covered, Mini (6) | 200 | 9 | 25 |
| White Choc Bites (23), 1.4 oz | 200 | 9 | 25 |
| *Pretzel Flipz* (Nestlé), 8 pieces, 1 oz | 130 | 5 | 20 |
| **Raisinets:** Milk Choc: | | | |
| 1.58 oz package | 190 | 8 | 32 |
| Movie Pack, 3.5 oz | 380 | 16 | 64 |
| Dark Chocolate, ¼ cup, 1.6 oz | 180 | 8 | 32 |
| *Reese's:* | | | |
| Clusters, 3 pieces, 1.5 oz | 220 | 12 | 24 |
| Crispy Crunchy Bar: 1.7 oz | 260 | 18 | 22 |
| 2 pieces, 1.2 oz | 170 | 10 | 19 |
| King Size, 3 oz | 480 | 32 | 40 |
| Fast Break, 2 oz bar | 260 | 12 | 35 |
| Peanut Butter Chips, 1 Tbsp, 0.5 oz | 80 | 4 | 8 |
| Peanut Butter Cups, Milk Chocolate: | | | |
| (2), 1.5 oz | 210 | 13 | 24 |
| Miniatures (5), 1.5 oz | 220 | 13 | 26 |
| Minis (11) | 200 | 12 | 23 |
| Big Cup, 1 cup, 1.4 oz | 200 | 12 | 22 |
| Sugar Free, Minis (5), 1.4 oz | 180 | 13 | 27 |
| Dark Chocolate (2), 1.5 oz | 210 | 14 | 23 |
| Pieces, Peanut Butter (51) | 200 | 9 | 25 |
| Sticks: 1.5 oz package | 220 | 13 | 23 |
| King Size, 3 oz package | 440 | 26 | 46 |
| Snack Size (1), 0.6 oz | 90 | 5 | 9 |
| Snacksters, 1 package, 0.8 oz | 100 | 4 | 14 |
| Whipps, 1.5 oz | 230 | 9 | 37 |
| *Rice Krispies Treats* (Kellogg's), | | | |
| 1 bar, average all varieties, 0.8 oz | 95 | 2.5 | 17 |
| *Riesen,* Choc. Chew, 4 pieces, 1.3 oz | 170 | 6 | 28 |
| **Rocky Road**, Milk/Dark, 1.8 oz bar | 240 | 11 | 34 |
| *Roca Thins,* 3 pieces, av. all varieties | 210 | 14 | 24 |
| *Rolo:* Regular, all varieties, 1.7 oz roll | 220 | 10 | 33 |
| Mini Chews, Caramel in milk choc. (11) | 190 | 9 | 26 |
| *Root Beer Barrels,* (3), 0.6 oz | 60 | 0 | 17 |

*Per Piece/Serving*

| | **C** | **F** | **Cb** |
|---|---|---|---|
| **Russell Stover Candy:** | | | |
| Boxed Chocolates: Chocolate Coated | | | |
| Assorted (2), 1.2 oz | 150 | 7 | 22 |
| Cherry Cordials (3), 0.4 oz | 150 | 5 | 25 |
| Dairy Cream Caramels (2), 1.2 oz | 160 | 7 | 22 |
| Elegant Collection (3), 1.6 oz | 210 | 10 | 25 |
| French Choc. Mints (4), 1.4 oz | 220 | 13 | 22 |
| Nut, Chewy & Crisp Centers (2) | 160 | 8 | 21 |
| Sugar Free: | | | |
| Assorted Hard Candies (3), 1.6 oz | 210 | 16 | 24 |
| Bags: Caramel (3), 1.3 oz | 180 | 8 | 25 |
| Coconut (3), 1.5 oz | 160 | 10 | 28 |
| Mint Patty (3), 1.5 oz | 180 | 12 | 26 |
| Peanut Butter Cups (2), 1.2 oz | 160 | 12 | 17 |
| Pecan Delight (2), 1.2 oz | 160 | 12 | 19 |
| Note: Carbohydrates include sugar alcohol | | | |
| **Salt Water Taffy** (Brach's), (5) | 170 | 2.5 | 36 |
| *Seashells* (Guylian), (4), 1.6 oz | 260 | 17 | 24 |
| **See's Candies:** | | | |
| Almond Royal (5), 1.3 oz | 190 | 13 | 18 |
| Butterscotch Chews (5), 1.5 oz | 210 | 12 | 27 |
| Krispy's: Caffe Latte (5), 1.3 oz | 180 | 8 | 27 |
| Mint (5), 1.3 oz | 170 | 8 | 27 |
| Little Pops: | | | |
| Butterscotch (4), 0.5 oz | 60 | 2 | 12 |
| Chocolate (4), 0.5 oz | 60 | 3 | 10 |
| Vanilla (4), 0.5 oz | 50 | 2 | 9 |
| Lollypops, average, 0.7 oz | 90 | 3 | 17 |
| Milk Molasses Chips, 6 pieces, 1.4 oz | 180 | 8 | 27 |
| Milk Peppermints, 2 pieces, 1.3 oz | 150 | 4 | 28 |
| Peanut Brittle Bar, 1 oz | 150 | 10 | 15 |
| Peanut Butter Patties, 2 pieces, 1.2 oz | 170 | 10 | 16 |
| Peppermint Twists (3), 0.5 oz | 60 | 0 | 15 |
| Toffee-ettes, 3 pieces, 1.6 oz | 270 | 21 | 18 |
| Sugar Free: Dark Bar, 1.5 oz | 180 | 16 | 24 |
| Dark Walnut Clusters (4), 1.5 oz | 230 | 21 | 17 |
| Peanut Brittle, 1.5 oz | 170 | 14 | 17 |
| *Skinny Cow:* | | | |
| Dreamy Clusters, all var., 1 pouch | 120 | 6 | 20 |
| Heavenly Crips, all varieties, 1 bar | 110 | 6 | 14 |
| *Skittles:* Original, 2 oz | 230 | 2.5 | 52 |
| Sour, 1.8 oz | 200 | 2 | 44 |
| Tropical; Wild Berry, 2.2 oz | 250 | 2.5 | 56 |
| Fun Size, 1 bag, 0.5 oz | 60 | 1 | 14 |
| Tear & Share, 4 oz bag | 420 | 4.5 | 93 |
| *Skor,* Toffee Bar (1), 1.4 oz | 200 | 12 | 25 |
| *Smarties:* Candy Rolls (1), 0.3 oz | 25 | 0 | 6 |
| Giant, 1 roll, 1 oz | 100 | 0 | 25 |

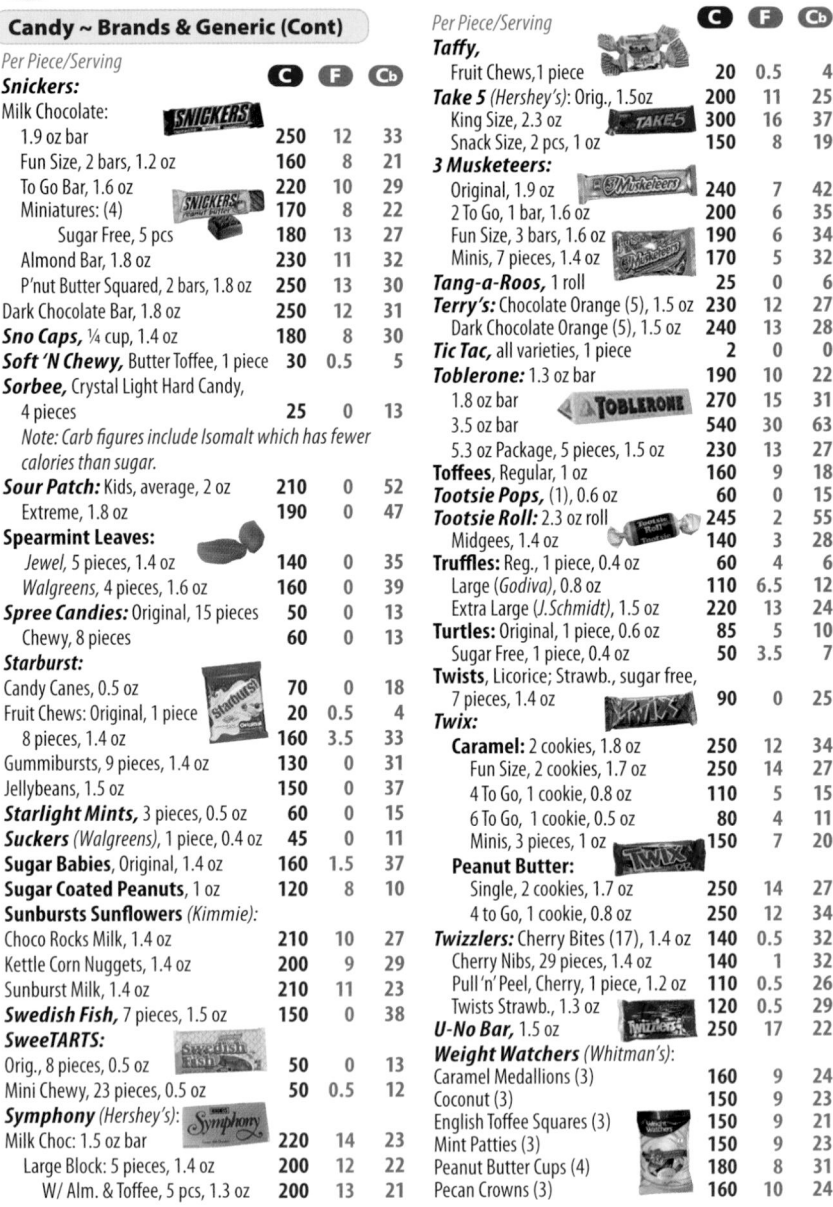

## Candy ~ Brands & Generic (Cont)

*Per Piece/Serving*

| | C | F | Cb |
|---|---|---|---|
| **Snickers:** | | | |
| Milk Chocolate: | | | |
| 1.9 oz bar | 250 | 12 | 33 |
| Fun Size, 2 bars, 1.2 oz | 160 | 8 | 21 |
| To Go Bar, 1.6 oz | 220 | 10 | 29 |
| Miniatures: (4) | 170 | 8 | 22 |
| Sugar Free, 5 pcs | 180 | 13 | 27 |
| Almond Bar, 1.8 oz | 230 | 11 | 32 |
| P'nut Butter Squared, 2 bars, 1.8 oz | 250 | 13 | 30 |
| Dark Chocolate Bar, 1.8 oz | 250 | 12 | 31 |
| **Sno Caps,** ¼ cup, 1.4 oz | 180 | 8 | 30 |
| **Soft 'N Chewy,** Butter Toffee, 1 piece | 30 | 0.5 | 5 |
| **Sorbee,** Crystal Light Hard Candy, | | | |
| 4 pieces | 25 | 0 | 13 |
| *Note: Carb figures include Isomalt which has fewer calories than sugar.* | | | |
| **Sour Patch:** Kids, average, 2 oz | 210 | 0 | 52 |
| Extreme, 1.8 oz | 190 | 0 | 47 |
| **Spearmint Leaves:** | | | |
| *Jewel,* 5 pieces, 1.4 oz | 140 | 0 | 35 |
| *Walgreens,* 4 pieces, 1.6 oz | 160 | 0 | 39 |
| **Spree Candies:** Original, 15 pieces | 50 | 0 | 13 |
| Chewy, 8 pieces | 60 | 0 | 13 |
| **Starburst:** | | | |
| Candy Canes, 0.5 oz | 70 | 0 | 18 |
| Fruit Chews: Original, 1 piece | 20 | 0.5 | 4 |
| 8 pieces, 1.4 oz | 160 | 3.5 | 33 |
| Gummibursts, 9 pieces, 1.4 oz | 130 | 0 | 31 |
| Jellybeans, 1.5 oz | 150 | 0 | 37 |
| **Starlight Mints,** 3 pieces, 0.5 oz | 60 | 0 | 15 |
| **Suckers** (Walgreens), 1 piece, 0.4 oz | 45 | 0 | 11 |
| **Sugar Babies,** Original, 1.4 oz | 160 | 1.5 | 37 |
| **Sugar Coated Peanuts,** 1 oz | 120 | 8 | 10 |
| **Sunbursts Sunflowers** (Kimmie): | | | |
| Choco Rocks Milk, 1.4 oz | 210 | 10 | 27 |
| Kettle Corn Nuggets, 1.4 oz | 200 | 9 | 29 |
| Sunburst Milk, 1.4 oz | 210 | 11 | 23 |
| **Swedish Fish,** 7 pieces, 1.5 oz | 150 | 0 | 38 |
| **SweeTARTS:** | | | |
| Orig., 8 pieces, 0.5 oz | 50 | 0 | 13 |
| Mini Chewy, 23 pieces, 0.5 oz | 50 | 0.5 | 12 |
| **Symphony** (Hershey's): | | | |
| Milk Choc: 1.5 oz bar | 220 | 14 | 23 |
| Large Block: 5 pieces, 1.4 oz | 200 | 12 | 22 |
| W/ Alm. & Toffee, 5 pcs, 1.3 oz | 200 | 13 | 21 |

*Per Piece/Serving*

| | C | F | Cb |
|---|---|---|---|
| **Taffy,** | | | |
| Fruit Chews, 1 piece | 20 | 0.5 | 4 |
| **Take 5** (Hershey's): Orig., 1.5oz | 200 | 11 | 25 |
| King Size, 2.3 oz | 300 | 16 | 37 |
| Snack Size, 2 pcs, 1 oz | 150 | 8 | 19 |
| **3 Musketeers:** | | | |
| Original, 1.9 oz | 240 | 7 | 42 |
| 2 To Go, 1 bar, 1.6 oz | 200 | 6 | 35 |
| Fun Size, 3 bars, 1.6 oz | 190 | 6 | 34 |
| Minis, 7 pieces, 1.4 oz | 170 | 5 | 32 |
| **Tang-a-Roos,** 1 roll | 25 | 0 | 6 |
| **Terry's:** Chocolate Orange (5), 1.5 oz | 230 | 12 | 27 |
| Dark Chocolate Orange (5), 1.5 oz | 240 | 13 | 28 |
| **Tic Tac,** all varieties, 1 piece | 2 | 0 | 0 |
| **Toblerone:** 1.3 oz bar | 190 | 10 | 22 |
| 1.8 oz bar | 270 | 15 | 31 |
| 3.5 oz bar | 540 | 30 | 63 |
| 5.3 oz Package, 5 pieces, 1.5 oz | 230 | 13 | 27 |
| **Toffees,** Regular, 1 oz | 160 | 9 | 18 |
| **Tootsie Pops,** (1), 0.6 oz | 60 | 0 | 15 |
| **Tootsie Roll:** 2.3 oz roll | 245 | 2 | 55 |
| Midgees, 1.4 oz | 140 | 3 | 28 |
| **Truffles:** Reg., 1 piece, 0.4 oz | 60 | 4 | 6 |
| Large (Godiva), 0.8 oz | 110 | 6.5 | 12 |
| Extra Large (J. Schmidt), 1.5 oz | 220 | 13 | 24 |
| **Turtles:** Original, 1 piece, 0.6 oz | 85 | 5 | 10 |
| Sugar Free, 1 piece, 0.4 oz | 50 | 3.5 | 7 |
| **Twists,** Licorice; Strawb., sugar free, | | | |
| 7 pieces, 1.4 oz | 90 | 0 | 25 |
| **Twix:** | | | |
| **Caramel:** 2 cookies, 1.8 oz | 250 | 12 | 34 |
| Fun Size, 2 cookies, 1.7 oz | 250 | 14 | 27 |
| 4 To Go, 1 cookie, 1.0 oz | 110 | 5 | 15 |
| 6 To Go, 1 cookie, 0.5 oz | 80 | 4 | 11 |
| Minis, 3 pieces, 1 oz | 150 | 7 | 20 |
| **Peanut Butter:** | | | |
| Single, 2 cookies, 1.7 oz | 250 | 14 | 27 |
| 4 to Go, 1 cookie, 0.8 oz | 250 | 12 | 34 |
| **Twizzlers:** Cherry Bites (17), 1.4 oz | 140 | 0.5 | 32 |
| Cherry Nibs, 29 pieces, 1 oz | 140 | 1 | 32 |
| Pull 'n' Peel, Cherry, 1 piece, 1.2 oz | 110 | 0.5 | 26 |
| Twists Strawb., 1.3 oz | 120 | 0.5 | 29 |
| **U-No Bar,** 1.5 oz | 250 | 17 | 22 |
| **Weight Watchers** (Whitman's): | | | |
| Caramel Medallions (3) | 160 | 9 | 24 |
| Coconut (3) | 150 | 9 | 23 |
| English Toffee Squares (3) | 150 | 9 | 21 |
| Mint Patties (3) | 150 | 9 | 23 |
| Peanut Butter Cups (4) | 180 | 8 | 31 |
| Pecan Crowns (3) | 160 | 10 | 24 |

## Candy ~ Brands & Generic (Cont)

*Per Piece/Serving* **C F Cb**

**Werther's:**

| | C | F | Cb |
|---|---|---|---|
| Hard Candy: Original (3), 0.5 oz | 70 | 1.5 | 14 |
| Sugar-Free Original (5) | 40 | 1.5 | 15 |

*Note: Carb figure includes 14g sugar alcohol*

| | C | F | Cb |
|---|---|---|---|
| Soft, Chocolate Caramel (4), 1.4 oz | 190 | 8 | 28 |
| **Whatchamacallit:** 1.5 oz Bar | 230 | 12 | 28 |
| King Size Bar, 2.5 oz | 370 | 20 | 45 |
| **Whitman's,** Boxed Chocolates: | | | |
| Sampler (4), 1.6 oz | 220 | 12 | 27 |
| 12 oz Box, 3 pieces, 1.2 oz | 170 | 9 | 21 |
| Reserve, 7 oz Box, 2 pieces, 1.2 oz | 160 | 9 | 21 |
| Sugar Free, 10 oz Box, 3 pcs, 1.5 oz | 190 | 13 | 25 |
| **Whoppers,** av. all varieties, 18 pcs | 190 | 7 | 31 |
| **Wonka:** | | | |
| Bar (1), 2.5 oz | 360 | 19 | 49 |
| Exceptional Bars, average, 4 pieces | 200 | 13 | 23 |
| Gobstopper, 9 pieces, 0.5 oz | 60 | 0 | 14 |
| Laffy Taffy: Ropes, all var., 0.8 oz | 80 | 1.5 | 18 |
| Stretchy & Tangy, all var., 1.5 oz | 150 | 3.5 | 29 |
| Nerds, Giant, Chewy, 1.8 oz package | 180 | 0 | 42 |
| **Yogurt Candy,** | | | |
| Coated Raisins, 27 pieces, 1.4 oz | 180 | 8 | 28 |
| **York:** Mints, (3) | 10 | 0 | 3 |
| Peppermint Pattie, reg, 1.4 oz | 140 | 2.5 | 31 |
| Pieces (50) | 170 | 8 | 28 |
| **Zagnut,** 1.75 oz bar | 220 | 9 | 35 |
| **Zero Bar:** 1.8 oz bar | 230 | 8 | 37 |
| King Size, 3.5 oz | 400 | 14 | 68 |

## Gum

*Per Piece* **C F Cb**

| | C | F | Cb |
|---|---|---|---|
| **Bazooka** | 15 | 0 | 4 |
| **Beechies** | 6 | 0 | 2 |
| **Big League Chews** | 10 | 0 | 2 |
| **Bubble Yum:** Original | 25 | 0 | 6 |
| Sugarless | 10 | 0 | 3 |
| Candilicious | 30 | 0 | 2 |
| **Carefree,** Sugarless/Regular | 5 | 0 | 2 |
| **Chiclet** | 5 | 0 | 1 |
| **Dentyne** | 5 | 0 | 0.5 |
| **Double Bubble Ball** | 20 | 0 | 5 |
| **Estee,** Bubble/Regular | 5 | 0 | 2 |
| **Extra** (Wrigley's), Sugar-Free | 5 | 0 | 2 |
| **Freshen-Up** | 10 | 0 | 3 |
| **Hubba Bubba:** Regular | 25 | 0 | 6 |
| Sugar-free, average | 14 | 0 | 0.5 |
| **Ice Breakers** | 5 | 0 | 2 |
| **Jolt Gum** | 5 | 0 | 2 |
| **Super Bubble** | 15 | 0 | 4 |
| **Trident,** Orig.; White | 5 | 0 | 1 |
| **Wrigley's,** all flavors | 10 | 0 | 2 |

## Carob Candy

**C F Cb**

*Per Piece/Serving*

| | C | F | Cb |
|---|---|---|---|
| **Carob**, Plain/Natural, 1 oz | 155 | 9 | 15 |
| **Carob Coated:** Raisins, 1 oz | 130 | 8 | 15 |
| Almonds/Peanuts, 1 oz | 150 | 10 | 14 |
| Caramels, 1 oz | 110 | 4 | 18 |
| Dates, 1 oz | 125 | 5 | 20 |
| Malt Balls, 1 oz | 135 | 8 | 15 |
| Soybeans | 145 | 9 | 16 |
| Trail/Party Mix, 1 oz | 150 | 9 | 15 |

## Cough Drops

*Per Drop/Piece*

| | C | F | Cb |
|---|---|---|---|
| **Beech Nut,** 1 drop | 10 | 0 | 2 |
| **CVS,** Honey Lemon Cough Drops | 15 | 0 | 4 |
| **Diabetic Tussin** | 0 | 0 | 0 |
| **Halls,** Defense Vitamin C: Regular | 15 | 0 | 4 |
| Sugar Free | 5 | 0 | 3 |
| Fruit Breezers | 15 | 0 | 4 |
| Menthol Drops: Regular | 15 | 0 | 4 |
| Sugar Free | 5 | 0 | 4 |
| Plus | 20 | 0 | 5 |
| **Listerine** (Amer. Chicle), Lozenge | 10 | 0 | 2 |
| **Luden's,** Throat Drops: Reg., all var. | 10 | 0 | 2 |
| Sugar Free | 0 | 0 | 0 |
| **Pine Bros,** Cough Drops | 10 | 0 | 2 |
| **Ricola,** Cough Drops: | | | |
| Natural Herbs | 10 | 0 | 3 |
| Sugar-Free Lemon Mint | 0 | 0 | 1 |
| **Rolaids,** Sodium Free | 5 | 0 | 1 |
| **Sathers,** Peppermint Lozenges | 15 | 0 | 3 |
| **Sucrets** (Beecham), Lozenges | 10 | 0 | 2.5 |
| **Wintergreen,** Lozenges | 15 | 0 | 3 |

**Eat at least 5 servings of fruit and vegetables every day . . . and Enjoy Better Health!**

### Quick Guide

**C F Cb**

#### Firm/Hard Cheeses
**American, Cheddar, Jack, Swiss:**
*Average All Brands*

| | C | F | Cb |
|---|---|---|---|
| **Regular Cheese:** | | | |
| Thin Deli slice, 0.8 oz | 80 | 6 | 0.5 |
| 1 oz slice/piece | 110 | 9 | 0.5 |
| 8 oz package | 880 | 72 | 3 |
| **Cubes:** 1" cube, 0.6 oz | 70 | 5.5 | 0.5 |
| 1¼" cube, 1 oz | 115 | 9 | 0.5 |
| **Diced**, 1 cup, 4.5 oz | 510 | 41 | 3 |
| **Melted**, ¼ cup, 2 oz | 245 | 20 | 1 |
| **Shredded:** ¼ cup, 1 oz | 110 | 9 | 0.5 |
| 1 cup, 4 oz | 440 | 36 | 2 |

### Cheese & Cheese Products

*Per 1 oz Unless Indicated*

| | C | F | Cb |
|---|---|---|---|
| **Almond** *(Lisanatti)*, Chunks, average | 50 | 1 | 3 |
| **American:** | | | |
| Regular: 1 slice, 1 oz | 105 | 9 | 0.5 |
| *Kraft,* Regular, 0.67 oz slice | 60 | 4.5 | 0 |
| *Land O'Lakes,* 1 oz slice | 100 | 9 | 2 |
| Reduced Fat: | | | |
| *Alpine Lace,* Yellow/White, 0.8 oz | 90 | 6 | 2 |
| *Borden,* 1 slice, 0.8 oz | 50 | 3 | 2 |
| *Kraft,* 2% Milk, 0.67 oz | 45 | 2.5 | 1 |
| *Land O Lakes,* 2% Milk, 1 oz | 90 | 6 | 1 |
| **Babybel** *(Laughing Cow),* Mini: | | | |
| Original (1), 0.8 oz | 70 | 6 | 0 |
| Light (1), 0.8 oz | 50 | 3 | 0 |
| Bonbel (1), 0.8 oz | 70 | 6 | 0 |
| Light Original (1), 0.8 oz | 50 | 3 | 0 |
| Gouda (1), 0.8 oz | 80 | 6 | 0 |
| **Blue/Bleu:** *Average all Brands* | | | |
| Crumbled, ¼ cup, 1 oz | 100 | 8 | 0 |
| Light, 0.8 oz | 35 | 1.5 | 2 |
| **Brie:** Average, 1 oz | 95 | 8 | 0 |
| *Alouette,* | | | |
| Baby Brie Wedge, 1 oz | 110 | 10 | 1 |
| **Camembert**, 1 oz | 85 | 7 | 0 |
| **Caraway**, 1 oz | 105 | 8 | 1 |
| **Castello,** 1 oz | 120 | 12 | 0 |
| **Cheddar:** | | | |
| Regular: Medium/Sharp, av., 1 oz | 110 | 9 | 1 |
| Shredded, ¼ cup, 1 oz | 110 | 9 | 1 |
| *Cracker Barrel:* Extra Sharp, 1 oz | 110 | 10 | 0 |
| Sharp, Shreds, 1 oz | 110 | 9 | 1 |

### Cheese & Cheese Products (Cont)

*Per 1 oz Unless Indicated*

| | C | F | Cb |
|---|---|---|---|
| **Cheddar (Cont):** | | | |
| Reduced Fat, 2% Milk, Shredded, | | | |
| *Kraft,* 1 oz | 80 | 6 | 1 |
| **Cheese Curds:** | | | |
| Fresh: ¼ cup, 1 oz | 110 | 9 | 0 |
| 1 cup, 4 oz | 440 | 36 | 0 |
| Breaded & Fried: | | | |
| *A&W,* 5 oz | 570 | 40 | 27 |
| *Culver's,* Wisconsin, 5.3 oz | 510 | 25 | 51 |
| **Cheese Logs** *(Kaukauna),* average | 100 | 7 | 4 |
| **Cheese Whiz:** | | | |
| Original, 2 Tbsp, 1 oz | 90 | 7 | 4 |
| Light, 2 Tbsp, 1 oz | 80 | 3.5 | 6 |
| Salsa Con Queso, | | | |
| 2 Tbsp, 1 oz | 90 | 7 | 4 |
| **Cheshire**, 1 oz | 110 | 9 | 1.5 |
| **Colby**, Regular, 1 oz | 110 | 8 | 0 |
| **Colby-Jack:** | | | |
| Big Slice, 0.8 oz | 90 | 7 | 0 |
| **Cottage Cheese:** *Average All Brands* | | | |
| Creamed (4% milk fat): | | | |
| 2 Tbsp, 1 oz | 30 | 1 | 1.5 |
| ½ cup, 4 oz | 110 | 5 | 4 |
| With fruit, ½ cup, 4 oz | 115 | 4 | 5 |
| Reduced-Fat (2%): 2 Tbsp, 1 oz | 25 | 0.5 | 1 |
| ½ cup, 4 oz | 100 | 3 | 4 |
| Low-Fat (1%): 2 Tbsp, 1 oz | 20 | 0.5 | 1 |
| ½ cup, 4 oz | 80 | 1 | 3 |
| Fat-Free/Non-Fat: 2 T., 1 oz | 20 | 0 | 1 |
| ½ cup, 4 oz | 80 | 0 | 5 |
| **Cottage Cheese:** *Brands* | | | |
| *Fiber One,* 1% Fat, ½ c., 4 oz | 80 | 2 | 8 |
| *Friendship:* | | | |
| 1% Low-Fat with Pineapple, 4 oz | 120 | 1 | 16 |
| Nonfat with Pineapple, ½ cup, 4 oz | 110 | 0 | 17 |
| Pot Style, 2%, ½ cup, 4 oz | 90 | 2.5 | 3 |
| *Hood,* Low Fat, 4 oz | 90 | 1 | 5 |
| *Knudsen/Breakstone's:* | | | |
| Free, Non-Fat, ½ cup, 4 oz | 70 | 0 | 7 |
| 2% Milk Fat, ½ cup, 4 oz | 100 | 2.5 | 6 |
| On the Go!, | | | |
| Low-Fat, 4 oz carton | 90 | 2.5 | 6 |
| *Lactaid,* Low-Fat, ½ cup, 4 oz | 80 | 1 | 7 |
| *Light n' Lively:* | | | |
| Fat-Free, ½ cup, 4.4 oz | 80 | 0 | 8 |
| Low-Fat, ½ cup, 4.4 oz | 80 | 1.5 | 6 |

# Cheese C

## Cheese & Cheese Products (Cont)

*Per 1 oz Unless Indicated*

| | C | F | Cb |
|---|---|---|---|
| **Cream Cheese:** *Average All Brands* | | | |
| Regular/Soft: | | | |
| 2 Tbsp, 1 oz | 95 | 10 | 1 |
| 3 oz package | 290 | 29 | 3.5 |
| 8 oz package | 780 | 78 | 9 |
| Light, Plain, 1 oz | 60 | 4.5 | 2.5 |
| Fat-Free, Plain, 1 oz | 30 | 0 | 2 |
| **Easy Cheese** *(Kraft),* | | | |
| American, 2 Tbsp, 1.2 oz | 90 | 6 | 2 |
| **Edam**, 1 oz | 100 | 8 | 0.5 |
| **Farmer**, Low-Fat, 1 oz | 40 | 2.5 | 0 |
| **Feta**: Regular, 1 oz | 75 | 6 | 1 |
| Crumbled, ½ cup, 2.5 oz | 190 | 15 | 3 |
| *Athenos*, Reduced-Fat, 1 oz | 60 | 4 | 1 |
| **Fontina**, 2 Tbsp, 1 oz | 110 | 9 | 0.5 |
| **Galaxy,** Cheese Substitute: | | | |
| Grated Parmesan Flavor, 2 tsp, 0.2 oz | 15 | 0 | 0 |
| Rice, Mozzarella flavor, 1 sl., 0.6 oz | 40 | 2.5 | 0.5 |
| Veggy, all varieties, 1 slice, 0.5 oz | 40 | 2.5 | 0.5 |
| **Goat's Milk Cheese:** | | | |
| Chevre: Original, 2 Tbsp | 75 | 6 | 0.5 |
| Semi-Soft, 1 oz | 100 | 8.5 | 1 |
| Hard, 1 oz | 130 | 10 | 0.5 |
| *Chavrie:* Regular, 2 Tbsp, 1 oz | 50 | 3.5 | 1 |
| Caramelized Onion, 2 Tbsp | 50 | 3 | 4 |
| Logs, average all varieties, 1 oz | 80 | 7 | 3 |
| Gjetost, fresh, 1 oz | 130 | 8 | 12 |
| Myzithra, grated, 1 oz | 80 | 4 | 2 |
| **Gorgonzola**, 1 oz | 100 | 8 | 0.5 |
| **Galbani,** Dolcelatte, 1 oz | 95 | 8 | 1 |
| **Gouda**, 1 oz slice | 100 | 8 | 0.5 |
| **Gruyere**, 1 oz | 115 | 9 | 1 |
| **Handi-Snacks** *(Kraft):* | | | |
| Breadsticks 'n Cheez Single, 1 oz | 110 | 4.5 | 14 |
| Ritz Crackers 'n Cheez Dip, 1 oz | 100 | 6 | 11 |
| **Havarti** *(Land O'Lakes)*, 0.8 oz | 80 | 7 | 0 |
| **Italian Pasta Blend** *(Sargento)*, 1 oz | 90 | 6 | 3 |
| **Jarlsberg**: Average, 1 oz | 100 | 8 | 0 |
| Reduced Fat, shredded, 1 oz | 70 | 3.5 | 0 |
| **Labneh**, (Lebanese Cream Chse), 1.8 oz | 70 | 4 | 4 |

## Cheese & Cheese Products (Cont)

*Per 1 oz Unless Indicated*

| | C | F | Cb |
|---|---|---|---|
| **Laughing Cow,** Wedges: | | | |
| Original Creamy Swiss (1) | 50 | 4 | 1 |
| Light Varieties, av., (1) | 35 | 2 | 2 |
| **Lifetime,** Cholesterol Reducing, | | | |
| Low Fat, all varieties, 1 Slice, 1 oz | 45 | 1.5 | 1 |
| **Limburger**, 1 oz | 95 | 8 | 0 |
| **Mascarpone**, av., 1 oz | 125 | 13 | 0.5 |
| **Mexican:** | | | |
| *Cacique:* Asadero, sliced | 70 | 5 | 1 |
| Cotija | 100 | 8 | 0 |
| Enchilado; Manchego | 90 | 7 | 0 |
| Panela | 80 | 6 | 0 |
| Queso Fresco | 80 | 6 | 0 |
| Queso Quesadilla | 90 | 7 | 0 |
| Ranchero | 80 | 6 | 0 |
| *Chi-Chi's,* Salsa Con Quéso, Mild | 45 | 3 | 4 |
| *El Mexicano:* Asadero, Regular | 90 | 7 | 0 |
| Cotija, Regular | 110 | 9 | 0 |
| *Kraft,* Mexican Four Cheese; Taco, Shredded, | 100 | 8 | 1 |
| *Sargento,* 4 Cheese Mexican | 110 | 9 | 1 |
| *Supremo:* Quéso Chihuahua, 1 oz | 100 | 8 | 0 |
| Quéso Oaxaca | 80 | 5 | 1 |
| **Monterey Jack:** | | | |
| Regular, shredded, 1 oz | 100 | 8 | 1 |
| *Alpine Lace,* Co-Jack, 1 oz | 70 | 5 | 0 |
| *Kraft,* 1 oz | 100 | 8 | 1 |
| **Mozzarella:** | | | |
| Regular: Average 1 oz | 85 | 6.5 | 0.5 |
| *Land O'Lakes/Polly-O:* | | | |
| Slice, average, 1 oz | 90 | 6 | 1 |
| Shredded, 1 oz | 90 | 6 | 1 |
| Fat-Free, | | | |
| *Kraft,* Shredded, 1 oz | 45 | 0 | 2 |
| Light: | | | |
| *Kraft,* 2% Milk Fat, Reduced Fat | 70 | 5 | 1 |
| *Polly-O Lite,* Shredded, 1 oz | 60 | 2.5 | 1 |
| Part Skim: | | | |
| *Borden/Kraft,* Shredded | 80 | 5 | 2 |
| *Kraft,* String | 80 | 6 | 0 |
| **Muenster:** | | | |
| Regular, 1 oz | 105 | 9 | 0.5 |
| Low-Fat, 1 oz | 85 | 5 | 1 |

Updated Nutrition Data ~ www.CalorieKing.com
Persons with Diabetes ~ See Disclaimer (Page 22)

**77**

## Cheese & Cheese Products (Cont)

*Per 1 oz Unless Indicated*    **C**   **F**   **Cb**

| | C | F | Cb |
|---|---|---|---|
| **Parmesan:** | | | |
| Fresh/Block, Dry, 1 oz | 110 | 7.5 | 1 |
| Grated (Packaged): 1 Tbsp | 20 | 1.5 | 0 |
| 1 oz | 120 | 8 | 1 |
| ½ cup, 1.8 oz | 215 | 14 | 2 |
| *Kraft,* Reduced-Fat Topping, 1 Tbsp | 20 | 1 | 2 |
| **Philadelphia:** | | | |
| **Cream Cheese:** Original, 2 T. 1 oz | 100 | 9 | 1 |
| 3 oz package | 300 | 27 | 3 |
| Regular, 1 oz | 90 | 9 | 2 |
| **Creme,** Cooking, av. all var., ¼ cup | 110 | 9 | 4 |
| **Flavored:** | | | |
| Blueberry, 1 oz | 80 | 6 | 5 |
| Honey Nut; Strawberry, av., 1 oz | 80 | 7 | 5 |
| Garden Vegetable, 1 oz | 80 | 7 | 2 |
| Salmon, 1 oz | 70 | 7 | 1 |
| **Light,** Plain, 1 oz | 70 | 5 | 2 |
| **⅓ Less Fat:** Plain, 2 T., 1 oz | 70 | 6 | 2 |
| Garden Veggie; Chive & On., 1 oz | 70 | 5 | 2 |
| Neufchatel, 2 T., 1 oz | 70 | 6 | 1 |
| **Fat-Free,** Plain, 1 oz | 30 | 0 | 2 |
| **Indulgence:** | | | |
| Milk/White Chocolate: | | | |
| 1 Tbsp, 0.6 oz | 60 | 3.5 | 6 |
| Mini Tub, 1.3 oz | 125 | 7 | 13 |
| 8 oz container | 800 | 47 | 80 |
| Dark Chocolate, 1 T., 0.6 oz | 55 | 3.5 | 6 |
| **Spread:** Regular, 1 oz | 80 | 7 | 2 |
| Flavors, average, 1.2 oz | 80 | 6 | 5 |
| **Whipped:** | | | |
| Regular, 0.8 oz | 60 | 5 | 2 |
| Mixed Berry, 0.7 oz | 70 | 5 | 3 |
| **Pizza Four Cheese**, shredded, | | | |
| *Kraft/Sargento,* Regular, av., 1 oz | 90 | 7 | 1 |
| **Port de Salut,** 1 oz | 100 | 8 | 0 |
| **Port Wine** *(Kaukauna/WisPride):* | | | |
| 8 oz Tub: Average, 1 oz | 85 | 7 | 3 |
| Lite, 2 Tbsp, average, 1 oz | 60 | 3 | 5 |
| Ball, 1 oz | 100 | 6 | 4 |
| Log, 1 oz | 100 | 7 | 4 |
| **Provolone:** Regular, 1 oz | 100 | 7.5 | 0.5 |
| *Alpine Lace,* Reduced-Fat, 0.8 oz | 60 | 4.5 | 0 |
| *Sargento,* Deli Style 1 slice, 0.67 oz | 50 | 3 | 0 |
| **Pub** *(Rondele),* average all varieties | 75 | 7 | 1 |
| **Quark:** 40% fat | 45 | 3 | 1 |
| 20% fat | 30 | 1.5 | 1 |
| Skim/Non-Fat | 20 | 0 | 1.5 |
| **Queso:** | | | |
| Anejo/Asadero/Blanco, 1 oz | 105 | 9 | 1 |
| Chichuahua/De Papa, 1 oz | 110 | 9 | 2 |
| **Rice Cheese Chunks** *(Lisanatti),* | | | |
| average, 1 oz | 60 | 3 | 2 |
| **Swiss** *(Lifetime),* Fat Free, 1 oz | 40 | 0 | 1 |

## Cheese & Cheese Products (Cont)

*Per 1 oz Unless Indicated*    **C**   **F**   **Cb**

| | C | F | Cb |
|---|---|---|---|
| **Ricotta Cheese:** | | | |
| Whole Milk: 1 oz | 50 | 3.5 | 1 |
| ½ cup, 4.5 oz | 215 | 16 | 4 |
| Part Skim: 1 oz | 40 | 2 | 1.5 |
| ½ cup, 4.5 oz | 170 | 10 | 6 |
| Light/Low-Fat: 1 oz | 25 | 1 | 1.5 |
| ½ cup, 4.5 oz | 125 | 5 | 6 |
| Fat-Free, ½ cup, 4.5 oz | 100 | 0 | 10 |
| Baked Ricotta, 2 oz | 130 | 9 | 3 |
| **Romano:** Block/Loaf | 110 | 8 | 1 |
| Grated: 1 oz | 120 | 9 | 1 |
| 1 Tbsp, 0.2 oz | 20 | 1.5 | 0 |
| **Roquefort,** 1 oz | 105 | 9 | 0.5 |
| **Sheep's Milk,** (Manchego), | | | |
| *Trader Joes/Wegman's,* 1 oz | 120 | 10 | 0 |
| **Soy Cheese:** | | | |
| *Trader Joe's,* Cheddar flavor, 0.7 oz | 45 | 2 | 3 |
| *Soy Kaas:* Cheddar, 1 oz | 50 | 2 | 8 |
| Monterey Jack, 1 oz | 60 | 4 | 0 |
| *Soy Sation,* Chunks, | | | |
| all varieties, 1 oz | 60 | 3 | 2 |
| **Smoked Cheddar,** average, 1 oz | 110 | 10 | 0 |
| **Stilton,** average, 1 oz | 110 | 10 | 0 |
| **String:** | | | |
| Regular, average all brands | 80 | 6 | 0.5 |
| *Kraft,* Twist-Ums & String-ums, | | | |
| Super Long, 1 stick, 1.1 oz | 90 | 6 | 1 |
| Light/Lite: | | | |
| *Frigo,* String | 60 | 2.5 | 0.5 |
| *Polly-O,* String, | | | |
| 2% Red-Fat, 0.8 oz | 60 | 2.5 | 0 |
| *Sargento:* 1 piece, 0.8 oz | 50 | 2.5 | 1 |
| Part Skim, 0.9 oz | 70 | 4.5 | 1 |
| **Swiss:** Regular, 1 oz | 110 | 8 | 1.5 |
| *Alpine Lace,* Reduced-Fat, 0.8 oz | 70 | 4.5 | 1 |
| *Kraft Singles,* 2% Milk, 0.67 oz | 45 | 2.5 | 2 |
| **Tilsit,** 1 oz | 100 | 7.5 | 0.5 |
| **Tybo,** 1 oz | 100 | 7 | 0.5 |
| **Tofutti,** Better Than Cream Cheese, | | | |
| all varieties, 1 oz | 85 | 5 | 9 |
| **Velveeta** *(Kraft):* | | | |
| Original, 1 oz | 80 | 5 | 3 |
| Reduced Fat, 2% Milk, 1 oz | 60 | 3 | 4 |
| Extra Thick, 1.2 oz | 100 | 7 | 3 |
| Mexican: Hot, 1 oz | 90 | 6 | 3 |
| Mild, 1 oz | 80 | 6 | 3 |

### Dips/Spreads  C  F  Cb

*Per 2 Tbsp, 1 oz, Unless Indicated*
***Average All Brands***

| | C | F | Cb |
|---|---|---|---|
| Avocado/Guacamole | 45 | 4 | 2 |
| Baba Ghanoush (Eggplant/Sesame) | 70 | 6 | 2 |
| Cheese Fondue, ½ cup, 4 oz | 260 | 15 | 4 |
| French Onion Dip | 60 | 4.5 | 3 |
| Hummus: 2 Tbsp | 50 | 1 | 5 |
| ½ cup, 4.5 oz | 220 | 4.5 | 23 |
| Tzatziki (Cucumber/Yogurt) | 30 | 2.5 | 2 |
| **Clearman's**, Original Spread | 150 | 16 | 0 |
| **De La Casa**, 5 Layer Party Dip | 45 | 2.5 | 4 |
| **Fritos:** *Per 2 Tbsp* | | | |
| **Dips:** | | | |
| Chili Cheese | 45 | 3 | 3 |
| Bean; Hot Bean w/ Jalap. | 35 | 1 | 5 |
| Jalapeno Cheddar Cheese | 50 | 3.5 | 3 |
| **Guiltless Gourmet**, | | | |
| Black Bean/Spicy Black Bean Dip | 40 | 0 | 7 |
| **Heluva Good Cheese**, | | | |
| French Onion Dip, 2 Tbsp | 50 | 4.5 | 2 |
| **Hidden Valley**, | | | |
| For Everything Topping, av. | 130 | 14 | 3 |
| **Kaukauna** *(Wisconsin):* | | | |
| Spreadable Cheddar: | | | |
| Sharp/Smokey Cheddar | 80 | 6 | 3 |
| Cheese Balls, all varieties | 100 | 6 | 4 |
| Cheese Logs, all varieties | 100 | 7 | 4 |
| **Kemps:** *Per 2 Tbsp* | | | |
| **Dips:** French Onion | 60 | 5 | 2 |
| Ranch Style | 60 | 5 | 2 |
| Top The Tater, | | | |
| Taco Fiesta; Veggie Ranch | 60 | 5 | 3 |
| **Kroger,** Dips, all varieties | 60 | 5 | 2 |
| **Kraft:** *Per 2 Tbsp* | | | |
| **Dips:** Average all varieties | 60 | 5 | 3 |
| Cheez Whiz: Orig., 1.2 oz | 90 | 7 | 4 |
| Light | 80 | 3.5 | 6 |
| Salsa Con Queso | 90 | 7 | 4 |
| **Spreads:** Olive & Pimento, 1.2 oz | 70 | 6 | 3 |
| Old English Sharp; Roka Blue, av | 85 | 8 | 2 |
| **Marzetti:** *Per 2 Tbsp* | | | |
| **Dips:** Choc Fruit, 1.4 oz | 110 | 1 | 25 |
| Caramel Apple, fat free, 1.4 oz | 110 | 0 | 26 |
| Veggie: Dill, Light, 1 oz | 60 | 5 | 2 |
| Ranch, 1 oz | 110 | 12 | 2 |
| Light Ranch, 1 oz | 60 | 4.5 | 4 |

### Dips/Spreads (Cont)  C  F  Cb

*Per 2 Tbsp, 1 oz, Unless Indicated*
**Marie's:**

| | C | F | Cb |
|---|---|---|---|
| **Dips:** Buttermilk Ranch; Crmy Dill. av. | 100 | 10 | 2 |
| Guacamole | 40 | 3 | 3 |
| **Naturally Fresh:** *Per 2 Tbsp* | | | |
| **Dips:** Chocolate | 90 | 0 | 23 |
| Cream Cheese Strawb. | 90 | 3 | 15 |
| Caramel | 100 | 4 | 16 |
| **Old Dutch:** | | | |
| **Dips:** French Onion, 1 oz | 50 | 3 | 5 |
| Mild Cheddar, 1 oz | 40 | 3 | 2 |
| Nacho Cheese: 1 oz | 35 | 2.5 | 2 |
| Microwave variety ,1 oz | 80 | 6 | 3 |
| **Old El Paso:** *Per 2 Tbsp* | | | |
| **Dips:** Cheese & Red Pepper, 1 oz | 40 | 3 | 3 |
| Thick N' Chunky Salsa | 10 | 0 | 2 |
| **Price's:** *Per 2 Tbsp* | | | |
| **Dips:** Pimiento Cheese | 85 | 7 | 3 |
| Light Pimiento | 55 | 3 | 3 |
| Zesty Jalapeno | 75 | 6 | 2.5 |
| **Stop & Shop:** *Per 2 Tbsp* | | | |
| **Dips:** Veggie | 100 | 10 | 3 |
| Sour Cream French Onion | 60 | 4.5 | 2 |
| **TGI Fridays,** | | | |
| Spinach, Cheese & Artichoke Dip | 30 | 2 | 2 |
| **Toby's,** Tofu Pate, 2 Tbsp | 80 | 8 | 2 |
| **Tostitos:** *Per 2 Tbsp* | | | |
| **Dips:** Creamy Spinach, 1 oz | 50 | 4 | 2 |
| Salsa Con Quéso | 45 | 3 | 4 |
| **Wise:** *Per 2 Tbsp* | | | |
| **Dips:** French Onion, 1.2 oz | 60 | 5 | 3 |
| Spinach, 1.2 oz | 50 | 4 | 3 |

***New Diet Aid
- The Refrigerator Air Bag!***

POOF!

## Condiments, Sauces | C | F | Cb

*Average of Brands & Homemade*

| | C | F | Cb |
|---|---|---|---|
| **Apple Sauce:** | | | |
| Sweetened, ¼ cup, 2.5 oz | 55 | 0 | 13 |
| Unsweetened, ¼ cup, 2 oz | 25 | 0 | 7 |
| **Barbecue Sauce:** | | | |
| Regular, av. all flavors, 2 Tbsp, 1 oz | 40 | 0 | 10 |
| *Bull's Eye,* Original, 1 oz | 60 | 0 | 14 |
| **Bearnaise Sauce**, ¼ cup, 2.5 oz | 190 | 19 | 5 |
| **Buffalo Wing Sce:** Hon. Mustard, 1 T. | 40 | 3 | 3 |
| Average other varieties, 1 Tbsp | 25 | 2 | 2 |
| **Cheese**, h/made, ¼ cup, 2.5 oz | 150 | 10 | 12 |
| **Chef-Mate**, Hot Dog, ¼ cup | 70 | 2.5 | 9 |
| **Chili Sauce** *(Heinz)*, 1 Tbsp | 20 | 0 | 5 |
| **Cocktail Sauce:** ¼ cup | 110 | 0 | 15 |
| *Walden Farms,* Fat-Free, 1 Tbsp | 0 | 0 | 0 |
| **Cranberry Sauce**, av. all varieties: 2 T. | 45 | 0 | 11 |
| ¼ cup, 2.5 oz | 110 | 0 | 27 |
| **Demi Glaze Gold**, 2 tsp | 30 | 0.5 | 3 |
| **Honey Mustard** *(French's)*, 2 Tbsp | 60 | 0.5 | 12 |
| **Horseradish:** 1 tsp | 2 | 0 | 0 |
| *Kraft,* 1 tsp | 15 | 1.5 | 1 |
| **Ketchup:** Regular, 1 Tbsp | 15 | 0 | 4 |
| *Heinz:* Reduced Sugar, 1 Tbsp | 5 | 0 | 1 |
| Simply Heinz, 1 Tbsp | 20 | 0 | 5 |
| **Mole:** | | | |
| *Dona Maria,* av. all varieties., 2 T. | 150 | 10 | 10 |
| *Rogelio Bueno,* 2 Tbsp, 1 oz | 160 | 11 | 12 |
| **Mushroom Sce**, ½ cup, 2 oz | 50 | 2 | 5 |
| **Mustard**, average, 1 tsp | 5 | 0 | 0.5 |
| **Pesto Sauce**, ¼ cup, 2 oz | 270 | 28 | 2 |
| **Pizza Sauce**, ¼ cup, 2 oz | 30 | 0 | 6 |
| **Seafood Cocktail Sce**, ¼ cup | 60 | 0 | 15 |
| **Soy Sauce:** Average all, 1 Tbsp | 10 | 0 | 1 |
| *Kikkoman,* Lite Soy, 1 Tbsp | 10 | 0 | 1 |
| **Spaghetti Sce**, ½ cup, 4.5 oz | 135 | 6 | 19 |
| **Steak Sauce:** | | | |
| *Kraft,* A1, 1 Tbsp, 0.5 oz | 15 | 0 | 3 |
| *Lea & Perrins,* 1 Tbsp, 0.5 oz | 20 | 0 | 5 |
| **Strawb. Puree Sauce**, Unsweet., 2 T. | 10 | 0 | 2 |
| **Sweet & Sour Sauce:** | | | |
| *Contadina,* 1.2 oz | 40 | 1 | 8 |
| *Kraft,* 1 Tbsp | 60 | 0 | 13 |
| **Tabasco Sauce**, 1 tsp | 2 | 0 | 0 |
| **Taco Sauce**, average all, 2 Tbsp, 1 oz | 10 | 0 | 1 |
| **Tartar Sauce:** *(Heinz)*, 2 Tbsp, 1 oz | 120 | 11 | 4 |
| *Hellmann's,* Regular, 2 Tbsp, 1 oz | 80 | 7 | 4 |
| *McCormick,* Fat-Free, 2 Tbsp, 1 oz | 30 | 0 | 7 |
| **Teriyaki Sauce** *(Kikkoman)*, 1 T., 0.5 oz | 15 | 0 | 2 |
| **Vinegar**, White or Wine, 2 T. | 4 | 0 | 1 |
| **White Sauce**, ½ cup, 5 oz | 130 | 7 | 10 |
| **Worcestershire Sauce**, 1 tsp | 5 | 0 | 1 |

## Pickles & Relish | C | F | Cb

*Average All Brands*

| | C | F | Cb |
|---|---|---|---|
| **Bread & Butter Pickles**, 4 sl.,1 oz | 25 | 0 | 6 |
| **Chutney**, 2 Tbsp, 1.25 oz | 50 | 0.5 | 11 |
| **Dill Pickles:** | | | |
| Slices, 4 slices, 1 oz | 4 | 0 | 1 |
| 1 large, (3¾"x 1¼" diam.), 2.25 oz | 12 | 0 | 3 |
| Extra large (4"x 1¾" diam.), 5 oz | 30 | 0 | 6 |
| Halves: Small, 1 oz | 3 | 0 | 0.5 |
| Large, 2.5 oz | 8 | 0 | 2 |
| **Gherkins**, sweet, 1 medium, 1 oz | 30 | 0 | 7 |
| **Green Chiles**, chopped, 2 Tbsp | 5 | 0 | 1 |
| **Horseradish**, 1 Tbsp | 10 | 0 | 2 |
| **Jalapenos**, pickled (2), 2 oz | 10 | 0.5 | 2 |
| **Jalapeno Relish**, 1 Tbsp, 0.5 oz | 5 | 0 | 1 |
| **Mustard**, av. all brands, 1 tsp | 5 | 0 | 0.5 |
| **Peppers**, Hot/Mild (1), 1.5 oz | 20 | 0 | 4 |
| **Pickled:** Beets, ½ cup, 4 oz | 75 | 0 | 19 |
| Cocktail Onion, 1 onion | 2 | 0 | 0 |
| Red Cabbage, ½ cup, 3 oz | 65 | 0 | 15 |
| **Pickles:** Sweet, 2 Tbsp, 1 oz | 35 | 0 | 8 |
| Large (3" x ¾ diam.),1.25 oz | 40 | 0 | 10 |
| Pickle in a Pouch, 1 large | 12 | 0 | 3 |
| **Relishes:** | | | |
| Cranberry-Orange, 1 Tbsp | 30 | 0 | 7 |
| Hot Dog *(Heinz)*, 1 T., 0.5 oz | 17 | 0 | 3 |
| S'wich Spread, 1 tsp | 20 | 1 | 5 |
| Sweet Pickle, 1 Tbsp, 0.5 oz | 20 | 0 | 5 |
| Sweet Cauliflower, 1 oz | 35 | 0 | 8 |
| Sugar Free Relish, 1 tsp | 5 | 0 | 1 |
| Sweet Gherkins (2), 1 oz | 5 | 0 | 1 |
| **Sauerkraut**, | | | |
| Drained, 1 cup, 5 oz | 25 | 0 | 6 |

## Salsa

*Average all Types:*

| | C | F | Cb |
|---|---|---|---|
| Regular, w/out oil, 2 T., 1 oz | 15 | 0 | 3.5 |
| Made with oil, 2 Tbsp, 1 oz | 40 | 3 | 8 |
| **La Victoria**, 2 Tbsp, 1 oz | 10 | 0 | 2 |
| **Old El Paso**, 1 Tbsp, 1 oz | 10 | 0 | 3 |
| **TGI Friday's**, 1.2 oz | 15 | 0 | 4 |

### Quick Guide    C F Cb

**Cookies:**
**Average All Brands:** *Per Cookie*

| | C | F | Cb |
|---|---|---|---|
| **Biscotti:** Small, 0.5 oz | 70 | 3 | 10 |
| Regular, 1 oz | 140 | 6.5 | 18 |
| **Chocolate Chip:** | | | |
| Small/Thin, 0.5 oz | 70 | 3.5 | 9 |
| Regular, 1 oz | 140 | 7 | 18 |
| Large (*Mrs Fields*), 3 oz | 350 | 17 | 45 |
| Extra Large, 4 oz | 555 | 28 | 73 |
| **Oatmeal/Oatmeal Raisin:** | | | |
| Small/Thin, 0.5 oz | 65 | 2.5 | 10 |
| Regular, 1 oz | 130 | 5 | 20 |
| Large (*Mrs Fields*), 2.5 oz | 330 | 14 | 44 |
| Extra Large, 4 oz | 510 | 20 | 78 |
| **Peanut Butter:** | | | |
| Small/Thin, 0.5 oz | 70 | 3.5 | 9 |
| Regular, 1 oz | 135 | 7 | 17 |
| Large (*Mrs Fields*), 2.5 oz | 330 | 17 | 41 |
| Extra Large, 4 oz | 540 | 27 | 67 |
| **Low-Fat Cookies:** | | | |
| Choc Chip (Low-Fat), (1), 0.5 oz | 65 | 2 | 10 |
| Oatmeal Raisin (Fat-Free), (1), 1 oz | 95 | 0.5 | 22 |
| Peanut Butter (Low-Fat), (1), 1 oz | 105 | 5 | 15 |

### Quick Guide

**Crackers**
**Average All Brands:** *Per Cracker Unless Indicated*

| | C | F | Cb |
|---|---|---|---|
| **Cheese Crackers:** | | | |
| Plain, 1" square | 5 | 0 | 0.5 |
| Bag, single serving, 1 oz | 140 | 7 | 16 |
| Cheese/P'nut Butter filled | 30 | 1.5 | 4 |
| **Crispbread**, Rye | 35 | 0 | 8 |
| **Grahams**, 2½" square | 30 | 0.5 | 5 |
| **Melba Toast**, Plain, 1 piece | 20 | 0 | 4 |
| **Matzo**, Plain, 1 oz | 110 | 0.5 | 23 |
| **Oyster/Soup**, ½ cup | 95 | 2 | 17 |
| **Rice:** 1 crackers | 70 | 1.5 | 11 |
| Oriental Style, 1 oz | 130 | 3.5 | 23 |
| **Saltines**, 5 crackers | 65 | 2 | 11 |
| **Snack-type**, 1 round cracker | 15 | 1 | 2 |
| **Soda Crackers** (*Saltine*), 2 | 25 | 1 | 4.5 |
| **Water Cracker** (*Carr's*), Original | 15 | 0.5 | 2.5 |
| **Wheat:** | | | |
| Wheat Thins | 10 | 0.5 | 1.5 |
| Cheese/Peanut Butter filled | 35 | 2 | 4 |

### Cookies & Crackers ~ Brands

*Per Cookie/Cracker, Unless indicated*   C F Cb

| | C | F | Cb |
|---|---|---|---|
| **Albertsons:** | | | |
| Animal Crackers (6), 1 oz | 130 | 3.5 | 22 |
| **Chocolate Chip:** | | | |
| Original (3), 1 oz | 150 | 7 | 20 |
| Chewy (2), 1 oz | 130 | 6 | 18 |
| Chunky (1), 0.5 oz | 80 | 3.5 | 10 |
| **Chocolate S'wich Cremes:** (3) 1 oz | 150 | 6 | 25 |
| Double Filled (2), 1 oz | 140 | 6 | 22 |
| Fudge Graham (3), 1 oz | 140 | 7 | 18 |
| Fudge Wafer (3), 1 oz | 140 | 8 | 18 |
| Fudge Marshmallow Ring | 120 | 5 | 19 |
| Pinwheels, Chocolate Marshmallow | 120 | 5 | 20 |
| Vanilla Wafers (9), 1 oz | 140 | 4 | 25 |
| **Graham:** Cinnamon (2) | 150 | 3 | 28 |
| Honey (2), 1 oz | 140 | 2 | 28 |
| **Annie's:** | | | |
| **Bunny Grahams:** | | | |
| Chocolate; Choc Chip, 1 oz | 130 | 4.5 | 21 |
| Cinnamon; Honey, 1 oz | 140 | 4.5 | 23 |
| Friends, 1 oz | 130 | 4.5 | 22 |
| Gluten Free: Cocoa & Vanilla, 1 oz | 120 | 3.5 | 22 |
| SnickerDoodles, 1 oz | 130 | 4 | 21 |
| **Cheddar Bunnie Crackers:** | | | |
| Regular: | | | |
| 1 oz Snack Pack | 140 | 6 | 19 |
| 7.5 oz Box | 1050 | 45 | 145 |
| Extra Cheesy, 1 oz | 150 | 7 | 18 |
| Sour Cream & Onion, 1 oz | 150 | 7 | 19 |
| White Cheddar; Whole Wheat, 1 oz | 140 | 6 | 19 |
| **Austin:** | | | |
| **Sandwich Crackers:** *Per Package* | | | |
| Cheese: With Cheddar Cheese | 190 | 10 | 23 |
| With Peanut Butter | 190 | 9 | 23 |
| Pepper Jack | 190 | 9 | 24 |
| Toasty, with Peanut Butter | 190 | 9 | 23 |
| **Barbara's Bakery:** | | | |
| **Fig Bars:** Raspberry, 1.4 oz | 120 | 0 | 27 |
| Wheat/Multigrain | 110 | 0.5 | 26 |
| **Snackimals:** | | | |
| Choc Chip, 1 oz | 120 | 4 | 19 |
| Double Chocolate, 1 oz | 140 | 4.5 | 23 |
| Vanilla, 1 oz | 110 | 4 | 17 |
| **Bear Naked:** | | | |
| **Soft-Baked Granola,** | | | |
| Double Choc.; Fruit & Nut, av. | 130 | 6 | 19 |

## Cookies & Crackers ~ Brands (Cont)

*Per Cookie/Cracker, Unless Indicated* **C** **F** **Cb**

**BelVita (Nabisco):**
**Breakfast Biscuits:**

| | C | F | Cb |
|---|---|---|---|
| Crunchy, 1 pack (4 biscuits), average | 230 | 8 | 36 |
| Soft Baked, 1 biscuit, average | 190 | 7 | 32 |
| **Bites**, (46), 1.8 oz | 230 | 8 | 36 |

**Blue Diamond:**

| | C | F | Cb |
|---|---|---|---|
| **Nut Thins**, (17), average all varieties | 130 | 3 | 23 |
| **Artisan Nut Thins**, (13), av. all var. | 130 | 3.5 | 22 |

**Brent & Sam's:**
**Natural:** *Per 2 Cookies*

| | C | F | Cb |
|---|---|---|---|
| Chocolate Chip Pecan | 130 | 7 | 14 |
| Key Lime White Chocolate | 120 | 6 | 16 |
| Triple Chocolate Bliss, 1 oz | 120 | 6 | 16 |

**Soft & Chewy:** *Per 1 Cookie*

| | C | F | Cb |
|---|---|---|---|
| Choc Chunk | 130 | 5 | 20 |
| Oatmeal Raisin | 140 | 6 | 20 |
| Snickerdoodle | 130 | 4 | 21 |

| | C | F | Cb |
|---|---|---|---|
| **Carr's:** Poppy & Sesame Crackers(4) | 80 | 4 | 10 |
| Rosemary Crackers(4) | 70 | 2.5 | 11 |
| Whole Wheat Crackers (2) | 80 | 4 | 10 |

**Cheez•It** ~ *See Sunshine, Page 87*
**Chips Ahoy!** ~ *See Nabisco, Page 85*
**Country Choice:**
Sandwich Cremes (2),

| | C | F | Cb |
|---|---|---|---|
| all varieties | 130 | 5 | 19 |

**Snacking:**

| | C | F | Cb |
|---|---|---|---|
| Ginger Snaps (5); Vanilla Wafers (7) | 140 | 5 | 22 |
| Iced Oatmeal (4) | 120 | 4 | 21 |

**Dr. Kracker:**
**Crispbread:**

| | C | F | Cb |
|---|---|---|---|
| 100% Whole Wheat (1) | 80 | 1 | 16 |
| Average other varieties (1) | 100 | 4 | 12 |
| **Snackers**, average all varieties (8) | 125 | 5 | 15 |

**Erin Baker's:**
**Original Breakfast:** *Per 3 oz*

| | C | F | Cb |
|---|---|---|---|
| Banana Walnut | 300 | 8 | 53 |
| Peanut Butter | 320 | 11 | 49 |

**Minis:** *Per 1 oz Cookie*

| | C | F | Cb |
|---|---|---|---|
| Peanut Butter | 110 | 3.5 | 16 |
| Dble Chocolate; Oatmeal Raisin, av. | 100 | 2 | 18 |

**Famous Amos:**
**Bite Size:** Choc. Chip,

| | C | F | Cb |
|---|---|---|---|
| 4 Cookies, 1 oz | 150 | 7 | 20 |
| Choc. Chip & Pecans (4) | 150 | 8 | 18 |
| Sandwich, Creme Filled, Choc.; Vanilla, 3 cookies, 1 oz | 170 | 7 | 25 |

*Per Cookie/Cracker, Unless Indicated* **C** **F** **Cb**

**Fig Newtons** ~ *See Nabisco, Page 85*

**Fifty50:**

| | C | F | Cb |
|---|---|---|---|
| Butter (4) | 190 | 9 | 24 |
| Average other varieties (4) | 165 | 9 | 22 |
| Wafers, average all varieties, (6) | 160 | 9 | 22 |

**Gamesa:**

| | C | F | Cb |
|---|---|---|---|
| Animalitos, 14 cookies, 1 oz | 110 | 1 | 25 |
| Arcoiris Marshmallow, 2 oz pkg, 6 cookies | 220 | 5 | 38 |
| Chocolatines Marshmallow, 2 cookies, 1 oz | 130 | 5 | 18 |
| Chokis, Chocolate Chip, 1.4 oz pkg | 190 | 9 | 27 |
| Emperador: Cream Cookie Sandwich Lemon Creme, 1 pkg, 6 cookies | 270 | 8 | 45 |
| Av. other flavors, 1 pkg, 6 cookies | 360 | 12 | 57 |
| Fruitbars, average, 1 cookie, 1 oz | 110 | 4.5 | 18 |
| Giro, 3 cookies, 1 oz | 140 | 6 | 20 |
| Mamut, Choc Marshmallow, 1 cookie, 1 oz | 130 | 5 | 19 |
| Marias, 8 cookies, 1 oz | 120 | 2 | 24 |
| Sugar Wafers, average, 3 wafers, 1.2 oz | 160 | 7 | 25 |

**Girl Scouts Cookies:**

| | C | F | Cb |
|---|---|---|---|
| Caramel DeLites/Samoas (2) | 130 | 6 | 19 |
| Do-si-dos (3) | 160 | 7 | 22 |
| Peanut Butter Patties (2) | 130 | 7 | 15 |
| Savannah Smiles (5) | 140 | 5 | 23 |

**Goya:**

| | C | F | Cb |
|---|---|---|---|
| **Lady Fingers**, 3 cookies | 65 | 0.5 | 13 |
| **Maria**, 5 cookies, 1 oz | 130 | 3 | 24 |
| **Wafers**, average all flavors, 4 wafers, 1 oz | 150 | 7 | 20 |

**Grandma's:**
**Frosted**,

| | C | F | Cb |
|---|---|---|---|
| average all flavors (1) | 230 | 9 | 34 |

**Homestyle:** *Per Cookie*

| | C | F | Cb |
|---|---|---|---|
| Chocolate Brownie | 160 | 7 | 23 |
| Chocolate Chip | 170 | 9 | 22 |
| Oatmeal Raisin | 150 | 6 | 23 |
| Peanut Butter | 170 | 9 | 19 |

**Sandwich Cremes:**

| | C | F | Cb |
|---|---|---|---|
| Peanut Butter (5) | 200 | 9 | 25 |
| Vanilla (5) | 190 | 9 | 27 |
| Mini's, Vanilla Flavored (9) | 150 | 7 | 22 |

## Cookies & Crackers ~ Brands (Cont)

*Per Cookie/Cracker, Unless Indicated*

| | C | F | Cb |
|---|---|---|---|
| **Great American Cookies:** | | | |
| Chewy Chocolate Supreme | 180 | 7 | 27 |
| Chewy Pecan Supreme | 230 | 12 | 31 |
| Double Fudge with Reese's | 230 | 11 | 33 |
| Original, w/ Reese's or M&M's | 240 | 12 | 31 |
| Peanut Butter w/ M&M's | 250 | 13 | 28 |
| White Chunk Macadamia | 250 | 14 | 30 |
| **Double Doozies:** | | | |
| Original, 5.3 oz | 690 | 34 | 94 |
| M&M Big Bite, 2.5 oz | 340 | 17 | 46 |
| **Cookie Cakes:** | | | |
| 16", 3.5 oz | 460 | 22 | 67 |
| 16" M&M, 4 oz | 500 | 24 | 73 |
| Heart Shaped, 3.5 oz | 440 | 21 | 64 |
| **Great Value** *(Walmart)*: | | | |
| Chocolate Chip (1) | 150 | 7 | 21 |
| Devil's Food (1) | 50 | 0 | 12 |
| Double Filled, Switch Aroos | | | |
| Chocolate & Vanilla (1) | 150 | 6 | 21 |
| Fudge Marshmallow (1) | 120 | 5 | 19 |
| Soft Cookies, Fudge & Cream (1) | 150 | 6 | 22 |
| Twist & Shout, Choc.; Vanilla (1), 1.3 oz | 160 | 6 | 25 |
| Buttery Rounds: Baked (5) | 80 | 4.5 | 10 |
| Reduced Fat (5) | 70 | 2 | 11 |
| Cheese Crackers, 1 oz | 150 | 8 | 18 |
| **Joseph's:** | | | |
| **Sugar Free:** *Per 4 Cookies* | | | |
| Almond; Chocolate Walnut, average | 95 | 3.5 | 14 |
| Chocolate Chip; Pecan Choc. Chip, av. | 95 | 5 | 14 |
| Average other varieties | 95 | 4 | 15 |
| *Carb figures include 6 grams Maltitol* | | | |
| **Kashi:** | | | |
| Chocolate Almond Butter | 130 | 5 | 19 |
| Happy Trail Mix, Chewy | 140 | 5 | 21 |
| Oatmeal: Dark Chocolate | 130 | 5 | 20 |
| Raisin Flax | 120 | 4.5 | 20 |
| **Crackers:** | | | |
| Original 7 Grain (15) | 120 | 3.5 | 19 |
| Fire Roasted Veggie (15) | 120 | 3.5 | 19 |
| Pita Crisps: | | | |
| Original 7 Grain with Salt (11) | 120 | 3 | 22 |
| Garlic Pesto (11) | 120 | 3 | 23 |

*Per Cookie/Cracker, Unless Indicated*

| | C | F | Cb |
|---|---|---|---|
| **Keebler:** | | | |
| **Animals**, Frosted (8) | 160 | 7 | 22 |
| **Chips Deluxe:** Original (2) | 160 | 8 | 19 |
| Chocolate Lovers (2) | 170 | 9 | 20 |
| Coconut (2) | 160 | 9 | 18 |
| Peanut Butter Cups (2) | 170 | 9 | 19 |
| Soft & Chewy (2) | 140 | 6 | 21 |
| **Rainbow:** Triple Choc. Chip (2) | 150 | 8 | 19 |
| Choc Chip Minis, 1.4 oz pkg | 200 | 10 | 27 |
| **Danish Wedding**, (4) | 140 | 7 | 19 |
| **E.L. Fudge:** Original (2) | 170 | 7 | 25 |
| Double Stuffed (2) | 180 | 9 | 24 |
| **Fudge Shoppe:** | | | |
| Cheesecake Middles, Orig. Grahams (3) | 130 | 7 | 17 |
| Deluxe Grahams (3) | 140 | 7 | 18 |
| Fudge Sticks: | | | |
| Original (3) | 150 | 8 | 20 |
| Jumbo (1) | 160 | 8 | 21 |
| Fudge Stripes: Original (2) | 150 | 7 | 21 |
| Dark Chocolate (3) | 170 | 9 | 20 |
| Filled Pretzel Bites, | | | |
| Peanut Butter & Fudge, | | | |
| average, 1 pkg | 170 | 9 | 21 |
| Grasshopper (4) | 140 | 7 | 20 |
| Mint Creme Middles, Choc. Graham (3) | 130 | 7 | 17 |
| **Gripz**, Chips Deluxe, 0.9 oz pouch | 120 | 5 | 18 |
| **Oatmeal**, (2), average all varieties | 140 | 6 | 20 |
| **Sandies Cookies:** | | | |
| Dark Choc. Almond; Pecan Shtbrd, av. | 170 | 10 | 19 |
| Fudge Dipped Shortbreads, | | | |
| 0.75 oz pkg | 100 | 4 | 15 |
| Average other varieites | 160 | 9 | 19 |
| **Vienna Fingers:** | | | |
| Creme Filled (2) | 150 | 6 | 23 |
| Reduced Fat (2) | 140 | 4.5 | 24 |
| **Wafers:** Vanilla (8) | 140 | 5 | 22 |
| Mini Vanilla (18) | 140 | 5 | 22 |
| **Crackers:** | | | |
| **Club:** Original (4) | 70 | 3 | 9 |
| Reduced Fat (5) | 70 | 2 | 12 |
| **Grahams:** Original (8) | 120 | 3.5 | 22 |
| Honey (8) | 140 | 4.5 | 23 |
| **Town House:** Original (5) | 90 | 5 | 9 |
| Reduced Fat (6) | 60 | 1.5 | 12 |

## Cookies & Crackers ~ Brands (Cont)

*Per Cookie/Cracker, Unless Indicated* **C** **F** **Cb**

| | C | F | Cb |
|---|---|---|---|
| **Kraft,** Macaroni & Cheese Crackers, av. all varieties, 1. oz | 150 | 7 | 18 |
| **Kroger:** | | | |
| **Chip Mates:** Orig. (3), 1.5 oz | 150 | 7 | 22 |
| Chunky (2), 1 oz | 120 | 6 | 17 |
| Peanut Butter (2), 1 oz | 120 | 7 | 15 |
| White Chip (2), 1 oz | 120 | 6 | 16 |
| **Chocolate Sandwich:** | | | |
| Original (3), 1.2 oz | 150 | 6 | 24 |
| Double Filled (2), 1 oz | 140 | 6 | 22 |
| Olde Southern Pecan Shortbread (2) | 150 | 9 | 16 |
| Vanilla Wafers (7) | 130 | 3.5 | 23 |
| **Crackers:** | | | |
| Grahams, Orig.; Honey, (4) | 120 | 3 | 20 |
| Saltines, Original (5), 0.5oz | 60 | 1.5 | 10 |
| **Lance:** | | | |
| **Cookies:** | | | |
| **6 Pack:** *Per Pack of 6 Cookies* | | | |
| Choc-O-Lunch/Van-O-Lunch, av. | 225 | 9 | 34 |
| Nekot, Peanut Butter | 240 | 11 | 32 |
| **Crackers:** | | | |
| **Cracker Sandwiches:** *Per 6 Crackers* | | | |
| Malt, with Peanut Butter Filling | 180 | 8 | 20 |
| Nip Chee, Cheddar Cheese | 190 | 9 | 24 |
| Toastchee, Peanut Butter | 210 | 10 | 25 |
| Toasty, Peanut Butter | 210 | 10 | 25 |
| Wholegrain, Cheddar Cheese | 200 | 9 | 26 |
| **Little Debbie:** | | | |
| Apple Oatmeal Pies (1) | 140 | 4.5 | 24 |
| Chocolate Chip Cream Pie (1) | 150 | 6 | 23 |
| Cookie Wreaths (1) | 100 | 5 | 12 |
| Marshmallow Puffs | 150 | 5 | 25 |
| Oatmeal Creme Pie (1) | 170 | 7 | 26 |
| Star Crunch(1) | 150 | 6 | 22 |

| | C | F | Cb |
|---|---|---|---|
| **Lu:** | | | |
| Petit Beurre (1), 1.2 oz | 140 | 4 | 24 |
| Petit Ecolier, av. all var., (1), 0.9 oz | 130 | 6 | 17 |
| Pim's, Raspberry (1), 0.9 oz | 100 | 3 | 16 |
| **Manischewitz:** | | | |
| **Crackers:** | | | |
| Tam Tams: Original (10) | 110 | 4 | 16 |
| Everything; Garlic (1), av. | 140 | 5 | 20 |
| **Mary's Gone Crackers:** | | | |
| **Cookies:** | | | |
| Chocolate Chip; Double Choc (2) | 130 | 6 | 19 |
| Ginger Snaps (3) | 140 | 5 | 23 |
| "N'Oatmeal" Raisin without Oats (2) | 120 | 4 | 20 |
| **Crackers,** all varieties (13), 1 oz | 140 | 5 | 21 |
| **Miss Meringue:** | | | |
| **Madeleines:** | | | |
| Traditional (2), 1.2 oz | 160 | 9 | 19 |
| Traditional & Dipped (2), 1.2 oz | 160 | 9 | 18 |
| **Meringue Classiques:** | | | |
| Cappuccino (4), 1 oz | 110 | 0 | 26 |
| Mint Choc. Chip (4), 1 oz | 120 | 1.5 | 25 |
| Triple Chocolate (4), 1 oz | 120 | 1.5 | 25 |
| Vanilla Rainbow/Van. (4), 1 oz | 110 | 0 | 27 |
| **Meringue Minis,** Low Fat: | | | |
| Mini: Choc. Chip (12), 1 oz | 130 | 1.5 | 27 |
| Mint Choc. Chip (12), 1 oz | 120 | 1.5 | 26 |
| **Meringue Minis,** Fat Free: | | | |
| Chocolate (12), 1 oz | 110 | 0 | 26 |
| Vanilla; Rainbow Vanilla (13), 1 oz | 110 | 0 | 27 |
| **Mother's:** | | | |
| Chocolate Chip (4), 1 oz | 150 | 7 | 20 |
| Circus Animal (7), 1 oz | 150 | 7 | 20 |
| Coconut Cocadas (5), 1.2 oz | 160 | 8 | 21 |
| Double Fudge (2), 1.3 oz | 190 | 8 | 27 |
| Iced: Lemonade (4), 1 oz | 150 | 7 | 19 |
| Oatmeal (4), 1.2 oz | 150 | 6 | 23 |
| Macaroons (2), 1 oz | 180 | 11 | 18 |
| Peanut Butter Gauchos (2), 1.3 oz | 190 | 9 | 26 |
| Taffy; Vanilla Cream (2), av., 1.3 oz | 195 | 9 | 27 |

**Mrs Fields Cookies** ~ *See Page 219*

## Cookies & Crackers ~ Brands (Cont)

*Per Cookie/Cracker, Unless Indicated* **C** **F** **Cb**

**Nabisco:**

| | C | F | Cb |
|---|---|---|---|
| **Cookies:** | | | |
| **100 Calorie Packs:** | | | |
| Chips A'hoy!, Thin Crisps, | | | |
| Baked, (6), 0.8 oz | 100 | 3 | 18 |
| Lorna Doone, | | | |
| Shortbread Cookie Crisps (6), 0.7 oz | 100 | 3 | 16 |
| Oreo, Thin Crisps (6), 0.8 oz | 100 | 2 | 19 |
| **Chips Ahoy!,** Chocolate Chip: | | | |
| Original: | | | |
| 2 cookies, 1.1 oz | 160 | 8 | 22 |
| Single Serve, 1.4 oz | 190 | 9 | 27 |
| Reduced Fat (2), 1.2 oz | 150 | 6 | 24 |
| Candy Blasts (2),1.2 oz | 180 | 9 | 22 |
| Chewy (2), av. all varieties, 1.1 oz | 140 | 6 | 21 |
| Chunky, Choc. Chunk (2), 1.2 oz | 160 | 8 | 20 |
| Ice Cream Creations, av., (2), 1 oz | 140 | 6 | 21 |
| Mini Choc. Chips: 1.1 oz | 150 | 7 | 21 |
| 3 oz Package | 450 | 21 | 63 |
| Go-Pak, 3.5 oz | 525 | 25 | 74 |
| **Lorna Doone,** Shorbread, 1.5 oz | 210 | 10 | 28 |
| **Mallomars,** (1), 1 oz | 120 | 5 | 18 |
| **Newtons:** | | | |
| **100% Whole Grain:** | | | |
| Fig (2), 1 oz | 110 | 2 | 23 |
| Other varieties (2), 1 oz | 100 | 1.5 | 21 |
| **Original Fig:** 2 cookies, 1 oz | 110 | 2 | 22 |
| Fat-Free, 2 cookies, 1 oz | 100 | 0 | 23 |
| **Fruit Thins,** Crispy (3), all var., 1 oz | 140 | 5 | 21 |
| **Nilla Wafers:** | | | |
| 8 wafers, 1 oz | 140 | 6 | 21 |
| Reduced-Fat (8), 1 oz | 120 | 2 | 24 |
| **Nutter Butter,** Peanut Butter Sandwich: | | | |
| 16 oz package, 1 cookie 1 oz | 130 | 5 | 20 |
| 4.8 oz package, 2 cookies, 0.9 oz | 120 | 5 | 17 |
| 1.9 oz package, 4 cookies | 250 | 10 | 37 |
| **Bites,** | | | |
| Big Bag; Go-Paks!, 3 oz pkg | 420 | 18 | 63 |
| **Oreo, Chocolate/Golden:** *Average all Fillings* | | | |
| 2 cookies | 140 | 7 | 21 |
| 3 cookies | 160 | 7 | 25 |
| Single Serve package (6), 2 oz | 270 | 11 | 41 |
| 5.25 oz package, 15 cookies | 800 | 35 | 125 |
| Reduced Fat (3), 1.2 oz | 150 | 5 | 26 |
| Thins (4), 1 oz | 140 | 6 | 21 |

*Per Cookie/Cracker, Unless Indicated* **C** **F** **Cb**

**Nabisco (Cont):**

| **Oreo, Choc./Golden (Cont):** *Average all Fillings* | C | F | Cb |
|---|---|---|---|
| Sugar Free, 1 cookie | 50 | 2.5 | 5 |
| Mini Bite: Single Sve pkg, 1.25 oz | 170 | 7 | 25 |
| Go-Paks, 3.5 oz | 455 | 21 | 74 |
| Double Stuf: 2 cookies, 1 oz | 140 | 7 | 21 |
| Single Serve, 1.5 oz | 210 | 10 | 30 |
| King Size (2), 1 oz | 140 | 7 | 21 |
| Fudge Cremes, average all varieties: | | | |
| 1 cookie | 60 | 3 | 8 |
| 3 cookies | 180 | 9 | 24 |
| **Teddy Grahams, 10 oz Box:** | | | |
| Snacks: Honey; Cinnamon (24), 1 oz | 130 | 4 | 23 |
| Chocolate (24), av. all var., 1 oz | 130 | 4 | 22 |
| **Crackers:** | | | |
| **Barnum's Animals:** | | | |
| 8 crackers, 1 oz | 120 | 3.5 | 22 |
| Snack Saks (17), 1 oz | 140 | 4 | 24 |
| **Cheese Nips:** | | | |
| Cheddar: 1 oz | 150 | 6 | 19 |
| Reduced Fat, 1 oz | 130 | 3.5 | 21 |
| Angry Birds; Avengers, 1 oz | 130 | 4.5 | 21 |
| Mini, Despicable Me, 1 oz Pack | 130 | 4 | 19 |
| **Honey Maid:** | | | |
| Grahamfuls, av. all var., 0.9 oz pkg | 115 | 5 | 18 |
| Grahams (8), average all var., 1 oz | 130 | 3 | 24 |
| **Premium:** | | | |
| Saltine: Original, 5 crackers, 0.5 oz | 70 | 1.5 | 12 |
| Unsalted Tops (5), 0.5 oz | 70 | 1.5 | 13 |
| Round; Unsalted Tops (6), 0.5 oz | 60 | 1.5 | 12 |
| **Triscuit:** | | | |
| Original, 6 crackers, 1 oz | 120 | 4 | 20 |
| Reduced Fat (7), 1.1 oz | 110 | 2.5 | 21 |
| Brown Rice (6), av. all varieties, 1 oz | 130 | 4.5 | 21 |
| Brown Rice & Wheat, | | | |
| Rstd Red Pepp. & Red Bean (6), 1 oz | 130 | 3 | 22 |
| Minis, | | | |
| Thin Crisps (10), all varieties, 1 oz | 130 | 3 | 23 |
| **Wheat Thins:** *Per 9 oz Box* | | | |
| Original (14), 1.1 oz | 140 | 5 | 22 |
| Av. other flav. (14), 1.1 oz | 140 | 5 | 21 |
| Multigrain (14), 1.1 oz | 130 | 4 | 22 |
| Flatbread, Garlic & Parsley, | | | |
| 0.5 oz serving | 60 | 1.5 | 12 |
| **Wheatsworth,** | | | |
| Stone Ground Wheat (5) | 80 | 4 | 10 |

*Per Cookie/Cracker, Unless Indicated* **C** **F** **Cb**

**Newman's Own Organics:**

| | C | F | Cb |
|---|---|---|---|
| **Alphabet:** Chocolate (10) | 110 | 3 | 21 |
| Other varieties (10) | 120 | 3 | 21 |
| **Chocolate Cups:** | | | |
| Milk/Dark: | | | |
| Peanut Butter (3), average | 180 | 13 | 17 |
| Dark Chocolate Peppermint (3) | 180 | 11 | 19 |
| **Family Recipe,** Ginger Snaps, | | | |
| 5 cookies, 1 oz | 130 | 3.5 | 24 |
| **Fig Newman's:** | | | |
| Fat-Free, 2 bars | 100 | 0 | 24 |
| Low-Fat, 2 bars | 110 | 1.5 | 23 |
| Wheat/Dairy-Free, 2 bars | 120 | 1.5 | 26 |
| **Newman-O's:** Original (2) | 130 | 5 | 20 |
| Chocolate/ Mint Creme, av., (2) | 125 | 5 | 20 |

**Nonni's:**

**Biscotti:**

| | C | F | Cb |
|---|---|---|---|
| Original; Decadence, | | | |
| average, 1 piece, 0.8 oz | 95 | 4 | 15 |
| Average other varieties, (1), 0.8 oz | 110 | 4 | 17 |
| Bites: Almond Dark Chocolate (3) | 120 | 6 | 16 |
| Berry Almond (3) | 110 | 4 | 18 |
| Double Choc. Salted Caramel (3) | 110 | 4 | 18 |

**Oreo Cookies** ~ See Nabisco, Page 85

**Payaso:**

| | C | F | Cb |
|---|---|---|---|
| **Animalitos,** 19 pieces | 120 | 1.5 | 23 |
| **Marias,** (8), 1 oz | 120 | 2.5 | 22 |
| **Orejitas Finas,** (4) | 100 | 5 | 13 |

**Pepperidge Farm:**

**Cookies:**

**100 Calorie Pouches,**

| | C | F | Cb |
|---|---|---|---|
| average all varieties, 1 pouch | 100 | 4.5 | 12 |

**American Collection:** *Per Cookie*

| | C | F | Cb |
|---|---|---|---|
| Chesapeake, Dark Chocolate Pecan | 130 | 7 | 16 |
| Lexington, Milk Chocolate, | | | |
| Toffee Almond | 130 | 6 | 17 |
| Nantucket: Dark Chocolate | 130 | 6 | 18 |
| Double | 140 | 7 | 19 |
| Sausalito, Milk Choc. Macadamia | 130 | 7 | 17 |
| Tahoe, | | | |
| White Choc. Macadamia | 130 | 7 | 17 |
| **Brussels,** (3) | 150 | 7 | 20 |
| **Classic Favorites,** (3) | 140 | 7 | 18 |
| **Geneva,** (3) | 160 | 7 | 19 |

*Per Cookie/Cracker, Unless Indicated* **C** **F** **Cb**

**Pepperidge Farm (Cont):**

**Cookies (Cont):**

| | C | F | Cb |
|---|---|---|---|
| **Milano:** Milk Chocolate (3) | 170 | 9 | 21 |
| Double Chocolate (2) | 140 | 8 | 17 |
| Mint; Orange; Raspb. (2), av. | 130 | 7 | 16 |
| Melts (2), av. all varieties | 145 | 8 | 18 |
| Slices (3), av. all varieties | 150 | 8 | 18 |
| **Pirouettes,** (2), av. all var. | 120 | 5 | 19 |
| **Tahiti,** Coconut (2) | 170 | 10 | 17 |

**Crackers:**

**Baked:**

| | C | F | Cb |
|---|---|---|---|
| Four Cheese Crisps (20) | 140 | 6 | 19 |
| Cracker Chips: | | | |
| Cheddar (27) | 130 | 3 | 23 |
| Cheddar & Sour Cream (25) | 130 | 4.5 | 21 |
| Classic BBQ (26) | 130 | 3.5 | 23 |
| Zesty Chili & Lime (24) | 130 | 4 | 23 |
| **Golden Butter,** (4) | 70 | 2 | 10 |
| **Harvest Wheat,** (4) | 100 | 4 | 14 |

**Ritz:**

| | C | F | Cb |
|---|---|---|---|
| Original (5), 0.5 oz | 80 | 4.5 | 10 |
| Reduced Fat (5), 0.5 oz | 70 | 2 | 11 |
| Bacon; Garlic Butter (5), 0.5 oz | 80 | 4 | 10 |
| Whole Wheat (5), 0.5 oz | 70 | 2.5 | 11 |
| **Toasted Chips:** | | | |
| Original (14), 1 oz | 130 | 4.5 | 21 |
| Cheddar; Sour Cream & Onion, | | | |
| (14), 1 oz | 140 | 6 | 19 |

**Safeway Select:**

| | C | F | Cb |
|---|---|---|---|
| **Homestyle,** Oatmeal Raisin, 1 oz | 130 | 6 | 18 |
| **Indulgent:** Double Choc Chunk, 1 oz | 130 | 7 | 18 |
| Milk Chocolate Macadamia Nut, 1 oz | 140 | 8 | 17 |

**Gourmet Sandwich Cremes:**

| | C | F | Cb |
|---|---|---|---|
| Maple Creme (2), 1 oz | 170 | 7 | 25 |
| Raspberry Swirl (2), 1 oz | 130 | 5 | 20 |
| Strawberry Swirl (2), 1 oz | 130 | 6 | 19 |

**Sedano's:**

| | C | F | Cb |
|---|---|---|---|
| **Cinnamon,** 5 cookies | 160 | 6 | 24 |
| **Maria,** 5 cookies, 1 oz | 120 | 3 | 22 |

**Shar Gluten Free** ~ See CalorieKing.com

**Special K:** *Per 1 oz Serving*

| | C | F | Cb |
|---|---|---|---|
| Crackers, Multigrain (24) | 120 | 3 | 23 |
| Cracker Chips, av. all varieties | 120 | 4 | 22 |

## Cookies & Crackers ~ Brands (Cont)

*Per Cookie/Cracker, Unless Indicated* **C** **F** **Cb**

**Stella D'Oro:**

| | C | F | Cb |
|---|---|---|---|
| Biscotti, av. all varieties, 0.8 oz | 100 | 4.5 | 13 |
| Breakfast Treats (1), av. all var. | 90 | 3 | 15 |
| Margherite: Chocolate (2) | 130 | 6 | 19 |
| Vanilla (2) | 120 | 4 | 20 |
| Roman Egg Biscuits, 1 oz | 130 | 4.5 | 19 |
| Swiss Fudge (3) | 170 | 9 | 22 |

**Toast & Sponge:**

| | C | F | Cb |
|---|---|---|---|
| Almond Toast (2) | 100 | 2 | 20 |
| Anisette Sponge (3) | 90 | 1 | 18 |
| Anisette Toast (3), 1 oz | 130 | 1 | 27 |

**Streit's:**

**Flavored Wafers:**

| | C | F | Cb |
|---|---|---|---|
| Chocolate (3) | 160 | 9 | 19 |
| Lemon (3) | 170 | 10 | 19 |
| Rolls, Chocolate Cream filled (3) | 105 | 6 | 12 |

**Sunshine:**

**Cheez-It Snack:**

| | C | F | Cb |
|---|---|---|---|
| Original (27), 1 oz | 150 | 8 | 17 |
| 1.25 oz bag | 180 | 9 | 20 |
| Colby (25) | 150 | 8 | 18 |
| Average other varieties (25), 1 oz | 145 | 8 | 18 |
| **Big:** Original,(13) | 150 | 8 | 17 |
| Monterey Jack (14), 1 oz | 150 | 8 | 17 |
| **Reduced Fat:** Original (29), 1 oz | 130 | 4.5 | 20 |
| White Cheddar (25), 1 oz | 130 | 4 | 22 |

**Trader Joe's:**

| | C | F | Cb |
|---|---|---|---|
| 100 Calorie Packs, average | 100 | 2.5 | 18 |
| Almond Windmill (2), 1 oz | 140 | 6 | 18 |
| Charmingly Chewy Choc Chip (2), 1 oz | 130 | 5 | 20 |
| Cherry Granola (2), 1 oz | 110 | 4 | 18 |
| **Chocolate Chip:** Small (4), 1 oz | 140 | 7 | 18 |
| Large, singles, 1.7 oz | 280 | 14 | 35 |
| Vegan (1), 1 oz | 130 | 6 | 18 |
| Caramel Cashew (3), 1 oz | 140 | 7 | 16 |
| Crispy Crunchy Choc Chip (12) | 150 | 9 | 19 |
| Crispy Oatmeal Choc Chip (12) | 150 | 7 | 19 |
| Dark Choc Chunks with almonds (3) | 140 | 7 | 17 |
| Dunkers: Chocolate Chip (2), 1.2 oz | 160 | 7 | 21 |
| Choc. Coated Choc. Chip (2), 1.3 oz | 190 | 9 | 25 |

*Per Cookie/Cracker, Unless Indicated* **C** **F** **Cb**

**Trader Joe's (Cont):**

| | C | F | Cb |
|---|---|---|---|
| Ginger Snaps, Gluten Free (5), 1 oz | 140 | 6 | 21 |
| Highbrow Chocolate (2) | 140 | 7 | 17 |
| Joe Joe's S'wich Cremes, Choc./ Vanilla (2), 1 oz | 130 | 6 | 19 |
| Macarons A La Parisienne (2) | 90 | 3 | 10 |
| Meringues, Vanilla (4) | 110 | 0 | 27 |
| Oatmeal Raisin, 1.8 oz | 270 | 12 | 35 |
| Pecan S'thrn Style (4), 1 oz | 150 | 9 | 15 |
| **Thins:** Meyer Lemon (9) | 130 | 4.5 | 22 |
| Toasted Coconut (8) | 130 | 4.5 | 22 |
| Triple Choc Chunk, 1 oz | 140 | 7 | 20 |
| Ultimate Vanilla Wafers (5) | 120 | 6 | 15 |
| Way More Chocolate Chip (3) | 160 | 11 | 14 |
| **Crackers,** Water (4) | 60 | 1 | 12 |

**Triscuits** ~ *See Page 85*

**Voortman:**

| | C | F | Cb |
|---|---|---|---|
| **Classics:** Almond Krunch (2), 1 oz | 140 | 6 | 20 |
| Chunky Chip (1), 0.8 oz | 100 | 4.5 | 14 |
| **Sugar Free:** Chocolate Chip (1), 0.7 oz | 80 | 5 | 13 |
| Shortbread Swirls (1) | 100 | 6 | 12 |
| **Wafers:** Coconut Creme (1) | 140 | 6 | 20 |
| Sugar Free, P'nut Buter Wafer (4) | 130 | 7 | 19 |

*Note: Carb figures include 4-6g of sugar alcohols*

**Whole Foods (365 Organic):**

| | C | F | Cb |
|---|---|---|---|
| Choc Chip (2), 1 oz | 150 | 7 | 21 |
| Classic Fig Bars (2), 1.3 oz | 140 | 2.5 | 27 |
| Lemon Wafers (7), 1 oz | 110 | 3 | 19 |
| Oatmeal (2), 1 oz | 130 | 4.5 | 20 |
| S'wich Cremes; Sugar (2), average | 130 | 5 | 20 |

**WhoNu?:**

| | C | F | Cb |
|---|---|---|---|
| Original Cookie (3), 1.3 oz | 160 | 7 | 22 |
| 2X Chocolate (2), 1.1 oz | 140 | 6 | 21 |
| Chocolate/Vanilla S'wich (3), 1.3 oz | 150 | 6 | 24 |
| Soft & Chewy, Chocolate Chip Cookie, (3) 1.5 oz | 150 | 6 | 24 |

## Cookie ~ Mixes

*Prepared as Directed*

**Betty Crocker:**

**Pouch Mix:** *Per 2 Cookies*

| | C | F | Cb |
|---|---|---|---|
| Double Choc. Chunk; P'nut Butter, av. | 140 | 6 | 21 |
| Walnut Chocolate Chip | 170 | 9 | 20 |
| Average other varieties | 145 | 6 | 22 |

**Duncan Hines,**

| | C | F | Cb |
|---|---|---|---|
| Chocolate Chip, 2 cookies, 1 oz | 180 | 9 | 23 |

## Thaw, Bake & Serve  **C** **F** **Cb**

*Per Cookie/Cracker Unless Indicated*

**Pillsbury Cookies:**

**Refrigerated Cookie Dough:** *Per Cookie*

| | C | F | Cb |
|---|---|---|---|
| Chocolate Chip Cookie | 130 | 6 | 18 |
| Create N Bake, | | | |
| Peppermint Sugar Cookies | 100 | 4.5 | 14 |
| Peanut Butter | 120 | 5 | 17 |
| Sugar, Regular | 120 | 5 | 18 |

**Ready To Bake:**

Big Deluxe Classics:

| | C | F | Cb |
|---|---|---|---|
| Chocolate Chip (1) | 170 | 8 | 23 |
| Oatmeal Raisin (1) | 150 | 6 | 24 |
| Peanut Butter Cup (1) | 160 | 7 | 22 |
| White Chunk Macadamia (1) | 170 | 9 | 22 |
| Simply Cookies: Choc. Chip (1) | 150 | 7 | 20 |
| Peanut Butter (1) | 140 | 6 | 19 |
| Chocolate Chip (2) | 170 | 8 | 23 |
| Choc. Chunk & Chip (2) | 170 | 8 | 23 |
| Holiday Cookies, Sugar, | | | |
| average all shapes, (2) | 120 | 6 | 15 |
| Oatmeal Chocolate Chip (2) | 160 | 7 | 24 |

**Refrigerated Sweet Buns/Rolls~** *See Page 67*

**Toll House (Nestle):**

**Refrigerated Dough Bars:** *Per Cookie*

| | C | F | Cb |
|---|---|---|---|
| Chocolate Chip | 90 | 4.5 | 11 |
| Oatmeal Raisin | 80 | 3 | 12 |
| P'B Chocolate Chip | 80 | 4.5 | 10 |
| Sugar Cookie | 80 | 3.5 | 12 |
| Walnut Chocolate Chip | 90 | 4.5 | 11 |

**Ultimates Refrigerated Dough:** *Per Cookie*

| | C | F | Cb |
|---|---|---|---|
| Chocolate Chip Lovers | 180 | 9 | 23 |
| Chocolate Pecan Deluxe | 190 | 10 | 22 |
| Choc. P'nut Butter Deluxe | 180 | 9 | 23 |
| Dark Chocolate Delight | 160 | 8 | 21 |
| Pecan Turtle Delight | 160 | 7 | 23 |

## Crispbreads  **C** **F** **Cb**

*Per Crispbread Unless Indicated*

**Finn Crisp:**

| | C | F | Cb |
|---|---|---|---|
| Classic: Traditional Rye | 40 | 0.5 | 7 |
| Hi-Fibre | 40 | 0.5 | 7 |
| Round: Original | 45 | 0.5 | 8 |
| Sesame | 50 | 1 | 8 |
| Thin Crisps, Original | 20 | 0 | 4 |

**Kavli Norwegian:**

| | C | F | Cb |
|---|---|---|---|
| Crispy Thin (3) | 50 | 0 | 10 |
| Golden Rye (2) | 60 | 0.5 | 12 |
| Hearty Thick (2) | 60 | 0 | 11 |
| Malsovit, Meal Wafers | 75 | 4 | 7 |

New York Flatbread Crisps,

| | C | F | Cb |
|---|---|---|---|
| Sesame, 0.4 oz | 50 | 1.5 | 7 |
| Ry-Krisp: Natural (2) | 50 | 0 | 11 |
| Seasoned (2) | 60 | 1 | 11 |
| Sesame (2) | 60 | 1.5 | 10 |

**Ryvita:**

| | C | F | Cb |
|---|---|---|---|
| Crackerbreads, Original; Wholegrain | 20 | 0 | 4 |
| Crispbreads, Original; Dark | 35 | 0 | 6.5 |

**WASA:**

| | C | F | Cb |
|---|---|---|---|
| Crisp'n Light 7 Grain (3) | 60 | 0 | 13 |
| Fiber (1), 0.35 oz | 40 | 1 | 7 |
| Hearty, 0.5 oz | 60 | 0 | 12 |
| Light Rye (2), 0.5 oz | 60 | 0 | 14 |
| Whole Grain, 0.5 oz | 50 | 0 | 11 |

## Matzos

**Manischewitz:**

| | C | F | Cb |
|---|---|---|---|
| Matzos: Egg 'n Onion, 1 oz | 80 | 0.5 | 17 |
| Thin Salted/Tea, average, 0.9 oz | 95 | 0 | 20 |
| Whole Wheat, 1 oz | 110 | 1 | 21 |
| Yolk Free, 1.2 oz | 100 | 0 | 20 |

**Crackers:**

| | C | F | Cb |
|---|---|---|---|
| Tam Tam: Original (10), 1 oz | 110 | 4 | 16 |
| Everything; Onion (10), 1 oz | 140 | 5 | 19 |
| Rye (10), 1 oz | 110 | 4 | 16 |

**Streit's:**

| | C | F | Cb |
|---|---|---|---|
| Mediterranean Matzos, 1 Matzo, 1 oz | 90 | 0.5 | 18 |
| Unsalted Matzos, 1 Matzo, 1 oz | 100 | 0 | 23 |

## Quick Guide  C  F  Cb

### Cream
#### Average All Brands
**Half & Half Cream:**

| | C | F | Cb |
|---|---|---|---|
| 1 Tbsp, 0.5 oz | 20 | 1.5 | 0.5 |
| 2 Tbsp, 1 oz | 40 | 3 | 1 |
| ¼ cup, 2 oz | 80 | 6 | 2 |
| **Light:** Coffee/table (20% fat): 1 Tbsp | 30 | 3 | 0.5 |
| 2 Tbsp, 1 oz | 60 | 6 | 0.5 |

**Sour Cream:**

| | | | |
|---|---|---|---|
| **Regular:** 1 Tbsp, 0.5 oz | 25 | 2.5 | 1 |
| 1 cup, 8 oz | 445 | 45 | 7 |
| **Low-Fat/Light:** 1 Tbsp, 0.5 oz | 20 | 1.5 | 1 |
| 2 Tbsp, 1 oz | 40 | 3 | 2 |
| **Fat-Free:** Av., 2 Tbsp, 1 oz | 20 | 0 | 4.5 |
| *Hood,* 2 Tbsp, 1 oz | 25 | 0 | 4 |
| *Knudsen,* 2 Tbsp, 1 oz | 30 | 0 | 5 |
| *Kroger,* 2 Tbsp, 1 oz | 20 | 0 | 3 |
| *Naturally Yours; Oak Farm,* 2 Tbsp | 20 | 0 | 3 |

**Sour Cream Substitute:**

| | | | |
|---|---|---|---|
| *Albertson's,* 2 Tbsp, 1 oz | 60 | 5 | 2 |
| *Tofutti,* Sour Supreme, 2 Tbsp, 1 oz | 85 | 5 | 9 |

#### Whipping Cream:
**Heavy,** (37% fat):

| | | | |
|---|---|---|---|
| 1 Tbsp fluid/2 Tbsp whipped | 50 | 5.5 | 0.5 |
| ¼ cup whipped | 105 | 11 | 1 |
| ½ cup fluid/1 cup whipped | 410 | 44 | 3.5 |
| **Light,** (30% fat): | | | |
| 1 Tbsp fluid/2 Tbsp whipped | 45 | 4.5 | 0.5 |
| ½ cup fluid/1 cup whipped | 350 | 37 | 3.5 |

### Coconut Cream/Milk

| | C | F | Cb |
|---|---|---|---|
| **Coconut Cream,** (Canned): | | | |
| **Plain/unsweetened:** 2 Tbsp, 1 oz | 75 | 6.5 | 3 |
| ½ cup, 4 oz | 285 | 26 | 12 |
| **Sweetened:** | | | |
| *Coco Lopez:* 1 oz | 130 | 5 | 21 |
| ½ cup, 4 oz | 520 | 20 | 84 |
| **Coconut Milk:** (Canned): | | | |
| *Thai Kitchen:* Lite, ⅓ cup, 2 fl.oz | 50 | 4.5 | 1 |
| Premium/Organic, 2 fl.oz | 115 | 10 | 4 |
| Unsweetened, ⅓ cup | 140 | 14 | 3 |
| **Coconut Water,** (Center), 1 cup | 45 | 0.5 | 9 |

## Whipped Toppings  C  F  Cb

#### Average All Brands

| | C | F | Cb |
|---|---|---|---|
| **Cream (Pressurized):** 2 Tbsp | 20 | 1.5 | 1 |
| ¼ cup | 40 | 3.5 | 2 |
| **Cream Topping,** Lite, 2 Tbsp | 20 | 1 | 3 |
| **Kraft:** | | | |
| **Cool Whip:** Regular, Original, ⅓ oz | 25 | 1.5 | 2 |
| Extra Creamy, 2 Tbsp | 25 | 2 | 2 |
| Lite, 2 Tbsp, ¼ oz | 20 | 1 | 3 |
| Free, 2 Tbsp, 0.3 oz | 20 | 0 | 3 |
| Seasons Delight, Fr. Vanilla, 0.3 oz | 25 | 1.5 | 2 |
| **Dream Whip,** 2 Tbsp | 10 | 0 | 2 |
| **Reddi wip:** | | | |
| **Original,** 2 Tbsp, 0.3 oz | 15 | 1 | 1 |
| **Extra Creamy,** 2 Tbsp, 0.3 oz | 15 | 1 | 1 |
| **Fat-Free,** 2 Tbsp, 0.3 oz | 5 | 0 | 1 |
| **Chocolate,** 2 Tbsp, 0.3 oz | 15 | 1 | 1 |

## Creamers (Non-Dairy)

**Powder:**
**Coffee-Mate/Cremora/N-Rich:**

| | C | F | Cb |
|---|---|---|---|
| **Original:** Unsweetened, 1 tsp | 10 | 0.5 | 1 |
| 1 heaping tsp | 25 | 2 | 2 |
| Lite, 1 tsp | 10 | 0 | 2 |
| Sweetened, 4 tsp | 60 | 2.5 | 9 |
| Flavors: Av., 4 tsp | 60 | 3 | 9 |
| Fat-Free, average, 4 tsp | 50 | 0 | 11 |

**Liquid/Refrigerated:**
*Per Tablespoon*

| | | | |
|---|---|---|---|
| **Bailey's:** Average all flavors | 35 | 1.5 | 5 |
| Fat Free, all flavors | 25 | 0 | 5 |
| **Coffee-Mate:** *Per Tablespoon* | | | |
| **Flavors:** Average all flavors | 35 | 1.5 | 5 |
| Fat-Free, all flavors | 25 | 0 | 5 |
| Sugar free, all flavors | 15 | 1 | 2 |
| **Unflavored:** Original | 20 | 1 | 2 |
| Fat-Free | 10 | 0 | 1 |
| Low-Fat | 10 | 0.5 | 2 |
| **Natural Bliss,** all flavors | 35 | 1.5 | 5 |
| **Hood,** Country Creamer, 1 Tbsp | 20 | 1.5 | 2 |
| **International Delight:** *Per Tbsp* | | | |
| **American/Classic/Coffee House:** | | | |
| Regular, all flavors | 35 | 1.5 | 6 |
| Fat-Free, all flavors | 30 | 0 | 7 |
| Fat-Free, Sugar-Free, all flav. | 15 | 0 | 3 |
| **Kroger:** *Per Tbsp* | | | |
| **Coffee Creamers:** Original | 20 | 1 | 3 |
| Caramel Vanilla; Hazelnut | 35 | 1.5 | 6 |
| Fat-free, Hazelnut | 30 | 0 | 6 |
| **Silk:** Almond, Vanilla | 20 | 1 | 3 |
| Soy: Original | 20 | 1.5 | 2 |
| Hazelnut | 30 | 1.5 | 4 |

## Ready-To-Serve

| | C | F | Cb |
|---|---|---|---|
| **Hunt's:** | | | |
| **Snack Pack Puddings:** | | | |
| **3.3 oz Container:** | | | |
| Butterscotch; Tapioca | 110 | 2.5 | 21 |
| Chocolate/ Chocolate Fudge | 120 | 3 | 21 |
| Vanilla | 100 | 2.5 | 20 |
| Fat Free: Chocolate | 90 | 0 | 20 |
| Tapioca | 80 | 0 | 19 |
| Sugar Free: Chocolate | 70 | 3 | 14 |
| Caramel; Vanilla | 60 | 3 | 10 |
| **Juicy Gels:** Lemon Lime, 5.5 oz | 150 | 0 | 38 |
| Strawberry, 5.5 oz | 170 | 0 | 41 |
| Sugar Free, Cherry, 3.25 oz | 10 | 0 | 2 |
| **Jell-O** *(Kraft):* | | | |
| **Gelatin,** av. all flavors, 3.4 oz | 70 | 0 | 17 |
| **Puddings & Mousse, 4 Pack:** | | | |
| Pudding Snacks, av. all flav., 3.9 oz | 110 | 1.5 | 23 |
| Mix Ins, Turtle Sundae, 3.4 oz | 150 | 6 | 23 |
| Pudding, Tapioca, 3.9 oz | 100 | 1.5 | 24 |
| Rice, Cinnamon/Vanilla, 3.6 oz | 110 | 3 | 20 |
| Temptations, Dble Choc. Pie, 3.4 oz | 110 | 3.5 | 18 |
| **Fat Free Puddings, 4 Pack:** | | | |
| Chocolate, 3.9 oz | 100 | 0 | 22 |
| Tapioca Pudding, 3.9 oz | 100 | 0 | 22 |
| **Red. Calorie Puddings, 4 Pack:** | | | |
| Boston Cream Pie, 3.6 oz | 60 | 1 | 10 |
| Chocolate, 3.6 oz | 60 | 1.5 | 13 |
| **Kozy Shack:** | | | |
| **Flan,** Creme Caramel, 1 cup, 4 oz | 160 | 4 | 28 |
| **Gluten Free Puddings:** | | | |
| Chocolate, 4.6 oz | 140 | 2.5 | 27 |
| Cinnamon Raisin, 4.6 oz | 140 | 2.5 | 26 |
| French Vanilla Rice, 4.6 oz | 140 | 2.5 | 24 |
| Original Rice, 4.6 oz | 130 | 2.5 | 24 |
| Tapioca, 4.6 oz | 130 | 2 | 25 |
| **Simply Well Puddings:** | | | |
| Chocolate, 4 oz | 90 | 2.5 | 13 |
| Rice; Tapioca, 4 oz | 90 | 1.5 | 14 |
| **Kroger:** *Per Container* | | | |
| **Puddings:** *Per 3.5 oz* | | | |
| Butterscotch | 110 | 2 | 22 |
| Chocolate | 110 | 2.5 | 21 |
| **Swiss Miss:** | | | |
| **Puddings:** *Per 4 oz Cup* | | | |
| Classic Butterscotch | 130 | 3.5 | 22 |
| Creamy : Milk Choc. | 150 | 3.5 | 27 |
| Vanilla | 140 | 3.5 | 24 |
| Old Fashioned Tapioca | 140 | 3.5 | 24 |
| Sugar Free: Chocolate | 70 | 3.5 | 15 |
| Vanilla | 60 | 3 | 11 |

## Homemade Puddings

| | C | F | Cb |
|---|---|---|---|
| Apple Tapioca, ½ cup | 150 | 0 | 32 |
| Bread Pudding, ½ cup | 250 | 8 | 40 |
| Blancmange, ½ cup | 140 | 5 | 19 |
| Chocolate, ½ cup | 190 | 6 | 30 |
| Crème Brûlée, ½ cup | 400 | 35 | 16 |
| Plum Pudding, ½ cup | 170 | 3 | 32 |
| Rice with Raisins, ½ cup | 200 | 4 | 38 |
| Sponge Pudding, 3.5 oz | 340 | 16 | 45 |
| Tapioca Cream, ½ cup | 110 | 4 | 15 |
| Trifle, ½ cup | 180 | 7 | 26 |

## Custards

| | C | F | Cb |
|---|---|---|---|
| **Custard Mix** *(Jello/Royal Flan),* average: | | | |
| Dry, ¼ of 2.9 oz package, 0.7 oz | 80 | 0 | 19 |
| Prepared: Whole milk, ½ cup | 155 | 4 | 25 |
| 2% milk, ½ cup | 140 | 2.5 | 25 |
| Non-Fat milk, ½ cup | 125 | 0 | 25 |
| **Home Made Egg Custard:** | | | |
| With Whole Milk, ½ cup | 170 | 8 | 18 |
| With 2% Milk, ½ cup | 155 | 6.5 | 18 |

## Gelatin • Parfait • Jell-O

| | C | F | Cb |
|---|---|---|---|
| **Jell-O:** | | | |
| **Gelatin Dessert Mix:** *Dry Mix Only* | | | |
| All flavors, 0.8 oz | 80 | 0 | 19 |
| Sugar free, all flavors, 0.3 oz | 10 | 0 | 0 |
| **Instant Pudding & Pie Filling:** *Dry Mix Only* | | | |
| Chocolate/Fudge, 1 oz | 100 | 0 | 25 |
| Devil's Food, 1 oz | 140 | 0 | 25 |
| Oreo, | | | |
| Cookies 'N Cream, 1 oz | 120 | 1 | 28 |
| White Chocolate, 0.8 oz | 90 | 0 | 23 |
| Sugar free, Fat-Free: | | | |
| Chocolate var., 0.3 oz | 35 | 0 | 8 |
| Other flavors, 0.3 oz | 25 | 0 | 6 |
| **No Bake Dessert Mix:** *Dry Mix Only* | | | |
| Cheesecake: Real, 2 oz | 290 | 15 | 39 |
| Cherry, 2.2 oz | 210 | 3.5 | 42 |
| Strawberry, 2.4 oz | 200 | 3.5 | 42 |
| Oreo, 2 oz | 280 | 8 | 48 |
| Peanut Butter Cup, 2 oz | 290 | 15 | 39 |
| Pumpkin Style Pie, 1.2 oz | 130 | 1.5 | 29 |
| **Ida Mae,** Strawberry Parfait | 90 | 2 | 18 |
| **Reser's,** Parfaits, av. all flavors, 3.9 oz | 100 | 2 | 19 |

## Meringues

| | C | F | Cb |
|---|---|---|---|
| Meringue Swirl, ½ cup | 50 | 0 | 8 |
| Meringue Shell, 1 oz | 100 | 0 | 16 |

## Chicken Eggs

| | C | F | Cb |
|---|---|---|---|
| **Fresh Eggs:** | | | |
| **Raw:** | | | |
| Small | 55 | 4 | 0 |
| Medium | 65 | 4 | 0 |
| Large | 70 | 5 | 0 |
| Extra Large | 80 | 5.5 | 0 |
| Jumbo | 90 | 6 | 0 |
| **Egg Yolk,** 1 extra large | 55 | 4.5 | 0 |
| **Egg White,** 1 extra large | 17 | 0 | 0 |
| **Dried Egg Powder:** | | | |
| **Whole Egg:** ¼ cup, 1 oz | 170 | 12 | 0 |
| 1 Tbsp | 30 | 2 | 0 |
| **Egg White,** ¼ cup, 1 oz | 105 | 0 | 0 |
| **Egg Yolk,** ¼ cup, 1 oz | 195 | 18 | 0 |

## Egg Substitutes

*¼ Cup (Equivalent to 1 Egg) ~ Zero Cholesterol*

| | C | F | Cb |
|---|---|---|---|
| **All Whites** (Crystal Farms), 1.6 oz | 25 | 0 | 0 |
| **Better 'n Eggs** (Crystal Farms): | | | |
| Regular, ¼ cup, 2 oz | 30 | 0 | 1 |
| **Egg Beaters** (ConAgra): | | | |
| Regular, 3 Tbsp, 1.6 oz | 25 | 0 | 1 |
| Southwestern Style, 3 Tbsp, 1.6 oz | 20 | 0 | 1 |
| Three Cheese, 3 Tbsp, 1.6 oz | 25 | 0.5 | 1 |
| **Egg Replacer** (Ener-g), 1.5 tsp, | 15 | 0 | 4 |
| **Eggs** (Second Nature), | | | |
| Egg Whites, Fat-Free, | | | |
| ¼ cup, 2 fl.oz | 35 | 0 | 1 |
| **Egg Substitute** (Albertson's), ¼ cup | 30 | 0 | 1 |
| **Naturegg** (Burnbrae Farms), | | | |
| Simply Egg White, ¼ cup, 2 oz | 30 | 0 | 0 |

## Other Eggs

| | C | F | Cb |
|---|---|---|---|
| Duck, 1 large, 2.5 oz | 130 | 9.5 | 0 |
| Goose, 1 large, 5 oz | 280 | 19 | 0 |
| Quail, 3 eggs, 1 oz | 42 | 3 | 0 |
| Turkey, 1 large, 3 oz | 135 | 9.5 | 0 |
| Turtle, 1 egg, 1.75 oz | 75 | 5 | 0 |

## Omega-3 Fat Enriched

| | C | F | Cb |
|---|---|---|---|
| **Eggland's Best,** 1 large | 60 | 4 | 0 |
| **Horizon Organic,** 1 large | 70 | 4.5 | 1 |

Note: Cholesterol content same as regular eggs, but Omega-3 fats inhibit blood cholesterol increase.

## Cooked Eggs

| | C | F | Cb |
|---|---|---|---|
| **Boiled Egg:** *Same as Raw Egg* | | | |
| **Hard-Cooked,** Small, peeled | 65 | 4 | 0 |
| **Fried Egg:** | | | |
| With fat: 1 large egg | 105 | 9 | 0.5 |
| 2 small eggs | 175 | 13 | 1 |
| No fat/nonstick pan, 1 large | 75 | 5 | 0.5 |
| **Deviled Egg,** 2 halves | 145 | 13 | 0.5 |
| **Eggs Benedict,** (2), | | | |
| on Toast or English Muffin | 860 | 56 | 25 |
| **Eggs Florentine,** (2), | | | |
| on Toast or English Muffin | 890 | 59 | 25 |
| **Pickled Egg,** 1 large | 80 | 5.5 | 0 |
| **Poached Egg,** 1 large | 65 | 4 | 0 |
| **Quiche** (Homemade): | | | |
| Egg & Bacon, 1 slice, 5.3 oz | 580 | 43 | 27 |
| Ham & Cheese, 1 slice, 5.3 oz | 475 | 33 | 29 |
| **Scotch Egg,** 1 egg | 300 | 21 | 16 |
| **Scrambled Eggs:** | | | |
| 1 large egg: | | | |
| With 1 Tbsp milk + 1 tsp fat | 120 | 9 | 1 |
| With 1 Tbsp skim milk/no fat | 85 | 5.5 | 1 |
| 2 large eggs: | | | |
| With 2 Tbsp milk + 2 tsp fat | 260 | 20 | 2 |
| With 2 Tbsp skim milk, w/o fat | 180 | 11 | 2 |

## Omelets

| | C | F | Cb |
|---|---|---|---|
| **1 Egg:** | | | |
| Plain (with 1 tsp fat) | 125 | 10 | 0.5 |
| With: ½ oz cheese | 175 | 15 | 0.5 |
| ½ oz cheese + ½ oz ham | 200 | 16 | 0.5 |
| **2 Eggs:** | | | |
| Plain (with 2 tsp fat) | 250 | 20 | 1 |
| With: 1 oz cheese | 360 | 29 | 2 |
| 1 oz cheese + 1 oz ham | 410 | 32 | 2 |
| **3 Eggs:** | | | |
| Plain (with 1 Tbsp fat) | 360 | 29 | 1.5 |
| With: 2 oz cheese | 580 | 47 | 2.5 |
| 2 oz cheese + 2 oz ham | 680 | 53 | 2.5 |
| **Extras,** Tomato/Onion/Veggies, 2 oz | 20 | 0 | 4.5 |
| **Egg Substitute** (EggBeaters): | | | |
| 2 eggs (½ cup) + 1 tsp fat | 100 | 4 | 2 |
| 3 eggs (¾ cup) + 2 tsp fat | 160 | 8 | 3 |
| Extras: 1 oz Cheese | 110 | 9 | 1 |
| 1 oz Ham | 50 | 3 | 1 |

## Egg Nog

| | C | F | Cb |
|---|---|---|---|
| *Average all Brands,* | | | |
| ½ cup, 4 oz | 170 | 9.5 | 17 |
| **Borden,** Regular, 4 fl.oz | 160 | 8 | 18 |
| **Hood,** Golden, ½ cup, 4 fl.oz | 180 | 9 | 22 |
| **Horizon/Hood,** Light/Low-Fat, | 140 | 4 | 22 |

### Breakfast Sides

| | C | F | Cb |
|---|---|---|---|
| **Toast:** | | | |
| Plain, 1 thick slice | 85 | 1 | 13 |
| With: 2 tsp butter/marg. | 155 | 9 | 13 |
| 3 tsp/1 Tbsp fat | 190 | 13 | 13 |
| **English Muffin:** | | | |
| Plain, 2 oz | 130 | 1 | 26 |
| With 3 tsp fat | 230 | 12 | 26 |
| **Bacon,** 2 strips | 70 | 5 | 0 |
| **Ham,** lean, 2 oz | 100 | 3 | 0 |
| **Hash Brown:** | | | |
| ½ cup, 3 oz | 125 | 6.5 | 14 |
| 1 cup serving, 6 oz | 250 | 13 | 28 |
| **Sausages,** 2 oz link | 180 | 16 | 1.5 |

### Frozen Egg Breakfasts

| | C | F | Cb |
|---|---|---|---|
| **Aunt Jemima:** | | | |
| **Breakfast Sandwich:** *Per Sandwich* | | | |
| Croissant, Sausage, Egg & Cheese | 350 | 23 | 23 |
| Griddlecake, Ham, Egg & Cheese | 240 | 8 | 33 |
| **Jimmy Dean:** | | | |
| **Breakfast Sandwich:** *Per Sandwich* | | | |
| Biscuit, Sausage, Egg & Cheese | 410 | 29 | 26 |
| Croissant, Egg, Red Peppers, Onions | | | |
| & Jack Cheese | 290 | 16 | 27 |
| Muffin, Sausage, Egg & Cheese | 350 | 21 | 26 |
| **Omelets:** *Per Omelet* | | | |
| Three Cheese | 290 | 23 | 4 |
| Ham & Cheese | 250 | 19 | 4 |
| **MorningStar Farms:** | | | |
| **Breakfast Sandwich:** *Each* | | | |
| Sausage, Egg & Cheese | 220 | 10 | 20 |
| Veggie Scramble with Cheese | 140 | 4.5 | 18 |
| **Pillsbury,** | | | |
| **Toaster Scrambles,** Cheese & Egg | 180 | 10 | 18 |
| **Red Baron:** | | | |
| **Scrambles:** *Each* | | | |
| Bacon, 5 oz | 370 | 18 | 38 |
| Sausage; Western, 5 oz | 360 | 17 | 38 |
| **Frozen Pancake/Waffles ~** *See Page 132* | | | |
| **Toaster Pastries ~** *See Page 64* | | | |

### Frozen Egg Rolls

| | C | F | Cb |
|---|---|---|---|
| **Kahiki:** *Each, without sauce* | | | |
| Chicken; Pork, av., 3.3 oz | 145 | 4 | 22 |
| Vegetable, 3.3 oz | 130 | 3 | 22 |
| **Lotus Restaurant:** | | | |
| Imperial, Chicken/Pork (1) | 160 | 6.5 | 24 |
| Vegetarian (1) | 120 | 5 | 20 |
| **Pagoda Express:** *Each, with Sauce* | | | |
| Chicken | 160 | 4 | 24 |
| Pork | 180 | 7 | 23 |
| Pork & Shrimp | 180 | 7 | 23 |
| Vegetable | 140 | 4 | 24 |

### Fast-Foods/Restaurants

| | C | F | Cb |
|---|---|---|---|
| **Arby's,** | | | |
| Bacon, Egg & Cheese Croissant | 400 | 26 | 25 |
| **Au Bon Pain,** 2 Egg on Plain Bagel | 430 | 12 | 58 |
| **Bob Evans:** | | | |
| **Omelets:** | | | |
| Border Scramble | 630 | 45 | 15 |
| Western | 495 | 35 | 7 |
| **Bojangles:** Egg & Cheese Biscuit | 515 | 34 | 35 |
| Bacon, Egg & Cheese Biscuit | 550 | 37 | 35 |
| **Bruegger's:** | | | |
| **Bagel:** With Egg & Cheese, 6.8 oz | 430 | 18 | 63 |
| With Egg, Cheese & Sausage, 8.3 oz | 590 | 34 | 63 |
| **Burger King:** | | | |
| **Breakfast Burrito:** Sausage | 310 | 19 | 22 |
| Southwestern | 600 | 38 | 43 |
| **Croissan'wich:** | | | |
| Bacon, Egg & Cheese | 370 | 21 | 31 |
| Ham, Egg & Cheese | 390 | 20 | 33 |
| Double, with Double Sausage | 630 | 45 | 32 |
| **Carl's Jr:** | | | |
| **Burrito:** Bacon & Egg | 570 | 34 | 38 |
| Big Country | 740 | 45 | 55 |
| Loaded Breakfast | 790 | 50 | 53 |
| Steak & Egg | 650 | 36 | 44 |
| **Chick-fil-A,** Chicken, Egg & Cheese, | | | |
| on Sunflower Multigrain Bagel | 480 | 20 | 48 |
| **Del Taco,** Egg & Cheese Burrito | 400 | 17 | 38 |
| **Denny's:** *With Hashbrowns, Without Bread* | | | |
| **Omelette:** | | | |
| Ultimate | 790 | 62 | 25 |
| Veggie-Cheese | 520 | 36 | 25 |
| **Dunkin Donuts:** | | | |
| Bagel, Ham, Egg & Cheese | 440 | 8 | 67 |
| Croissant, Bacon, Egg & Cheese | 480 | 27 | 40 |
| **Eat 'N Park:** | | | |
| **Omelette:** | | | |
| Ham & Cheese | 535 | 35 | 5 |
| Meat Lovers | 725 | 55 | 4 |
| **Hardee's:** | | | |
| **Biscuit:** Loaded Omelet | 490 | 28 | 40 |
| Sausage & Egg | 560 | 37 | 39 |
| **IHOP:** T-Bone Steak & Eggs, 12 oz | 1180 | 63 | 64 |
| Omelette, Spinach & Mushroom | 980 | 82 | 21 |
| **Jack in the Box:** | | | |
| **Biscuit:** Bacon, Egg & Cheese | 410 | 25 | 26 |
| Sausage, Egg & Cheese | 535 | 38 | 27 |
| **McDonald's:** | | | |
| Biscuit, Bacon, Egg & Cheese, regular | 460 | 26 | 38 |
| McMuffin, Egg | 300 | 13 | 31 |
| **Whataburger,** Breakfast Platter, | | | |
| with Bacon | 630 | 41 | 37 |

## Quick Guide

| | **C** | **F** | **Cb** |
|---|---|---|---|

### Butter
*Average All Brands*

| | C | F | Cb |
|---|---|---|---|
| **Regular:** 1 tsp, 0.2 oz | 35 | 4 | 0 |
| 1 Tbsp, 0.5 oz | 100 | 11 | 0 |
| 2 Tbsp, 1 oz | 205 | 23 | 0 |
| 1 Stick, ½ cup, 4 oz | 810 | 92 | 0 |
| 1 Pound, 2 cups, 16 oz | 3255 | 368 | 0 |
| **Light:** Regular, 40% Fat | | | |
| 1 tsp, 0.2 oz | 30 | 3 | 0 |
| 1 Tbsp, 0.5 oz | 70 | 7.5 | 0 |
| 2 Tbsp, 1 oz | 140 | 15 | 0 |
| **Whipped Butter:** Regular | | | |
| 1 tsp, 0.1 oz | 20 | 2.5 | 0 |
| 1 Tbsp, 0.3 oz | 65 | 7.5 | 0 |
| 1 Stick, 2 .7 oz | 545 | 62 | 0 |
| **Whipped Light Butter** *(Land O Lakes):* | | | |
| 1 tsp, 0.15 oz | 15 | 1.5 | 0 |
| 1 Tbsp, 0.4 oz | 45 | 5 | 0 |
| 2 Tbsp, 0.8 oz | 90 | 10 | 0 |

**Unsalted ~** *Same as Salted*

### Flavored Butter/Spreads

*Average All Brands*

| | C | F | Cb |
|---|---|---|---|
| **Honey Butter,** (60% Fat): | | | |
| 1 Tbsp, 0.5 oz | 90 | 8 | 4 |
| *Downey's,* 2% Fat, | | | |
| 1 Tbsp, 0.5 oz | 60 | 1 | 11 |
| **Garlic Butter,** (80% Fat): | | | |
| 1 Tbsp, 0.5 oz | 100 | 11 | 0 |
| **Sweet Cream Butter:** | | | |
| *Land O Lakes:* Reguar, 1 Tbsp | 100 | 11 | 0 |
| Honey Butter Spread, 1 Tbsp | 70 | 6 | 4 |

### Butter & Butter Blends

*Per 1 Tablespoon*

| | C | F | Cb |
|---|---|---|---|
| **Challenge:** Stick, 0.5 oz | 100 | 11 | 0 |
| Tub, Whipped, 0.3 oz | 70 | 7 | 0 |
| **Brummel & Brown,** | | | |
| Spread Made with Yogurt, 0.5oz | 45 | 5 | 0 |
| **Land O'Lakes:** | | | |
| **Sticks:** Original, 0.5oz | 100 | 11 | 0 |
| Light, 0.5 oz | 50 | 6 | 0 |
| **Tubs:** Butter With Olive Oil, 0.5 oz | 90 | 10 | 0 |
| Light, with Canola Oil, 0.5 oz | 50 | 5 | 0 |
| **Smart Balance:** | | | |
| Original Buttery Spread, 0.5 oz | 90 | 10 | 0 |
| Butter & Canola, 0.5 oz | 100 | 11 | 0 |

### Ghee (Clarified Butter)

| | **C** | **F** | **Cb** |
|---|---|---|---|

(Example ~ *Purity Farms*)
Note: Ghee is 100% fat compared to regular butter (80% fat + 20% water)

| | C | F | Cb |
|---|---|---|---|
| 1 tsp, 0.2 oz | 45 | 5 | 0 |
| 1 Tbsp, 0.5 oz | 120 | 14 | 0 |

### Light & Reduced Fat Spreads

*Per Tablespoon*

| | C | F | Cb |
|---|---|---|---|
| **bestlife,** Buttery Spread, 0.5 oz | 60 | 6 | 0 |
| **Benecol:** Regular, 0.5 oz | 70 | 8 | 0 |
| Light, 0.5 oz | 50 | 5 | 0 |
| **Blue Bonnet:** | | | |
| Stick, Light Spread, 0.5 oz | 50 | 5 | 1 |
| Tub, Original Soft Spread, 0.5 oz | 60 | 6 | 1 |
| **Country Crock** *(Shedd's)* | | | |
| **Tubs:** Original Spread, 0.5 oz | 70 | 7 | 0 |
| Light Spread, 0.5 oz | 50 | 5 | 0 |
| Churn Style, 0.5 oz | 60 | 7 | 0 |
| **Fleischmann's:** | | | |
| **Original:** Soft Spread, 0.4 oz | 60 | 7 | 0 |
| Spread, 0.5 oz | 80 | 9 | 0 |
| Light Spread, 0.5 oz | 40 | 4.5 | 0 |
| **I Can't Believe It's Not Butter!:** | | | |
| **Tubs:** Original Spread, 0.5 oz | 60 | 6 | 0 |
| Light, 0.5 oz | 40 | 4 | 0 |
| Olive Oil Spread, 1 Tbsp | 60 | 6 | 0 |
| **Parkay:** | | | |
| Original Spread, 0.4 oz | 70 | 7 | 0 |
| Spray, 5 sprays | 0 | 0 | 0 |
| Squeeze Bottle, 0.5 oz | 70 | 8 | 0 |
| **Promise:** | | | |
| Activ, Spread, 0.5 oz | 45 | 5 | 0 |
| Buttery Spread, 0.5 oz | 80 | 8 | 0 |
| Light Spread, 0.5 oz | 45 | 5 | 0 |
| **Smart Balance:** | | | |
| **Tubs,** Buttery Spread: | | | |
| Original, 0.5 oz | 90 | 10 | 0 |
| HeartRight, Light, 0.5 oz | 50 | 5 | 0 |
| HeartRight, Light, 0.5 oz | 50 | 5 | 0 |
| Light with Flaxseed Oil. 0.5 oz | 50 | 5 | 0 |
| Omega 3: Reg., 0.5 oz | 80 | 9 | 0 |
| Light, 0.5 oz | 50 | 5 | 0 |

### Butter Substitutes

| | C | F | Cb |
|---|---|---|---|
| **Butter Buds:** | | | |
| **Butter Flavored:** Mix, 1 tsp | 5 | 0 | 2 |
| Sprinkles, 1 tsp | 5 | 0 | 2 |
| **Earth Balance,** | | | |
| Original, 1 Tbsp | 100 | 11 | 0 |
| **Molly McButter,** 1 tsp | 5 | 0 | 1 |
| **Sunsweet,** (Butter/Oil Replacement), | | | |
| Lighter Bake, 1 Tbsp, 0.7 oz | 35 | 0 | 9 |

Updated Nutrition Data ~ www.CalorieKing.com
Persons with Diabetes ~ See Disclaimer (Page 22)

## Animal Fats/Lards   **C** **F** **Cb**

*Average All Types*

**Beef Tallow/Drippings, Lard (Pork),
Chicken, Duck, Goose, Turkey:**

| | | | |
|---|---|---|---|
| 1 Tbsp, 0.5 oz |  | **115** | 13 | 0 |
| 2.25 Tbsp, 1 oz | | **255** | 28 | 0 |
| 1 cup, 7.3 oz | | **1850** | 205 | 0 |
| ½ pound, 8 oz | | **2040** | 227 | 0 |

**Ghee/Butter/ Oil ~** *See Page 93*

## Vegetable Shortening

*Average All Types*

| | | | |
|---|---|---|---|
| 1 Tbsp, 0.5 oz | | **115** | 13 | 0 |
| 2.25 Tbsp, 1 oz | | **250** | 28 | 0 |
| 1 cup, 7.3 oz | | **1810** | 205 | 0 |

## Vegetable Oils

Includes almond, avocado, canola, corn, coconut, flaxseed, grapeseed, linseed, mustard, olive, palm, peanut, rice bran, safflower, sesame, sunflower, soybean, wheat germ. Note: Oil is 100% fat.

| | | | |
|---|---|---|---|
| 1 tsp, 0.2 oz | | **45** | 5 | 0 |
| 1 Tbsp, 0.5 oz | | **120** | 14 | 0 |
| 2 Tbsp, 1 oz | | **240** | 28 | 0 |
| 1 cup, 7.3 oz | | **1930** | 205 | 0 |

## Fish Oils

*Average All Types*
(Includes Cod Liver, Herring,
Salmon, Sardines): 1 Tbsp, 0.5 oz     **125**  14  0

## Cooking Sprays/Squeezes

Cooking Sprays: (PAM, Mazola, I Can't Believe It's Not Butter, Weight Watchers, Wesson):

| | | | |
|---|---|---|---|
| *Pam:* ¼ second spray | **2** | 0 | 0 |
| 1-3 second spray | **6** | 1 | 0 |
| *I Can't Believe It's Not Butter,* | | | |
| Original Spray | **0** | 0 | 0 |
| *Parkay,* Buttery Spray | **0** | 0 | 0 |

## Olestra (Olean)   **C** **F** **Cb**

**Olestra** *(Olean)*     **0**  0  0

Note: Olean is Proctor & Gamble's brand name for Olestra – a no-calorie cooking oil that gives snacks (like potato chips, tortilla chips and crackers) taste and texture without adding fat or calories.

**Examples:**
- *Frito-Lay,* Light Products
  (*Lays, Ruffles, Tostitos, Doritos*)
- *Pringles,* Fat-Free Potato Crisps

## Quick Guide   **C** **F** **Cb**

### Mayonnaise:

**Regular:** *Per 1 Tbsp, 0.5 oz Unless Indicated*

| | | | |
|---|---|---|---|
| Average All Brands | **90** | 10 | 0 |
| ***Best Foods; Hellman's; Kraft:*** | | | |
| Original/Real | **90** | 10 | 0 |
| ½ cup, 4 oz | **720** | 80 | 0 |
| ***Hain,*** Safflower Mayonnaise | **100** | 11 | 0 |
| ***Spectrum,*** Canola Mayo | **100** | 11 | 0 |

**Light/Reduced Fat:** *Per 1 Tbsp, 0.5 oz*

| | | | |
|---|---|---|---|
| ***Best Foods/Hellman's*** | **35** | 3.5 | 1 |
| ***Kraft,*** Light/Olive Oil | **35** | 3 | 1 |
| ***Smart Balance,*** Omega | **50** | 5 | 0 |
| ***Spectrum,*** Light Canola Mayo, | | | |
| Eggless | **35** | 3.5 | 0.5 |

**Fat Free:**

| | | | |
|---|---|---|---|
| ***Kraft:*** Original, 1 Tbsp | **10** | 0 | 2 |
| ½ cup, 4 oz | **80** | 0 | 16 |

**Sugar Free:**

| | | | |
|---|---|---|---|
| ***Dukes Mayo,*** 1 Tbsp | **100** | 12 | 0 |

### Mayonnaise Style Dressing:
*Per 1 Tbsp, 0.5 oz*

| | | | |
|---|---|---|---|
| ***Best Foods,*** Sandwich Spread | **60** | 5 | 2 |
| ***Kraft:*** | | | |
| Miracle Whip Dressing: | | | |
| Original | **40** | 3.5 | 1 |
| Light | **20** | 1.5 | 1 |
| Fat Free | **15** | 0 | 3 |
| Mayo: | | | |
| Chipotle | **35** | 3 | 1 |
| Horseradish-Dijon | **35** | 3 | 1 |
| Sandwich Shop, Hot & Spicy | **100** | 11 | 0 |
| ***Nasoya,*** Egg & Dairy Free: | | | |
| Nayonaise: Regular/Whipped | **40** | 3.5 | 1 |
| Light | **20** | 1.5 | 1 |

## Quick Guide | C | F | Cb

### Fresh Fish
**Low Oil:** *Less than 2.5% fat*
**White/Lightly-colored flesh. Examples:**
Cod, Flounder, Haddock, Halibut, Mahi Mahi, Perch, Pike,
Pollock, Snapper, Sole, Whiting.

| | C | F | Cb |
|---|---|---|---|
| **Raw,** without bones, 4 oz | 100 | 1 | 0 |
| **Steamed,** Broiled, Baked, 4 oz | 140 | 1.5 | 0 |
| **Fried:** Lightly Floured, 4 oz | 210 | 8 | 3.5 |
| Breaded, 4 oz | 260 | 12 | 8 |
| In Batter, 4 oz | 320 | 16 | 27 |

**Medium Oil:** *2.5-5% fat*
**Lightly-colored flesh. Examples:**
Bluefin Tuna, Catfish, Kingfish, Orange Roughy, Salmon
(Pink), Swordfish, Rainbow Trout, Yellowtail.

| | C | F | Cb |
|---|---|---|---|
| **Raw,** without bones, 4 oz | 145 | 7 | 0 |
| **Baked/Broiled,** 4 oz | 195 | 8 | 0 |
| **Fried,** 4 oz | 230 | 11 | 8 |

**High Oil:** *Over 5% fat*
**Darker-colored flesh. Examples:**
Albacore Tuna, Mackerel,
Salmon (Atlantic/Chinook/Sockeye), Sardines, Trout.

| | C | F | Cb |
|---|---|---|---|
| **Raw,** without bones, 4 oz | 220 | 14 | 0 |
| **Baked,** Broiled, 4 oz | 275 | 17 | 0 |
| **Fried,** 4 oz | 340 | 23 | 12 |

### Cooking Yields (Fin Fish):
4 oz Raw wt. = 3.5 oz Cooked weight
4 oz Cooked wt. = 5 oz Raw weight

### Calorie & Fat Variations:
The amount of fat/oil in fish varies with the species, season
and locality. Within the same fish, fat/oil content is generally
higher towards the head.

### Fish & Shellfish
*Edible Weights: (no bones/shell)*

| | C | F | Cb |
|---|---|---|---|
| **Abalone:** Raw, 3 oz | 90 | 0.5 | 5 |
| Fried, 3 oz | 160 | 6 | 9.5 |
| **Ahi Tuna,** grilled, 6 oz fillet (w/o fat) | 235 | 2 | 0 |
| **Anchovy:** Paste, 1 Tbsp, 0.5 oz | 45 | 3 | 0 |
| Canned in oil, drained, (5 ), 0.7 oz | 40 | 2 | 0 |
| **Barracuda (Pacific),** raw, 4 oz | 130 | 3 | 0 |
| **Basa/Swai,** raw, 4 oz fillet | 70 | 2 | 0 |
| **Bass:** | | | |
| Sea: Raw, 4.6 oz fillet | 125 | 2.5 | 0 |
| Baked, 3 oz | 105 | 2 | 0 |
| Striped: Raw, 1 fillet, 5.5 oz | 150 | 3.5 | 0 |
| Baked, 3 oz | 105 | 3 | 0 |
| Freshwater: Raw, 3 oz | 95 | 3 | 0 |
| Baked, 3 oz | 125 | 4 | 0 |

### Fish & Shellfish (Cont) | C | F | Cb

*Edible Weights: (no bones/shell)*

| | C | F | Cb |
|---|---|---|---|
| **Calamari/Squid:** | | | |
| Raw, 4 oz | 100 | 1.5 | 3.5 |
| Baked, 1 cup | 190 | 6.5 | 5.5 |
| Fried, 3 oz | 150 | 6 | 7 |
| **Catfish:** | | | |
| Farmed: Raw, 1 fillet 5.6 oz | 190 | 9.5 | 0 |
| Baked, 1 fillet 5 oz | 205 | 10 | 0 |
| Wild: Raw, 1 fillet, 5.6 oz | 150 | 4.5 | 0 |
| Baked, 1 fillet, 5 oz | 150 | 4 | 0 |
| Breaded, fried, 1 fillet, 3 oz | 200 | 12 | 0 |
| **Caviar,** black/red, 1 Tbsp, 16g | 40 | 3 | 0.5 |
| **Clams:** Raw (4 large/9 small), 3 oz | 70 | 1 | 3 |
| Breaded, Fried (20 small), 6.6 oz | 380 | 21 | 20 |
| Canned, drained, ½ cup, 2.8 oz | 115 | 1 | 0 |
| Steamed (10 small), 3.3 oz | 140 | 2 | 5 |
| **Clam Juice** *(Snow's)*, 1 Tbsp | 0 | 0 | 0 |
| **Cod:** | | | |
| Atlantic: Raw, 4 oz | 95 | 1 | 0 |
| Baked, 3 oz | 90 | 1 | 0 |
| Canned, solids & liquid | 90 | 0.5 | 0 |
| Pacific: Raw, 4 oz | 80 | 0.5 | 0 |
| Baked, 3 oz | 70 | 0.5 | 0 |
| **Crab:** | | | |
| Alaska King, | | | |
| 1 leg, cooked, 4.7 oz | 130 | 2 | 0 |
| Blue: Raw, 1 crab, 6 oz | 150 | 1 | 0 |
| Steamed, 3 oz | 70 | 0.5 | 0 |
| Canned, drained, 6.5 oz can | 105 | 0.5 | 0 |
| Dungeness: Raw, 1 crab, 5.8 oz | 140 | 1.5 | 0 |
| Steamed, 4.45 oz | 140 | 1.5 | 0 |
| **Crab Cakes** *(Capt. D's)*, (1), 2.8 oz | 250 | 16 | 16 |
| **Crayfish:** | | | |
| Farmed: Raw, 3 oz | 60 | 1 | 0 |
| Steamed, 3 oz | 75 | 1 | 0 |
| Wild: Raw 3 oz | 65 | 1 | 0 |
| Steamed, 3 oz | 70 | 1 | 0 |
| **Cuttlefish,** raw, 3 oz | 70 | 1 | 1 |
| **Dolphinfish** ~ *See Mahi-Mahi* | | | |
| **Eel:** Raw, 3 oz | 155 | 10 | 0 |
| Baked, 3 oz | 200 | 13 | 0 |
| **Fish & Chips** *(Red Lobster)*, | | | |
| battered, without condiments | 630 | 26 | 54 |
| **Fish Sandwich** *(Burger King)*, | | | |
| without Tartar Sauce | 410 | 12 | 53 |
| **Fish Oil,** 1 Tbsp, 0.5 oz | 125 | 14 | 0 |
| **Flounder/Sole:** | | | |
| Raw, 4 oz | 80 | 2 | 0 |
| Baked, 3 oz | 75 | 2 | 0 |
| **Frozen Fish** ~ *See Pages 114-122* | | | |

| Fish & Shellfish (Cont) | C | F | Cb |
|---|---|---|---|
| *Edible Weights: Without Bones or Shell* | | | |
| **Haddock:** Raw, 4 oz | 85 | 0.5 | 0 |
| Baked, 3 oz | 75 | 0.5 | 0 |
| Smoked, 3 oz | 100 | 1 | 0 |
| **Halibut:** | | | |
| Atlantic: Raw, 4 oz | 105 | 1.5 | 0 |
| Baked, ½ fillet, 5.6 oz | 175 | 2.5 | 0 |
| **Herring:** | | | |
| Atlantic, raw, 4 oz | 180 | 10 | 0 |
| Canned: Plain, drained, 3 oz | 130 | 8 | 0 |
| In Tomato Sauce, 3.5 oz | 140 | 8 | 2 |
| Pickled, 2 pieces, 1 oz | 75 | 5 | 3 |
| Smoked, kippered, 4 oz | 245 | 14 | 0 |
| **Jellyfish:** Raw, 1 oz | 30 | 0 | 0 |
| Dried, Salted, 1 cup, 2 oz | 20 | 1 | 0 |
| **Ling,** raw, 4 oz | 100 | 0.5 | 0 |
| **Lobster,** Northern: | | | |
| 1.5 lb Whole Lobster, edible portion: | | | |
| Raw, 6.3 oz | 140 | 1.5 | 0 |
| Boiled, 5 oz | 140 | 1 | 0 |
| Lobster Salads, average, ½ cup | 220 | 13 | 5 |
| Lobster Newberg, average, ¾ cup | 360 | 20 | 9 |
| Lobster Thermidor, av., 1 serving | 370 | 22 | 15 |
| **Lobster Tail,** | | | |
| *Red Lobster,* grilled/roasted | 170 | 1 | 1 |
| **Lox,** Regular/Nova, 2 oz | 65 | 2.5 | 0 |
| **Mackerel,** Atlantic: Raw, 4 oz | 230 | 16 | 0 |
| Baked, 3 oz fillet | 225 | 15 | 0 |
| Pacific/Jack: Raw, 4 oz | 180 | 9 | 0 |
| Baked, 3 oz | 170 | 9 | 0 |
| Spanish: Raw, 4 oz | 160 | 7 | 0 |
| Baked, 3 oz | 135 | 5.5 | 0 |
| **Mahi-Mahi/Dolphinfish:** | | | |
| Raw, 4 oz | 95 | 1 | 0 |
| Baked, 4 oz | 125 | 1 | 0 |
| **Monkfish:** Raw, 4 oz | 85 | 1.5 | 0 |
| Baked, 3 oz | 80 | 2 | 0 |
| **Mullet, Striped:** Raw, 4 oz | 135 | 4.5 | 0 |
| Baked, 3 oz | 130 | 4 | 0 |
| **Mussels:** | | | |
| Raw: 4 oz (edible wt) | 100 | 2.5 | 4 |
| 1 cup, 5.3 oz (edible weight) | 130 | 3.5 | 5 |
| Cooked, moist heat, 3 oz | 150 | 4 | 6 |
| **Ocean Perch:** | | | |
| Atlantic: Raw, 4 oz | 90 | 2 | 0 |
| Baked, 3 oz | 80 | 1.5 | 0 |
| **Octopus:** | | | |
| Common: Raw, 4 oz | 95 | 1 | 2.5 |
| Boiled, 3 oz | 140 | 2 | 4 |
| **Orange Roughy:** | | | |
| Raw, 4 oz | 85 | 1 | 0 |
| Baked, 3 oz | 90 | 1 | 0 |

| Fish & Shellfish (Cont) | C | F | Cb |
|---|---|---|---|
| *Edible Weights: Without Bones or Shell* | | | |
| **Oysters,** Common, Raw, 3 oz | 70 | 2 | 4 |
| Eastern: | | | |
| Farmed: Raw, 6 medium, 3 oz | 50 | 1.5 | 4.5 |
| Cooked, dry heat, 6 med., 2 oz | 45 | 1.5 | 4.5 |
| Wild: Raw, 6 medium, 3 oz | 45 | 1.5 | 2.5 |
| Cooked, dry heat, 6 med., 2 oz | 45 | 1.5 | 2.5 |
| Breaded & Fried, 6 med., 3 oz | 175 | 11 | 10 |
| Pacific: Raw, 1 medium, 1.8 oz | 40 | 1 | 2.5 |
| Steamed, 1 medium, 0.8 oz | 40 | 1 | 2.5 |
| **Perch ~** *See Ocean Perch* | | | |
| **Pike:** Northern: Raw, 4 oz | 100 | 1 | 0 |
| Baked, 3 oz | 95 | 1 | 0 |
| Walleye: Raw, 4 oz | 105 | 1.5 | 0 |
| Baked, 3 oz | 100 | 1.5 | 0 |
| **Pollock,** Atlantic: Raw, 4 oz | 105 | 1 | 0 |
| Baked, 3 oz | 100 | 1 | 0 |
| **Pompano,** Florida, raw, 4 oz | 185 | 11 | 0 |
| **Red Snapper ~** *See Snapper* | | | |
| **Roe,** raw, 2 Tbsp, 1 oz | 40 | 2 | 0.5 |
| **Sablefish:** Raw, 4 oz | 220 | 17 | 0 |
| Smoked, 3 oz | 220 | 17 | 0 |
| **Salmon:** | | | |
| Atlantic, Farmed: Raw, 4 oz | 235 | 15 | 0 |
| Baked, 3 oz | 175 | 10 | 0 |
| Steaks: Raw, 7 oz | 410 | 27 | 0 |
| Baked, 6 oz | 365 | 22 | 0 |
| Atlantic, Wild: Raw, 4 oz | 160 | 7 | 0 |
| Baked, 3 oz | 155 | 7 | 0 |
| Steaks: Raw, 7 oz | 280 | 13 | 0 |
| Baked, 6 oz | 310 | 14 | 0 |
| Chinook: Raw, 4 oz | 205 | 12 | 0 |
| Baked, 3 oz | 195 | 11 | 0 |
| Smoked, 3 oz | 100 | 3.5 | 0 |
| King: Raw, 3.5 oz | 185 | 12 | 0 |
| Kippered, 3.5 oz piece | 265 | 16 | 0 |
| Smoked & canned, 3.5 oz | 150 | 6 | 0 |
| Coho: | | | |
| Farmed: Raw, 4 oz | 180 | 8.5 | 0 |
| Baked, 3 oz | 150 | 7 | 0 |
| Wild: Raw, 4 oz | 165 | 6.5 | 0 |
| Steamed, 3 oz | 155 | 6.5 | 0 |
| Pink/Chum: Raw, 4 oz | 145 | 5 | 0 |
| Baked, 3.5 oz | 155 | 5.5 | 0 |
| Canned: Drained solids, 11 oz | 435 | 16 | 0 |
| Without skin & bones, 8.5 oz | 330 | 10 | 0 |
| Sockeye: Raw, 4 oz | 160 | 6.5 | 0 |
| Baked, 3 oz | 145 | 5.5 | 0 |
| Canned, Drained solids, 3 oz | 140 | 6.5 | 0 |
| Smoked, 3.5 oz | 205 | 7.5 | 0 |
| Salmon Cake (1), 3 oz | 240 | 15 | 6 |

## Fish & Shellfish (Cont)

**Sardines:** *Canned, Average all Brands*

| | | | |
|---|---|---|---|
| Drained of Oil: | | | |
| ¼ cup drained, 2.2 oz | 130 | 9 | 0 |
| 3.75 oz can, drained, 3.3 oz | 190 | 11 | 0 |
| 1 large/2 medium, ⅗", 0.8 oz | 50 | 3 | 0 |
| In Tomato Sauce, 3.8 oz | 150 | 8 | 3 |
| **Sashimi** ~ *See Japanese Foods, Page 171* | | | |
| **Scallops:** Raw, 6 lge/15 small, 3 oz | 65 | 0.5 | 3 |
| Breaded, Fried (6), 5 oz | 385 | 20 | 39 |
| Steamed, 3 oz | 95 | 0.5 | 0 |
| **Sea Bass** ~ *See Bass* | | | |
| **Seafood Salad**, Deli Style, | | | |
| ½ cup, 3.5 oz | 250 | 21 | 11 |
| **Shark:** Raw, 4 oz | 145 | 5 | 0 |
| Baked, 4 oz | 185 | 7 | 0 |
| Batter-dipped, fried, 4 oz | 260 | 16 | 7 |
| **Shrimp:** | | | |
| Raw: Small/Medium (4), 0.8 oz | 15 | 0 | 0 |
| Large (4), 1 oz | 20 | 0 | 0 |
| Breaded & Fried, 4.8 oz | 395 | 24 | 27 |
| Steamed, in shell, 3 oz | 100 | 1.5 | 0 |
| Canned, 1 can, 4.5 oz | 130 | 2 | 0 |
| **Snapper:** Raw, 4 oz | 115 | 1.5 | 0 |
| Baked: 3 oz | 110 | 1.5 | 0 |
| 6 oz fillet | 220 | 3 | 0 |
| **Sole:** Raw, 4 oz | 80 | 2 | 0 |
| Baked, 3 oz | 75 | 2 | 0 |
| **Squid** ~ *see Calamari* | | | |
| **Surimi**, (Imitation Crab), 4 oz | 110 | 0.5 | 17 |
| **Swai/Basa**, raw, 4 oz | 70 | 2 | 0 |
| **Swordfish:** Raw, 4 oz | 165 | 7.5 | 0 |
| Medium Steak, 6 oz | 250 | 11 | 0 |
| Baked: Small Steak, 4 oz | 205 | 7 | 0 |
| Medium Steak, 6 oz | 290 | 13 | 0 |
| **Tilapia:** Raw, 4 oz | 110 | 2 | 0 |
| Baked: 3 oz | 110 | 2.5 | 0 |
| **Trout**, Rainbow: | | | |
| Farmed: Raw, 4 oz | 160 | 7 | 0 |
| Baked, 3 oz | 145 | 6.5 | 0 |
| Wild: Raw, 4 oz | 135 | 4 | 0 |
| Baked, 3 oz | 130 | 5 | 0 |
| **Tuna:** | | | |
| **Raw:** Bluefin, 4 oz | 165 | 5.5 | 0 |
| Skipjack, Yellowfin, av., 4 oz | 120 | 1 | 0 |
| **Baked:** Bluefin, 3 oz | 155 | 5.5 | 0 |
| Skipjack, Yellowfin, av., 3 oz | 110 | 1 | 0 |
| **Canned:** In Water, drained | | | |
| Chunk Light: 2 oz | 50 | 1 | 0 |
| 3 oz can | 75 | 1.5 | 1 |
| 5 oz can | 125 | 2.5 | 1.5 |

| **Tuna (Cont):** | **C** | **F** | **Cb** |
|---|---|---|---|
| In Water, drained (Cont): | | | |
| Solid White: 2 oz | 60 | 0.5 | 0 |
| 5 oz can | 150 | 1.5 | 0 |
| 7 oz can | 210 | 2 | 0 |
| In Oil, drained: | | | |
| Chunk Light: 2 oz can | 80 | 4 | 0 |
| 5 oz can | 200 | 10 | 0 |
| Solid White: 2 oz can | 90 | 4 | 0 |
| 6 oz can | 270 | 12 | 0 |
| **Tuna Salad**, Deli Style, ½ cup, 4oz | 280 | 20 | 8 |
| **Whitefish:** Raw, 4 oz | 150 | 6.5 | 0 |
| Baked, 3 oz | 145 | 6.5 | 1 |
| Smoked, 3 oz | 90 | 1 | 0 |
| **Whiting:** Raw, 4 oz | 100 | 1.5 | 0 |
| Baked, 3 oz | 100 | 1.5 | 0 |
| **Yellowtail:** Raw, 4 oz | 165 | 6 | 0 |
| Grilled, 3 oz | 160 | 6 | 0 |

## Other Canned/Packaged Fish

| | | | |
|---|---|---|---|
| **Bumble Bee:** | | | |
| **Jack Mackerel**, drained, 2 oz | 90 | 4 | 0 |
| **Pink Salmon**, Skinless & Boneless, | | | |
| drained, 5 oz | 60 | 1.5 | 0 |
| **Red Salmon**, 2.2 oz | 100 | 5 | 0 |
| **Sardines**, in Soya Oil, drained, 1.7 oz | 110 | 6 | 0 |
| **Tuna Ready-To-Eat Kits:** *With Crackers:* | | | |
| Sensations, Tuna Medley: | | | |
| Sundried Tomato & Basil, | | | |
| 3 oz can | 110 | 4.5 | 2 |
| Thai Chili, 3 oz can | 130 | 4.5 | 8 |
| **Tuna, Snack on the Run!:** *With Crackers Kit* | | | |
| Tuna Salad, 2.9 oz can | 220 | 19 | 7 |
| Tuna, Fat Free w/ Wheat Crackers, | | | |
| 2.9 oz can | 70 | 0 | 11 |
| **Tuna, White Albacore:** | | | |
| Pouch, in water, 2 oz | 70 | 1.5 | 0 |
| Solid, in Oil, drained, 2 oz | 80 | 2.5 | 0 |
| **Chicken of the Sea:** | | | |
| Pink Salmon, skinless/boneless, | | | |
| 2.5 oz pouch | 70 | 2 | 0 |
| Sardines, in Olive Oil, 3.75 oz cans | 200 | 16 | 0 |
| Tuna: | | | |
| Lunch Solutions, | | | |
| Tuna Salad Cup & Crackers, 3.4 oz | 80 | 0.5 | 7 |
| To-Go-Cups, Tuna Salad, 2.8 oz | 80 | 0.5 | 7 |
| **Starkist:** | | | |
| **Autentico**, average all, 2 oz drained | 85 | 5 | 3.5 |
| **Pouch:** *Per 2.6 oz Pouch* | | | |
| Albacore White Tuna in water | 80 | 1.5 | 0 |
| Chunk, Light, Tuna in water | 70 | 0.5 | 0 |
| **Lunch-To-Go Kit**, Chunk Light Tuna | | | |
| With Light Mayo & Crackers, 4 oz | 230 | 9 | 20 |
| **Tuna Creations:** *Per 2.6 oz* | | | |
| Herb & Garlic | 110 | 4 | 2 |
| Lemon Pepper | 80 | 0.5 | 1 |

| Flours & Grains | C | F | Cb |
|---|---|---|---|
| **Amaranth Flour**, ½ cup, 3.5 oz | 365 | 6.5 | 65 |
| **Arrowroot Flour**, ½ cup, 2.3 oz | 230 | 0 | 56 |
| **Barley:** Grain, regular, ½ cup, 2.6 oz | 255 | 1 | 55 |
| Pearled, raw, 3.5 oz | 350 | 1 | 78 |
| **Buckwheat:** Grain, ½ cup, 3 oz | 290 | 3 | 61 |
| Flour, whole-groat, ½ cup, 2 oz | 200 | 2 | 42 |
| Groats: Rstd, dry, ½ cup, 3 oz | 285 | 2 | 62 |
| Roasted, cooked, 3.5 oz | 80 | 0.5 | 17 |
| **Bulgur:** Dry, ½ cup, 2.5 oz | 240 | 1 | 53 |
| Cooked, ½ cup, 3.2 oz | 75 | 0.5 | 17 |
| **Carob Flour**, ½ cup, 1.8 oz | 115 | 0.5 | 46 |
| **Corn Kernels**, cooked, av., ½ cup | 80 | 0.5 | 18 |
| **Corn Bran**, ½ cup, 1.3 oz | 85 | 0.5 | 33 |
| **Corn Flour/Masa**, ½ cup, 2 oz | 215 | 2.5 | 43 |
| **Corn Grits:** | | | |
| Dry, ½ cup, 2.8oz | 290 | 1 | 62 |
| Cooked, ½ cup, 4.3 oz | 70 | 0.5 | 15 |
| **Corn Germ**, toasted, ½ cup, 4 oz | 100 | 1.5 | 22 |
| **Cornmeal**, average all varieties: | | | |
| 3 Tbsp, 1 oz | 105 | 0.5 | 22 |
| ½ cup, 2.5 oz | 255 | 1 | 54 |
| Mixes, same as above | 230 | 1 | 48 |
| **Cornstarch:** 1 Tbsp, 0.3 oz | 30 | 0 | 8 |
| ½ cup, 2.3oz | 245 | 0 | 58 |
| **Couscous:** Dry, 1 oz | 110 | 0 | 22 |
| 1 cup cooked, 5.5 oz | 175 | 0.5 | 37 |
| **Farina:** Dry, ½ cup, 3 oz | 325 | 0.5 | 69 |
| Cooked, ½ cup, 4 oz | 55 | 0 | 12 |
| **Flaxseed:** Whole, 1 T., 0.3 oz | 45 | 3.5 | 2 |
| Ground, 2 Tbsp, 0.3 oz | 60 | 4.5 | 4 |
| **Garbanzo**, (Chick Pea), ½ cup, 1.6 oz | 180 | 3 | 27 |
| **Gluten Free Flour**, 3 Tbsp | 100 | 0 | 24 |
| **Matzo Meal**, ½ cup, 2.2 oz | 230 | 0.5 | 48 |
| **Millet:** Raw, ½ cup, 3.5 oz | 380 | 4 | 73 |
| Cooked, ½ cup, 3 oz | 105 | 1 | 21 |
| **Oat Bran:** Raw, ⅓ cup, 1 oz | 75 | 2 | 21 |
| Cooked, ½ cup, 3.8 oz | 45 | 1 | 13 |
| **Oats**, Rolled/Oatmeal: | | | |
| Dry/Groats, ½ cup, 1.5 oz | 160 | 3 | 28 |
| Cooked, ½ cup, 4.2 oz | 75 | 1 | 13 |
| **Polenta** ~ *See Cornmeal* | | | |
| **Potato Flour**, ½ cup, 2.8 oz | 285 | 0.5 | 66 |
| **Psyllium Husks**, 1 Tbsp, 0.2 oz | 10 | 0 | 4 |
| **Quinoa:** Dry ½ cup, 3 oz | 320 | 5 | 59 |
| Cooked, ½ cup, 3.8 oz | 130 | 2 | 24 |
| **Rice Bran**, ½ cup, 2 oz | 180 | 12 | 28 |
| **Rice Flour**, ½ cup, 2.8 oz | 290 | 1 | 63 |

| Flours & Grains (Cont) | C | F | Cb |
|---|---|---|---|
| **Rice Polish**, ½ cup, 3.5 oz | 360 | 0.5 | 80 |
| **Rye Flour:** | | | |
| Dark, ½ cup, 2.3 oz | 210 | 2 | 44 |
| Light, ½ cup, 1.8 oz | 190 | 1 | 41 |
| Medium, ½ cup, 1.8 oz | 180 | 1 | 40 |
| **Rye Grain:** ½ cup, 3 oz | 280 | 2 | 59 |
| Flakes, ¼ cup, 1 oz | 100 | 0.5 | 21 |
| **Semolina Flour**, ½ cup, 3 oz | 300 | 1 | 61 |
| **Sorghum**, ½ cup, 3.4 oz | 325 | 3 | 72 |
| **Soy Flour:** | | | |
| Defatted, 1 cup, 3.5 oz | 330 | 1 | 38 |
| Low-Fat, 1 cup, 3 oz | 325 | 6 | 33 |
| Full-Fat, 1 cup, 3 oz | 365 | 17 | 29 |
| **Soy Meal**, defatted, 1 cup, 4.3 oz | 415 | 3 | 49 |
| **Spelt Flour**, ½ cup, 2 oz | 190 | 1 | 41 |
| **Tapioca Pearl:** | | | |
| Dry, ½ cup, 2.7 oz | 270 | 0 | 67 |
| 3 Tbsp, 1 oz | 100 | 0 | 25 |
| **Teff Seed Flour**, 2 oz | 215 | 2 | 42 |
| **Tortilla Flour Mix**, | | | |
| ½ cup, 2 oz | 220 | 6 | 37 |
| **Triticale:** | | | |
| ½ cup, 3.4 oz | 325 | 2 | 70 |
| Flour, wholegrain, ½ cup, 2.3 oz | 220 | 1 | 48 |
| **Wheat Bran**, unprocessed, ½ cup, 1 oz | 65 | 1 | 19 |
| **Wheat Flakes**, ½ cup, 1.5 oz | 160 | 1 | 35 |
| **Wheat Germ:** | | | |
| Raw, ¼ cup, 1 oz | 105 | 3 | 15 |
| Toasted, ¼ cup, 1 oz | 110 | 3 | 14 |
| **Wheat Flour:** | | | |
| White, All Purpose/Self-Rising: | | | |
| 1 level Tbsp, 0.3 oz | 30 | 0 | 6 |
| ½ cup, 2.2 oz | 230 | 0.5 | 48 |
| 1 cup, 4.4 oz | 455 | 1.5 | 95 |
| Whole Wheat, 1 cup, 4.2 oz | 405 | 2 | 87 |

FRUIT
TIME

## Fruit ~ Fresh

*Weights As Purchased*

| | C | F | Cb |
|---|---|---|---|
| **Apples**, all varieties, average: | | | |
| Whole, with skin: | | | |
| 1 small, 4 oz | 55 | 0 | 14 |
| 1 medium, 5.5 oz | 75 | 0 | 19 |
| 1 large, 8 oz | 110 | 0 | 28 |
| 1 extra large, 11 oz | 145 | 0 | 36 |
| Flesh only, no skin or core: 1 oz | 15 | 0 | 3.5 |
| Slices, 1 cup, 4 oz | 55 | 0 | 14 |
| Candy/Caramel Apple, 1 med., 6.5 oz | 245 | 4 | 54 |
| *Chiquita,* Apple Bites, 14 slices, 5 oz | 80 | 0 | 20 |
| **Apricots:** 1 small, 1.5oz | 20 | 0 | 4 |
| 1 medium, 2 oz | 25 | 0 | 6 |
| 1 large, 3 oz | 40 | 0 | 10 |
| 1 extra large, 4 oz | 50 | 0 | 12 |
| **Asian Pear**, (Nashi Fruit), 1 med., 7 oz | 85 | 0 | 21 |
| **Avocado:** | | | |
| Fuerte (Florida) variety: | | | |
| ¼ medium, 2.7 oz pulp | 90 | 7.5 | 6 |
| ½ medium, 5.4 oz pulp | 180 | 15 | 12 |
| Mashed, 1 Tbsp, 1 oz | 35 | 3 | 2 |
| Hass variety (Californian/Mexican): | | | |
| Cubes, ½ cup, 2.5 oz | 120 | 11 | 6 |
| Mashed: 2 Tbsp, 1 oz | 50 | 4 | 2 |
| ¼ cup, 2 oz | 95 | 8 | 5 |
| Pulp: ¼ medium, 1.5 oz | 70 | 6.5 | 3 |
| ½ medium, 3 oz | 140 | 13 | 7 |
| 1 medium (8.5 oz whole), 6 oz | 280 | 26 | 14 |
| Salad slices (3), 1 oz | 50 | 4 | 2 |

Note: The fat of avocados is heart-healthy. Avocados are very low in sugars; and most of the carbohydrate is fiber. This benefits blood sugar and cholesterol levels. Use in place of butter and other high-fat spreads.

| | C | F | Cb |
|---|---|---|---|
| **Banana:** | | | |
| Weight with skin: | | | |
| 1 baby, 3 oz | 50 | 0 | 12 |
| 1 small (5"), 4 oz | 65 | 0 | 16 |
| 1 medium (7"), 5 oz | 80 | 0 | 20 |
| 1 large (8"), 8 oz | 120 | 0 | 30 |
| 1 extra large (9"), 9 oz | 135 | 0 | 34 |
| Flesh only, weight without skin: | | | |
| Mashed, ½ cup, 4 oz | 100 | 0 | 25 |
| Slices, ½ cup, 2.5 oz | 65 | 0 | 16 |
| Green Bananas, weight with skin: | | | |
| 1 medium (7"), 5 oz | 75 | 0 | 18 |
| 1 large (8"), 7 oz | 110 | 0 | 27 |
| **Blackberries**, 1 cup, 5 oz | 60 | 0.5 | 14 |
| **Blueberries:** ¼ cup, 1 oz | 15 | 0 | 4 |
| 1 cup or ½ pint container, 5 oz | 80 | 0 | 20 |
| 1 pint container, 10 oz | 160 | 0 | 40 |

*Weights As Purchased*

| | C | F | Cb |
|---|---|---|---|
| **Boysenberries**, 1 cup, 4.5 oz | 60 | 4.5 | 14 |
| **Breadfruit**, ½ cup, 4 oz | 115 | 0 | 30 |
| **Cactus Fruit:** | | | |
| 1 small, 2 oz | 15 | 0 | 4 |
| 1 medium, 5 oz | 40 | 0 | 9 |
| 1 large, 7 oz | 55 | 0 | 13 |
| Pulp, no skin, 1 cup, 5.3 oz | 60 | 0 | 14 |
| **Cantaloupe:** Flesh, without skin, 1 oz | 10 | 0 | 2 |
| Pieces/Balls, 1 cup, 5.5 oz | 55 | 0 | 13 |
| Slices, ½ circle, without rind: | | | |
| 1 thin (buffet), (⅛"), 0.5 oz | 5 | 0 | 1 |
| 1 medium (¼"), 1 oz | 10 | 0 | 2 |
| 1 thick (½"), 2 oz | 20 | 0 | 5 |
| Wedges, length cut, without skin: | | | |
| 1 thin, 1/16 medium, 2 oz | 20 | 0 | 5 |
| 1 thick, ⅛ medium, 4 oz | 40 | 0 | 9 |
| Whole, weight with seeds and skin: | | | |
| ½ small, 20 oz | 195 | 1 | 46 |
| ½ medium, 28 oz | 270 | 1.5 | 65 |
| ½ large, 2.5 lb | 370 | 2 | 90 |
| **Cape Gooseberries**, 1 cup, 5 oz | 70 | 1 | 15 |
| **Cherimoya:** Pulp, ½ cup, 3 oz | 60 | 0 | 14 |
| 1 Fruit (11 oz), 8 oz edible | 170 | 1 | 40 |
| **Cherries**, (Red/White), sweet, raw: | | | |
| 6 medium or 4 large, 2 oz | 30 | 0 | 7 |
| 1 cup, 4.5 oz | 75 | 0 | 18 |
| ½ lb quantity | 130 | 0 | 32 |
| Sour, red, raw, 1 cup, 4 oz | 50 | 0 | 12 |
| **Clementine**, 1 medium, 2.6 oz | 35 | 0 | 9 |
| **Coconut**, raw: | | | |
| Young, sweet, | | | |
| Pieces: 1 piece (2" x 2"), 1.5 oz | 35 | 2 | 4 |
| ½ cup, 3.5 oz | 80 | 5 | 9 |
| Mature, hard, 1 piece (2"x 2"), 1.5 oz | 160 | 15 | 6 |
| **Crabapples**, slices, ½ cup, 2 oz | 40 | 0 | 11 |
| **Cranberries**, fresh, ¼ cup, 1 oz | 25 | 0 | 6.5 |
| **Custard Apple** ~ *See Cherimoya* | | | |
| **Dates:** Medium (1), 0.3 oz | 20 | 0 | 5 |
| Large Medjool (1), 0.5 oz | 40 | 0 | 10 |
| Extra Large Medjool (1), 0.9 oz | 65 | 0 | 16 |
| Chopped, ½ cup, 3 oz | 240 | 0 | 58 |
| **Dragon Fruit**, (Pitahaya): | | | |
| 1 medium, 4"long, 12 oz | 60 | 0 | 12 |
| 1 large, 5"long, 16 oz | 80 | 0 | 18 |
| **Durian**, pulp, 4 oz | 165 | 6 | 31 |
| **Elderberries**, ½ cup, 2.5 oz | 55 | 0.5 | 13 |

| Weights As Purchased | C | F | Cb |
|---|---|---|---|
| **Feijoa**, (Pineapple Guava), | | | |
| 1 medium, 2 oz | 30 | 0.5 | 5.5 |
| **Figs**, green/black: | | | |
| 1 medium, 2 oz | 40 | 0 | 10 |
| 1 large, 3 oz | 60 | 0 | 15 |
| **Gooseberries**, raw, 1 cup, 5 oz | 65 | 1 | 15 |
| **Grapefruit**, all varieties, average: | | | |
| ½ fruit, 10 oz (6 oz flesh) | 55 | 0 | 13 |
| 1 cup sections w/ juice, 8 oz | 75 | 0 | 18 |
| **Grapes:** Average, 1 cup, 5.5 oz | 105 | 0 | 28 |
| 1 small bunch, 4 oz | 80 | 0 | 20 |
| 1 medium bunch, 7 oz | 140 | 0 | 36 |
| 1 large bunch, 16 oz | 315 | 0 | 82 |
| **Granadilla**, pulp, ½ cup, 4 oz | 110 | 0 | 27 |
| **Guanabana**, pulp, ½ cup, 4 oz | 75 | 0 | 19 |
| **Guava**, 1 medium, 4 oz | 80 | 1 | 16 |
| **Honeydew:** | | | |
| 1 slice, ¾" thick, 3 oz | 30 | 0 | 7 |
| 1 wedge (⅛ of 7" diameter), | | | |
| 12 oz (with rind) | 80 | 0 | 20 |
| Cubes/Balls, 1 cup, 6 oz | 60 | 0 | 14 |
| ½ small (4½ lb whole) | 180 | 0.5 | 42 |
| ½ medium (6lb whole) | 230 | 1 | 56 |
| **Honey Murcots**, 1 only, 5 oz | 45 | 0 | 11 |
| **Jaboticaba**, 1 cup, 5.5 oz | 55 | 0 | 14 |
| **Jackfruit**, flesh, ⅛, 4 oz | 105 | 0 | 27 |
| **Kiwano**, ½ medium, 5 oz | 35 | 0 | 8 |
| **Kiwifruit:** | | | |
| 1 Medium, 2.7 oz | 45 | 0 | 11 |
| 1 Large, 3.2 oz | 55 | 0 | 13 |
| **Langsat**, Duku, 1 medium, 2 oz | 25 | 0 | 5 |
| **Lemons:** 1 medium, 5oz | 20 | 0 | 4 |
| 1 wedge, 1 oz | 5 | 0 | 1 |
| **Limes:** 1 medium, 2.4 oz | 20 | 0 | 7 |
| **Loganberries**, frozen, ½ cup, 2.5 oz | 40 | 0 | 9 |
| **Longans**, 5 fruit, 0.5oz | 10 | 0 | 2.5 |
| **Loquats**, 4 fruit, 2.3 oz | 30 | 0 | 8 |
| **Lychees**, 4 fruit, 2.3 oz | 30 | 0 | 7 |
| **Mamey Apple**, Cubes, 1 cup, 6 oz | 85 | 1 | 20 |
| **Mandarin Orange:** | | | |
| 1 small, 3 oz | 35 | 0 | 9 |
| 1 medium, 4 oz | 45 | 0 | 11 |
| 1 large, 6 oz | 50 | 0 | 13 |
| **Mango:** | | | |
| Slices, ½ cup, 3 oz | 55 | 0 | 14 |
| 1 small mango, 7 oz | 90 | 0.5 | 24 |
| 1 medium: 10 oz | 130 | 0.5 | 34 |
| Side cheek, 4 oz | 60 | 0 | 14 |
| 1 large, 17 oz | 220 | 1 | 58 |
| 1 extra large, 24 oz | 310 | 1.5 | 82 |
| **Marionberries**, 1 cup, 5 oz | 75 | 1 | 15 |

| Weights As Purchased | C | F | Cb |
|---|---|---|---|
| **Melons**, all varieties, average, | | | |
| cubes/balls, 1 cup, 6 oz | 60 | 0 | 14 |
| **Mulberries**, 20 fruit, 1 oz | 15 | 0 | 3 |
| **Nashi Fruit/Asian Pear**, 1 med. 7 oz | 85 | 0 | 21 |
| **Nectarines:** 1 medium, 5oz | 60 | 0 | 14 |
| 1 large, 7 oz | 80 | 0 | 18 |
| **Oheloberries**, ½ cup, 2.5 oz | 20 | 0 | 5 |
| **Olives**, Pickled: Green, 10 lge, 1.5 oz | 60 | 6.5 | 1.5 |
| Ripe, Greek Style, 10 medium, 1 oz | 70 | 6 | 4 |
| Ripe (Black) Californian: | | | |
| 1 small/medium | 5 | 0 | 0.2 |
| 1 large/extra large | 6 | 0.5 | 0.5 |
| 1 jumbo | 7 | 0.5 | 0.5 |
| 1 colossal | 11 | 1 | 0.5 |
| **Oranges**, all varieties, average, weights with skin: | | | |
| 1 small, (2.5" diam.), 5 oz | 45 | 0 | 11 |
| 1 medium (3") 7 oz | 75 | 0 | 18 |
| 1 large, (3.5") 10 oz | 105 | 0 | 25 |
| 1 extra large, (4"), 14 oz | 130 | 0 | 30 |
| Flesh/Pulp only, 1 cup, 6 oz | 85 | 0 | 21 |
| Peel, 1 Tbsp | 0 | 0 | 0 |
| California Navel (3"), 7 oz | 70 | 0 | 17 |
| Californian Valencia, | | | |
| 1 medium (2¾" diam.) 6 oz | 60 | 0 | 14 |
| Florida Orange, 1 med., 7 oz | 70 | 0 | 17 |
| Sunkist Navel, large, 14 oz | 130 | 0 | 30 |
| **Papaya:** | | | |
| 1" pieces, 1 cup, 5 oz | 60 | 0 | 15 |
| 1 medium, 16 oz | 120 | 0 | 30 |
| Green (unripe), ½ cup, 3.5 oz | 20 | 0 | 5 |
| **Passionfruit:** | | | |
| 1 small, 1.5 oz | 15 | 0 | 3 |
| 1 large, 2.7 oz | 30 | 0 | 6 |
| Pulp, ½ cup, 4 oz | 110 | 0 | 27 |
| **Peaches:** 1 baby/donut, 3 oz | 30 | 0 | 7 |
| 1 small, 5 oz | 50 | 0 | 12 |
| 1 medium, 6 oz | 60 | 0 | 14 |
| 1 large, 7 oz | 70 | 0 | 16 |
| 1 extra large, 9 oz | 90 | 0 | 21 |
| **Pears**, all varieties, average: | | | |
| 1 mini, 2.5 oz | 35 | 0 | 8 |
| 1 small, 5 oz | 75 | 0 | 18 |
| 1 medium, 7 oz | 100 | 0 | 25 |
| 1 large, 9 oz | 130 | 0 | 33 |
| 1 extra large, 12 oz | 170 | 0 | 42 |
| **Pepino**, ½ medium, 4 oz | 20 | 0 | 4 |
| **Persimmons:** Native, 1 oz | 35 | 0 | 9 |
| Japanese (2½"d. x 2½"h), 7 oz | 120 | 0 | 30 |
| Seedless (Maui), 1 medium, 5 oz | 100 | 0 | 25 |

### Weights As Purchased

| | C | F | Cb |
|---|---|---|---|
| **Pineapple,** average all varieties: | | | |
| Weights without skin: | | | |
| 1 thin slice (½"), 2 oz | 30 | 0 | 7 |
| 1 thick slice (¾"), 3 oz | 40 | 0 | 10 |
| 1 cup, chunks, 6 oz | 80 | 0 | 20 |
| Whole fruit, wt with skin: | | | |
| Baby/Mini, 16 oz | 150 | 0 | 39 |
| Medium size, 3 lbs | 450 | 1 | 118 |
| **Canned ~** *See Page 102* | | | |
| **Pitanga,** (Surinam-Cherry) (5), 1.2 oz | 10 | 0 | 2 |
| **Plantains:** | | | |
| Fresh/Raw, weight with skin: | | | |
| 1 medium, 10 oz | 220 | 0 | 55 |
| Slices, 1 cup, 5 oz | 180 | 0 | 44 |
| Cooked: | | | |
| Mashed, ½ cup, 3.5 oz | 115 | 0 | 30 |
| Slices, 1 cup, 5.5 oz | 180 | 0 | 47 |
| Fried in oil: 10 slices (¼"), 2 oz | 160 | 6 | 26 |
| 1 cup, 4.2 oz | 360 | 14 | 58 |
| **Plums,** all varieties, average: | | | |
| 1 mini/Damson, (1" diam), 0.5 oz | 10 | 0 | 1.5 |
| 1 small (2"), 2.3oz | 30 | 0 | 7 |
| 1 medium (2½"), 3.5 oz | 45 | 0 | 10 |
| 1 large (3"), 5 oz | 60 | 0 | 14 |
| **Plumcot,** 1 medium, 6 oz | 75 | 0 | 18 |
| **Pomegranates:** | | | |
| 1 small (3"), 5.5 oz | 70 | 1 | 15 |
| 1 medium (3½"), 10 oz | 125 | 2 | 27 |
| 1 large (4"), 16 oz | 230 | 3 | 50 |
| Seeds/Arils, ¼ cup, 2 oz | 40 | 1 | 10 |
| **Pomelo,** flesh, ½ cup, 3.5 oz | 35 | 0 | 9 |
| **Prickly Pear ~** *See Cactus Fruit* | | | |
| **Quince,** 1 medium, 3.5 oz | 55 | 0 | 14 |
| **Rambuta/Rambotang,** | | | |
| Red/Yellow, 1 medium, 2 oz | 15 | 0 | 4 |
| **Raspberries:** ½ cup, 2 oz | 30 | 0 | 7 |
| 10 Raspberries, 0.8 oz | 10 | 0 | 2 |
| 1 Cup, 4.3 oz | 65 | 1 | 15 |
| 1 Pint, 11 oz | 160 | 2 | 37 |
| **Sapodilla:** 1 medium, 6 oz | 140 | 2 | 34 |
| Pulp, 1 cup, 8.5 oz | 200 | 2.5 | 45 |
| **Sapote:** | | | |
| Black: 1 medium, 4.5 oz | 60 | 0 | 14 |
| Pulp only, ½ cup, 4 oz | 100 | 1 | 22 |
| Mamey, piece, 1 cup, 6 oz | 220 | 1 | 50 |
| **Satsuma Tangerine,** 1 medium, 3 oz | 45 | 0 | 11 |
| **Soursop,** pulp, 1 cup, 8 oz | 150 | 0.5 | 38 |
| **Starfruit,** (Carambola): | | | |
| 1 medium, (3½" long), 3 oz | 30 | 0 | 6 |
| 1 large (4½"), 4.5 oz | 40 | 0 | 8 |
| **Strawberries:** 1 cup, 5.5 oz | 50 | 0.5 | 12 |
| 6 medium/3 large, 2 oz | 20 | 0 | 4 |
| 1 pint container, heaping, 16 oz | 130 | 0 | 32 |
| Chocolate Dipped, 1 large | 45 | 2.5 | 6 |

### Weights As Purchased

| | C | F | Cb |
|---|---|---|---|
| **Sugar-Apple (Sweetsop),** | | | |
| pulp, ½ cup, 4 oz | 120 | 0 | 28 |
| **Sugar Cane:** | | | |
| Unpeeled, 1 baton (7" long), 4 oz | 30 | 0 | 7 |
| Peeled, 1 small stick (3"), 2 oz | 35 | 0 | 8 |
| **Tamarillo,** 1 medium, 3 oz | 20 | 0 | 3 |
| **Tamarind:** 1 fruit (3"x1") | 5 | 0 | 1.5 |
| Pulp, ½ cup, 2 oz | 140 | 0.5 | 37 |
| **Tangelo:** 1 small, 4 oz | 55 | 0 | 13 |
| 1 medium, 5 oz | 70 | 0 | 17 |
| 1 large, 7 oz | 95 | 0 | 23 |
| **Tangerine,** 1 med., (2½" diam.), 4 oz | 50 | 0 | 13 |
| **Tangor,** 1 medium, 4 oz | 35 | 0 | 7 |
| **Tomatillos:** | | | |
| 3 medium, 3.5 oz | 35 | 0.5 | 6 |
| 1lb (16 oz) quantity | 160 | 2 | 27 |
| **Tomatoes:** | | | |
| 1 small (2¼" diameter), 3 oz | 15 | 0 | 3 |
| 1 medium (2¾"), 5 oz | 25 | 0 | 5 |
| Sliced: 2 thin slices, 1 oz | 5 | 0 | 1 |
| 2 thick (⅜"), 2 oz | 10 | 0 | 2 |
| Wedge, ¼, 1.3 oz | 6 | 0 | 1 |
| 1 large (3½"), 8 oz | 40 | 0.5 | 9 |
| 1 extra large (4"), 12 oz | 60 | 0.5 | 14 |
| Cherry: 4 medium, 2 oz | 10 | 0 | 2 |
| 1 cup, 5 oz | 25 | 0 | 6 |
| Grape, 5 medium, 2 oz | 10 | 0 | 2 |
| Yellow Tear Drop, 3 medium, 1 oz | 5 | 0 | 2 |
| **Canned Tomatoes/Products ~** *See Page 144* | | | |
| **Tree Tomato/Tamarillo,** 3 oz | 20 | 0 | 5 |
| **Ugli Fruit,** Tangelo type, 5 oz | 40 | 0 | 8 |
| **Watermelon:** | | | |
| Flesh only, weights without skin: | | | |
| 1 thin slice (½"), ¼ circle, 3 oz | 25 | 0 | 6 |
| 1 thick slice (1"): ¼ circle, 6 oz | 50 | 0 | 12 |
| ½ circle, 12 oz | 100 | 1 | 24 |
| Buffet Slice, small, thin, 1 oz | 8 | 0 | 2 |
| Cubes or Balls, 1 cup, 5.5 oz | 45 | 0 | 11 |
| Round Seedless Melon, weight with skin: | | | |
| Medium size, 13 lb, (8" diam.): | | | |
| Whole melon, 13 lb | 1160 | 5 | 280 |
| Wedge, ⅛ whole, 26 oz | 145 | 1 | 35 |
| Mini size, 6 lb, (6.5" diam.): | | | |
| Whole melon, 6 lb | 480 | 2.5 | 110 |
| Wedge, ⅛ whole, 12 oz | 60 | 0 | 14 |

### Dried Fruit

| | C | F | Cb |
|---|---|---|---|
| **Apples**, 5 rings, 1 oz | 80 | 0 | 19 |
| **Apricots**, 8 halves, 1 oz | 65 | 0 | 16 |
| **Banana Chips**, ⅓ cup, 1 oz | 180 | 9 | 16 |
| **Banana Flakes**, 4 Tbsp, 1 oz | 80 | 0 | 20 |
| **Cranberries** *(Craisins)*: | | | |
| Original, ¼ cup | 130 | 0 | 33 |
| Reduced Sugar, ¼ cup | 100 | 0 | 31 |
| Chocolate Covered, ¼ cup, 2 oz | 180 | 8 | 28 |
| **Dates** ~ *See Dates in Fresh Fruit* | | | |
| **Figs**, 3 medium figs, 1 oz | 90 | 0 | 23 |
| **Goji Berries**, 3 Tbsp, 1 oz | 100 | 1 | 20 |
| **Mango Slices**, 5 pieces, 1.4 oz | 25 | 0 | 6 |
| **Papaya Spears**, 2 pieces, 1.4 oz | 120 | 0 | 30 |
| **Peaches**, 2 halves, 1 oz | 60 | 0 | 15 |
| **Pears**, 3 halves, 2 oz | 140 | 0.5 | 34 |
| **Plums** *(Sunsweet)*, (5), 1.4 oz | 100 | 0 | 24 |
| **Prunes/Dried Plums**: | | | |
| With pits, 3 medium, 1 oz | 70 | 0 | 17 |
| Without pits, 4 medium, 1 oz | 70 | 0 | 17 |
| Cooked: With sugar, ½ cup, 5 oz | 155 | 0 | 38 |
| Without sugar, ½ cup, 4.5 oz | 135 | 0 | 33 |
| **Raisins:** 2 Tbsp, 1 oz pack | 85 | 0 | 20 |
| ½ cup, 2.8 oz | 220 | 0.5 | 56 |

### Candied/Glazed Fruit

| | C | F | Cb |
|---|---|---|---|
| **Apricot**, 1 medium, 1 oz | 70 | 0 | 17 |
| **Cherry**, Maraschino (1) | 8 | 0 | 2 |
| **Citron/Fruit Peel**, 1 oz | 85 | 0 | 20 |
| **Ginger**, 1 oz | 90 | 0 | 21 |
| **Pineapple**, 1 slice, 1.3 oz | 120 | 0 | 29 |
| **Tamarind**, dried, sweetened, 1 oz | 70 | 0 | 17 |

### Fruit Leather Rolls

| | C | F | Cb |
|---|---|---|---|
| *Betty Crocker:* Fruit By The Foot, | | | |
| 1 roll, 0.8 oz | 80 | 0 | 17 |
| Fruit Gushers, 1 oz | 90 | 1 | 20 |
| Fruit Roll-Ups, 1 roll | 50 | 1 | 12 |
| *Stretch Island*, Leathers, 1 pouch, 0.5 oz | 45 | 0 | 12 |

### Canned/Bottled Fruit

*Solids & Liquids:*
*Per ½ Cup, 4½ oz Unless indicated*

| | C | F | Cb |
|---|---|---|---|
| **Apricots/Peaches/Pears:** | | | |
| In juice, light | 60 | 0 | 15 |
| In heavy syrup | 105 | 0 | 28 |
| In water/diet | 35 | 0 | 8 |
| **Black/Blueberries:** | | | |
| In heavy syrup | 120 | 0 | 30 |
| In light syrup | 110 | 0 | 26 |

### Canned/Bottled Fruit (Cont)

| | C | F | Cb |
|---|---|---|---|
| **Cherries**, pitted: | | | |
| In heavy syrup | 105 | 0 | 27 |
| In light syrup | 85 | 0 | 22 |
| In water | 55 | 0 | 15 |
| Maraschino, 1 oz | 50 | 0 | 12 |
| **Fruit Cocktail/Salad:** | | | |
| In heavy syrup | 95 | 0 | 25 |
| In juice, light | 60 | 0 | 16 |
| In water/diet | 35 | 0 | 10 |
| **Gooseberries**, light syrup | 90 | 0 | 24 |
| **Grapefruit**, in light syrup | 75 | 0 | 20 |
| **Lychees**, ½ cup, 4.5 oz | 105 | 0 | 26 |
| **Mixed Fruit:** In fruit juices/light syrup | 70 | 0 | 18 |
| In heavy syrup | 90 | 0 | 24 |
| In water/diet | 40 | 0 | 10 |
| **Pineapple**, all varieties: | | | |
| In heavy syrup, 4.3 oz | 110 | 0 | 26 |
| In own juice, 4 oz | 60 | 0 | 15 |
| **Prunes:** With syrup, 3 oz | 90 | 0 | 23 |
| Stewed in water, ½ cup | 135 | 0 | 35 |

### Fruit Snack Cups

| | C | F | Cb |
|---|---|---|---|
| **Deli/Take-Out:** Small, 6 oz | 70 | 0 | 16 |
| Large, 12 oz | 140 | 0 | 32 |
| Yogurt and Fruit Cup, 15 oz | 380 | 4.5 | 75 |
| **Del Monte:** | | | |
| **Fruit Natural:** All varieties, av., 7 oz | 100 | 0 | 24 |
| No Sugar Added, all varieties, 6.5 oz | 55 | 0 | 12 |
| **Snack Cups In Light Syrup:** Av., 4 oz | 70 | 0 | 18 |
| No Added Sugar, Peaches, 3.8 oz | 30 | 0 | 7 |
| **Snack Cups In Gel:** | | | |
| Mixed Fruit in Cherry Flav. Gel, 4.5 oz | 80 | 0 | 20 |
| Peaches in Peach Flavored Gel, 4.5 oz | 80 | 0 | 19 |
| **Dole:** | | | |
| **Fruit Bowls:** *Per 4 oz Container* | | | |
| Cherry Mixed Fruit; Tropical Fruit, av. | 65 | 0 | 17 |
| Diced Pears | 90 | 0 | 21 |
| **Fruit in Gel:** *Per 4.3 oz Container* | | | |
| Mixed Fruit, in Cherry Gel | 100 | 0 | 24 |
| Average other fruits, in various Gels | 95 | 0 | 24 |

### Apple & Fruit Sauces

| | C | F | Cb |
|---|---|---|---|
| **Apple Sauce:** | | | |
| Regular/sweetened, 2 Tbsp, 1 oz | 20 | 0 | 6 |
| 4 oz package | 90 | 0 | 22 |
| **Cranberry**, Jellied, ¼ cup | 110 | 0 | 25 |
| **Fruit Sauces & Purees:** | | | |
| All fruit types, average: 2 Tbsp, 1 oz | 25 | 0 | 6 |
| ½ cup, 4 oz | 100 | 0 | 24 |
| **Mott's:** | | | |
| Apple Sauce: Original, 4 oz | 90 | 0 | 24 |
| Fruit Flavored, 4 oz | 90 | 0 | 23 |
| Healthy Harvest, all flavors, 4 oz | 50 | 0 | 13 |
| **Ocean Spray**, Cranberry, ¼ cup | 110 | 0 | 25 |

## Quick Guide  **C** **F** **Cb**

### Ice Cream
*Average all Flavors:*

**Regular (10% fat):**
*Examples: Dreyer's Grand, Hood, Friendly's*

| | C | F | Cb |
|---|---|---|---|
| ½ cup, 4 fl.oz | 140 | 7 | 16 |
| 1 cup, 8 fl.oz | 280 | 14 | 32 |
| 1 pint, 16 fl.oz | 560 | 28 | 64 |

**Rich/Premium (16-17% fat):**
*Examples: Baskin Robbins, Ben & Jerry's, Haagen-Dazs*

| | C | F | Cb |
|---|---|---|---|
| ½ cup, 4 fl.oz | 250 | 16 | 24 |
| 1 cup, 8 fl.oz | 500 | 32 | 48 |
| 1 pint, 16 fl.oz | 1000 | 64 | 96 |

**Reduced-Fat/Light (5% fat):**
*Examples: Breyers ½ The Fat, Friendly's Light, Hood Light*

| | C | F | Cb |
|---|---|---|---|
| ½ cup, 4 fl.oz | 140 | 5 | 21 |
| 1 cup, 8 fl.oz | 280 | 10 | 42 |
| 1 pint, 16 fl.oz | 560 | 20 | 84 |

**Fat-Free:**
*Example: Breyers*

| | C | F | Cb |
|---|---|---|---|
| ½ cup, 4 fl.oz | 90 | 0 | 21 |
| 1 cup, 8 fl.oz | 180 | 0 | 42 |
| 1 pint, 16 fl.oz | 360 | 0 | 84 |

### Scoop Shops:
*Average all Brands*
Add extra for cone (see next column)

| | C | F | Cb |
|---|---|---|---|
| **Kids,** 3 fl.oz | 125 | 8 | 12 |
| **Regular,** 6 fl.oz | 250 | 16 | 24 |
| **Large,** 9 fl.oz | 375 | 24 | 36 |

### Soft Serve:
*Average all Brands*

| | C | F | Cb |
|---|---|---|---|
| **Regular:** ½ cup, 4 fl.oz | 255 | 15 | 25 |
| 1 cup, 8 fl.oz | 510 | 30 | 50 |
| **Light:** ½ cup, 4 fl.oz | 145 | 3 | 25 |
| 1 cup, 8 fl.oz | 290 | 6 | 50 |

## Quick Guide

### Frozen Yogurt
*Average all Brands*

| | C | F | Cb |
|---|---|---|---|
| **Hard:** Low-Fat, ½ cup | 110 | 3 | 19 |
| Non-Fat, ½ cup | 110 | 0 | 24 |
| **Soft:** Low-Fat, ½ cup | 120 | 4 | 17 |
| Non-Fat, ½ cup | 100 | 0 | 30 |

**Brands** ~ *See Ice Cream & Novelties Section*

## Quick Guide  **C** **F** **Cb**

### Gelato/Ices/Frozen Custard

**Gelato:** *Per ½ Cup*

| | C | F | Cb |
|---|---|---|---|
| Milk base: Vanilla | 160 | 6 | 25 |
| Chocolate Hazelnut | 230 | 15 | 21 |
| Water base, ½ cup | 100 | 0 | 26 |

**Frozen Custard**, Choc./Vanilla, av:

| | C | F | Cb |
|---|---|---|---|
| ½ cup | 210 | 11 | 23 |
| Single Scoop, 5 oz wt | 300 | 15 | 38 |
| Double Scoop, 10 oz wt | 600 | 30 | 76 |

**Ice (Milk base):** *Average all flavors*

| | C | F | Cb |
|---|---|---|---|
| Hard (4% fat), ½ cup | 100 | 3 | 15 |
| Soft Serve (3% fat), ½ cup | 110 | 2 | 19 |
| **Shaved Ice**, average, 12 fl.oz | 160 | 0 | 40 |
| **Sherbet**, average, ½ cup | 110 | 1.5 | 22 |
| **Sorbet**, Fruit, fat free, ½ cup | 70 | 0 | 19 |
| **Fruit Ice Pops** | 80 | 0 | 20 |

## Sundaes

**Baskin Robbins:**

| | C | F | Cb |
|---|---|---|---|
| **Classic:** Banana Royale | 620 | 28 | 87 |
| Banana Split | 1010 | 34 | 173 |
| Brownie | 920 | 47 | 119 |

**Denny's,**

| | C | F | Cb |
|---|---|---|---|
| Banana Split, 15 oz | 810 | 31 | 125 |

**Toppings** ~ *See Page 195*

**McDonald's:**

| | C | F | Cb |
|---|---|---|---|
| **Sundaes:** Hot Caramel, 6.4 oz | 340 | 8 | 60 |
| Hot Fudge, 6.3 oz | 330 | 9 | 53 |
| Strawberry, 6.4 oz | 280 | 6 | 49 |
| **Toppings**, Peanuts, 0.3 oz | 40 | 3.5 | 1 |

## Ice Cream Cones & Cups

*Average all Brands*

| | C | F | Cb |
|---|---|---|---|
| **Wafer Cone/Cup**, average | 20 | 0 | 4 |
| **Sugar Cone**, average | 50 | 0 | 14 |

**Waffle Cone:**

| | C | F | Cb |
|---|---|---|---|
| Small | 50 | 1 | 10 |
| Large | 90 | 0.5 | 19 |

**Brands:**

| | C | F | Cb |
|---|---|---|---|
| *Comet*, Sugar Cone | 50 | 0 | 11 |
| *Keebler*, Sugar Cone | 50 | 0 | 10 |
| *Oreo*, Chocolate Cone | 50 | 1 | 10 |

## Ice Cream ~ Brands  C  F  Cb

**Amy's:**

**Non Dairy Frozen Dessert:** *Per ½ Cup*

| | C | F | Cb |
|---|---|---|---|
| Chocolate; Vanilla, average, 3.3 oz | 175 | 12 | 15 |
| Choc./Mocha Choc. Chip, av., 3.5 oz | 230 | 15 | 23 |

**Baskin-Robbins** ~ *See Fast-Foods Section*

**Ben & Jerry's:**

**Scoop Shop Ice Cream:** *Hand Scooped, per ½ Cup*

| | C | F | Cb |
|---|---|---|---|
| Americone Dream | 260 | 14 | 29 |
| Butter Pecan | 270 | 19 | 19 |
| Choc. Chip Cookie Dough | 250 | 13 | 28 |
| Chocolate Fudge Brownie | 230 | 12 | 27 |
| Chocolate Peanut Buttery Swirl | 270 | 18 | 22 |
| Chocolate Therapy | 240 | 13 | 26 |
| Chunky Monkey | 260 | 16 | 26 |
| Coconut Seven Layer Bar | 270 | 17 | 27 |
| Mint Chocolate Chunk | 240 | 15 | 24 |
| NY Super Fudge Chunk | 260 | 17 | 24 |
| Strawberry Cheesecake | 220 | 13 | 24 |
| Sweet Cream & Cookies | 230 | 13 | 25 |
| Vanilla Toffee Bar Crunch | 280 | 19 | 24 |

**Ice Cream, 1 Pint Tubs:** *Per ½ Cup*

| | C | F | Cb |
|---|---|---|---|
| Banana Split | 250 | 14 | 28 |
| Boston Cream Pie | 260 | 14 | 30 |
| Cake Batter | 270 | 16 | 27 |
| Cherry Garcia | 260 | 15 | 27 |
| Chocolate Chip Cookie Dough | 280 | 15 | 32 |
| Chubby Hubby | 340 | 21 | 33 |
| Everything But The... | 310 | 19 | 29 |
| Hazed & Confsed; Milk & Cookies, av. | 280 | 17 | 29 |
| Peanut Butter Cup | 370 | 26 | 29 |
| Peanut Butter Fudge | 300 | 19 | 28 |
| Salted Caramel | 270 | 14 | 31 |
| Phish Food | 290 | 14 | 38 |
| Red Velvet Cake | 260 | 14 | 29 |
| S'mores | 310 | 16 | 36 |
| That's My Jam | 260 | 13 | 31 |
| Triple Caramel Chunk | 270 | 15 | 32 |
| What a Cluster | 320 | 19 | 31 |

**Frozen Yogurt:** *Per ½ Cup*

| | C | F | Cb |
|---|---|---|---|
| **Fro Yo:** Cherry Garcia | 170 | 3 | 32 |
| Chocolate Fudge Brownie | 180 | 2.5 | 35 |
| Half Baked | 180 | 3 | 35 |
| Pfish Food, 3.6 oz | 250 | 7 | 42 |
| **Greek:** Peach Melba | 150 | 5 | 23 |
| Raspberry Fudge Chunk | 190 | 7 | 26 |
| Strawberry Shortcake | 170 | 5 | 26 |
| **Sorbet,** average all flavors | 95 | 0 | 23 |

**Blue Bunny:**  C  F  Cb

**Premium Ice Cream (Pint Ctn):** *Per ½ Cup*

| | C | F | Cb |
|---|---|---|---|
| Banana Split | 160 | 7 | 21 |
| Bunny Tracks | 190 | 11 | 21 |
| Chocolate | 130 | 6 | 17 |
| Cookies 'n Cream | 150 | 7 | 20 |

**Fat Free, No Sugar Added:** *Per ½ Cup*

| | C | F | Cb |
|---|---|---|---|
| Brownie Sundae | 80 | 0 | 23 |
| Caramel Toffee Crunch | 90 | 0 | 23 |
| Vanilla | 80 | 0 | 20 |

*Carb figures include 4-8 g sugar alcohols*

**Hi Lite:** *Per ½ Cup*

| | C | F | Cb |
|---|---|---|---|
| Homemade Vanilla | 110 | 3.5 | 18 |
| Vanilla, 2.3 oz | 100 | 3 | 17 |

**Frozen Yogurt:** *Per ½ Cup*

| | C | F | Cb |
|---|---|---|---|
| Bordeaux Cherry Chocolate | 120 | 3 | 21 |
| Caramel Praline Crunch | 120 | 4 | 20 |

**Bars/Pops ~** *See Page 108*

**Breyers:**

**Original Ice Cream:** *Per ½ Cup*

| | C | F | Cb |
|---|---|---|---|
| Butter Pecan | 130 | 6 | 17 |
| Cherry Vanilla; Cookies & Cream | 125 | 3.5 | 23 |
| Chocolate Truffle | 170 | 9 | 21 |
| Mint Chocolate Chip | 150 | 8 | 18 |
| Natural Strawberry | 110 | 5 | 14 |
| Salted Caramel | 130 | 3.5 | 23 |
| Vanilla, Chocolate | 130 | 7 | 16 |

**Fat Free,** average all flavors | 90 | 0 | 21

**Half The Fat:** *Per ½ Cup*

| | C | F | Cb |
|---|---|---|---|
| Cookies & Cream | 120 | 4 | 20 |
| Creamy, Chocolate or Vanilla, av. | 105 | 3 | 18 |

**No Added Sugar:**

| | C | F | Cb |
|---|---|---|---|
| Butter Pecan; Mini Chip Swirl, av. | 100 | 5 | 14 |
| Salted Crmel Swirl; Strawb & Crm, av. | 85 | 4 | 15 |
| Vanilla; Vanilla, Choc., Strawberry | 80 | 4 | 13 |

*Carb figures include 1-5g sugar alcohol and 0-4g fiber*

**Blasts!:** *Per ½ Cup*

| | C | F | Cb |
|---|---|---|---|
| Girl Scout Cookies Thin Mint | 140 | 4.5 | 23 |
| Mrs Field's Choc Fudge Brownie | 140 | 4 | 25 |
| Oreo Cookies and Cream Mint | 120 | 4 | 20 |
| Strawberry Waffle Cone | 130 | 4 | 22 |

**CarbSmart,** average all flav., ½ cup | 115 | 6 | 14

*Carb figures includes 5g sugar alcohol and 4g fiber*

**Bruster's:**

**Ice Cream,** Choc./Vanilla, av., ½ cup | 210 | 12 | 24

**Fat Free, No Added Sugar:** *Per ½ Cup*

| | C | F | Cb |
|---|---|---|---|
| Chocolate | 100 | 0 | 26 |
| Chocolate Caramel/Fudge Swirl | 120 | 0 | 31 |
| Cinnamon; Coffee; Vanilla, av. | 100 | 0 | 23 |

**Frozen Yogurt,**

| | C | F | Cb |
|---|---|---|---|
| Chocolate; Vanilla, average, ½ cup | 150 | 4.5 | 24 |

## Ice Cream ~ Brands (Cont)

| | **C** | **F** | **Cb** |
|---|---|---|---|
| **Clemmy's:** *Per ½ Cup* | | | |
| Chocolate; Chocolate Chip, average | 175 | 13 | 22 |
| Coffee; Vanilla Bean, av. | 160 | 11 | 21 |
| Orange Cream | 120 | 6 | 23 |
| Toasted Almond | 170 | 11 | 26 |
| *Carb figures include 13-15g sugar alcohol* | | | |

**Carvel Ice Cream** ~ *See Fast-Foods Section*
**Coldstone Creamery** ~ *See Fast-Foods Section*
**Dairy Queen/Brazier** ~ *See Fast-Foods Section*
**Dannon:**

| **Oikos Greek Frozen Yogurt:** *Per ½ Cup* | | | |
|---|---|---|---|
| Cookies & Cream; Strawberry, av. | 140 | 3 | 24 |
| Salted Caramel | 160 | 3 | 28 |
| Average other flavors | 150 | 3 | 26 |

**Dippin' Dots:**

| **Original Dots:** *Per ½ Cup* | | | |
|---|---|---|---|
| Banana Split | 160 | 8 | 20 |
| Caramel Brownie Sundae | 190 | 9 | 23 |
| Cookies 'n Cream | 200 | 11 | 22 |
| Mint Chocolate | 170 | 8 | 21 |
| Rocky Road | 200 | 10 | 22 |
| Strawberry | 160 | 8 | 18 |
| Vanilla | 160 | 8 | 18 |

**Dove:**

| **Ice Cream:** *Per ½ Cup* | | | |
|---|---|---|---|
| Mint/Vanilla Choc. Chunk | 180 | 11 | 17 |
| Unconditional Chocolate | 200 | 12 | 23 |

**Dreyer's/Edy's:**

| **Ice Cream:** *Per ½ Cup* | | | |
|---|---|---|---|
| **Grand:** Chocolate | 140 | 7 | 17 |
| Mint Chocolate Chip | 150 | 8 | 18 |
| Neapolitan | 130 | 6 | 16 |
| Real Strawberry | 120 | 5 | 16 |
| Vanilla | 140 | 7 | 16 |

| **Slow Churned, ½ The Fat:** *Per ½ Cup* | | | |
|---|---|---|---|
| Chocolate | 100 | 3.5 | 15 |
| Double Fudge Brownie | 120 | 3 | 19 |
| Fudge Tracks | 120 | 3.5 | 19 |
| Mint Chocolate Chip | 120 | 4.5 | 17 |
| Peanut Butter Cup | 130 | 5 | 18 |

**Friendly's:**

| **Rich & Creamy Ice Cream:** *Per ½ Cup* | | | |
|---|---|---|---|
| Butter Crunch; Classic Chocolate, av. | 150 | 7 | 18 |
| Chocolate Almond Chip | 160 | 9 | 17 |
| Coffee | 130 | 7 | 15 |
| Strawberry; Vanilla, av. | 140 | 7 | 16 |
| Vienna Mocha Chunk | 170 | 9 | 19 |

| **Friendly's** (Cont): | **C** | **F** | **Cb** |
|---|---|---|---|
| **Smooth Churned Ice Cream:** *Per ½ Cup* | | | |
| Light: Black Raspberry | 110 | 3 | 18 |
| Chocolate Chip Cookie Dough | 140 | 5 | 21 |
| Fudge Swirl | 130 | 4 | 21 |
| Mint Chocolate Chip | 120 | 4.5 | 19 |
| Purely Pistachio | 120 | 4.5 | 18 |
| Vanilla Bean | 100 | 3.5 | 16 |

| **Sundae Cup:** *Per Container* | | | |
|---|---|---|---|
| Original Fudge | 290 | 14 | 38 |
| Choc. Chip Cookie Dough | 330 | 15 | 45 |
| Reese's P'nut Butter Cup | 430 | 25 | 42 |

| **Sherbet**, all flavors, ½ cup | 130 | 1.5 | 28 |
|---|---|---|---|

| **Yogurt Frozen:** *Per ½ Cup* | | | |
|---|---|---|---|
| Regular, average all flavors | 145 | 5 | 24 |
| Fat Free, all flavors | 110 | 0 | 23 |

**Gelati-da:**

| **Gelato:** *Per ½ Cup* | | | |
|---|---|---|---|
| Amaretto Chocolate | 150 | 4.5 | 23 |
| Choc Mint Milano | 120 | 2.5 | 22 |
| Coffee Fudge Latte | 130 | 2 | 22 |
| Limoncello; Vanilla Marsala, average | 120 | 3 | 21 |
| Red Raspberry | 130 | 1.5 | 25 |

**Great Value** *(Walmart):*

| **Ice Cream:** *Per ½ cup* | | | |
|---|---|---|---|
| Chocolate Chip Cookie Dough | 150 | 8 | 19 |
| Coffee | 130 | 7 | 15 |
| Decadent Fudge Tracks | 180 | 10 | 20 |
| Homestyle Vanilla | 140 | 7 | 17 |
| Peanut Butter Cup | 160 | 9 | 17 |
| **Sherbet**, average all flav. | 110 | 0 | 26 |

**Haagen-Dazs:**

| **Regular:** *Tubs, Per ½ Cup* | | | |
|---|---|---|---|
| Butter Pecan | 300 | 22 | 20 |
| Chocolate Peanut Butter | 340 | 23 | 26 |
| Dulce de Leche | 270 | 16 | 27 |
| White Chocolate Raspberry Truffle | 280 | 16 | 31 |

| **Gelato:** *Per ½ Cup* | | | |
|---|---|---|---|
| Black Cherry Amaretto | 240 | 9 | 35 |
| Sea Salt Caramel | 270 | 11 | 38 |

**Healthy Choice,**

| **Greek Frozen Yogurt,** | | | |
|---|---|---|---|
| average all varieties, | 100 | 2 | 18 |

**Bars ~** *See Page 109*

## Ice Cream ~ Brands (Cont)

**Hood:** | | C | F | Cb |
|---|---|---|---|
| **Ice Cream:** *Per ½ Cup* | | | |
| Chocolate | 140 | 6 | 18 |
| Classic Trio | 140 | 7 | 17 |
| Cookie Dough | 170 | 8 | 21 |
| Cookies 'N Cream | 150 | 8 | 19 |
| Creamy Coffee | 140 | 7 | 16 |
| Fudge Twister | 140 | 6 | 20 |
| Golden/Natural Vanilla; Patchwork | 140 | 7 | 17 |
| Maple Walnut | 150 | 9 | 17 |
| **Churned, Light:** *Per ½ Cup* | | | |
| Chocolate Chip | 120 | 4.5 | 18 |
| Coffee | 100 | 3 | 16 |
| Moosehead Lake Fudge | 160 | 7 | 21 |
| Under The Stars | 160 | 8 | 18 |
| Vanilla | 110 | 3 | 16 |
| **Frozen Fat-Free Yogurt:** *Per ½ Cup* | | | |
| Chocolate; Strawberry, av. | 85 | 0 | 19 |
| Chocolate Chip | 110 | 1.5 | 20 |
| Mocha Fudge | 100 | 0 | 22 |

**New England Creamery ~** *www.CalorieKing.com*

**Jerseymaid (Vons):** *Per ½ Cup*

| **Ice Cream:** | | | |
|---|---|---|---|
| Cookies & Cream | 160 | 8 | 18 |
| Choc Chip; Mint Choc Chip | 150 | 9 | 16 |
| Heavenly Hash | 165 | 9 | 19 |
| Mocha Almond Fudge; Chocolate | 150 | 9 | 16 |
| Neapolitan; Real Vanilla | 140 | 8 | 15 |
| Strawberry | 130 | 6 | 17 |

**Oberweis:**

| **Super Premium Ice Cream:** *Per 6 oz Scoop* | | | |
|---|---|---|---|
| Chocolate | 480 | 31 | 43 |
| Chocolate Peanut Butter | 550 | 39 | 42 |
| Cookie Dough | 500 | 28 | 56 |
| Vanilla | 460 | 31 | 40 |

**Oikos ~** *see Dannon*

**Pinkberry:**

| **Frozen Yogurt:** *Without Toppings* | | | |
|---|---|---|---|
| Original: Mini, 3.2 oz wt | 90 | 0 | 19 |
| Small, 5 oz wt | 140 | 0 | 29 |
| Medium, 8 oz wt | 230 | 0 | 48 |
| Large, 13 oz wt | 380 | 0 | 78 |
| Chocolate Hazelnut, 13 oz | 590 | 15 | 96 |
| Cookies & Cream, 13 oz | 520 | 7.5 | 96 |
| Mango, 13 oz | 405 | 0 | 89 |

**Red Mango:** | | C | F | Cb |
|---|---|---|---|
| **Frozen Yogurt:** *No Toppings Included* | | | |
| Original: 3.3 oz wt | 80 | 0 | 18 |
| Small, 4.7 oz wt | 120 | 0 | 26 |
| Regular, 7.5 oz wt | 190 | 0 | 42 |
| Large, 11.4 oz wt | 290 | 0 | 64 |
| Blueberry: 3.3 oz wt | 100 | 0 | 23 |
| Small, 4.7 oz wt | 150 | 0 | 33 |
| Regular, 7.5 oz wt | 230 | 0 | 53 |
| Large, 11.4 oz wt | 350 | 0 | 81 |
| Dulce de Leche: 3.3 oz wt | 80 | 0 | 18 |
| Small, 4.7 oz wt | 120 | 0 | 27 |
| Regular, 7.5 oz wt | 190 | 0 | 43 |
| Large, 11.4 oz wt | 290 | 0 | 65 |
| Pomegranate: 3.3 oz wt | 90 | 0 | 21 |
| Small, 4.6 oz wt | 130 | 0 | 30 |
| Regular, 7.5 oz wt | 210 | 0 | 48 |
| Large, 11.4 oz wt | 320 | 0 | 73 |

**Rice Dream:**

| **Frozen Dessert:** *Per ½ Cup* | | | |
|---|---|---|---|
| Carob Chip | 180 | 7 | 28 |
| Cocoa Marble Fudge | 170 | 6 | 31 |
| Strawberry | 170 | 6 | 30 |
| Vanilla | 160 | 6 | 26 |

**Bars ~** *See Page 110*

**Skinny Cow:**

**Bars/Sandwiches/Cones ~** *See Page 110*

**So Delicious:**

| **Coconut Based:** *Per ½ Cup* | | | |
|---|---|---|---|
| Cherry Amaretto | 130 | 5 | 23 |
| Chocolate | 140 | 7 | 21 |
| Choc. P'Nut Butter Swirl | 200 | 14 | 22 |
| Coconut | 140 | 8 | 20 |

| **Soy Based:** *Per ½ Cup* | | | |
|---|---|---|---|
| Chocolate Obsession | 180 | 7 | 31 |
| Chocolate Velvet | 130 | 3.5 | 23 |
| Creamy Vanilla | 120 | 3 | 24 |
| Mocha Fudge | 130 | 3 | 27 |
| Neapolitan | 120 | 3.5 | 24 |
| Peanut Butter Zig Zag | 210 | 11 | 28 |

**Soy Dream:**

| **Frozen Dessert:** *Per ½ Cup* | | | |
|---|---|---|---|
| Butter Pecan | 190 | 11 | 23 |
| French Vanilla; Vanilla | 170 | 9 | 21 |
| Vanilla Fudge | 170 | 9 | 21 |

## Ice Cream ~ Brands (Cont)

| | **C** | **F** | **Cb** |
|---|---|---|---|
| **Stonyfield Farm:** | | | |
| **Frozen Yogurt:** *Per ½ Cup* | | | |
| After Dark Chocolate | 100 | 0 | 21 |
| Creme Caramel | 130 | 1.5 | 26 |
| Gotta Have Vanilla | 100 | 0 | 21 |
| **Stop & Shop:** | | | |
| **Ice Cream:** *Per ½ Cup* | | | |
| Chocolate | 150 | 8 | 18 |
| Neapolitan; Vanilla, average | 140 | 7.5 | 17 |
| Vanilla Fudge Swirl | 140 | 7 | 18 |
| Light: Moose Tracks | 130 | 5 | 18 |
| Vanilla | 100 | 3 | 17 |
| **Premium:** | | | |
| Cookies & Cream | 170 | 9 | 21 |
| Mint Chocolate Chip | 160 | 9 | 18 |
| **Simply Enjoy:** | | | |
| Chocolate | 210 | 12 | 22 |
| Strawberry; Vanilla, average | 225 | 13 | 25 |
| **Tasti D-Lite:** | | | |
| **Soft Serve:** *Per 4 fl.oz* | | | |
| Banana, 2.5 oz | 70 | 1 | 13 |
| Blueberry Cheesecake, 2.6 oz | 80 | 1.5 | 15 |
| Brownie Batter, 2.6 oz | 70 | 1.5 | 13 |
| Buttercrunch Mania, 2.5 oz | 90 | 3.5 | 13 |
| Coffee 'n Cream, 2.5 oz | 70 | 1.5 | 12 |
| Marshmallow, 2.6 oz | 80 | 1 | 14 |
| **Tofutti:** | | | |
| **Premium Pints:** *Per ½ Cup* | | | |
| Better Pecan | 250 | 15 | 27 |
| Chocolate | 210 | 13 | 20 |
| Vanilla | 210 | 13 | 21 |
| Vanilla Almond Bark | 240 | 15 | 24 |
| Vanilla Fudge; Wild Berry Supreme | 190 | 9 | 25 |
| **TCBY** ~ *See Page 250* | | | |
| **Turkey Hill:** | | | |
| **All Natural:** *Per ½ Cup* | | | |
| Chocolate Chip | 170 | 10 | 18 |
| Mint Chocolate Chip | 180 | 10 | 18 |
| **Light:** *Per ½ Cup* | | | |
| Moose Tracks | 140 | 6 | 20 |
| Vanilla Bean | 100 | 2 | 17 |

| **Turkey Hill (Cont)** | **C** | **F** | **Cb** |
|---|---|---|---|
| **No Sugar Added:** *Per ½ Cup* | | | |
| Dutch Chocolate; Vanilla Bean, av. | 70 | 0 | 20 |
| Moose Tracks | 120 | 5 | 22 |
| **Premium Ice Cream:** *Per ½ Cup* | | | |
| Black Cherry | 130 | 6 | 18 |
| Butter Pecan; Choco Mint Chip, av. | 160 | 10 | 16 |
| Chocolate Peanut Butter Cup | 180 | 11 | 18 |
| Cookies 'n Cream; Tin Roof Sundae | 150 | 8 | 19 |
| Rocky Road | 170 | 8 | 23 |
| Vanilla Bean | 130 | 7 | 16 |
| **Frozen Yogurt:** *Per ½ Cup* | | | |
| Mint Cookies 'n Cream | 110 | 1.5 | 22 |
| Fat-Free: Chocolate Marshmallow | 110 | 0 | 24 |
| Other flavors | 90 | 0 | 19 |
| **Gelato:** *Per ½ Cup, 3.1 oz* | | | |
| Chocolate Chocolate Chip | 220 | 12 | 26 |
| Chocolate Peanut Butter | 230 | 15 | 21 |
| Hazelnut | 240 | 14 | 24 |
| Sea Salted Caramel | 220 | 11 | 27 |
| **Sherbet**, Fruit Rainbow | 120 | 1 | 26 |
| **Wawa:** | | | |
| **Premium Ice Cream:** *Per ½ Cup* | | | |
| Butter Pecan; Mint Choc. Chip, av. | 180 | 10 | 20 |
| Chocolate; Vanilla Bean, average | 160 | 8 | 20 |
| Cookies & Cream | 180 | 9 | 21 |
| Strawberry Shortcake | 160 | 7 | 22 |
| **Wegmans:** *Per ½ Cup* | | | |
| Chocolate | 130 | 7 | 15 |
| French Van./ Vanilla, av. | 145 | 7 | 19 |
| **Yoplait:** | | | |
| **Go-Gurt!**, Frozen Yogurt, tube, 2.3 oz wt | 60 | 0.5 | 12 |
| **Frozen Yogurt:** *Per ½ Cup* | | | |
| Original Fruit flavors, average | 115 | 2 | 21 |
| Vanilla | 110 | 2.5 | 19 |
| **Greek:** | | | |
| Fruit Flavors, average | 130 | 2 | 21 |
| Honey Caramel | 140 | 2.5 | 22 |
| Vanilla | 120 | 2.5 | 17 |

# 1 Ice Cream Bars & Pops

## Ice Cream Bars & Pops ~ Brands

*Per Bar/Serving Unless Indicated*

| | C | F | Cb |
|---|---|---|---|
| **Ben & Jerry's:** | | | |
| **Bars:** Cherry Garcia | 270 | 17 | 26 |
| Half Baked | 340 | 20 | 34 |
| **Big Bear** ~ *See Klondike* | | | |
| **Blue Bunny:** | | | |
| **Bars:** | | | |
| Caramel Crunch, 1.4 oz | 120 | 8 | 12 |
| Chocolate Sundae Crunch, 2.2 oz | 170 | 7 | 24 |
| Cookies 'n Cream, 2.4 oz | 180 | 9 | 25 |
| English Toffee, 1.4 oz | 130 | 8 | 13 |
| Fudge Bar, 2.4 oz | 90 | 1 | 18 |
| Orange Dream: 1.7 oz Bar | 70 | 1 | 13 |
| 2.6 oz Bar | 100 | 1.5 | 19 |
| Root Beer Float, 1.9 oz | 60 | 1 | 12 |
| Star Bar, 1.5 oz | 110 | 7 | 11 |
| King Size: Chocolate Eclair, 2.8 oz | 210 | 9 | 30 |
| Crunch with Candy Center, 3 oz | 350 | 28 | 25 |
| Strawberry Shortcake, 2.8 oz | 200 | 10 | 27 |
| **Champ Cones:** | | | |
| 6 Pack: Caramel Lovers, 3.4 oz | 310 | 16 | 37 |
| Chocolate Lovers, 3.2 oz | 270 | 13 | 35 |
| Cookies 'n Cream, 3.2 oz | 270 | 13 | 37 |
| King Size: | | | |
| Bunny Tracks, 5.9 oz | 490 | 27 | 57 |
| Vanilla Brownie, 5.8 oz | 460 | 22 | 60 |
| **FrozFruit:** | | | |
| Chunky: Mango | 140 | 0 | 35 |
| Pineapple | 120 | 0 | 30 |
| Strawberry | 130 | 0 | 33 |
| Creamy Coconut | 210 | 5 | 39 |
| Double Lime | 120 | 0 | 32 |
| **Jolly Rancher**, Cool Tubes, 3 oz | 110 | 1 | 23 |
| **Ice Cream Sandwiches:** | | | |
| Birthday Party, 2.5 oz | 180 | 5 | 30 |
| Cookies-N-Cream, 3 oz | 250 | 10 | 36 |
| Simply Vanilla, 2.5 oz | 160 | 5 | 27 |
| **Big:** Bopper, 5 oz | 470 | 23 | 61 |
| Double Strawberry, 3.9 oz | 250 | 7 | 42 |
| Mississippi Mud, 4 oz | 280 | 9 | 46 |
| Neapolitan, 3.7 oz | 240 | 7 | 40 |
| **Breyers:** | | | |
| **Carb Smart:** | | | |
| Fudge Bar | 100 | 7 | 9 |
| *Carb figure includes 3g sugar alcohol sweetener* | | | |
| Vanilla Ice Cream Bar | 180 | 14 | 11 |
| Vanilla Almond Ice Cream Bar | 190 | 15 | 11 |
| *Carb figures include 2g sugar alcohol sweetener* | | | |

*Per Bar/Serving Unless Indicated*

| | C | F | Cb |
|---|---|---|---|
| **Butterfinger** *(Nestle):* | | | |
| **Ice Cream Bar:** | | | |
| King Size | 280 | 18 | 27 |
| Loaded | 270 | 17 | 28 |
| **Clemmy's,** | | | |
| **Bars,** average all flavors, 2 oz | 70 | 3 | 16 |
| **Cool Classics:** | | | |
| **Arctic Blasters:** | | | |
| Crispy Bar | 160 | 11 | 15 |
| Fudge Bar | 100 | 1 | 21 |
| Ice Cream Bar | 150 | 10 | 13 |
| Orange Cream | 100 | 2.5 | 18 |
| Strawberry Shortcake | 150 | 8 | 20 |
| Toffee Bar | 160 | 11 | 14 |
| **Icepix:** Grape; Cherry; Orange | 35 | 0 | 8 |
| Honeydew; Watermelon; Cantelope | 35 | 0 | 9 |
| **Swirl Pops**, Mango-Cherry | 80 | 0 | 20 |
| **Creamsicles:** 100 Calorie Bar | 100 | 2 | 20 |
| Sugar-Free, all flavors | 40 | 0.5 | 12 |
| *Note: Sugar-Free carb figure includes 5g Sucralose sweetener* | | | |
| **Diana's Bananas:** | | | |
| **Banana Babies:** | | | |
| Milk/Dark Chocolate (1) | 130 | 6 | 18 |
| Milk Choc. & Peanuts (1) | 215 | 13 | 21 |
| **Banana Bites**, (5), 2 oz | 130 | 8 | 16 |
| **Dove:** | | | |
| **Bars:** *Per 2.6 oz Bar* | | | |
| Vanilla: | | | |
| With Milk Chocolate | 250 | 16 | 24 |
| And Almonds | 250 | 17 | 21 |
| Caramel Swirl & Cashews | 250 | 16 | 23 |
| Vanilla, | | | |
| with Dark Chocolate | 250 | 17 | 24 |
| **Miniatures**, Variety Pack, | | | |
| w/ Milk/Dark Choc., 5 pcs, 3.2 oz, av. | 330 | 21 | 32 |
| **Dreyer's/Edy's:** | | | |
| **Outshine Fruit Bars:** | | | |
| Coconut Waters, av. all flav. | 60 | 0 | 15 |
| Creamy Coconut | 120 | 3 | 20 |
| Mango; Pineapple | 80 | 0 | 20 |
| Strawberry | 70 | 0 | 18 |
| Average other varieties | 70 | 0 | 20 |

## Ice Cream Bars/Pops ~ Brands (Cont)

| Per Bar/Serving | C | F | Cb |
|---|---|---|---|
| **Drumstick** *(Nestlé):* | | | |
| **Classic Cones:** Chocolate | 310 | 17 | 34 |
| Vanilla | 290 | 16 | 33 |
| Vanilla Caramel | 310 | 16 | 38 |
| Super Nugget: Van. Fudge | 330 | 18 | 37 |
| Other flavors | 310 | 18 | 34 |
| **Lil' Drums,** av. all flavors | 120 | 6 | 18 |
| **Simply Dipped:** Mint | 270 | 13 | 37 |
| Vanilla | 270 | 13 | 37 |
| *Edy's ~ See Dreyer's* | | | |
| **Eskimo Pie** *(Nestle):* | | | |
| Milk Chocolate, Vanilla | 150 | 10 | 14 |
| Dark Chocolate, No Sugar Added | 150 | 10 | 13 |
| **Fat Boy:** | | | |
| **Sundae On A Stick:** | | | |
| Nut Sundae | 270 | 20 | 23 |
| Toffee Crunch | 280 | 20 | 26 |
| Vanilla Dipped | 260 | 19 | 22 |
| **Sandwiches:** Chocolate, 3 oz | 210 | 9 | 31 |
| Cookies n' Cream, 3 oz | 220 | 8 | 34 |
| Mint Chocolate Chip, 3 oz | 220 | 9 | 33 |
| Premium Vanilla, 3 oz | 210 | 8 | 31 |
| Rasp. Cheesecake, 3 oz | 210 | 7 | 35 |
| Strawberry, 3 oz | 210 | 7 | 35 |
| **Fresh & Easy,** Vanilla Sundae Cone | 260 | 15 | 29 |
| **Fudge Bar** *(Nestle),* | | | |
| Regular, 2.8 oz | 110 | 2 | 21 |
| **Fudgesicle:** | | | |
| **Fudge Bar:** Original, 2 bars, 2.9 oz | 80 | 1.5 | 19 |
| 100 Calorie (1), 2.3 oz | 100 | 2 | 17 |
| Low Fat (1), 1.5 oz | 60 | 1.5 | 12 |
| **Good Humor:** | | | |
| **Dessert Bars, Single:** | | | |
| Orig. Vanilla, Choc. Coated, 2.8 oz | 250 | 15 | 27 |
| Birthday Cake | 180 | 9 | 25 |
| Chocolate Eclair | 200 | 10 | 27 |
| Oreo Bar | 220 | 12 | 26 |
| Toasted Almond | 190 | 10 | 24 |
| **Cones, Singles:** | | | |
| Giant King Cone, | | | |
| Vanilla ;Chocolate | 330 | 16 | 44 |
| King Cone, Vanilla | 230 | 11 | 30 |
| Multi-Packs, | | | |
| King Cones, Choc.; Vanilla, av. | 270 | 15 | 31 |
| **Dessert Cups:** | | | |
| Mounds, multi-pack, (1) | 180 | 11 | 21 |
| Reeses, Peanut Butter, 4 count, (1) | 260 | 17 | 25 |
| **Sandwiches:** Choc. Chip Cookie | 270 | 11 | 42 |
| Giant, Neapolitan; Vanilla, av. | 250 | 9 | 38 |

| Per Bar/Serving | C | F | Cb |
|---|---|---|---|
| **Haagen-Dazs:** | | | |
| **Dark Chocolate Bar,** Chocolate | 280 | 20 | 22 |
| **Milk Chocolate Bars:** | | | |
| Salted Caramel | 300 | 19 | 28 |
| Vanilla & Almonds | 300 | 22 | 21 |
| Vanilla | 280 | 20 | 21 |
| Vanilla Chocolate Peanut Butter | 310 | 23 | 21 |
| **Snack Size:** | | | |
| Coffee & Almond Crunch | 190 | 14 | 15 |
| Vanilla & Almonds | 195 | 15 | 13 |
| **Healthy Choice:** Fudge Bar | 80 | 1.5 | 13 |
| Mocha Swirl | 90 | 1 | 17 |
| Frozen Yogurt Bars, av. | 85 | 1 | 16 |
| **Hershey's:** | | | |
| **Cones:** Candy Bar Overload | 320 | 12 | 48 |
| Incredible | 250 | 13 | 28 |
| Moose Tracks | 430 | 27 | 43 |
| P-Nutty | 210 | 13 | 20 |
| Low fat, Cookies & Cream; Crazy, av. | 120 | 2 | 25 |
| **Pops,** all flavors | 35 | 0 | 10 |
| **Sandwiches:** | | | |
| 99 Cent Vanilla Ice Cream | 210 | 9 | 30 |
| Giant: Andes Creme de Menthe | 350 | 16 | 48 |
| Neopolitan | 320 | 14 | 43 |
| Vanilla, 6 oz | 300 | 12 | 43 |
| **Signature Bars:** Chocolate Eclair | 230 | 10 | 30 |
| Cookies & Cream | 290 | 15 | 33 |
| Cotton Candy | 280 | 15 | 33 |
| Strawb. Shortcake | 230 | 9 | 34 |
| **Hood:** | | | |
| **Bars:** Ice Cream Bar | 130 | 7 | 14 |
| Orange Cream | 90 | 1.5 | 18 |
| **Hoodsie:** | | | |
| Cups, Chocolate; Vanilla, 3 oz | 100 | 5 | 12 |
| Sundae Cups, 3 oz | 120 | 5 | 19 |
| **Sandwich,** av., 2.2 oz | 175 | 6 | 29 |
| **Klondike:** | | | |
| **Bars:** *Multipacks, Per Bar* | | | |
| 100 Calorie, av.erage all flavors | 100 | 6 | 13 |
| Original Vanilla | 250 | 14 | 29 |
| Krunch | 250 | 14 | 29 |
| Mint Chocolate Chip | 230 | 14 | 27 |
| Oreo Cookies & Cream | 250 | 15 | 27 |
| **Choco Taco,** Original | 230 | 11 | 31 |
| **Sandwiches:** *Each* | | | |
| Mrs Fields | 210 | 8 | 34 |
| Vanilla | 180 | 5 | 31 |

# Ice Cream Bars & Pops

## Ice Cream Bars/Pops ~ Brands (Cont)

*Per Bar/Serving* | **C** | **F** | **Cb**

**Luigi's:**
| | | | |
|---|---|---|---|
| Real Italian Ice: Cherry | 100 | 0 | 26 |
| Chocolate Fudge | 150 | 0 | 36 |
| Lemon; Mango | 100 | 0 | 26 |
| Watermelon; Blue Raspberry | 160 | 0 | 39 |

**M&M's:**
| | | | |
|---|---|---|---|
| Cone, Single, 2.6 oz | 240 | 11 | 32 |
| Cookie Ice Cream Sandwich, 2.9 oz | 250 | 12 | 33 |

**Magnum:**
| | | | |
|---|---|---|---|
| Almond, 2.8 oz | 270 | 18 | 24 |
| Dark, 3.2 oz | 240 | 17 | 20 |
| Double Caramel, 3.6 oz | 320 | 20 | 32 |
| Gold, 3 oz | 290 | 20 | 25 |
| White, 2.7 oz | 250 | 16 | 23 |
| Minis: Almond (2), 3.7 oz | 320 | 22 | 28 |
| Double Caramel (2), 3.8 oz | 380 | 22 | 38 |

**Minute Maid:**
| | | | |
|---|---|---|---|
| **Bars:** Juice, all flavors, 2.25 oz | 40 | 0 | 10 |
| Soft Frozen Lemonade/Limeade, all flavors, 3 fl.oz | 70 | 0 | 19 |

**Nestlé:**
| | | | |
|---|---|---|---|
| **Bars:** Crunch, 1.7 oz | 160 | 10 | 16 |
| Orange & Cream | 80 | 2 | 16 |
| Strawberry Shortcake | 220 | 10 | 31 |
| **Dibs,** av. all flavors, 4 oz container | 340 | 24 | 30 |

**Drumsticks ~ See Page 109**
| | | | |
|---|---|---|---|
| **Ice Pop,** Wildberry & Zesty Lemon | 90 | 0 | 22 |
| **Sandwiches:** Neapolitan | 240 | 7 | 40 |
| Vanilla | 160 | 4 | 29 |
| **Toll House,** Choc. Chip Cookie S'wich | 380 | 16 | 54 |

**Popsicle:**
| | | | |
|---|---|---|---|
| Firecracker, all flavors (1) | 35 | 0 | 9 |
| Hello Kitty (2) | 60 | 0 | 14 |
| Marvel Avengers Assemble (1) | 40 | 0 | 10 |
| Scribblers (2) | 60 | 0 | 15 |
| SpongeBob Pop-Ups (1) | 80 | 1 | 11 |
| Slow Melts, Mighty Minis, 5 pieces | 60 | 0 | 11 |

**Reese's,** P'nut Butter Ice Cream Cup, 2.5 oz | 280 | 19 | 22

**Skinny Cow:**
| | | | |
|---|---|---|---|
| **Bars:** Fudge | 110 | 1 | 22 |
| Truffle, all flavors | 100 | 2.5 | 19 |
| Vanilla Almond Crunch | 190 | 11 | 19 |
| **Cones,** average all flavors (1) | 155 | 3 | 28 |

**Snickers:**
| | | | |
|---|---|---|---|
| **Bars:** Regular, 1.8 oz | 180 | 11 | 18 |
| Mini Bar, 1 piece, 0.9 oz | 90 | 6 | 9 |
| **Cone,** 2.9 oz | 250 | 13 | 29 |
| **Ice Cream Brownie,** 3.3 oz | 300 | 13 | 41 |

*Per Bar/Serving* | **C** | **F** | **Cb**
| | | | |
|---|---|---|---|
| Snow Cone *(Wonder)*, av. all, 7 fl.oz | 60 | 0 | 15 |

**So Delicious** *(Turtle Mountain):*

**Almond Based Minis:**
| | | | |
|---|---|---|---|
| Bars, all varieties (1), 1.8 oz | 150 | 10 | 14 |
| Sandwich, Vanilla, 1.3 oz | 90 | 3.5 | 13 |

**Coconut Based Minis:**
| | | | |
|---|---|---|---|
| Bars: Almond, 1.8 oz | 180 | 13 | 17 |
| Simply Strawberry, 2 oz | 80 | 3.5 | 14 |

**Soy Based:**
| | | | |
|---|---|---|---|
| Mini Sandwiches: Neapolitan, 1.4 oz | 90 | 2 | 18 |
| Vanilla, 1.4 oz | 90 | 2 | 17 |

**Soy Dream,**
| | | | |
|---|---|---|---|
| Lil' Dreamers, Vanilla | 100 | 4 | 15 |
| **Tampico,** Freezer Pops, all var., 1.4 oz | 30 | 0 | 7 |

**Tofutti:**
**Bars:**
| | | | |
|---|---|---|---|
| Chocolate Fudge/Coffee Break Treats | 30 | 0 | 6 |
| Hooray Hooray Bar | 120 | 8 | 8 |
| Marry Me Bar | 170 | 8 | 22 |
| Totally Fudge Pops | 95 | 1.5 | 19 |

*Note: Carb figures include 0-7g sugar alcohols*
| | | | |
|---|---|---|---|
| **Cones,** (1), all flavors | 220 | 13 | 24 |
| **Cuties,** average all flavors | 130 | 6 | 18 |

**Turkey Hill:**
| | | | |
|---|---|---|---|
| **Cups,** Vanilla & Chocolate, (1), 3.6 oz | 130 | 7 | 15 |
| **Sandwiches:** Double Decker, 2.5 oz | 190 | 7 | 30 |
| Vanilla Bean, 2.5 oz | 190 | 7 | 29 |
| **Sundae Cone,** Van. Fudge | 320 | 18 | 33 |
| **Twix Bar,** 2.4 oz | 250 | 14 | 28 |

**Wegmans:**
| | | | |
|---|---|---|---|
| **Bars:** Fudge, low fat | 100 | 1.5 | 19 |
| Peanut Butter Sundae Crunch | 200 | 11 | 22 |
| Vanilla, Choc Coated, 2 oz | 160 | 11 | 14 |
| **Cones:** Nutty Sundae, 2.5 oz | 210 | 11 | 25 |
| Sundae Nut, 3 oz | 260 | 15 | 29 |

**Weight Watchers:**
**Bars:**
| | | | |
|---|---|---|---|
| Dark Chocolate: Dulce de Leche | 120 | 4.5 | 19 |
| Raspberry | 170 | 10 | 22 |
| Giant: Chocolate/Cookies & Cream | 140 | 4.5 | 26 |
| Fudge Bar | 100 | 1 | 24 |
| **Cones,** Double Caramel Swirl, snack | 90 | 2 | 17 |
| **Cups,** Chocolate Chip Cookie Dough | 140 | 3 | 26 |
| **Sandwiches:** Giant Vanilla | 140 | 2 | 31 |
| Mint | 140 | 1.5 | 31 |
| Red Velvet, snack size | 100 | 1.5 | 20 |
| **Sundae,** Peanut Butter Cup | 130 | 3 | 23 |

**Yoplait ~ *See Frozen Yogurt***
| | | | |
|---|---|---|---|
| **Yosicle,** Swirlz, average all flavors, (1) | 45 | 1 | 7 |

## Canned & Packaged Meals ~ Brands

### Amy's: *Per Serve*

| | C | F | Cb |
|---|---|---|---|
| **Frozen:** | | | |
| **Asian Meals:** | | | |
| Stir-Fry: Asian Noodle,10 oz | 300 | 7 | 50 |
| Thai, 9.5 oz | 310 | 11 | 45 |
| **Bowls:** Baked Ziti, 9.5 oz | 390 | 12 | 62 |
| Broccoli & Cheddar Bake, 9.5 oz | 430 | 20 | 44 |
| Pesto Tortellini, 9.5 oz | 440 | 20 | 50 |
| **Burritos:** Bean & Cheese, 6 oz | 310 | 9 | 46 |
| Bean & Rice, 6 oz | 320 | 8 | 52 |
| Breakfast Burrito, 6 oz | 270 | 8 | 38 |
| **Entrees:** Cheese Enchilada, 4.5 oz | 240 | 14 | 18 |
| Cheese Lasagna, 10.3 oz | 410 | 16 | 46 |
| Macaroni & Cheese, 9 oz | 400 | 16 | 47 |
| Roasted Vegetable Lasagna, 9.8 oz | 350 | 11 | 47 |
| **Light & Lean:** *Per 8 oz Serve* | | | |
| Black Bean & Cheese Enchilada | 250 | 5 | 44 |
| Mattar Paner | 260 | 6 | 42 |
| Soft Taco Fiesta | 220 | 4.5 | 40 |
| **Pot Pies:** | | | |
| Broccoli, 7.5 oz | 460 | 24 | 50 |
| Mex. Tamale; Shephd's Pie, av., 8 oz | 165 | 3.5 | 27 |
| Vegetable, 7.5 oz | 430 | 20 | 54 |
| **Snacks:** Nacho, Chse & Bean, 5-6 pcs | 220 | 9 | 25 |
| Cheese Pizza, 5-6 pieces | 210 | 9 | 25 |
| **Whole Meals:** | | | |
| Black Bean Enchil., 10 oz | 330 | 8 | 53 |
| Veggie Loaf, 10 oz | 340 | 10 | 47 |
| Veggie, Steak & Gravy, 11 oz | 380 | 16 | 50 |
| **Wraps:** | | | |
| Indian Samosa, 5 oz | 250 | 9 | 35 |
| Teriyaki, 5.5 oz | 310 | 7 | 51 |
| Tofu Scramble, 5.5 oz | 300 | 13 | 35 |

### Atkins: *Per 9 oz Tray/Bowl*

| | C | F | Cb |
|---|---|---|---|
| **Frozen:** | | | |
| Beef Merlot | 310 | 21 | 9 |
| Chicken & Broccoli Alfredo | 330 | 20 | 9 |
| Chili Con Carne | 320 | 21 | 8 |
| Crustless Chicken Pot Pie | 330 | 22 | 8 |
| Italian Style Pasta Bake | 360 | 21 | 10 |
| Meatloaf with Portob. Mshrm Gravy | 340 | 23 | 11 |

### Bagel Bites:

| | C | F | Cb |
|---|---|---|---|
| **Frozen:** | | | |
| Cheese, Sausage & Pepperoni, 4 pcs | 200 | 6 | 28 |
| Supreme; Three Cheese, av., 4 pcs, 3 oz | 195 | 5 | 31 |

### B&M:

| | C | F | Cb |
|---|---|---|---|
| **Baked Beans:** *Per 16 oz Can, ½ cup, 4.6 oz* | | | |
| Original | 170 | 2 | 31 |
| Boston's Best | 170 | 1.5 | 32 |
| Maple Flavor | 150 | 1 | 28 |
| Vegetarian | 160 | 1 | 25 |
| **Brown Bread,** Raisin, ½ slice, 2 oz | 130 | 0.5 | 29 |

### Banquet:

| | C | F | Cb |
|---|---|---|---|
| **Homestyle Bakes:** *1 Cup, Prepared* | | | |
| Cheeseburger Mac | 240 | 6 | 36 |
| Creamy Cheesy Chicken Alfredo | 330 | 15 | 37 |
| Creamy Turkey & Stuffing | 270 | 12 | 32 |
| Pasta & Meatballs in Marinara Sce | 290 | 8 | 43 |
| **Frozen:** | | | |
| **Dinners:** Boneless Pork Rib, 10 oz | 310 | 11 | 37 |
| Cheesy Smothered Meat Patty, 7 oz | 280 | 16 | 20 |
| Chicken: Fingers, 7 oz | 480 | 21 | 56 |
| Nuggets, 6.7 oz | 320 | 15 | 31 |
| Pasta Marinara, 6.5 oz | 290 | 14 | 30 |
| Sesame, 8 oz | 350 | 15 | 40 |
| Double Meat: | | | |
| Meat Loaf Patties, 12.5 oz | 380 | 21 | 27 |
| Pork Rib, 12.5 oz | 480 | 23 | 48 |
| Salisbury Steak | 460 | 29 | 30 |
| Fettuccine Alfredo, 8 oz | 290 | 11 | 39 |
| Fish Sticks, 7.5 oz | 310 | 9 | 47 |
| Homestyle Charbroiled Patty | 310 | 17 | 25 |
| Lasagna, w/- Meat Sce | 270 | 7 | 38 |
| Meat Loaf, 9.5 oz | 250 | 11 | 26 |
| Pepperoni Pizza, 5.8 | 330 | 11 | 48 |
| Rigatoni & Italian Sausage, 8 oz | 280 | 8 | 42 |
| Salisbury Steak, 9.5 oz | 230 | 9 | 26 |
| Spaghetti & Meatballs, 9 oz | 360 | 16 | 43 |
| Spaghetti & Popcorn Chicken, 7 oz | 300 | 10 | 40 |
| Sweet & Sour Chicken, 8 oz | 390 | 14 | 56 |
| Turkey, 9.3 oz | 230 | 6 | 31 |
| **Family:** | | | |
| Broccoli Chkn & Cheese, with Rice & Sce, 7.7 oz | 210 | 7 | 26 |
| Chicken Alfredo, with Broccoli & Noodles, 8 oz | 210 | 6 | 29 |
| Salisbury Steak & Gravy, 4.5 oz | 180 | 12 | 11 |
| **Pies:** *Per 7 oz* | | | |
| Deep Dish: B'fast Ham & Potato | 410 | 22 | 44 |
| Breakfast Sausage Gravy | 450 | 28 | 39 |
| Pot Pie: Chicken; Turkey, average | 400 | 24 | 37 |
| Chicken with Broccoli | 380 | 23 | 34 |

| Barilla: | C | F | Cb |
|---|---|---|---|
| **Microwaveables:** *Per 9 oz Container* | | | |
| Ital. Ssg; Meat Sauce Gemelli, av | 350 | 7 | 60 |
| Marinara/tomato & Basil Penne, av. | 310 | 4 | 60 |
| **Betty Crocker:** | | | |
| **Bowl Appetit:** | | | |
| Herb Chicken Flavored Veggie Rice | 250 | 3 | 51 |
| Pasta Alfredo | 350 | 9 | 55 |
| Three-Cheese Rotini | 340 | 7 | 59 |
| **Hamburger Helper:** *Per 1 Cup, Prepared* | | | |
| Bacon Cheeseburger | 320 | 14 | 27 |
| Beef Pasta | 280 | 12 | 24 |
| Cheeseburger Macaroni | 320 | 13 | 30 |
| Cheesy Baked Potatoes | 310 | 12 | 30 |
| Cheesy Italian Shells | 310 | 12 | 27 |
| Crunchy Taco | 330 | 14 | 33 |
| Salisbury | 280 | 11 | 27 |
| **Helper Complete Meals:** *Per 1 Cup, Prepared* | | | |
| Cheesy Beef Taco | 220 | 5 | 35 |
| Chicken & Buttermilk Biscuits | 260 | 9 | 39 |
| Chicken with Cheesy Rice & Broccoli | 230 | 6 | 36 |
| Stroganoff | 230 | 8 | 33 |
| **Potatoes:** *Per Serving, Prepared* | | | |
| Casserole: Au Gratin, ½ cup | 150 | 5 | 24 |
| Cheddar & Bacon, ½ c. | 150 | 5 | 24 |
| Roasted Garlic, ½ cup | 120 | 3 | 21 |
| Scalloped, ⅔ cup | 130 | 3 | 23 |
| Sour Cream and Chives, ⅔ cup | 130 | 3 | 24 |
| Flavored Potatoes, prepared, | | | |
| av. all varieties, ⅔ cup | 145 | 6 | 18 |
| Seasoned Skillet: | | | |
| Hash Brown, ½ cup | 120 | 4 | 18 |
| Rstd Garlic & Herb Potatoes, ⅔ c. | 170 | 9 | 21 |
| Trad'nl Recipe Potatoes, ½ cup | 180 | 9 | 22 |
| **Tuna Helper:** *Per 1 Cup, Prepared* | | | |
| Creamy Parmesan | 270 | 10 | 30 |
| Average other varieties | 265 | 10 | 30 |
| **Biggest Loser:** | | | |
| **Refrigerated:** | | | |
| **Simply Sensible:** *Per ½ Package* | | | |
| Beef Pot Roast & Gravy | 220 | 5 | 16 |
| Beef Tips & Gravy | 200 | 3.5 | 21 |
| Lasagna | 200 | 5 | 28 |
| Mediterranean-Style Chicken | 250 | 6 | 36 |
| Zing Chicken | 230 | 1.5 | 38 |

| Birds Eye: | C | F | Cb |
|---|---|---|---|
| **Frozen:** | | | |
| **Voila!:** *Per 1 Cup Prepared Unless Indicated* | | | |
| Alfredo Chicken, 1½ cups | 280 | 12 | 37 |
| Beef & Broccoli Stir Fry | 160 | 6 | 13 |
| Chicken Florentine | 230 | 6 | 27 |
| Chicken Parmesan | 360 | 11 | 50 |
| Garlic Shrimp | 230 | 9 | 30 |
| Shrimp Scampi | 190 | 2.5 | 31 |
| Sweet & Sour Chicken | 200 | 1 | 38 |
| **Boca:** | | | |
| **Frozen:** | | | |
| **Burger:** | | | |
| All American Flame Grilled, 2.5 oz | 120 | 5 | 6 |
| Cheeseburger, 2.5 oz | 100 | 4.5 | 6 |
| Grilled Vegetables, 2.5 oz | 80 | 1 | 7 |
| Original Vegan, 2.5 oz | 70 | 0.5 | 6 |
| **Chik'n:** Orig. Nuggets, 3 oz | 180 | 7 | 17 |
| Patties (1), 2.5 oz | 160 | 6 | 15 |
| Spicy Patties (1), 2.5 oz | 160 | 6 | 15 |
| **Boston Market:** | | | |
| **Frozen:** | | | |
| **Dinners:** Beef Steak & Pasta, 14 oz | 470 | 14 | 52 |
| Chicken Parmesan, 13 oz | 500 | 13 | 70 |
| Oven Roasted Chicken, 13 oz | 280 | 7 | 31 |
| Salisbury Steak, 14.5 oz | 530 | 32 | 38 |
| Swedish M'balls, 13 oz | 660 | 30 | 67 |
| **Buitoni:** | | | |
| **Refrigerated:** | | | |
| **Ravioli:** Crab, 3.8 oz | 300 | 11 | 36 |
| Four Cheese, 3.7 oz | 330 | 12 | 42 |
| **Tortelloni:** | | | |
| Cheese & Rstd Garlic, 3.7 oz | 310 | 9 | 43 |
| Chicken & Proscuitto, 3.8 oz | 330 | 9 | 46 |
| **Other Pasta Dishes** ~ *See Page 133* | | | |
| **Bush's Best:** *Per ½ Cup, 4.6 oz* | | | |
| **Baked Beans:** Original | 140 | 1 | 29 |
| Vegetarian | 130 | 0 | 29 |
| Average other varieties | 150 | 1 | 32 |
| Black Beans | 105 | 0.5 | 23 |
| Chili Pinto Beans, with sauce | 110 | 1 | 20 |
| Dark Red Kidney Beans | 100 | 0 | 22 |
| Garbanzo Beans | 120 | 2 | 20 |
| **Grillin' Beans:** | | | |
| Black Bean Fiesta | 110 | 1 | 21 |
| Sweet Mesquite | 160 | 1 | 32 |
| Texas Ranchero | 120 | 2 | 20 |
| Average other varieties | 165 | 0.5 | 35 |
| **Refried Beans:** Traditional | 150 | 3 | 24 |
| Fat Free | 130 | 0 | 24 |

## Campbell's:

| | C | F | Cb |
|---|---|---|---|
| **Pork & Beans,** 11 oz can, | | | |
| 4.6 oz | 140 | 1.5 | 25 |
| **Chunky Microwaveable Bowls:** | | | |
| Firehouse; Roadhouse, | | | |
| Chunky Beef & Beans Chili, 1 cup | 220 | 6 | 28 |
| **Spaghetti O's:** *Per Cup* | | | |
| Original | 170 | 1 | 35 |
| With Meatballs | 260 | 9 | 33 |
| With Sliced Franks | 220 | 6 | 32 |

## Chef Boyardee: *Per 1 Cup*

**Canned (15 oz can):**

| | C | F | Cb |
|---|---|---|---|
| Beefaroni, 8.8 oz | 250 | 10 | 30 |
| Lasagna, | | | |
| with Tomato & Meat Sce, 8.8 oz | 250 | 9 | 32 |
| Ravioli: | | | |
| Beef, in Tomato & Meat Sauce: | | | |
| Regular, 8.7 oz | 220 | 7 | 31 |
| 99% Fat Free, 8.6 oz | 170 | 2 | 31 |
| Overstuffed, 9.2 oz | 230 | 5 | 37 |
| Cheese Ravioli, | | | |
| in Meat & Tomato Sce, 8.7 oz | 230 | 6 | 34 |
| Italian Sausage Ravioli, | | | |
| Overstuffed, 9.2 oz | 260 | 7 | 37 |
| Pepperoni Pizza Ravioli, | | | |
| in Zesty Sauce, 9.1 oz | 210 | 4 | 36 |
| Spaghetti & Meatballs, | | | |
| in Tomato Sauce, 9 oz | 260 | 11 | 31 |

**Microwaveable:** *Per 7.5 oz Cup*

| | C | F | Cb |
|---|---|---|---|
| Beef Ravioli, in Tomato & Meat Sce | 190 | 6 | 28 |
| Mini Beef Ravioli, | | | |
| in Tomato & Meat Sauce | 240 | 9 | 32 |

**Boxed Pizza Maker Kits:** *Single Kits*

| | C | F | Cb |
|---|---|---|---|
| Cheese, ¼ package, 4 oz | 260 | 4.5 | 47 |
| Pepperoni, ¼ package, 4 oz | 280 | 8 | 42 |
| Pizza Sauce, w/- Chse, ¼ c., 2 oz | 35 | 1.5 | 4 |

## Country Crock *(Hormel)*:

**Side Dishes:**

| | C | F | Cb |
|---|---|---|---|
| 4 Cheese Penne Pasta, | | | |
| with Broccoli, 8.3 oz | 340 | 16 | 36 |
| Bacon Ranch Mashed Potatoes 5 oz | 160 | 7 | 21 |
| Cheddar Brocc. Rice, 7 oz | 260 | 11 | 33 |
| Elbow Mac. & Cheese, 8 oz | 330 | 14 | 38 |
| Garlic Mashed Potato, 5 oz | 120 | 4 | 19 |
| Loaded Mashed Potatoes, 5 oz | 190 | 11 | 18 |
| Mashed Sweet Potatoes, 7 oz | 170 | 6 | 27 |
| Tomato Basil Penne, 8.6 oz | 280 | 13 | 34 |

## Dennison's Chili: *Per Cup*

**Chili Con Carne:**

| | C | F | Cb |
|---|---|---|---|
| Original: W/- Beans, 9 oz | 350 | 15 | 31 |
| Without Beans, 8.8 oz | 310 | 16 | 20 |
| **Chili:** Original, with Beans, 9 oz | 360 | 14 | 38 |
| Chunky, with Beans, 8.8 oz | 300 | 10 | 32 |
| Hot, with Beans, 9 oz | 350 | 14 | 36 |
| Vegetarian, 99% fat free, 9 oz | 190 | 1.5 | 34 |

## Dinty Moore:

**Big Bowl (Microwave):** *Approx. ½ of 15 oz Bowl*

| | C | F | Cb |
|---|---|---|---|
| Beef Stew, 8.3 oz | 200 | 10 | 17 |
| Chicken & Dumplings, 8.5 oz | 220 | 7 | 29 |
| Scalloped Potatoes & Ham, 8.7 oz | 280 | 16 | 23 |

**Hearty Meals:** *Approx. ½ of 20 oz Can*

| | C | F | Cb |
|---|---|---|---|
| Beef Stew, 8.3 oz | 200 | 10 | 17 |
| Chicken & Dumplings, 8.5 oz | 230 | 8 | 28 |
| Chicken Pot Pie, 8.6 oz | 240 | 11 | 24 |
| Turkey Stew, 8.5 oz | 140 | 3 | 19 |

## Dr. McDougall's: *Per 2 oz Package*

| | C | F | Cb |
|---|---|---|---|
| **Asian Noodle Entree Cups,** | | | |
| average all varieties | 200 | 1.5 | 41 |
| **Quinoa Cups:** Black Bean | 280 | 3 | 51 |
| Curry Almond and Rice | 260 | 3 | 51 |
| Tomato Pine Nut | 260 | 5 | 44 |

## Eden Organics: *Per ½ Cup, 4.6 oz*

| | C | F | Cb |
|---|---|---|---|
| Baked Navy Beans, | | | |
| w/ Sorghum, Mstrd | 150 | 0 | 27 |
| Chili Beans, w/- Jalap. & Chili Peppers | 130 | 0 | 21 |
| Lentils, with Onions & Bay Leaf | 90 | 0 | 13 |
| Refried: Black Beans | 110 | 1.5 | 18 |
| Pinto; Kidney Beans, average | 85 | 1 | 17 |

## Farmhouse:

**Rice:** *Per 1 Cup, Prepared*

| | C | F | Cb |
|---|---|---|---|
| Long Grain & Wild Herb | | | |
| & Butter | 250 | 7 | 44 |
| Mexican, 6 oz | 230 | 5 | 42 |
| Roasted Chicken Flavor, 6 oz | 230 | 5 | 44 |

## French's:

**French Fried Onions:**

| | C | F | Cb |
|---|---|---|---|
| Original; Cheddar: | | | |
| 2 Tbsp, 0.3 oz | 45 | 3.5 | 3 |
| ¼ cup, 0.5 oz | 90 | 7 | 6 |
| 1 cup, 2 oz | 360 | 28 | 24 |

## GardenBurger:

**Veggie Burger:**

| | C | F | Cb |
|---|---|---|---|
| Original, 3 oz | 110 | 3 | 16 |
| Black Bean Chipotle, 2.5 oz | 90 | 3 | 16 |

| | C | F | Cb |
|---|---|---|---|
| **Garden Lites:** | | | |
| **Bakes:** *Per 7 oz Serving* | | | |
|   Cheddar Broccoli | 210 | 6 | 29 |
|   Fiesta; Italian, av. | 180 | 8 | 21 |
| **Bites:** | | | |
|   Broccoli & Brown Rice (4) | 130 | 5 | 16 |
|   Kale & Brown Rice (4) | 130 | 5 | 17 |
| **Casserole,** Cheesy Veggie | 210 | 10 | 20 |
| **Melt,** Veggie, Chili & Cornbread, 7 oz | 200 | 4.5 | 33 |
| **Souffle:** *Per 7 oz Serving* | | | |
|   Kale & Quinoa | 200 | 6 | 23 |
|   Loaded Potato | 200 | 5.5 | 27 |
|   Pizza | 200 | 4 | 31 |
|   Pumpkin Spice | 190 | 2.5 | 34 |
|   Roasted Vegetable | 170 | 3 | 28 |
|   Spinach | 170 | 3 | 25 |
|   Zucchini | 180 | 3 | 28 |
| **Gorton's:** | | | |
| **Battered Pollock Fillets:** | | | |
|   Beer Battered (2), 3.6 oz | 230 | 14 | 20 |
|   Crispy Battered (2), 3.8 oz | 240 | 14 | 20 |
| **Breaded Pollock Fillets:** | | | |
|   Crunchy (2), 3.8 oz | 250 | 13 | 23 |
|   Lemon Herb Crunchy (2), 3.7 oz | 240 | 13 | 21 |
| **(Grilled Fillets)** | | | |
|   Garlic Butter Pollock (1), 3.5 oz | 80 | 3 | 0 |
|   Lemon Butter Pollock (1), 3.5 oz | 90 | 3 | 0 |
|   Signature Tilapia (1), 3.2 oz | 80 | 2 | 2 |
| **Shrimp:** | | | |
|   Crispy Beer Battered (9), 3.5 oz | 240 | 12 | 25 |
|   Crunchy Butterfly Shrimp (5), 3.5 oz | 220 | 8 | 27 |
|   Garl. Butter Shrimp Scampi (6), 4 oz | 120 | 5 | 8 |
| **Great Value** *(Walmart):* | | | |
| **Breakfast Bowls:** *Per 8 oz* | | | |
|   Sausage | 390 | 25 | 22 |
|   Sausage & Gravy | 360 | 24 | 21 |
| **Complete Skillet Meals:** *Per ½ Package* | | | |
|   Chicken Florentine & Farfalle | 575 | 32 | 40 |
|   Grilled Chicken Alfredo | 710 | 44 | 55 |
|   Shrimp Scampi & Linguini | 550 | 23 | 58 |
| **Meals:** | | | |
|   Chicken Enchilada Casserole, 7 oz | 230 | 7 | 30 |
|   Lasagna, 7.5 oz | 290 | 14 | 26 |
| **Party Size:** Lasagna, 7.5 oz | 270 | 9 | 32 |
|   Mexican Style Lasagna, 8 oz | 380 | 17 | 38 |
| **Health Valley:** | | | |
| **Vegetarian Chili:** *Per 8.7 oz Cup* | | | |
|   3 Bean Chipotle | 200 | 3 | 37 |
|   Black Bean Mango | 210 | 3 | 41 |
|   Average other varieties | 200 | 3 | 37 |

| | C | F | Cb |
|---|---|---|---|
| **Healthy Choice:** *Per Meal* | | | |
| **100% Natural Cafe Steamers:** *Per Container* | | | |
|   Asian Potstickers | 330 | 3.5 | 67 |
|   Portabella Spin. Parmesan | 230 | 5 | 38 |
|   Pumpkin Squash Ravioli | 260 | 6 | 44 |
|   Tortellini Primavera Parmesan | 250 | 4.5 | 42 |
| **Asian Cafe Steamer,** | | | |
|   Beef Teriyaki, 9.5 oz | 270 | 5 | 39 |
| **Baked:** 4 Cheese Ziti Marin., 9.2 oz | 310 | 5 | 46 |
|   Italian Sausage Pasta, 8.5 oz | 270 | 6 | 40 |
|   Roasted Chicken & Potatoes, 9.7 oz | 180 | 3.5 | 21 |
| **Complete Meals:** *Per Container* | | | |
|   Beef Pot Roast | 260 | 7 | 32 |
|   Chicken Parmigiana | 330 | 10 | 43 |
|   Lemon Pepper Fish | 340 | 4 | 59 |
| **Simply Cafe Steamers:** *Per Container* | | | |
|   Chicken & Vegetable Stir Fry | 190 | 4 | 15 |
|   Grilled Chicken & Broccoli Alfredo | 190 | 6 | 8 |
|   Grilled Chicken Pesto & Vegetables | 200 | 6 | 11 |
| **Extra Product Listings ~** *www.CalorieKing.com* | | | |
| **Heinz,** Vegetarian Beans, | | | |
|   ½ cup, 4 oz | 140 | 0.5 | 27 |
| **Hormel:** | | | |
| **Chili with Beans:** *Per 8.7 oz Serving* | | | |
|   Regular | 260 | 7 | 29 |
|   Hot; Chunky | 260 | 7 | 33 |
|   Turkey | 210 | 3 | 28 |
|   Vegetarian | 190 | 1 | 35 |
| **Chili without Beans:** *Per 8.3 oz Serving* | | | |
|   Chunky/Hot Chili, average | 215 | 9 | 19 |
|   Turkey | 190 | 3 | 16 |
| **Compleats, Comfort Classics:** *7.5 oz Serving* | | | |
|   Beefy Mac & Cheese | 220 | 4 | 35 |
|   Chicken & Dumplings | 170 | 4 | 25 |
|   Chicken & Noodles | 180 | 6 | 20 |
|   Noodles & Beef | 150 | 2 | 26 |
|   Scalloped Potatoes & Beef | 170 | 5 | 24 |
| **Compleats, Homesyle:** | | | |
|   Beef Pot Roast | 230 | 6 | 22 |
|   Chicken Alfredo, 10 oz | 340 | 18 | 28 |
|   Chkn Breast & Msh'd Pot., 10 oz | 210 | 4.5 | 26 |
|   Meatloaf & Mashed Pot., 9 oz | 280 | 12 | 27 |
|   Salisbury Steak, 9 oz | 300 | 17 | 23 |
|   Swedish Mtballs, 9 oz | 270 | 12 | 27 |
| **Refrigerated Meals:** | | | |
|   H'style Meat Loaf & Tom. Sce, 5 oz | 220 | 9 | 14 |
|   Rstd Chicken Breasts & Gravy, 5 oz | 120 | 2.5 | 4 |
|   Sliced Rst Tukey Brst & Gravy, 5 oz | 110 | 2 | 3 |
|   Sweet chicken Teriyaki, 4.5 oz | 180 | 2.5 | 25 |

| Hot Pockets: | C | F | Cb |
|---|---|---|---|
| **Sandwiches:** *Per Sandwich* | | | |
| Crispy Buttery Crust: BBQ Rcpe Beef | 320 | 13 | 43 |
| Cheddar Cheeseburger | 300 | 12 | 40 |
| Hickory Ham & Chse | 280 | 11 | 38 |
| Crispy Crust: | | | |
| Five Cheese Pizza | 350 | 18 | 37 |
| Signature Pepp. Pizza | 340 | 19 | 35 |
| Croissant Crust: | | | |
| Chkn, Brocc. & Chedd. | 300 | 14 | 35 |
| Hickory Ham & Cheese | 310 | 15 | 35 |
| Garlic Buttery Seasoned Crust | | | |
| Four Cheese Pizza | 320 | 13 | 39 |
| Four Meat & Four Cheese | 310 | 14 | 35 |
| Italian Style Meatballs & Mozz. | 310 | 13 | 38 |
| Pepperoni Pizza, Reduced Fat | 290 | 7 | 42 |
| Signature Pepperoni & Sausage | 320 | 14 | 35 |
| Pretzel Bread: | | | |
| Appwd Bacon Chedd. Chse Melt | 310 | 13 | 35 |
| Queso Chicken | 280 | 10 | 34 |
| Seasoned Crust: | | | |
| Beef Taco | 280 | 12 | 35 |
| Philly Steak & Cheese, Red. Fat | 270 | 8 | 40 |
| Spicy Beef Nacho | 260 | 10 | 34 |
| **Hungry Jack:** | | | |
| **Hungry Jack:** *Prepared As Per Directions* | | | |
| Casserole Potatoes, | | | |
| average all varieties, ½ cup | 165 | 7 | 21 |
| Easy Mash'd Cheesy, | | | |
| average all varieties, ⅔ cup | 110 | 1.5 | 21 |
| Hashbrowns: Original, ⅓ cup | 100 | 4.5 | 14 |
| Cheesy, ½ cup | 140 | 7 | 17 |
| Mashed Potatoes, average, ⅓ cup | 80 | 0 | 19 |
| **Hungry Man:** | | | |
| **Dinners:** | | | |
| Boneless Fried Chicken | 790 | 37 | 88 |
| Boneless Pork Rib Shaped Patties | 730 | 33 | 85 |
| Country Fried Chicken | 580 | 26 | 56 |
| Grilled Beef Patty | 450 | 22 | 39 |
| Home-Style Meatloaf | 530 | 22 | 64 |
| Roasted Carved White Meat Turkey | 430 | 11 | 62 |
| Salisbury Steak | 540 | 28 | 49 |
| **Pub Favorites:** | | | |
| Beer Battered Chkn | 760 | 38 | 75 |
| Honey Bourbon Chicken Strips | 600 | 25 | 69 |

| Hungry Man (Cont): | C | F | Cb |
|---|---|---|---|
| **Selects:** *Per Package* | | | |
| Classic Fried Chicken | 840 | 41 | 77 |
| Spicy Classic Fried Chicken | 700 | 34 | 61 |
| **XXL Sandwiches:** *Per Box* | | | |
| Angus Beef Charbroil | 740 | 47 | 52 |
| BBQ Pork Ribs | 690 | 39 | 62 |
| Buffalo Fried Chicken | 650 | 27 | 73 |
| Chicken Parmesan | 610 | 29 | 63 |
| Crispy Fried Chicken | 670 | 32 | 64 |
| **José Olé:** | | | |
| **Breakfast Burritos:** | | | |
| Egg & Bacon, 4 oz | 260 | 9 | 33 |
| Egg & Sausage, 4 oz | 270 | 10 | 34 |
| **Premium Burritos:** | | | |
| Chicken Monterey (1) | 270 | 6 | 41 |
| Steak & Cheese (1) | 300 | 10 | 40 |
| **Premium Chimichangas:** | | | |
| Chicken & Cheese (1), 5 oz | 330 | 11 | 45 |
| Steak & Cheese (1), 5 oz | 350 | 14 | 41 |
| **Snacks:** | | | |
| Mini: Chimichangas, | | | |
| Steak & Cheddar (3) | 370 | 20 | 37 |
| Quesadillas, | | | |
| Grilled Chicken & 3 Cheese (4) | 210 | 8 | 25 |
| Tacos, Beef & Cheese (4) | 230 | 12 | 23 |
| **Taquitos:** Chicken, Corn Tortillas, (3) | 200 | 8 | 26 |
| Steak & Cheese, Flour Tortillas, (2) | 250 | 12 | 26 |
| **Kashi:** | | | |
| **Entrees:** *Per 10 oz Pkg* | | | |
| Black Bean Mango | 340 | 8 | 58 |
| Chicken Enchilada | 280 | 9 | 38 |
| Chicken Florentine | 290 | 9 | 31 |
| Chicken Pasta Pomodoro | 280 | 6 | 38 |
| Mayan Harvest Bake | 340 | 9 | 58 |
| Pesto Pasta Primavera | 290 | 11 | 37 |
| Southwest Style Chicken | 310 | 5 | 49 |
| **Kid Cuisine:** *Per Meal* | | | |
| Cheese Stuffed Crust Pizza | 330 | 7 | 54 |
| Chicken Breast Nuggets, 8 oz | 400 | 13 | 55 |
| Fish Sticks, 7.6 oz | 320 | 11 | 45 |
| Fried Chicken, 10 oz | 530 | 22 | 53 |
| Hot Dog, 7.2 oz | 320 | 5 | 55 |
| Mac. & Cheese, 10.6 oz | 420 | 11 | 69 |
| Pancakes, 7.2 oz | 400 | 15 | 59 |
| Popcorn Chicken, 8.6 oz | 370 | 12 | 53 |
| Spaghetti w/- Mini Meatballs, 10.2 oz | 290 | 6 | 45 |

| Knorr: Sides, Prepared as Directed | C | F | Cb |
|---|---|---|---|
| **Asian:** Chicken Fried Rice | 290 | 7 | 48 |
| Teriyaki Noodles | 280 | 9 | 45 |
| Teriyaki Rice | 280 | 7 | 48 |
| **Cajun,** Garlic Butter Rice | 260 | 4 | 48 |
| **Fiesta:** Mexican Rice | 280 | 6 | 48 |
| Spanish Rice | 280 | 6 | 49 |
| Taco Rice | 270 | 6 | 46 |
| **Pasta:** Alfredo | 290 | 10 | 39 |
| Alfredo Broccoli | 300 | 10 | 39 |
| Butter | 260 | 8 | 39 |
| Butter & Herb | 260 | 7 | 39 |
| Cheesy Cheddar | 270 | 7 | 39 |
| Parmesan | 290 | 10 | 39 |
| Stroganoff | 260 | 7 | 39 |
| **Rice:** Cheddar Broccoli | 280 | 6 | 48 |
| Chicken Flavor Broccoli | 270 | 5 | 48 |
| Chicken Flavor | 280 | 6 | 48 |
| **Kraft:** | | | |
| **Macaroni & Cheese Dinner:** Per Cup, Prepared | | | |
| Original flavor, 2.5 oz | 400 | 19 | 47 |
| Thick 'N Creamy, 2.5 oz | 410 | 17 | 50 |
| White Cheddar, 2.5 oz | 380 | 15 | 48 |
| **Deluxe:** Four Cheese, 3.5 oz | 320 | 10 | 46 |
| Sharp Cheddar, 3.5 oz | 320 | 9 | 46 |
| **Velveeta Potatoes:** Per ½ Cup, Prepared | | | |
| Cheesy: Au Gratin | 190 | 7 | 24 |
| Bacon Scalloped | 200 | 7 | 27 |
| Mashed, Twin Pack | 180 | 9 | 21 |
| Shells & Cheese, Original, 4 oz | 360 | 12 | 49 |
| **Kroger:** | | | |
| **Kitchen Creation Skillet Dinners:** Per Cup, Prepared | | | |
| Creamy Broccoli | 300 | 12 | 33 |
| Creamy Pasta | 300 | 13 | 33 |
| Double Cheeseburger | 320 | 13 | 30 |
| Lasagna | 280 | 12 | 26 |
| Stroganoff | 320 | 14 | 27 |
| **Frozen:** | | | |
| **Healthy Meals Made Simple:** Refrigerated, Per Cup | | | |
| Braised Beef Pot Roast & Gravy | 220 | 5 | 15 |
| Lean Beef Tips & Gravy | 210 | 4 | 20 |
| Lem. Herb Chkn w/ Rice | 170 | 1.5 | 23 |
| Sweet & Spicy Chicken | 270 | 1.5 | 48 |

| Kroger (Cont): | C | F | Cb |
|---|---|---|---|
| **Frozen (Cont):** | | | |
| **Meals Made Simple:** | | | |
| Beef Stir Fry, 1¾ cups | 180 | 4 | 26 |
| Chicken Florentine, | | | |
| 2¼ cups, 6.9 oz | 320 | 18 | 22 |
| Chicken Stir Fry, 1½ cups | 180 | 2 | 25 |
| Shrimp Fried Rice, 1¼ cups, 8 oz | 240 | 0 | 44 |
| **Oven Ready:** | | | |
| Breaded Calamari Rings (10), 3 oz | 200 | 10 | 21 |
| Coconut Shrimp (5), | | | |
| with 1 oz sweet chili sauce | 350 | 20 | 34 |
| **La Choy:** | | | |
| **Family Meals, Canned:** Per 1 Cup | | | |
| Beef Pepper Oriental, 8.9 oz | 80 | 1 | 11 |
| Beef Chow Mein, 8.7 oz | 80 | 0 | 11 |
| Chicken Chow Mein, 8.8 oz | 100 | 4 | 11 |
| Sweet & Sour Chicken, 8.9 oz | 180 | 1.5 | 35 |
| **Lean Cuisine:** | | | |
| **Culinary Collection:** Per Complete Meal | | | |
| Asparagus & Cheese Ravioli | 260 | 7 | 40 |
| Beef Chow Fun | 320 | 5 | 54 |
| Broccoli Cheddar Dip with Pita Bread | 200 | 6 | 29 |
| Chicken Pecan | 320 | 7 | 49 |
| Chkn in Peanut Sauce | 280 | 6 | 35 |
| Chicken with Almonds | 270 | 4 | 44 |
| Chicken with Basil Cream Sauce | 230 | 5 | 28 |
| Chili Lime Chicken | 240 | 2 | 38 |
| Fiesta Grilled Chicken | 260 | 6 | 33 |
| Lemon Pepper Fish | 300 | 8 | 40 |
| Mushroom Mezzaluna Ravioli | 290 | 9 | 39 |
| Orange Chicken | 310 | 8 | 46 |
| Parmesan Crusted Fish | 300 | 8 | 43 |
| Ranchero Braised Beef | 240 | 5 | 32 |
| Roasted Chicken & Garden Veggies | 230 | 3 | 35 |
| Sesame Chicken | 330 | 9 | 47 |
| Spinach Artichoke Ravioli | 280 | 7 | 41 |
| Sweet & Sour Chicken | 300 | 3 | 51 |
| Spring Rolls: | | | |
| Fajita Style Chicken (2) | 220 | 8 | 22 |
| Garlic/Thai Chicken (2), average | 200 | 7 | 24 |

continued next page...

| Lean Cuisine (Cont): | C | F | Cb |
|---|---|---|---|
| **Market Collections:** | | | |
| Chicken Pot Stickers | 280 | 7 | 43 |
| Garlic Chicken | 290 | 5 | 38 |
| Roasted Turkey Breast | 290 | 7 | 38 |
| Salisbury Steak | 260 | 6 | 38 |
| Shanghai Style Shrimp | 250 | 3 | 41 |
| Shrimp Scampi | 250 | 7 | 32 |
| Sweet & Spicy Ginger Chicken | 290 | 2 | 45 |
| **Simple Favorites:** | | | |
| BBQ Chicken Quesadilla | 280 | 6 | 37 |
| Chicken Chow Mein | 200 | 2 | 34 |
| French Bread Cheese Pizza | 340 | 6 | 53 |
| Spaghetti with Meat Sauce | 310 | 4 | 53 |
| **Spa Collection:** | | | |
| Butternut Squash Ravioli | 260 | 7 | 40 |
| Lemongrass Chicken | 240 | 4 | 38 |
| Salmon with Basil | 250 | 2 | 38 |
| **Pizzas** ~ See Page 136 | | | |
| **Extra Product Listings** ~ www.CalorieKing.com | | | |
| **Lean Pockets** | | | |
| **Sandwiches:** *Per Single Pocket* | | | |
| Garlic Buttery Crust, Pepp. Pizza | 320 | 15 | 35 |
| Pretzel Bread: BBQ Recipe Chicken | 250 | 5 | 41 |
| Chicken Japalpeno Cheddar | 260 | 8 | 35 |
| Three Cheese & Spinach | 250 | 7 | 37 |
| Seasoned Crust, | | | |
| Four Cheese Pizza | 260 | 6 | 42 |
| Whole Grain Crust: | | | |
| Bacon, Egg & Cheese | 260 | 8 | 35 |
| Garlic Chicken White Pizza | 260 | 8 | 37 |
| Hickory Ham & Cheddar | 270 | 8 | 39 |
| Supreme Pizza | 220 | 7 | 33 |
| Three Cheese & Broccoli | 250 | 6 | 40 |
| **Lightlife (Meatless):** | | | |
| **Beef:** | | | |
| Gimme Lean Beef, 2 oz | 60 | 0 | 7 |
| Smart Grounds: | | | |
| Mexican Crumbles, 2 oz | 60 | 0 | 6 |
| Original Crumbles, 2 oz | 70 | 0 | 6 |
| **Burgers:** | | | |
| Orig., with Quinoa (1) | 100 | 2.5 | 10 |
| Black Bean (1) | 100 | 2.5 | 11 |
| **Chick'n:** | | | |
| Smart Cutlets/Tenders, 3 oz | 110 | 1 | 7 |
| Smart Strips, 3 oz | 80 | 0 | 5 |
| Smart Wings, 4 wings, 3 oz | 110 | 0 | 6 |
| **Tempeh:** | | | |
| Fakin' Bacon Strips, 4 slices | 140 | 5 | 10 |
| Flax, 3 oz | 160 | 7 | 9 |

| Lunchables: | C | F | Cb |
|---|---|---|---|
| **Crackers Stackers:** *Without Drink* | | | |
| Ham & Swiss, 3.4 oz | 320 | 10 | 42 |
| Light Bologna & Am. Cheese, 2.8 oz | 310 | 16 | 34 |
| Turkey & Cheddar, 2.9 oz | 340 | 14 | 42 |
| Extra Cheesy Pizza | 270 | 9 | 30 |
| Ham & Cheddar, | | | |
| with Crackers, 3.2 oz | 260 | 13 | 22 |
| Nachos, Cheese Dip & Salsa, 4.7 oz | 500 | 23 | 65 |
| Pizza, with Pepperoni | 300 | 13 | 32 |
| Turkey & Cheddar, w/- Crackers, 3.2 oz | 260 | 13 | 22 |
| **Lunchmakers** *(Armour): Per Package* | | | |
| Bologna Cracker Crunchers | 350 | 14 | 46 |
| Cheese Pizza | 340 | 12 | 51 |
| Nachos | 480 | 17 | 77 |
| Pepperoni Pizza | 330 | 10 | 55 |
| Turkey Cracker Crunchers | 350 | 14 | 45 |
| **Marie Callender's:** | | | |
| **Beef:** *Per Container* | | | |
| Beef & Broccoli | 370 | 9 | 50 |
| Beef Pot Roast | 320 | 11 | 35 |
| Country Fried Beef Steak & Gravy | 660 | 31 | 75 |
| **Chicken:** *Per Container* | | | |
| Chicken Parmigiana | 530 | 27 | 47 |
| Country Fried Chicken & Gravy | 560 | 27 | 61 |
| Fettuccini with Chicken & Broccoli | 500 | 24 | 41 |
| Sweet & Sour Chicken | 560 | 13 | 93 |
| **Pasta:** *Per Container* | | | |
| Fettuccini Alfredo & Garlic Bread | 610 | 31 | 59 |
| Grilled Chicken Alfredo Bake | 480 | 21 | 45 |
| **Pot Pies:** *Per 1 Cup, 7 oz* | | | |
| Beef | 410 | 23 | 39 |
| Cheesy Chicken & Bacon | 520 | 31 | 43 |
| Chicken | 380 | 21 | 38 |
| Chicken Corn Chowder | 470 | 27 | 44 |
| Creamy: | | | |
| Mushroom Chicken | 450 | 27 | 41 |
| Parmesan Chicken | 420 | 24 | 35 |
| Turkey | 480 | 28 | 46 |
| **Under 500 Calories:** | | | |
| Country Fried Pork Chop & Gravy | 460 | 19 | 55 |
| Golden Battered Fish Filet | 410 | 11 | 58 |
| Herb Roasted Chicken | 470 | 17 | 46 |
| Meat Loaf & Gravy | 450 | 17 | 43 |
| Spaghetti & Meatballs | 420 | 13 | 52 |
| Steak & Roasted Potatoes | 350 | 11 | 40 |
| **Family size:** *Per 1 Cup* | | | |
| Cheesy Chicken Lasagna, 8 oz | 320 | 14 | 33 |
| Vermont White Cheddar | | | |
| Mac & Cheese, 6.3 oz | 350 | 20 | 31 |

| Maruchan: | C | F | Cb |
|---|---|---|---|
| **Bowls,** all varieties, 3.3 oz | 380 | 16 | 50 |
| **Ramen,** Noodle Soup, average all, 3 oz pkg | 380 | 16 | 52 |
| **Instant Lunch,** average, 1 package | 290 | 11 | 39 |
| **Yakisoba:** *Per 4 oz Pkg* | | | |
| Chicken/Teriyaki Beef Flavor, av. | 520 | 21 | 72 |
| Sweet & Sour Chicken | 560 | 22 | 78 |
| **Michael Angelo's:** | | | |
| **Organic:** Chicken Parmesan, 10 oz | 350 | 6 | 47 |
| Four Cheese Lasagna, 10 oz | 380 | 11 | 46 |
| Lasagna with Meat Sauce, 10 oz | 390 | 16 | 38 |
| Manicotti, with Sauce, 10 oz | 410 | 18 | 35 |
| **Signature:** Chicken Alfredo, 11 oz | 410 | 12 | 47 |
| Meat Lasagna, 11 oz | 420 | 13 | 51 |
| Shrimp Scampi, 10 oz | 540 | 28 | 46 |
| **Minute Rice:** | | | |
| **Ready To Serve:** *Per 4.4 oz Container, Prepared* | | | |
| Brown/Chicken Rice Mix, average | 230 | 5 | 42 |
| Fried/Yellow Rice Mix, average | 225 | 2.5 | 46 |
| **Morningstar Farms (Meatless):** | | | |
| **Breakfast,** Hot & Spicy Ssg Patty (1) | 70 | 3 | 3 |
| **Burgers:** *Per Patty* | | | |
| Grillers Original (1) | 130 | 6 | 5 |
| Mushroom Lovers (1) | 110 | 5 | 6 |
| Spicy Black Bean (1) | 110 | 4 | 13 |
| **Chik'n:** | | | |
| Buffalo Wings (5) | 200 | 9 | 19 |
| Chik'n Nuggets (4) | 180 | 8 | 18 |
| Patties: | | | |
| Chik, Original (1) | 160 | 6 | 19 |
| Grillers Chik'n Veggie (1) | 80 | 3 | 7 |
| Hot & Spicy Sausage (1) | 70 | 3 | 3 |
| **Entree:** Baja Black Bean Pizza (1) | 380 | 11 | 59 |
| Mediterranean Chickpea Pizza (1) | 380 | 12 | 59 |
| **Newman's Own:** | | | |
| **Comp[lete Skillets:** *Per ½ Package, 11-12 oz* | | | |
| Chicken: Fettuccini Alfredo | 410 | 12 | 49 |
| Florentine & Farfalle | 370 | 10 | 42 |
| Parmigiana & Penne | 490 | 25 | 47 |
| Garlic Chicken Lo Mein Noodles | 320 | 7 | 42 |
| Italian Ssge & Rigatoni | 510 | 28 | 48 |
| Steak Fajita | 290 | 6 | 47 |
| Sweet & Sour Chicken | 330 | 10 | 46 |

| Nissin: | C | F | Cb |
|---|---|---|---|
| **Chow Mein:** *Per 4 oz Package* | | | |
| Chicken Flavor | 480 | 18 | 70 |
| Spicy Chicken Flavor | 560 | 28 | 66 |
| Teriyaki Beef | 520 | 20 | 68 |
| With Shrimp | 540 | 24 | 68 |
| **Cup Noodles,** | | | |
| Beef/Chicken/Shrimp Flav., 1 cup | 280 | 11 | 40 |
| **Top Ramen,** average, 3 oz package | 380 | 14 | 52 |
| **Old El Paso:** | | | |
| **Dinner Kits:** *Per Serving, Prepared with Chicken* | | | |
| Chicken Soft Taco | 300 | 10 | 30 |
| Enchilada | 390 | 16 | 27 |
| **Frozen Meals:** *Per ½ Pkg* | | | |
| Chicken Burritos (1) | 480 | 17 | 59 |
| Chicken Quesadillas (1) | 620 | 30 | 57 |
| Shredded Beef Burritos (1) | 490 | 16 | 63 |
| **Pasta Roni:** *Per Cup, Prepared* | | | |
| Angel Hair Pasta varieties, average | 310 | 14 | 40 |
| Butter & Herb Italiano | 300 | 11 | 41 |
| Chicken & Broccoli | 360 | 15 | 49 |
| Chicken Flavor | 300 | 12 | 40 |
| Fettuccine Alfredo | 450 | 24 | 44 |
| Four Cheese Corkscrew | 370 | 15 | 49 |
| Stroganoff | 350 | 13 | 48 |
| Tomato Parmesan | 270 | 9 | 40 |
| White Cheddar & Broccoli | 300 | 13 | 39 |
| **P.F. Chang's:** *Per ½ Package, 11 oz* | | | |
| **Meals:** Beef with Broccoli | 360 | 17 | 30 |
| General Chang's Chicken | 350 | 14 | 35 |
| King Pao Chicken | 360 | 17 | 27 |
| Mongolian Style Beef | 340 | 11 | 41 |
| Mongolian Style Chicken | 310 | 9 | 40 |
| Orange Chicken | 430 | 18 | 44 |
| Sweet & Sour Chicken | 335 | 12 | 40 |
| Shrimp Lo Mein | 390 | 12 | 52 |

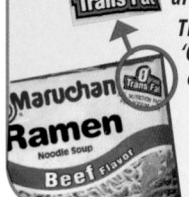

*Most packaged noodle soups are high in calories and fat.*

*Their promotion of '0 Grams Trans Fat' does not make them heart-healthy.*

*They are still high in saturated fat as well as salt/sodium.*

| Rice-A-Roni: | C | F | Cb |
|---|---|---|---|
| **Classic Favorites:** *Per Cup, Prepared* | | | |
| Beef; Herb & Butter; Rice Pilaf, av. | 310 | 9 | 52 |
| Broccoli Au Gratin | 350 | 16 | 46 |
| Chicken Flavor | 300 | 9 | 50 |
| Chicken & Broccoli | 220 | 5 | 40 |
| Spanish Rice | 260 | 8 | 44 |
| **Whole Grain Blends:** | | | |
| Roasted Garlic Italiano | 270 | 9 | 41 |
| Spanish | 250 | 8 | 42 |
| **Rosarita:** | | | |
| Kidney Beans, ½ cup, 4.5 oz | 110 | 0 | 20 |
| Chili Beans, ½ cup, 4.5 oz | 130 | 0.5 | 24 |
| **Refried Beans:** | | | |
| Traditional, ½ cup, 4.5 oz | 120 | 2 | 18 |
| No Fat, ½ cup, 4.5 oz | 100 | 0 | 18 |
| **Safeway Select:** | | | |
| **Frozen:** | | | |
| Beef Salisbury Steak, 9.4 oz | 410 | 28 | 23 |
| Chicken Cacciatore, 8.8 oz | 290 | 10 | 34 |
| Fettucini Alfredo, 11.5 oz | 380 | 12 | 55 |
| Five Vegetable Lasagna, 10.6 oz | 330 | 8 | 48 |
| Homestyle Baked Chicken, 9 oz | 260 | 11 | 31 |
| Orange Chicken, 9 oz | 360 | 7 | 61 |
| Penne Pasta, 8 oz | 300 | 11 | 42 |
| Pot Roast, 9 oz | 270 | 11 | 23 |
| Spaghetti with Meat Sauce, 12 oz | 450 | 16 | 61 |
| Swedish Meat Balls, 11.5 oz | 470 | 24 | 43 |
| Three Cheese Tortellini, 7.5 oz | 350 | 16 | 38 |
| **S & W:** *Per ½ Cup* | | | |
| Black Beans, 4.5 oz | 110 | 0.5 | 22 |
| Chili Beans, | | | |
| in Zesty Tomato Sauce, 4.6 oz | 130 | 1.5 | 23 |
| Kidney Beans, 4.7 oz | 110 | 0 | 22 |
| White Beans, 4.5 oz | 110 | 0.5 | 21 |
| **Seapak** ~ *See www.calorieking.com* | | | |
| **Simply Asia:** | | | |
| **Noodle Bowls:** *Per 8.5oz Bowl* | | | |
| Roasted Peanut | 460 | 12 | 75 |
| Sesame Teriyaki | 390 | 13 | 82 |
| Soy Ginger | 420 | 6 | 84 |
| Spicy Mongolian | 430 | 6 | 86 |

| Simply Asia: | C | F | Cb |
|---|---|---|---|
| **Noodle Bowls:** *Per 8.5oz Bowl* | | | |
| Roasted Peanut | 460 | 12 | 75 |
| Sesame Teriyaki | 390 | 13 | 82 |
| Soy Ginger | 420 | 6 | 84 |
| Spicy Mongolian | 430 | 6 | 86 |
| **Noodles & Sauce:** *Per ⅓ Package* | | | |
| Sesame Teriyaki | 300 | 3 | 60 |
| Soy Ginger | 320 | 4.5 | 60 |
| Spicy Kung Pao | 350 | 7 | 63 |
| **Quick Noodles:** *Per 8.8 oz Tray* | | | |
| Honey Teriyaki | 430 | 3.5 | 85 |
| Pad Thai | 460 | 3 | 93 |
| Szechwan Garl. Chow Mein | 460 | 7 | 83 |
| **Smart Ones** *(Weight Watchers):* | | | |
| **Classic Favorites:** *Per Meal* | | | |
| Angel Hair Marinara | 180 | 2 | 34 |
| Chkn Enchiladas Suiza | 290 | 6 | 46 |
| Lasagna Bake with Meat Sauce | 250 | 5 | 39 |
| Lasagna Florentine | 320 | 10 | 43 |
| Lemon Herb Chicken Piccata | 210 | 2.5 | 32 |
| Macaroni & Cheese | 260 | 2 | 51 |
| Pasta Primavera | 200 | 2.5 | 35 |
| Pasta with Ricotta & Spinach | 290 | 5 | 44 |
| Ravioli Florentine | 210 | 3.5 | 37 |
| Spaghetti with Meat Sauce | 280 | 3.5 | 50 |
| Swedish Meatballs | 290 | 7 | 38 |
| Three Cheese Macaroni | 300 | 6 | 48 |
| Traditional Lasagna w/ Meat Sauce | 310 | 8 | 45 |
| Tuna Noodle Gratin | 250 | 3 | 44 |
| **Smart Beginnings:** *Per Meal* | | | |
| Breakfast Quesadilla | 230 | 7 | 29 |
| Canadian Bacon English Muffin | 210 | 6 | 27 |
| English Muffin S'wich, | | | |
| Egg White & Cheese | 210 | 5 | 28 |
| Three Cheese Omelet | 200 | 7 | 20 |
| **Smart Creations:** *Per Meal* | | | |
| Chicken Fettucini | 300 | 4 | 45 |
| Chicken Parmesan | 280 | 5 | 37 |
| Homestyle Turkey Breast, | | | |
| with Stuffing | 280 | 6 | 36 |
| Meatloaf | 270 | 9 | 25 |
| Teriyaki Chicken & Vegetables | 250 | 2.5 | 41 |

## Stagg Chili:

| | C | F | Cb |
|---|---|---|---|
| **Chili with Beans:** *15 oz Can, 1 cup, 8.7 oz* | | | |
| Classic | 290 | 13 | 30 |
| Chunkero | 320 | 16 | 28 |
| Dynamite Hot | 320 | 15 | 30 |
| Fiesta Grille | 280 | 13 | 25 |
| Ranch House Chicken | 240 | 8 | 26 |
| Turkey Ranchero | 250 | 5 | 32 |
| Vege Garden Four-Bean | 200 | 1 | 37 |
| White Chicken Chili | 260 | 12 | 20 |
| **No Beans,** Steakhouse | 320 | 22 | 14 |

## Stouffer's:

| | C | F | Cb |
|---|---|---|---|
| **Satisfying Servings For One:** *Per Package* | | | |
| Baked Ziti | 520 | 18 | 68 |
| Bourbon Steak Tips | 490 | 17 | 61 |
| Chicken Fettuccini Alfredo | 840 | 38 | 94 |
| Five Cheese Lasagna | 330 | 14 | 33 |
| Lasagna Italiano | 290 | 12 | 30 |
| Macaroni & Cheese | 340 | 16 | 36 |
| Meatloaf | 530 | 26 | 40 |
| Meat Lovers Lasagna | 310 | 14 | 31 |
| Monterey Chicken | 530 | 21 | 54 |
| Savory Beef & Vegetables | 360 | 16 | 34 |
| White Meat Chicken Pot Pie | 590 | 34 | 54 |
| **Signature Classics For One:** *Per Package* | | | |
| Baked Chicken Breast | 240 | 8 | 17 |
| Beef Pot Roast | 320 | 8 | 41 |
| Beef Stroganoff | 380 | 17 | 34 |
| Creamed Chipped Beef | 140 | 7 | 11 |
| Fettuccini Alfredo | 630 | 35 | 63 |
| Green Pepper Steak | 240 | 4 | 32 |
| Meatloaf | 320 | 16 | 23 |
| Spaghetti with Meat Sauce | 350 | 12 | 44 |
| White Meat Chicken Pot Pie | 670 | 38 | 64 |
| **Simple Dishes For One:** *Per ½ Package* | | | |
| Cheddar Potato Bake | 270 | 17 | 21 |
| Garlic Parmesan Mac & Cheese | 340 | 15 | 36 |
| Macaroni & Cheese | 340 | 16 | 33 |
| Spinach Souffle | 150 | 10 | 9 |

## Stouffer's (Cont):

| | C | F | Cb |
|---|---|---|---|
| **Family Size Meals:** *Per Serving* | | | |
| Cheese Manicotti | 340 | 16 | 33 |
| Cheesy Chicken & Broccoli Rice Bake | 330 | 15 | 30 |
| Chicken & Broccoli Pasta Bake | 300 | 14 | 24 |
| Chicken & Vegetable Rice | 360 | 15 | 37 |
| Chicken Cordon Bleu | 330 | 15 | 28 |
| Chicken Enchiladas | 290 | 9 | 38 |
| Lasagna Italiano | 250 | 9 | 30 |
| Lasagna with Meat Sauce | 320 | 12 | 32 |
| Macaroni & Cheese | 350 | 17 | 34 |
| Meatloaf in Gravy | 190 | 10 | 9 |
| Meat Lovers Lasagna | 330 | 16 | 31 |
| Rigatoni with Chicken & Pesto | 270 | 12 | 25 |
| Salisbury Steak | 220 | 15 | 7 |
| Stuffed Green Peppers | 190 | 8 | 20 |

## Swanson:

| | C | F | Cb |
|---|---|---|---|
| **Dinners:** *Per Package* | | | |
| Chicken Nuggets | 590 | 25 | 71 |
| Rib Style Bnless Pork | 540 | 23 | 71 |
| Salisbury Steak | 450 | 22 | 44 |
| **Skillets:** *For Two* | | | |
| Alfredo Chicken | 370 | 12 | 42 |
| Beef Lo Mein | 360 | 6 | 55 |
| Chicken Parmesan | 430 | 14 | 60 |
| Garlic Chicken | 420 | 15 | 51 |
| Teriyaki Chicken | 290 | 2.5 | 51 |

## Tasty Bite:

| | C | F | Cb |
|---|---|---|---|
| **Vegetarian Entrees:** *Per ½ Package, 5 oz* | | | |
| Bengal Lentils | 160 | 6 | 20 |
| Bombay Potatoes | 130 | 4 | 19 |
| Jaipur Vegetables | 180 | 11 | 12 |
| Jodhpur Lentils | 110 | 2.5 | 16 |
| Madras Lentils | 150 | 6 | 18 |
| Punjab Eggplant | 150 | 9 | 13 |

## TGI Friday's:

| | C | F | Cb |
|---|---|---|---|
| Cheese & Bacon Loaded Fries, 3 oz | 220 | 14 | 14 |
| Chicken Parmesan Sliders, 3 oz | 260 | 13 | 27 |
| Chicken Wings, Buffalo Style Sce, 3.4 oz | 180 | 13 | 4 |
| Cream Cheese Stuffed Jalap., 2.7 oz | 200 | 11 | 20 |
| Crispy Green Bean Fries & Sce, 3 oz | 190 | 9 | 26 |
| Dill Pickle Chips, w/ Horseradish Sce | 200 | 11 | 22 |
| Mozzarella Sticks (1), w/ Marinara Sce, | 100 | 4.5 | 10 |
| Potato Skins, Cheddar & Bacon (3) | 200 | 10 | 21 |

| Thai Kitchen: | C | F | Cb |
|---|---|---|---|
| **Take-Out Meals:** *Per ½ Package* | | | |
| Original Pad Thai | 250 | 2 | 54 |
| Thai Basil & Chili | 250 | 3 | 50 |
| Thai Peanut | 270 | 5 | 51 |
| **Noodle Carts:** *Per 9 oz Tray* | | | |
| Pad Thai | 460 | 2 | 104 |
| Thai Peanut | 510 | 9 | 96 |
| **Rice Noodle Soup Bowls,** | | | |
| average all varieties, 2.5 oz | 240 | 2 | 50 |
| **Stir-Fry Rice Noodles:** *Per ½ Package* | | | |
| Original Pad Thai | 390 | 3.5 | 84 |
| Thai Peanut | 390 | 2 | 87 |
| **Tofurky:** | | | |
| **Chick'n:** | | | |
| BBQ Style, 3.2 oz | 200 | 5 | 14 |
| Sesame, 3.2 oz | 210 | 9 | 10 |
| Tandoori, 3.2 oz | 180 | 6 | 9 |
| **Pies:** | | | |
| Chick'N Pot Pie (1), 8 oz | 520 | 33 | 45 |
| Sausage & Veggie Quiche (1), 7.5 oz | 520 | 28 | 43 |
| **Pockets:** BBQ Chick'N (1), 4.5 oz | 290 | 4 | 50 |
| Broccoli Cheddar (1), 4.5 oz | 240 | 5 | 40 |
| Pepp. Pizza (1), 4.5 oz | 300 | 5 | 43 |
| **Trader Joe's:** | | | |
| **Baked Beans,** Organic, | | | |
| average all varieties, ½ cup | 140 | 0 | 29 |
| **Black Beans:** | | | |
| Regular, ½ cup | 110 | 0 | 19 |
| Cuban Style, ½ cup | 100 | 0.5 | 19 |
| Chicken Chili with Beans, 1 cup | 290 | 9 | 32 |
| Pasta, Shells & White Cheddar, 1 cup | 280 | 6 | 47 |
| **Potatoes:** Garlic Mashed, ½ cup | 150 | 7 | 19 |
| Cheddar Cheese Au Gratin, ½ cup | 140 | 5 | 21 |
| Turkey Chili w/ Beans, 1 cup | 240 | 4.5 | 30 |
| **Frozen:** | | | |
| Butter Chicken w/ Basmati Rice, 1 cup | 270 | 8 | 33 |
| Chicken Chow Mein, ⅓ package, 6.7 oz | 210 | 2 | 35 |
| Chicken Quesadilla (1), 6 oz | 320 | 16 | 26 |
| Citrus Glazed Chicken with Rice, 8 oz | 270 | 5 | 40 |
| Mac & Cheese: Regular, 1 cup, 7 oz | 360 | 15 | 42 |
| Reduced Guilt, 7 oz | 270 | 6 | 40 |
| Shrimp Stir Fry, 6.4 oz | 70 | 0.5 | 6 |
| Spag. & Beef Meatballs, | | | |
| 1 cup, 9 oz | 380 | 13 | 48 |
| Spicy Beef & Broccoli, | | | |
| 1¾ cups | 430 | 13 | 64 |
| Thai Vegetable Kao Soi, 12.6 oz | 430 | 20 | 55 |
| Vegetable Pad Thai, 10.5 oz tray | 520 | 21 | 74 |
| **Pies:** Chicken Pot Pie, ½ pie, 8 oz | 360 | 22 | 28 |
| Shepherd's Pie, 1 cup, 8 oz | 170 | 3 | 22 |

| Tyson: | C | F | Cb |
|---|---|---|---|
| **Any'tizers Snacks:** | | | |
| H'style Chicken Fries (7), 3.2 oz | 230 | 13 | 14 |
| Stuffed Chicken Cordon Bleu, | | | |
| Minis, 3 pieces, 3 oz | 200 | 12 | 11 |
| Chicken Wings: Buffalo Style Hot Wings | | | |
| bone-in, 3 oz | 190 | 13 | 3 |
| Honey BBQ, 3 oz | 190 | 12 | 8 |
| Hot & Spicy, 3 oz | 190 | 13 | 1 |
| Chicken Wyngz, Boneless: | | | |
| Buffalo Style, 3 pcs | 150 | 7 | 8 |
| Honey BBQ, 3 oz | 200 | 8 | 20 |
| **Better For You:** *Per 3 oz Serving* | | | |
| Grilled & Ready Chicken Breast Strips: | | | |
| 100% Natural | 100 | 2.5 | 1 |
| Fajita | 110 | 4 | 1 |
| Southwestern | 120 | 3 | 5 |
| **Breaded Chicken:** | | | |
| 100% All Natural: | | | |
| Breast Patties (1), 2.7 oz | 200 | 13 | 10 |
| Chicken Nuggets (5), 3.2 oz | 270 | 17 | 15 |
| Crispy Chicken Strips, 3 oz | 190 | 9 | 12 |
| Breast Nuggets (5), 3.1 oz | 220 | 13 | 15 |
| Buffalo Chicken Strips, 3 oz | 190 | 9 | 17 |
| **Fully Cooked Beef:** | | | |
| Country Fried Steak, 1 pattie, 2.6 oz | 250 | 17 | 13 |
| Steak Fingers, 2 pieces, 2.5 oz | 250 | 18 | 14 |
| **To Go Products:** | | | |
| Mini Chicken Sandwich: | | | |
| Original, breaded | 390 | 16 | 46 |
| With Cheese | 440 | 20 | 47 |
| **Uncle Ben's:** | | | |
| **Country Inn:** *Per Cup, Prepared with Water Only* | | | |
| Broccoli Rice Au Gratin | 200 | 2 | 41 |
| Chicken & Vegetable Rice | 200 | 1 | 43 |
| Chicken Flavored Rice | 200 | 1 | 42 |
| Rice Pilaf | 200 | 1 | 43 |
| **Flavored Grains:** *1 Cup cooked As Directed* | | | |
| 5 Grain Medley Quinoa Pilaf | 200 | 1.5 | 41 |
| Basmati Medley Savory Herb | 200 | 0.5 | 43 |
| Brown Rice Medley, | | | |
| Roasted Garlic & Herbs, 2 oz | 200 | 2 | 40 |
| **Ready Rice:** *Per Package, Heat & Serve* | | | |
| Butter & Garlic Flavored | 220 | 4 | 41 |
| Garden Vegetable | 200 | 2.5 | 41 |
| Roasted Chicken Flavored | 210 | 3 | 42 |
| Teriyaki Style | 220 | 3 | 42 |
| **Ready Whole Grain Medley,** | | | |
| average all varieties, 1 pkt | 210 | 3 | 41 |

| Van Camp's: | C | F | Cb |
|---|---|---|---|
| Baked Beans, Original, ½ cup, 4.8 oz | 160 | 1 | 30 |
| Hickory Baked Beans, ½ cup, 4.8 oz | 170 | 1 | 32 |
| Pork & Beans, 28 oz can, ½ cup, 4.6 oz | 110 | 1 | 23 |
| **Van De Kamp's:** | | | |
| Beer Battrd Fillets, 3.8 oz | 210 | 10 | 21 |
| Crispy Fish Tenders, 3.6 oz | 230 | 2.5 | 21 |
| Cracked Blk Pepper & Sea Salt Salmon, 4.3 oz | 230 | 8 | 20 |
| Crunchy Fish Fillets, 1.8 oz | 90 | 4 | 13 |
| Garlic Herb Cod, 5 oz | 260 | 10 | 26 |
| Parmesan & Rsted Garlic Tilapia, 5 oz | 280 | 10 | 26 |
| **Whole Foods (365):** | | | |
| Chickenless Nuggets, breaded (4), 2.8 oz | 180 | 7 | 16 |
| Meatless Meatballs (4), 2 oz | 110 | 4 | 9 |
| Meatless Burgers (1), 2.5 oz | 120 | 4.5 | 7 |
| Pasta Rings in Tomato Sauce, 1 cup | 150 | 1 | 31 |
| Vegetarian Chili, 1 cup | 130 | 2 | 25 |
| **Worthington/Loma Linda:** | | | |
| Big Franks: 1 link, 1.8 oz | 110 | 6 | 3 |
| Low-fat, 1 link, 1.8 oz | 80 | 2.5 | 3 |
| Chili, 1 cup, 8.10 oz | 280 | 10 | 25 |
| Choplets, 2 slices, 3.2 oz | 90 | 1 | 4 |
| Diced Chik, 2 oz | 50 | 0 | 2 |
| FriChik, Original, low fat, 2 pieces, 3 oz | 80 | 2.5 | 4 |
| Linketts (1), 1.3 oz | 70 | 4 | 1 |
| Little Links (2), 1.6 oz | 90 | 5 | 3 |
| Redi-Burger, ⅝" slice, 3 oz | 120 | 2.5 | 7 |
| Super Links (1), 1.5 oz | 110 | 8 | 2 |
| Tender Rounds (6), 2.8 oz | 120 | 4.5 | 6 |
| Vegetable Skallops, ½ cup, 3 oz | 90 | 1 | 4 |
| Vegetarian Burger, ¼ cup, 1.9 oz | 70 | 1.5 | 3 |
| Veja-Links (1), 1 oz | 50 | 3 | 1 |
| **Frozen:** | | | |
| Chic-ketts, 2 slices | 110 | 5 | 3 |
| Dinner Roast, ¾" slice | 180 | 11 | 6 |
| FriPats, 1 pattie, 2.3 oz | 130 | 6 | 5 |
| Leanies, 1 link, 1.4 oz | 100 | 7 | 2 |
| Meatless: | | | |
| Chicken Style Roll, ⅜" slice | 90 | 4.5 | 2 |
| Smoked Turkey Roll, ⅜" slice | 130 | 8 | 4 |
| Prosage Links (2), 1.6 oz | 80 | 3 | 3 |
| Stakelets, 2.5 oz piece | 150 | 7 | 7 |
| Stripples, 2 strips, 0.6 oz | 60 | 4.5 | 2 |

| Yves Veggie Cuisine: | C | F | Cb |
|---|---|---|---|
| **Brats:** *Per Brat* | | | |
| Veggie Classic, 3.5 oz | 160 | 5 | 9 |
| Zesty Italian, 3.5 oz | 150 | 5 | 9 |
| **Burgers:** Meatless Beef Burger (1) | 110 | 4 | 8 |
| Meatless Chicken (1) | 100 | 3 | 5 |
| **Deli Slices:** | 80 | 2.5 | 2 |
| Meatless: Bologna, 4 slices | 80 | 2.5 | 2 |
| Ham, 4 slices | 100 | 2 | 5 |
| Pepperoni, 6 slices | 80 | 1 | 4 |
| Roast without the Beef, 4 slices | 110 | 2.5 | 4 |
| Salami, 4 slices | 80 | 0 | 4 |
| Smoked Chicken, 4 slices | 100 | 1.5 | 5 |
| Turkey, 4 slices | 100 | 1.5 | 5 |
| **Ground Rounds:** | | | |
| Meatless: Taco Stuffers, ⅓ cup, 2 oz | 90 | 2.5 | 5 |
| Turkey, ⅓ cup, 2 oz | 60 | 1 | 4 |
| **Hot Dog:** | | | |
| Good Dog (1), 2 oz | 70 | 3.5 | 1 |
| Hot Dog (1), 1.5 oz | 50 | 0.5 | 2 |
| Jumbo Hot Dog (1), 2.8 oz | 110 | 3 | 5 |
| Tofu Dog (1), 1.5 oz | 45 | 1 | 2 |
| **Skewers & Strips:** | | | |
| Chicken Skewers (1) | 100 | 1 | 7 |
| Meatless Beef/Chicken Strips, average, 2.8 oz | 115 | 1 | 4 |
| **Veggie Seafood:** | | | |
| Shrimp, 3 oz | 50 | 1.5 | 8 |
| Shrimp Scampi, 3.5 oz | 100 | 7 | 8 |
| Tuna Steak, with Sesame Ginger Sce, 3.5 oz | 250 | 20 | 8 |
| **Zatarain's:** | | | |
| **New Orleans Style:** *Per Dry Mix Only* | | | |
| Black Beans & Rice, Original, 2.3 oz | 230 | 1 | 47 |
| Caribbean Rice Mix, 2.5 oz | 250 | 2 | 52 |
| Chicken Creole Rice Mix, 1.5 oz | 140 | 1 | 29 |
| Chicken Flavor Rice, 2 oz | 210 | 0.5 | 45 |
| Garlic & Herb & Rice Mix, 1.5 oz | 130 | 0.5 | 29 |
| Rice Pilaf, 2 oz | 210 | 0.5 | 45 |
| Smothered Chicken Rice Mix, 1.6 oz | 160 | 0.5 | 34 |
| Yellow Rice, 2 oz | 200 | 0.5 | 43 |
| **Frozen:** | | | |
| **Meals:** *Per Meal* | | | |
| Blackened Chicken Alfredo, 10.5 oz | 500 | 21 | 56 |
| Dirty Rice with Beef & Pork, 10 oz | 430 | 13 | 64 |
| Jambalaya Flavored w/ Ssge, 12 oz | 490 | 10 | 86 |
| Red Beans & Rice w/ Sausage, 12 oz | 540 | 17 | 79 |
| Shrimp Scampi with Pasta, 10.5 oz | 350 | 10 | 49 |

Note: Cooking reduces weight of meat by 20-45% due to water and fat losses. Average weight loss is 30%. Actual loss depends on cooking method and cooking time.

Examples:

4 oz raw weight = approx. 3 oz cooked weight

4 oz cooked weight = approx. 5½ oz raw weight

**What 3 oz Cooked Meat Looks Like:**
- Rectangular piece (4" x 2½" x ½" thick)
- Deck of cards (3½" x 2½" x ⅝" thick)

### Quick Guide

**Sirloin (Choice Grade):**
**External fat trimmed to ⅛"**
*Broiled, Edible Portion (no bone)*

**Small/Regular Serving, 3 oz, cooked weight:**
(from 4-4½ oz raw)

| | | | |
|---|---|---|---|
| Lean + external fat (⅛"), 3 oz | 220 | 13 | 0 |
| Lean + marbling, 3 oz | 185 | 9 | 0 |
| Lean only, 3 oz | 160 | 6 | 0 |

(No external fat or marbling)

**Medium Serving, 5 oz, cooked weight:**
(from approximately 7 oz raw)

| | | | |
|---|---|---|---|
| Lean + external fat (⅛"), 5 oz | 365 | 22 | 0 |
| Lean + marbling, 5 oz | 310 | 15 | 0 |
| Lean only, 5 oz | 265 | 10 | 0 |

**Large Serving, 8 oz, cooked weight:**
(from approximately11-12 oz raw)

| | | | |
|---|---|---|---|
| Lean + external fat (⅛"), 8 oz | 585 | 36 | 0 |
| Lean + marbling, 8 oz | 500 | 24 | 0 |
| Lean only, 8 oz | 425 | 15 | 0 |

**Extra Large Serving, 12 oz, cooked weight:**
(from approximately 16-17 oz raw)

| | | | |
|---|---|---|---|
| Lean + external fat (⅛"), 12 oz | 875 | 54 | 0 |
| Lean + marbling, 12 oz | 745 | 36 | 0 |
| Lean only, 12 oz | 640 | 22 | 0 |

**Pan Fried:**
Sirloin (Choice), medium serving,

| | | | |
|---|---|---|---|
| Lean + external fat (⅛"), 5 oz | 445 | 30 | 0 |

### Other Steaks

**Filet Mignon (Tenderloin):**
1 Medium steak, 6 oz raw weight:
Broiled, with ¼" fat trim:

| | | | |
|---|---|---|---|
| Lean + fat (¼"), 4 oz | 360 | 27 | 0 |
| Lean only, 3.5 oz | 230 | 12 | 0 |

**New York/Club Steak:**
Top Loin/Short Loin:
1 steak, regular (9.25 oz raw, ¼" fat):

| | | | |
|---|---|---|---|
| Broiled: Lean + fat (¼"), 6.3 oz | 580 | 43 | 0 |
| Lean + marbling, 5.5 oz | 400 | 25 | 0 |
| Lean only, 5.25 oz | 360 | 20 | 0 |

**Porterhouse Steak:**
1 Medium, 6 oz raw weight, without bone, broiled:

| | | | |
|---|---|---|---|
| Lean + fat (¼"), 4.3 oz | 410 | 33 | 0 |
| Lean only, 3.5  oz | 210 | 11 | 0 |

1 Large ,12 oz raw weight, without bone, broiled:

| | | | |
|---|---|---|---|
| Lean + fat (¼") 8.5 oz cooked | 820 | 66 | 0 |
| Lean only, 7 oz cooked | 420 | 22 | 0 |

**T-Bone Steak:** *Broiled or Grilled*
**Medium Size:** *8 oz raw weight, without bone*
Approximately 6 oz cooked:

| | | | |
|---|---|---|---|
| Lean + Fat (¼"), 5 oz | 400 | 28 | 0 |
| Lean only, 4 oz | 265 | 12 | 0 |

**Large Size:** *12 oz raw weight*
Approximately 9 oz cooked:

| | | | |
|---|---|---|---|
| Lean + fat (¼"), 7 oz, without bone | 560 | 39 | 0 |
| Lean only, 6 oz, without bone | 400 | 18 | 0 |

**Extra Large Size:** *20 oz raw weight*
Approximately 16 oz cooked:

| | | | |
|---|---|---|---|
| Lean + Fat (¼"), 12 oz, without bone | 960 | 66 | 0 |
| Lean Only, 10 oz, without bone | 660 | 30 | 0 |

**Also See Fast-Foods & Restaurants Section ~**
*Lone Star Steakhouse; Outback Steakhouse*

### Beef – Individual Cuts  C  F  Cb

*Average All Grades*
Edible Weight, Without Bone

**Brisket, whole, braised:**

| | C | F | Cb |
|---|---|---|---|
| Lean + fat (¼" trim), 3 oz | 330 | 27 | 0 |
| Lean + marbling, 3 oz | 250 | 17 | 0 |
| Lean only, 3 oz | 185 | 9 | 0 |

**Chuck blade, braised:**

| | | | |
|---|---|---|---|
| Lean + fat (¼"), 3 oz | 310 | 24 | 0 |
| Lean + marbling, 3 oz | 295 | 22 | 0 |
| Lean only, 3 oz | 245 | 13 | 0 |

**Flank:** Raw, 4 oz

| | | | |
|---|---|---|---|
| Flank: Raw, 4 oz | 175 | 8 | 0 |
| Braised, 3 oz | 225 | 14 | 0 |
| Broiled, 3 oz | 155 | 6 | 0 |

**Round, bottom, braised:**

| | | | |
|---|---|---|---|
| Lean + marbling, 3 oz | 190 | 7.5 | 0 |
| Lean only, 3 oz | 185 | 6.5 | 0 |

**Round, eye/tip, rstd:**

| | | | |
|---|---|---|---|
| Lean + fat (¼"), 3 oz | 205 | 11 | 0 |
| Lean, w/ marbling, 3 oz | 150 | 5 | 0 |

**Round, top:** *Per 3 oz, Cooked Weight*

| | | | |
|---|---|---|---|
| Braised, Lean + fat | 210 | 10 | 0 |
| Lean only | 170 | 4 | 0 |
| Broiled, Lean + fat | 180 | 8 | 0 |
| Lean only | 160 | 5 | 0 |
| Pan-fried, Lean + fat | 235 | 13 | 0 |
| Lean only | 195 | 7 | 0 |

### Beef Ribs

**Back Ribs:** *7" long, visible fat trimmed to ¼"*
10.3 oz raw w/ bone or 3.5 oz cooked, braised, w/o bone

| | | | |
|---|---|---|---|
| 1 average rib | 410 | 34 | 0 |
| 3 ribs | 1230 | 102 | 0 |

**Short Ribs:** *2½" long, visible fat trimmed to ¼"*
6 oz raw with bone or 2.52 oz cooked, braised, w/o bone

| | | | |
|---|---|---|---|
| 1 average rib | 320 | 28 | 0 |
| 3 ribs | 960 | 85 | 0 |

### Ground Beef

**Ground Beef, Raw:** *Per 4 oz*

| | | | |
|---|---|---|---|
| 70% lean (30% fat) | 380 | 34 | 0 |
| 75% lean (25% fat) | 335 | 29 | 0 |
| 80% lean (20% fat) | 290 | 23 | 0 |
| 85% lean (15% fat) | 245 | 17 | 0 |
| 90% lean (10% fat) | 200 | 12 | 0 |
| 95% lean (5% fat) | 155 | 6 | 0 |

**Baked/Broiled:**

| | | | |
|---|---|---|---|
| Regular (70%), 3 oz | 230 | 16 | 0 |
| Lean (80%), 3 oz | 215 | 14 | 0 |
| Extra lean (90%), 3 oz | 185 | 10 | 0 |

**Pan-Broiled:**

| | | | |
|---|---|---|---|
| Regular (70%), 3 oz | 230 | 15 | 0 |
| Lean (80%), 3 oz | 210 | 14 | 0 |
| Extra lean (90%), 3 oz | 195 | 10 | 0 |

**Ground Beef Patties:** *Average, 23% Fat*

| | | | |
|---|---|---|---|
| Raw, 4 oz | 330 | 25 | 0 |
| Broiled, 3 oz (from 4 oz raw) | 250 | 19 | 0 |

### Quick Guide  C  F  Cb

**Roast Beef**
**Round (Eye/Tip, average):** *Average All Cuts*

**Small/Regular Serving:** *3 oz*
(2 thin slices/1 thick slice)

| | C | F | Cb |
|---|---|---|---|
| Lean + fat (⅛" fat trim) | 180 | 9 | 0 |
| Lean only | 145 | 5 | 0 |

**Medium Serving:** *5 oz*
(3-4 thin slices)

| | | | |
|---|---|---|---|
| Lean + fat (⅛" fat trim) | 300 | 15 | 0 |
| Lean only | 245 | 6.5 | 0 |

**Large Serving, 8 oz:** *3 thick slices*

| | | | |
|---|---|---|---|
| Lean + fat (⅛" fat trim) | 480 | 24 | 0 |
| Lean only | 385 | 11 | 0 |

### Roast Dinner Extras

**Gravy:**

| | C | F | Cb |
|---|---|---|---|
| Thin, 2 Tbsp | 20 | 0.5 | 3.5 |
| Thick, 2 Tbsp | 50 | 2 | 0.5 |
| 1 Ladle/4 Tbsp | 100 | 4 | 1 |

**Veggies:**

| | | | |
|---|---|---|---|
| Beans, green, ½ cup | 20 | 0 | 5 |
| Cauliflower with cheese sauce, 4 oz | 135 | 9 | 15 |
| Corn, kernels, ¼ cup | 35 | 0 | 9 |
| Carrots, ¼ cup | 20 | 0 | 3 |
| Peas, ¼ cup | 35 | 0 | 6 |

**Potato:**

| | | | |
|---|---|---|---|
| Baked in jacket: Plain, 1 large | 280 | 0 | 63 |
| With sour cream, 2 Tbsp | 270 | 5 | 64 |
| With whipped butter, 1 Tbsp | 350 | 8 | 63 |
| Roasted with fat, 1 small | 155 | 8 | 30 |

| | | | |
|---|---|---|---|
| **Sweet Potato/Yam,** 1 medium | 105 | 1 | 24 |
| **Yorkshire Pudding,** 1 oz | 90 | 3.5 | 11 |

**Beef Kebab:** *Cooked*

| | | | |
|---|---|---|---|
| Beef & Veggies, 2 oz | 160 | 10 | 4 |
| If very lean meat | 100 | 4 | 4 |

*"347 ~ 348 ~ 349…"*

## Lamb

**C · F · Cb**

**Choice Grade:**

**Leg (Whole), roasted:**
| | C | F | Cb |
|---|---|---|---|
| Lean + fat, 3 oz | 220 | 14 | 0 |
| Lean only, 3 oz | 160 | 7 | 0 |

**Leg (Sirloin Half), roasted:**
| | | | |
|---|---|---|---|
| Lean + fat, 3 oz | 250 | 18 | 0 |
| Lean only, 3 oz | 175 | 8 | 0 |

**Leg (Shank Half), roasted:**
| | | | |
|---|---|---|---|
| Lean + fat, 3 oz | 190 | 11 | 0 |
| Lean only, 3 oz | 155 | 6 | 0 |

**Loin Chop, broiled:**
1 chop (raw weight, 4.25 oz):
| | | | |
|---|---|---|---|
| Lean + fat (2.25 oz edible) | 180 | 12 | 0 |
| Lean only (1.6 oz edible) | 85 | 3.5 | 0 |

**Rib Chop, broiled:**
1 chop (raw wt., 3.5 oz):
| | | | |
|---|---|---|---|
| Lean + fat (2.5 oz edible) | 255 | 21 | 0 |
| Lean only (1.75 oz edible) | 105 | 6 | 0 |

**Shoulder (Arm/Blade):**
| | | | |
|---|---|---|---|
| Braised: Lean + fat, 3 oz | 295 | 21 | 0 |
| Lean only, 3 oz | 240 | 12 | 0 |
| Broiled: Lean + fat, 3 oz | 240 | 17 | 0 |
| Lean only, 3 oz | 170 | 8 | 0 |
| Roasted: Similar to Broiled | | | |

**Cubed Lamb (Leg/Shoulder):**
For stew or kebab:
| | | | |
|---|---|---|---|
| Braised, lean only, 3 oz | 190 | 8 | 0 |
| Broiled, lean only, 3 oz | 160 | 6 | 0 |

## Veal

**Edible Weights:**
**Leg (Top Round):**
| | | | |
|---|---|---|---|
| Braised: Lean + fat, 3 oz | 180 | 6 | 0 |
| Lean only, 3 oz | 175 | 5 | 0 |
| Pan-fried, breaded: | | | |
| Lean + fat, 3 oz | 195 | 8 | 9 |
| Lean only, 3 oz | 185 | 6 | 9 |
| Pan-fried, not breaded: | | | |
| Lean + fat, 3 oz | 180 | 7 | 0 |
| Lean only, 3 oz | 155 | 4 | 0 |
| Roasted: Lean + fat, 3 oz | 135 | 4 | 0 |
| Lean only, 3 oz | 130 | 3 | 0 |

## Veal (Cont)

**C · F · Cb**

**Loin Chop:** *1 chop, 7 oz raw weight*
| | C | F | Cb |
|---|---|---|---|
| Braised: Lean + fat, 3 oz | 240 | 15 | 0 |
| Lean only, 3 oz | 190 | 8 | 0 |
| Roasted: Lean + fat, 3 oz | 185 | 11 | 0 |
| Lean only, 3 oz | 150 | 6 | 0 |

**Rib, roasted:** *Lean + fat, 3 oz*
| | | | |
|---|---|---|---|
| | 195 | 12 | 0 |
| Lean only, 3 oz | 150 | 7 | 0 |

**Shoulder, Arm/Blade, roasted:**
| | | | |
|---|---|---|---|
| Lean + fat, 3 oz | 155 | 7 | 0 |
| Lean only, 3 oz | 140 | 5 | 0 |

**Sirloin, roasted:**
| | | | |
|---|---|---|---|
| Lean + fat, 3 oz | 170 | 9 | 0 |
| Lean only, 3 oz | 145 | 6 | 0 |

**Cubed for Stew, braised:**
| | | | |
|---|---|---|---|
| Leg/Shoulder, lean only, 3 oz | 160 | 4 | 0 |
| (1 lb raw yields approximately 9.25 oz cooked) | | | |

## Pork

**Fresh Pork:** *Cooked Weight, without bone):*
*4 oz raw weight = approx. 3 oz cooked weight*

**BBQ, Pulled:**
| | | | |
|---|---|---|---|
| 2 oz | 90 | 2.5 | 10 |
| 4 oz | 180 | 5 | 20 |
| 8oz | 360 | 10 | 40 |

**Blade Steak, broiled:**
| | | | |
|---|---|---|---|
| Lean + fat, 3 oz | 220 | 15 | 0 |
| Lean only, 3 oz | 190 | 11 | 0 |

**Country Style Ribs, broiled/roasted:**
| | | | |
|---|---|---|---|
| Lean + fat, 3 oz | 280 | 22 | 0 |
| Lean only, 3 oz | 210 | 13 | 0 |

**Spareribs, braised:** *Lean & fat, 6 oz*
| | | | |
|---|---|---|---|
| (from 1 lb raw weight) | 675 | 52 | 0 |

**Leg (Ham), whole, roasted:**
| | | | |
|---|---|---|---|
| Lean + fat, 3 oz | 230 | 15 | 0 |
| Lean only, 3 oz | 180 | 8 | 0 |

**Loin Chops, broiled:** *Average*
(From 1 chop: 5 oz raw weight with bone
or 4 oz raw weight, without bone)
| | | | |
|---|---|---|---|
| Lean + fat, 3 oz | 200 | 11 | 0 |
| Lean only, 3 oz | 165 | 7 | 0 |

**Loin Roast, roasted:**
| | | | |
|---|---|---|---|
| Lean + fat, 3 oz | 210 | 13 | 0 |
| Lean only, 3 oz | 180 | 8 | 0 |

**Rib Chops, (Boneless), broiled:**
| | | | |
|---|---|---|---|
| Lean + fat, 3 oz | 220 | 14 | 0 |
| Lean only, 3 oz | 185 | 9 | 0 |

**Rib Roast:**
| | | | |
|---|---|---|---|
| Lean + fat, 3 oz | 215 | 13 | 0 |
| Lean only, 3 oz | 180 | 9 | 0 |

## Pork (Cont)

| | C | F | Cb |
|---|---|---|---|
| **Sirloin Chop, broiled:** | | | |
| Lean + fat, 3 oz | 180 | 8 | 0 |
| Lean only, 3 oz | 165 | 6 | 0 |
| **Sirloin Roast, roasted:** | | | |
| Lean + fat, 3 oz | 175 | 8 | 0 |
| Lean only, 3 oz | 170 | 7 | 0 |
| **Tenderloin (Boneless), roasted:** | | | |
| Lean + fat, 3 oz | 125 | 4 | 0 |
| Lean only, 3 oz | 120 | 3 | 0 |
| **Ground Pork:** | | | |
| Raw, average, ¼ lb, 4 oz | 300 | 24 | 0 |
| Broiled, 3 oz | 250 | 18 | 0 |
| Pan-fried, drained, 3 oz | 260 | 19 | 0 |

### Bacon

| | C | F | Cb |
|---|---|---|---|
| **Raw:** 1 med. slice, 0.75 oz | 95 | 9 | 0 |
| 1 thick slice, 1.3 oz | 175 | 17 | 0 |
| (1 lb raw yields approximately 5 oz cooked) | | | |
| **Broiled/Pan-Fried:** | | | |
| 1 medium slice, 0.3 oz | 40 | 3 | 0 |
| 3 medium slices, 0.8 | 125 | 10 | 0 |
| 2 thin slices, 0.5 oz | 75 | 6 | 0 |
| 1 thick slice, 0.9 oz | 65 | 5 | 0 |
| **Canadian Bacon:** | | | |
| Cooked: 1 slice, 1 oz | 45 | 2 | 0.5 |
| 2 slices, 2 oz | 90 | 4 | 1 |
| **Bacon Bits,** 1 Tbsp, 0.3 oz | 35 | 2 | 0 |
| **Breakfast Strips,** Broiled, 1 sl., 0.4 oz | 50 | 4 | 0 |

### Ham

| | C | F | Cb |
|---|---|---|---|
| **Boneless Ham,** cooked: | | | |
| Regular, (approximately 13% fat): | | | |
| Roasted, 3 oz | 150 | 8 | 0 |
| Extra Lean (5% fat), | | | |
| Roasted, 3 oz | 125 | 5 | 0 |
| **Whole Ham,** cooked: | | | |
| Lean + fat (as purchased) | | | |
| Roasted, 3 oz | 210 | 15 | 0 |
| Lean only, Roasted, 3 oz | 135 | 5 | 0 |
| **Canned Ham:** *Similar to boneless ham* | | | |
| Chopped, canned, 3 oz | 200 | 16 | 0 |
| **Ham Patties,** cooked, (1), 2.3 oz | 220 | 20 | 1 |
| **Ham Steak,** extra lean, 2 oz | 70 | 2.5 | 0 |
| **Lunch Slices ~** *See Deli Meats, Page 128* | | | |

## Game & Other Meats

| | C | F | Cb |
|---|---|---|---|
| **Bison Steak,** | | | |
| lean, 6 oz (raw) | 205 | 4 | 0 |
| **Boar (wild),** roasted, 3 oz | 140 | 4 | 0 |
| **Buffalo Steak,** | | | |
| *New West Foods,* 4 oz | 70 | 3 | 0 |
| **Caribou,** roasted, 3 oz | 140 | 4 | 0 |
| **Deer/Venison,** roasted 3 oz | 135 | 3 | 0 |
| **Goat (Capretto):** | | | |
| Raw, 3 oz | 95 | 2 | 0 |
| Roasted, 3 oz | 120 | 2.5 | 0 |
| **Ostrich:** | | | |
| *Blackwing Ostrich Meats:* | | | |
| Sausage Patties (2) 2 oz | 60 | 0.5 | 0 |
| Sport Jerky, 0.5 oz piece | 25 | 0 | 0 |
| *New West Foods:* | | | |
| Ground Ostrich, 4 oz | 165 | 7 | 0 |
| Ostrich Steak, 4 oz steak | 130 | 2.5 | 0 |
| **Rabbit:** Roasted, 3 oz | 165 | 7 | 0 |
| Stewed, 1 cup, diced, 5 oz | 290 | 12 | 0 |

## Variety & Organ Meats

| | C | F | Cb |
|---|---|---|---|
| **Brain (Lamb):** Braised, 3 oz | 125 | 9 | 0 |
| Pan-fried, 3 oz | 230 | 19 | 0 |
| **Chitterlings,** pork, simmered, 3 oz | 260 | 25 | 0 |
| **Ears,** pork, simmered, 1 ear, 4 oz | 185 | 12 | 0 |
| **Feet,** Pork: Simmered, 3 oz | 200 | 14 | 0 |
| Cured, pickled, 3 oz | 170 | 14 | 0 |
| *Hormel,* 2 oz | 80 | 6 | 0 |
| **Head Cheese (Pork Snouts/Ears/Vinegar/Spices),** | | | |
| 1 oz slice | 50 | 4 | 0 |
| **Heart,** Beef, braised, 3 oz | 140 | 4 | 0 |
| **Jowl,** pork, raw, 4 oz | 750 | 80 | 0 |
| **Kidneys,** braised, 3 oz | 140 | 5 | 0 |
| **Liver (beef):** Raw, 4 oz | 150 | 4 | 4 |
| Braised, 3 oz | 140 | 4 | 3 |
| Pan-fried, 3 oz | 185 | 7 | 7 |
| **Pancreas,** pork, braised, 3 oz | 185 | 8 | 0 |
| **Pork Cracklins,** 0.5 oz | 80 | 6 | 0 |
| **Pork Hocks,** 1 piece, 6 oz | 340 | 23 | 0 |
| **Scrapple,** pork, 2 oz | 120 | 8 | 8 |
| **Spleen,** pork, braised, 3 oz | 130 | 3 | 0 |
| **Stomach,** pork, raw, 4 oz | 185 | 12 | 0 |
| **Sweetbreads:** | | | |
| Beef,/Lamb, cooked, 3 oz | 125 | 9 | 0 |
| **Tail,** pork, simmered, 3 oz | 340 | 31 | 0 |
| **Tongue:** Raised Veal, 3 oz | 170 | 9 | 0 |
| Beef/Lamb/Pork, av., 3 oz | 235 | 17 | 0 |
| **Tripe,** beef, raw, 3 oz | 85 | 3.5 | 0 |

## Quick Guide    C   F   Cb

### Franks & Weiners
*Average All Brands*

| | C | F | Cb |
|---|---|---|---|
| **Regular (Pork Mix):** *Per Frank* | | | |
| Regular, 1.5 oz | 140 | 13 | 1 |
| Bun Length/Jumbo, 2 oz | 185 | 17 | 2 |
| Extra Long, 2.75 oz | 255 | 24 | 2 |
| Small/Cocktail, each | 30 | 3 | 0.5 |
| **Beef Franks:** *Per Frank* | | | |
| Regular, 1.5 oz | 140 | 13 | 2 |
| Bun Length/Jumbo, 2 oz | 175 | 17 | 2.5 |
| ¼ lb Dog, 4 oz | 375 | 33 | 5 |

### Franks & Weiners

*Ball Park: Per 2 oz Frank Unless Indicated*

| | C | F | Cb |
|---|---|---|---|
| **Angus Beef:** | | | |
| Original; Bun Size, 2 oz | 170 | 15 | 3 |
| Lean, 1.8 oz | 70 | 5 | 2 |
| **Beef:** Original, Bun Size, 2 oz | 190 | 16 | 4 |
| Deli Style: Regular, 1.8 oz | 150 | 12 | 2 |
| BunSize, 1.8 oz | 150 | 12 | 2 |
| Park's Finest, Chili Beef, 2 oz | 180 | 15 | 4 |
| **Better For You,** Turkey, 2 oz | 110 | 7 | 6 |
| **Foster Farms,** Chicken; Turkey, 2 oz | 140 | 12 | 1 |
| **Hebrew National:** *Per Frank* | | | |
| Beef: Regular, 1.7 oz | 150 | 14 | 1 |
| ¼ Pounder, 4 oz | 360 | 33 | 3 |
| Jumbo, 3 oz | 270 | 25 | 2 |
| 97% Fat-Free, 1.6 oz | 40 | 1 | 3 |
| Beef Frank in a Blanket, 5 pcs, 3 oz | 300 | 24 | 12 |
| **Jennie-O:** *Per Frank* | | | |
| Turkey Franks: 1.2 oz | 70 | 6 | 1 |
| Jumbo, 2 oz | 120 | 10 | 2 |
| **Oscar Mayer:** *Per Frank* | | | |
| Beef: Classic, 1.6 oz | 140 | 13 | 0 |
| Lean, 1.8 oz | 60 | 3.5 | 1 |
| Turkey: Classic, 1.6 oz | 100 | 8 | 1 |
| Classic Bun Length, 2 oz | 120 | 10 | 3 |
| **Shelton's:** *Per Frank* | | | |
| Chicken, uncured, 1.2 oz | 80 | 7 | 1 |
| Turkey, Regular, 1.2 oz | 60 | 4.5 | 1 |
| **Zacky Farms,** Chkn; Turkey, av, 2 oz | 115 | 10 | 4 |

## Quick Guide    C   F   Cb

### Fresh Sausages
**Pork/Beef:** *Average All Types*

| | C | F | Cb |
|---|---|---|---|
| **Small:** Raw, 4" link, 1 oz | 85 | 7.5 | 0 |
| Broiled/Pan-fried | 80 | 7 | 0 |
| **Medium:** Raw, 2 oz | 170 | 15 | 0 |
| Broiled/Pan-fried | 165 | 14 | 0 |
| **Large:** Raw, 3 oz | 255 | 22 | 0 |
| Broiled/Pan-fried | 245 | 21 | 0 |
| **Italian:** Raw, 3.2 oz | 315 | 28 | 1 |
| Cooked, 2.4 oz | 230 | 18 | 3 |
| **Chorizo:** Beef Chorizo, 2.5 oz piece | 250 | 23 | 5 |
| Pork Chorizo, 2 oz piece | 250 | 23 | 5 |

**Note:** Fat is lost in broiling/pan frying.
Cooked weight = approx. 60-70% raw weight

### Smoked Sausages

*Per Link:*

| | C | F | Cb |
|---|---|---|---|
| **Butterball,** Turkey, 2 oz | 100 | 6 | 4 |
| **Eckrich:** | | | |
| **Grillers:** Original, 2 oz | 180 | 15 | 4 |
| Cheese | 190 | 17 | 1 |
| **Hillshire Farm:** | | | |
| Angus Beef, 2 oz | 170 | 15 | 3 |
| Cheddar Wurst, 2 oz | 180 | 16 | 2 |
| Chicken Hardwood, 2 oz | 100 | 7 | 3 |
| **Johnsonville** ~ *See CalorieKing.Com* | | | |

### Breakfast Sausages/Patties

| | C | F | Cb |
|---|---|---|---|
| **Butterball:** *Fully Cooked* | | | |
| Turkey: | | | |
| B'fast Sausage Links (3), 2.5 oz | 110 | 6 | 2 |
| Sausage Patties (2), 2.5 oz | 110 | 6 | 2 |
| **Jimmy Dean:** *Fully Cooked* | | | |
| **Heat 'N Serve Sausage Links:** | | | |
| Pork, Regular (3), 1.9 oz | 210 | 19 | 2 |
| Turkey (3), 2 oz | 130 | 8 | 2 |
| **Maple Pork Sausages,** (3), 2.4 oz | 260 | 22 | 3 |
| **Heat 'N Serve Sausage Patties:** | | | |
| Pork, Original (2), 1.8 oz | 200 | 17 | 2 |
| Turkey (2), 1.8 oz | 120 | 8 | 1 |
| **Maple Pork Patties,** (2), 2.4 oz | 260 | 22 | 3 |
| **Breakfast Sandwiches** ~ *See Page 92* | | | |
| **Jones Dairy Farm:** | | | |
| **All Natural Golden Brown Sausages:** *Fully Cooked* | | | |
| Mild Pork Sausages (3), 2 oz | 250 | 24 | 1 |
| Pork Sausage Patty (1),1.2 oz | 120 | 12 | 0 |
| **Vegetarian Patties:** | | | |
| Boca ~ *See Page 117* | | | |
| GardenBurer ~ *See Page 114* | | | |

## Bagel, Corn & Hot Dogs   **C** **F** **Cb**

### Hot Dogs, Ready-To-Go:
*Includes Ketchup/Relish*

| | C | F | Cb |
|---|---|---|---|
| **Regular,** 1.5 oz frank, 1.5 oz bun | 260 | 15 | 22 |
| **Bun Length,** 2 oz frank, 1.5 oz bun | 290 | 18 | 21 |
| **Jumbo Dog,** 2 oz frank, 2 oz bun | 360 | 20 | 36 |
| **¼ lb Beef Dog,** 2 oz bun | 480 | 15 | 36 |
| **Mile Long Dog,** 2.6 oz dog, 1.5 oz bun | 360 | 24 | 23 |

### Corn Dogs:
| | C | F | Cb |
|---|---|---|---|
| Beef/Pork Frank, average, 2.6 oz | 170 | 10 | 16 |

**Foster Farms:**
**Corn Dogs:**
| | C | F | Cb |
|---|---|---|---|
| Chili Cheese: (1), 2.7 oz | 180 | 9 | 19 |
| Honey Crunchy: | | | |
| Regular (1), 2.7 oz | 180 | 9 | 19 |
| Jumbo (1), 4 oz | 280 | 15 | 27 |
| Mini (4), 2.7 oz | 210 | 12 | 18 |

**State Fair:**
| | C | F | Cb |
|---|---|---|---|
| Beef Corn Dog (1), 2.7 oz | 230 | 11 | 26 |
| Classic Corn Dog (1), 2.7 oz | 190 | 8 | 23 |
| Fiesta (1), 2.7 oz | 180 | 9 | 19 |

### Bagel Dogs:
**Einstein Bros/Noah's:**
| | C | F | Cb |
|---|---|---|---|
| **N.Y. Bagels:** Asiago | 620 | 33 | 58 |
| Original | 610 | 32 | 57 |

**Vienna Beef:**
| | C | F | Cb |
|---|---|---|---|
| **Bageldog:** 5.5 oz | 400 | 1 | 64 |
| 6.5 oz | 470 | 18 | 56 |
| Mini (4), 3 oz | 220 | 13 | 16 |

### Hot Dog Toppings/Extras:
| | C | F | Cb |
|---|---|---|---|
| **American Cheese,** 1 slice, 1 oz | 110 | 9 | 1 |
| **Chili Con Carne,** ¼ cup | 50 | 2 | 5.5 |
| **Ketchup,** 1 Tbsp | 15 | 0 | 4 |
| **Mustard,** 1 Tbsp | 20 | 0 | 1 |
| **Onions,** chopped, 1 Tbsp | 5 | 0 | 1 |
| **Pickle Relish,** 1 Tbsp | 20 | 0 | 5 |
| **Sauerkraut,** ½ cup | 20 | 0 | 5 |

## Deli/Lunch Meats & Sausage

| | C | F | Cb |
|---|---|---|---|
| **Beef Jerky/Meat Snacks,** | | | |
| Berliner (pork/beef), 1 oz | 65 | 5 | 1 |
| **Beerwurst (Beef):** | | | |
| Small (2¾"diam), ¹⁄₁₆" slice | 20 | 2 | 0 |
| Large (4"diam), ⅛" slice | 75 | 7 | 0.5 |
| **Beerwurst (Pork):** | | | |
| Small (2.75"diameter), ¹⁄₁₆" slice | 15 | 1 | 0 |
| Large (4"diameter), ⅛" Slice | 55 | 4 | 0.5 |
| **Blood Sausage,** 1 oz | 100 | 9 | 0.5 |

## Deli/Lunch Meats & Sausages (Cont)

| | C | F | Cb |
|---|---|---|---|
| **Bologna:** | | | |
| Beef Bologna: 1 slice, 1 oz | 90 | 8 | 1 |
| Light, 1 slice, 1 oz | 60 | 4 | 2 |
| *Oscar Mayer:* Regular, 1 oz | 90 | 8 | 1 |
| 98% Fat Free, 1 oz | 25 | 0.5 | 3 |
| Light, 1 slice, 1 oz | 60 | 4 | 2 |
| *Boar's Head,* Ring, 2 oz | 150 | 13 | 1 |
| Pork Bologna: 1 Slice, 1 oz | 65 | 6 | 1 |
| Fat-Free, 1 slice, 1 oz | 20 | 0 | 2 |
| Turkey Bologna, average, 1 oz | 60 | 5 | 0.5 |
| **Bratwurst:** Average, 1 oz | 80 | 7 | 1 |
| *Bob Evan's,* Beer B'wurst, 2.2 oz link | 170 | 14 | 0 |
| **Braunschweiger,** (Pork/Liver/Sausage), | | | |
| *Oscar Mayer,* 2 oz slice | 190 | 17 | 1 |
| **Chicken,** average: | | | |
| 1 thick or 2 thin slices, 1 oz | 30 | 1 | 1 |
| 2 oz slice | 60 | 2 | 2 |
| *Hillshire Farm,* | | | |
| Rotiss. Seas'nd Chicken Breast, 2 oz | 50 | 0.5 | 2 |
| **Corned Beef,** average, full fat, 1 oz | 60 | 5 | 0.5 |
| **Ham, Sliced:** | | | |
| Baked/Broiled, 1 oz slice | 35 | 1 | 1 |
| *Oscar Mayer,* Baked, Lean, | | | |
| 3 slices, 2.3 oz | 80 | 2.5 | 1 |
| Honey/Brown Sugar, av., 1 oz | 35 | 1 | 1 |
| Prosciutto, average, 1 oz | 70 | 5 | 0 |
| **Ham & Cheese Loaf,** average, 1 oz | 70 | 5 | 1 |
| **Italian Sausage,** 2.6 oz | 250 | 20 | 3 |
| **Kielbasa:** Polish Sausage, 2 oz | 65 | 5 | 1 |
| Beef, 2 oz link | 190 | 17 | 1 |
| *Hillshire Farm,* | | | |
| Polska Kielbasa, 2 oz | 180 | 16 | 3 |
| **Knockwurst,** av., 1 oz | 90 | 8 | 0.5 |
| **Linguica** *(Gaspar's),* 2 oz | 130 | 9 | 1 |
| **Liverwurst,** 1 oz | 65 | 5 | 2 |
| **Liver Pate,** fresh, average, 1 oz | 90 | 8 | 1 |
| **Mortadella,** 1 oz | 105 | 9 | 0 |
| **Olive Loaf:** Average, 1 oz | 70 | 5 | 3 |
| *Oscar Mayer,* 1 oz | 80 | 6 | 3 |
| **Pancetta,** *Boars Head,* 1 slice | 50 | 4.5 | 0 |

## Deli/Lunch Meats & Sausages (Cont)

| | C | F | Cb |
|---|---|---|---|
| **Pastrami (Beef):** | | | |
| *Boar's Head:* | | | |
| 1st cut Brisket, 2 oz | 90 | 4 | 2 |
| Cap-Off Top Round, 2 oz | 80 | 3 | 1 |
| *Hillshire*, Deli Select, | | | |
| Ultra Thin, 7 slices., 2 oz | 60 | 1.5 | 1 |
| **Peppered Beef,** 1 oz slice | 40 | 2 | 1 |
| **Pepperoni,** 5 slices, 1 oz | 140 | 13 | 0 |
| **Pickle Loaf,** average, 1 oz | 70 | 5 | 5 |
| **Pickle & Pepper Loaf,** | | | |
| *Boars Head,* 2 oz | 150 | 13 | 2 |
| **Proscuitto/Proscuitti,** av., 1 oz | 70 | 5 | 1 |
| **Roast Beef,** Lean, 1 oz | 40 | 2 | 0 |
| **Salami:** Beef, av., 1 oz | 80 | 7 | 1 |
| *Oscar Mayer,* Hard, 1 slice, 1.8 oz | 100 | 8 | 1 |
| Beer Salami, average, 1 oz | 50 | 4 | 0.5 |
| *Oscar Mayer,* Cotto, 1 slice, 1 oz | 70 | 6 | 1 |
| Dry, Hard, average, 4 slices, 1 oz | 100 | 8 | 1 |
| Genoa: Average, 1 oz | 100 | 8 | 1 |
| Stick, 1.8 oz | 175 | 14 | 2 |
| *Bridgford,* Italian, 1 oz | 120 | 11 | 0 |
| **SPAM (Hormel):** *Per 2 oz* | | | |
| Classic: 2 oz serving | 180 | 16 | 1 |
| 7 oz can | 630 | 56 | 3.5 |
| 12 oz can | 1080 | 96 | 6 |
| Spam Lite: 2 oz | 110 | 8 | 1 |
| 12 oz can | 660 | 48 | 6 |
| **Other Spam Products:** *Per 2 oz* | | | |
| Hickory Smoked | 170 | 16 | 2 |
| Hot & Spicy | 180 | 16 | 2 |
| Oven Roasted Turkey | 80 | 4 | 2 |
| Spam Spresd | 140 | 12 | 0 |
| Spam with Bacon | 180 | 16 | 1 |
| Spam with Cheese | 170 | 15 | 2 |
| 25% Less Sodium | 180 | 16 | 1 |
| **Spam Singles:** *Per 3 oz* | | | |
| Classic, 3 oz package | 210 | 16 | 0 |
| Lite, 3 oz package | 160 | 11 | 2 |

## Deli/Lunch Meats & Sausages (Cont)

| | C | F | Cb |
|---|---|---|---|
| **Summer Sausage:** | | | |
| Armour, 2 oz | 190 | 17 | 2 |
| Hillshire Farm, 2 oz | 190 | 16 | 1 |
| **Treet** *(Armour),* Luncheon Loaf, | | | |
| Original, 2 oz | 140 | 11 | 4 |
| **Turkey**, average: 1 oz slice | 30 | 1 | 0.5 |
| 0.8 oz slice | 22 | 0.5 | 0.5 |
| **Turkey Breast:** | | | |
| *Butterball,* Oven Roasted: | | | |
| Thick Slice, 1 slice 1 oz | 30 | 0.5 | 2 |
| Deli Inspirations, | | | |
| Extra Thin Slices, 4 slices, 2 oz | 50 | 1 | 3 |
| *Hillshire,* Deli Select, | | | |
| Oven Roasted, 6 slices, 2 oz | 50 | 0.5 | 2 |
| **Turkey Ham,** 1 slice, 1 oz | 35 | 1.5 | 0.5 |
| **Turkey Loaf,** 1 oz | 30 | 1 | 0.5 |
| **Turkey Pastrami,** 1 oz | 35 | 1.5 | 1 |
| **Turkey Roll,** 1 oz | 40 | 2 | 0.5 |
| **Vegetarian Deli** ~ See Page 118 | | | |

### Meat Spreads

**Average All Brands:** *Per 2 oz*

| | C | F | Cb |
|---|---|---|---|
| Chicken, white meat | 130 | 10 | 2 |
| Ham, Deviled | 140 | 11 | 0 |
| Liverwurst | 190 | 16 | 2 |
| Roast Beef | 130 | 10 | 2 |
| Sandwich Spread | 140 | 10 | 9 |
| Turkey | 110 | 7 | 2 |
| **Underwood:** *Per 2 oz* | | | |
| Chicken, White Meat | 140 | 11 | 2 |
| Deviled Ham | 180 | 15 | 1 |
| Liverwurst | 160 | 13 | 4 |
| Roast Beef | 130 | 10 | 2 |

### Paté

**Les Trois Petit Cochons:** *Per 2 oz*

| | C | F | Cb |
|---|---|---|---|
| **Pate:** de Campagne 2 oz | 240 | 22 | 2 |
| de Canard a l'Orange; Forestier, 2 oz | 210 | 18 | 3 |
| Paysan, 2 oz | 150 | 12 | 2 |
| Rustique, 2 oz | 240 | 22 | 2 |
| Venison, 2 oz | 200 | 16 | 4 |
| Wild Boar, 2 oz | 180 | 15 | 4 |
| **Old Wisconsin Pate,** | | | |
| Braunschweiger, 2 oz | 210 | 18 | 3 |

**Nuts**

*Per 1 oz Unless Indicated*

| | C | F | Cb |
|---|---|---|---|
| **Acorns,** raw 1 oz | 110 | 7 | 12 |
| **Almonds:** Dried/Dry Roasted: | | | |
| Whole: 12 medium size, 0.5 oz | 85 | 7.5 | 3 |
| 23-25 medium size, 1 oz | 170 | 15 | 6 |
| ½ cup, 2.5 oz | 420 | 37 | 13 |
| Ground, 1 cup, 3.4 oz | 545 | 47 | 20 |
| Sliced, ½ cup, 1.6 oz | 260 | 22 | 10 |
| Slivered, ½ cup, 2 oz | 310 | 27 | 12 |
| Chocolate Coated (5-6), 1 oz | 150 | 10 | 15 |
| Honey Roasted, 1 oz | 170 | 14 | 8 |
| Oil Roasted (*Blue Diamond*), 1 oz | 170 | 16 | 5 |
| **Brazil Nuts,** 8 medium, 1 oz | 185 | 19 | 3.5 |
| **Cashews,** dry or oil roasted: | | | |
| 14 large/18 med./26 small: 1 oz | 165 | 14 | 9 |
| ½ cup, 2.4 oz | 375 | 31 | 20 |
| Honey Roasted, 1 oz | 165 | 13 | 10 |
| **Chestnuts:** | | | |
| Average, dried, 1 oz | 105 | 1 | 22 |
| Raw/Fresh, 5-6 nuts, 1 oz | 60 | 0 | 13 |
| Canned, water chestnuts, | | | |
| sliced/whole/drained, 1 oz | 30 | 0 | 7 |
| **Coconut, Fresh:** | | | |
| 1 piece, 2″x2″x ½″, 1 oz | 185 | 18 | 7 |
| Shredded, fresh, ½ cup, 1.4 oz | 140 | 13 | 6 |
| Dried (Desiccated): | | | |
| Sweetened: Shredded, 1 oz | 145 | 10 | 14 |
| Grated, ½ cup, 1.3 oz | 185 | 13 | 18 |
| Unsweetened, 1 oz | 185 | 18 | 7 |
| Cream (canned), ½ cup, 5.2 oz | 285 | 26 | 12 |
| Milk (canned), unsweetened, | | | |
| ¼ cup, 2 fl.oz | 100 | 10 | 3 |
| Water (center liquid), ½ cup, 4.3 oz | 25 | 0 | 4.5 |
| **Filberts or Hazelnuts:** | | | |
| Shelled, 18-20 nuts | 180 | 17 | 4.5 |
| Chopped, ¼ cup, 1 oz | 180 | 18 | 5 |
| Ground, ¼ cup, 0.6 oz | 120 | 12 | 3 |
| **Ginkgo Nuts,** canned, 14 med., 1 oz | 32 | 0.5 | 6.5 |
| **Hickory,** | | | |
| 30 small nuts, 1 oz | 200 | 18 | 5 |
| **Macadamia Nuts,** Shelled: | | | |
| Raw or Dry Roasted, avg: | | | |
| 12 small or 8 med., 1 oz | 200 | 21 | 4 |
| 6-7 large, 1 oz | 200 | 21 | 4 |
| ½ cup, 2.3 oz | 480 | 51 | 10 |
| **Mixed Nuts:** Raw, 18-22 nuts, 1 oz | 170 | 15 | 7 |
| Oil Roasted, all types | 170 | 16 | 6 |
| Sweet Roasts, 26 pieces, 1 oz | 160 | 12 | 10 |
| *Planters*, Dry Roasted/Honey | 160 | 12 | 9 |
| **Nut Toppings,** chopped, 1 Tbsp, 0.3 oz | 40 | 4 | 1.5 |

*Per 1 oz Unless Indicated*

| | C | F | Cb |
|---|---|---|---|
| **Peanuts,** dry or oil roasted, average: | | | |
| Small handful, 0.5 oz | 85 | 7 | 3 |
| ⅕ cup, 1 oz | 165 | 14 | 6 |
| ½ cup, 2.5 oz | 415 | 35 | 15 |
| 3 oz bag | 500 | 42 | 18 |
| 7 oz bag | 1160 | 98 | 42 |
| *Planters:* | | | |
| Cocktail, all varieties | 170 | 14 | 5 |
| Honey Roasted | 160 | 13 | 7 |
| Spanish Redskins | 170 | 15 | 4 |
| Sweet N' Crunchy | 140 | 8 | 15 |
| Japanese Style Peanuts, | | | |
| Coated in Crunchy Shell | 150 | 8 | 13 |
| Raw: Shelled, 1 oz | 160 | 14 | 4.5 |
| In shell, 1 oz | 115 | 110 | 3 |
| **Pecans,** roasted: | | | |
| 10 halves, 0.5 oz | 95 | 10 | 2 |
| 20 Halves, 1 oz | 195 | 20 | 4 |
| 1 cup, halves, 3.5 oz | 680 | 71 | 14 |
| **Pilinuts,** dried, 1 oz | 215 | 24 | 1 |
| **Pine Nuts,** | | | |
| dried, 1 Tbsp, 0.3 oz | 70 | 7 | 1.5 |
| **Pistachios,** raw: | | | |
| Shelled, 45 nuts, 1 oz | 160 | 13 | 8 |
| Unshelled, 2 oz | 165 | 14 | 7 |
| *Lance*, Roasted, 1.5 oz | 120 | 9 | 6 |
| **Sesame Nut Mix,** 1 oz | 160 | 13 | 9 |
| **Soy Nuts:** Dry Roasted | 130 | 6 | 9 |
| ½ cup, 3 oz | 390 | 18 | 28 |
| *Dr Soy*, Chocolate coated, 1 oz pkg | 140 | 7 | 13 |
| **Trail Mix** *(Planters):* | | | |
| Daybreak, Berry Almond, 1.5 oz | 180 | 7 | 27 |
| Energy Mix, 1.5 oz | 250 | 20 | 14 |
| Fruit & Nut | 140 | 9 | 14 |
| Nut & Chocolate, 1.3oz | 150 | 9 | 14 |
| Nuts, Seeds & Raisins, 1 oz | 160 | 11 | 11 |
| Spicy Nuts & Cajun Sticks | 150 | 11 | 10 |
| Sweet & Nutty, 1 oz | 150 | 9 | 13 |
| **Walnuts,** average all types: | | | |
| 7-10 halves, 0.5 oz | 90 | 9 | 2 |
| 15-20 halves, 1 oz | 175 | 17 | 3 |
| Chopped, ½ cup, 2.2 oz | 380 | 36 | 6 |
| Ground, ¼ cup, 0.7 oz | 130 | 13 | 3 |

## Quick Guide | C | F | Cb

**Peanut Butter:** *Average All Brands*

| | C | F | Cb |
|---|---|---|---|
| 1 level tsp, 0.2 oz | 35 | 3 | 1 |
| 1 level Tbsp, 0.6 oz | 100 | 8.5 | 3.5 |
| 1 oz Quantity | 165 | 14 | 6 |
| ½ cup, 5 oz | 835 | 72 | 29 |

## Peanut Butter ~ Brands

| | C | F | Cb |
|---|---|---|---|
| **Jif:** Regular, all varieties, 2 Tbsp | 190 | 16 | 8 |
| Natural, average all varieties, 2 Tbsp | 190 | 16 | 9 |
| Reduced Fat, all varieties, 2 Tbsp | 190 | 12 | 15 |
| To Go: Crmy/Crunch, 1.5 oz cup | 250 | 22 | 11 |
| Reduced Fat, 1.7 oz cup | 250 | 16 | 20 |
| Whipped: Creamy, 2 Tbsp | 140 | 12 | 6 |
| Chocolate flavored, 2 Tbsp | 150 | 11 | 11 |
| **Laura Scudder's**, Natural, Smooth; Nutty, 2 Tbsp | 200 | 16 | 6 |
| **Peanut Wonder**, Original, 2 Tbsp | 100 | 2 | 13 |
| **Peter Pan:** | | | |
| **Natural**, Creamy/Crunchy, 2 Tbsp | 210 | 17 | 6 |
| **Creamy/Crunchy**, Red.-Fat, 2 Tbsp | 200 | 13 | 14 |
| **Creamy**, Whipped, 2 Tbsp | 150 | 12 | 5 |
| **Planters**, Creamy/Crunchy, 2 Tbsp | 180 | 15 | 8 |
| **Smucker's**, Goober, Grape/Srawberry, 3 Tbsp. 2 oz | 240 | 13 | 24 |
| **Skippy:** Natural, Creamy/Chunky, 2 T. | 190 | 16 | 6 |
| Reduced Fat, all varieties, 2 Tbsp | 180 | 12 | 15 |
| Dark Chocolate Spread, 2 Tbsp | 200 | 14 | 12 |

## Peanut Butter & Jelly Sandwich

**1 sandwich:** *With 2 oz Bread*

| | C | F | Cb |
|---|---|---|---|
| Thin Spread, 1 Tbsp Peanut Butter + 1 Tbsp Jelly | 310 | 10 | 48 |
| Thick Spread, 2 Tbsp Peanut Butter + 2 Tbsp Jelly | 480 | 19 | 67 |

## Nut & Chocolate Spread

**Nutella:**

| | C | F | Cb |
|---|---|---|---|
| 1 Tbsp, 0.7 oz | 110 | 6 | 11 |
| 2 Tbsp, 1.3 oz | 200 | 11 | 22 |

Note: Nutella contains approx. 50% sugar & 13% hazelnuts

## Other Nut & Seed Butters

*Per 1 Tbsp, 0.5 oz*

| | C | F | Cb |
|---|---|---|---|
| Almond Butter | 100 | 10 | 3.5 |
| Cashew Butter | 95 | 8 | 4.5 |
| Hazelnut Butter; Pecan Butter | 110 | 10 | 2 |
| Pistachio Butter | 90 | 6.5 | 4.5 |
| Sesame Butter (Tahini) | 90 | 8 | 3 |
| Soy Nut Butter | 75 | 5 | 4 |

## Seeds | C | F | Cb

| | C | F | Cb |
|---|---|---|---|
| **Alfalfa Seeds,** sprouted, ½ cup, 0.5 oz | 5 | 0 | 1 |
| **Caraway/Fennel,** 1 tsp | 7 | 0.5 | 1 |
| **Chia Seeds:** 1 Tbsp, 0.4 oz | 45 | 3 | 4 |
| 3 Tbsp, 1 oz | 140 | 8.5 | 12 |
| **Cottonseed Kernels,** roasted, 1 Tbsp | 50 | 3.5 | 2 |
| **Flax Seeds,** 3 Tbsp, 1 oz | 140 | 9 | 9 |
| **Lotus Seeds,** dried, ½ cup, 0.5 oz | 55 | 0.5 | 10 |
| **Poppy Seeds,** 1 tsp | 15 | 1 | 1 |
| **Pumpkin/Pepita Seeds,** whole: | | | |
| Roasted/Tamari: 1 oz | 150 | 12 | 4 |
| ½ cup, 4 oz | 590 | 48 | 15 |
| Dried (hulled), ¼ cup, 1 oz | 155 | 13 | 5 |
| **Safflower Kernels,** dried, 1 oz | 150 | 11 | 10 |
| **Sesame Seeds:** | | | |
| Dried, 1 Tbsp, 0.3 oz | 50 | 4.5 | 2 |
| Roasted/Toasted, 1 oz | 160 | 14 | 7.5 |
| **Sunflower Kernels/Seeds:** | | | |
| Dried, ¼ cup w/out hulls, 0.3 oz | 200 | 18 | 7 |
| Dry Roasted: 1 Tbsp, 0.3 oz | 45 | 4 | 2 |
| ¼ cup, 1 oz | 165 | 14 | 7 |
| Oil Roasted, ⅕ cup, 1 oz | 170 | 14 | 6.5 |
| **Watermelon Seeds,** dried, ¼ cup, 1 oz | 150 | 13 | 4 |

*N*ut eaters are healthier and live longer, say scientists.

Nuts are a nutritious source of protein, vitamins, minerals, fiber, healthy fats, and antioxidants.

The fat and fiber of nuts can help reduce blood cholesterol. Their protein and fiber also promotes meal satiety (fullness) and reduces hunger levels – of benefit in weight control.

Eat nuts instead of high-sugar snacks, candy and soft drinks. Add chopped nuts to breakfast cereals.

# P Pancakes & Waffles

## Quick Guide  **C** **F** **Cb**

### Pancakes:
**Plain:** *Average All Types*

| | C | F | Cb |
|---|---|---|---|
| Small (3" diameter), 0.8 oz | 50 | 2 | 6 |
| Medium (4" diameter), 1.3 oz | 85 | 3.5 | 11 |
| Large (6" diameter), 2.5 oz | 175 | 7.5 | 22 |

*Add Extra for Syrups/Butter*

| | C | F | Cb |
|---|---|---|---|
| **Pancake Syrup:** Regular, 1 Tbsp | 50 | 0 | 12 |
| ¼ cup, 4 Tbsp | 185 | 0 | 49 |
| Lite, 1 Tbsp | 25 | 0 | 6.5 |
| ¼ cup, 4 Tbsp | 100 | 0 | 27 |
| **Butter/Margarine:** | | | |
| Regular, 1 Tbsp | 100 | 11 | 0 |
| Whipped, 1 Tbsp | 65 | 7.5 | 0 |

### Waffles:

| | C | F | Cb |
|---|---|---|---|
| **Homemade,** 7" waffle, 2.5 oz | 220 | 11 | 25 |
| **Frozen + Toasted,** (4" diam.), 1 oz | 105 | 3 | 16 |

## Pancake Brands

*Prepared As Directed*
**Aunt Jemima:** *Prepared*
**Mixes:** *Per 4" Pancake*

| | C | F | Cb |
|---|---|---|---|
| Original (4) | 250 | 8 | 36 |
| Original Complete (2) | 160 | 1.5 | 32 |
| Buttermilk (4) | 160 | 3 | 27 |
| Whole Wheat Blend (3) | 200 | 6.5 | 30 |

**Bisquick:** *Prepared*
**Pancake/Waffle Mix:**

| | C | F | Cb |
|---|---|---|---|
| Complete, Simply Buttermilk, with Whole Grain (3) | 210 | 4 | 39 |
| Shake 'n Pour, Buttermilk (3) | 220 | 3 | 43 |

**Hungry Jack:**
**Pancake & Waffle Mixes:** *Per 4" Pancake*
Complete Mixes: Just Add Water

| | C | F | Cb |
|---|---|---|---|
| Blueberry Wheat, 1.9 oz | 190 | 2 | 39 |
| Chocolate Chip, 1.9 oz | 190 | 2.5 | 39 |
| Cinnamon spice, 1.9 oz | 190 | 1 | 41 |

**Easy Packs:** *Dry Mix Only*

| | C | F | Cb |
|---|---|---|---|
| Blueberry Wheat, 1.9 oz | 190 | 2 | 39 |
| Buttermilk, 1.6 oz | 150 | 1.5 | 31 |

**Traditional:** *Dry Mix Only*

| | C | F | Cb |
|---|---|---|---|
| Original, 1.7 oz | 160 | 1 | 34 |
| Buttermilk, 1.7 oz | 160 | 1 | 34 |
| Extra Light & Fluffy, 1.6 oz | 150 | 1 | 32 |

**Northern Pines,**

| | C | F | Cb |
|---|---|---|---|
| Premium Mix (3), 4", 3.5 oz, prep'd | 200 | 3.5 | 38 |

## Frozen Breakfasts  **C** **F** **Cb**

**Aunt Jemima:**

| | C | F | Cb |
|---|---|---|---|
| **French Toast:** Cinnamon, 2 slices | 210 | 4 | 35 |
| Homestyle, 2 slices | 210 | 4 | 34 |
| Sticks, Cinnamon (4) | 260 | 2.5 | 39 |
| **Pancakes:** Blueberry (3) | 260 | 6 | 45 |
| Buttermilk (3) | 250 | 6 | 41 |
| Low-Fat (3) | 210 | 2 | 42 |
| Homestyle (3) | 240 | 6 | 41 |
| Mini Pancakes (10) | 280 | 8 | 45 |

**Eggo** *(Kellogg's)*:

| | C | F | Cb |
|---|---|---|---|
| **French Toaster Sticks,** (2), average | 225 | 6 | 37 |
| **Pancakes:** Blueberry (3) | 260 | 8 | 42 |
| Buttermilk (3) | 280 | 9 | 45 |

**Krusteaz:**

| | C | F | Cb |
|---|---|---|---|
| **French Toast,** Cinnamon Swirl, Regular Cut, 3 slices | 320 | 7 | 53 |
| **Pancakes:** | | | |
| Blueberry (3) | 290 | 4 | 55 |
| Buttermilk (3) | 290 | 3.5 | 57 |

**Pillsbury:**

| | C | F | Cb |
|---|---|---|---|
| **Pancakes:** | | | |
| Buttermilk (3) | 230 | 4 | 45 |
| Mini Buttermilk (11) | 230 | 4 | 45 |

## Frozen Waffles

| | C | F | Cb |
|---|---|---|---|
| **Aunt Jemima:** Buttermilk (2) | 190 | 5 | 29 |
| Homestyle (2) | 170 | 5 | 28 |

**Eggo** *(Kellogg's)*:

| | C | F | Cb |
|---|---|---|---|
| Blueberry (2) | 180 | 6 | 29 |
| Chocolatey Chip (2) | 200 | 7 | 31 |
| Homestyle (2) | 190 | 7 | 27 |
| Nutri-Grain: | | | |
| Blueberry (2) | 180 | 6 | 30 |
| Whole Wheat (2) | 170 | 6 | 27 |

| | C | F | Cb |
|---|---|---|---|
| **Kashi,** all varieties (2) | 150 | 5 | 25 |

**Nature's Path:**

| | C | F | Cb |
|---|---|---|---|
| Ancient Grains; Maple Cinn., av, (2) | 180 | 6 | 29 |
| Buckwheat Wildberry (2) | 190 | 7 | 33 |
| Chia Plus; Homestyle, (2) | 210 | 7 | 34 |
| Flax Plus (2) | 200 | 8 | 30 |
| **Van's:** 8 Whole Grains, Berry (2) | 170 | 6 | 27 |
| Belgian, Homestyle (2) | 250 | 10 | 37 |
| **Wheat Gluten Free,** Apple Cinnamon (2) | 200 | 6 | 35 |
| **Mini,** Chocolate Chip (8) | 160 | 5 | 29 |

### Spaghetti/Pasta **C** **F** **Cb**

- Pasta includes all shapes and sizes; (e.g. spaghetti, fettuccini, elbows, shells, twists, sheets, cannelloni, linguini, tubes, ziti).
- All regular pasta products have the same cals/fat/carbs on a weight basis.
- 1 oz Dry = approximately 2.5 -3 oz cooked.

### Dry Spaghetti/Pasta

| | C | F | Cb |
|---|---|---|---|
| **1 oz quantity** | 105 | 0.5 | 21 |
| **1lb box/pkg,** 16 oz | 1685 | 7 | 339 |
| **Elbows,** 1 cup, 4 oz | 380 | 2 | 80 |
| **Shells,** small, 1 cup, 3.3 oz | 330 | 1.5 | 69 |
| **Spirals,** 1 cup, 3 oz | 305 | 1.5 | 64 |

### Cooked Spaghetti/Pasta

**Plain, All Types (no added fat):**

| | C | F | Cb |
|---|---|---|---|
| Firm/Al Dente (8-10 minutes), 1 oz | 42 | 0.5 | 8.5 |
| Medium (11-13 minutes), 1 oz | 37 | 0.5 | 7.5 |
| Tender (14-20 minutes), 1 oz | 32 | 0.5 | 7 |

Longer cooking increases water absorbed

| | C | F | Cb |
|---|---|---|---|
| **Spaghetti:** ½ cup, 2.5 oz | 90 | 0.5 | 18 |
| Medium serving, 1 cup, 5 oz | 225 | 1.5 | 44 |
| Large serving, 2 cups, 10 oz | 450 | 3 | 88 |
| Extra large, 3 cups, 15 oz | 675 | 5 | 132 |
| **Elbows/Spirals,** 1 cup, 5 oz | 220 | 1.5 | 43 |
| **Small Shells,** 1 cup, 4 oz | 180 | 1 | 36 |
| **Protein-fortified:** Dry, 1 c., 3.4 oz | 350 | 2 | 63 |
| Cooked, 1 cup, 5 oz | 230 | 0.5 | 45 |
| **Spinach/Vegetable:** Dry, 1 cup, 3 oz | 310 | 1 | 61 |
| Cooked, 1 cup, 5 oz | 180 | 0.5 | 38 |
| **Whole-wheat:** Dry, 1 cup, 3.8 oz | 365 | 1.5 | 79 |
| Cooked, 1 cup, 5 oz | 175 | 1 | 37 |

### Fresh Pasta (Refrigerated)

*Average All Brands:*

**Plain/Spinach/Tomato:**

| | C | F | Cb |
|---|---|---|---|
| As purchased, 4.5 oz | 370 | 3 | 70 |
| Cooked, 1 cup, 5 oz | 185 | 1.5 | 35 |
| **Home-made,** w/o egg, cooked, 1 c. 5 oz | 175 | 1 | 35 |

**Buitoni:**

**Cut Pasta:**

| | C | F | Cb |
|---|---|---|---|
| Angel Hair, 3 oz | 230 | 2 | 43 |
| Fettuccine/Linguine, 3 oz | 240 | 2 | 45 |

**House Foods:**

**Tofu Shirataki Noodles:**

| | C | F | Cb |
|---|---|---|---|
| Traditional, 1.6 oz | 0 | 0 | 1 |
| Angel Hair/Fettuccini, | | | |
| Macaroni/Spaghetti, 4 oz | 15 | 0.5 | 3 |

**Nasoya,**

| | C | F | Cb |
|---|---|---|---|
| Shirataki Spaghetti, | | | |
| Pasta Zero, ⅔ cup, 4 oz | 20 | 0 | 4 |

---

**Buitoni:** *Per 1 Cup Unless Indicated* **C** **F** **Cb**

| | C | F | Cb |
|---|---|---|---|
| **Agnolotti:** Butternut Squash, 3.7 oz | 300 | 12 | 37 |
| Wild Mushroom, 3.8 oz | 280 | 10 | 34 |
| **Ravioli:** Beef & Sausage, 3.8 oz | 260 | 8 | 33 |
| Chicken Marsala, 3.9 oz | 280 | 8 | 36 |
| Light 4-Cheese, 1¼ cups, 3.3 oz | 260 | 6 | 39 |
| **Tortellini:** Herb Chicken, 3.9 oz | 330 | 8 | 52 |
| Mixed Cheese, 3.7 oz | 320 | 8 | 48 |
| **Tortelloni:** Italian Sausage, 4 oz | 350 | 10 | 51 |
| Spinach & Ricotta, 3.7 oz | 270 | 7 | 39 |

**Other Varieties ~** *See Page 112*
**Pasta Sauces ~** *See Page 144*

### Macaroni & Cheese

**Packaged (Kraft) ~** *See Page 116*
**Restaurant:** *Average*

| | C | F | Cb |
|---|---|---|---|
| Side Serve, 6 oz | 265 | 13 | 26 |
| Medium serve, 1 cup, 9 oz | 350 | 17 | 34 |
| Large serve, 2 cups, 18 oz | 700 | 34 | 68 |

### Noodles

| | C | F | Cb |
|---|---|---|---|
| **Plain/Egg:** Dry, 1 oz | 110 | 1.5 | 20 |
| 1 cup, 1.4 oz | 145 | 1.5 | 27 |
| **Cooked:** 1 oz | 40 | 0.5 | 7 |
| ½ cup, 2.8 oz | 110 | 1.5 | 20 |
| 1 cup, 5.5 oz | 220 | 3.5 | 40 |
| **Stir-Fried:** 1 cup, 5.5 oz | 270 | 9 | 40 |
| 2 cup serving, 11 oz | 540 | 18 | 80 |
| **Low Carb Noodles,** | | | |
| *Quest Pasta,* 4 oz | 10 | 0 | 3 |

*Note: Carbs are from glucomannan fiber*

**Yolk Free (Cooked):**

| | C | F | Cb |
|---|---|---|---|
| *Manischewitz,* Yolk Free, 2 oz | 200 | 1 | 41 |
| **Chinese:** Cellophane/Rice, dry, 1 oz | 100 | 0 | 25 |
| Chow Mein/hard, dry, 1 oz | 150 | 9 | 16 |
| **Japanese:** Soba: Dry, 1 oz | 95 | 0.5 | 21 |
| Cooked, 1 cup, 4 oz | 115 | 0.5 | 24 |
| Somen: Dry, 1 oz | 100 | 0.5 | 21 |
| Cooked, 1 cup, 6 oz | 230 | 0.5 | 49 |
| **Japanese Style Pan Fried,** | | | |
| Yaki-Soba (*Maruchan's*), av., 5.6 oz | 260 | 3 | 50 |

**Ramen Noodles ~** *See Page 117*

| | C | F | Cb |
|---|---|---|---|
| **Rice Noodles:** Dry, 3.5 oz | 365 | 0.5 | 83 |
| Cooked, 1 cup, 6.2 oz | 190 | 0.5 | 44 |
| *Yakisoba,* Stir Fry, 3.5 oz | 430 | 6 | 52 |
| *House Foods,* Tofu Shirataki, 4 oz | 20 | 0.5 | 3 |
| *Chikara,* Udon, average, 7.5 oz pkt | 250 | 1 | 52 |

*Simply Asia/Thai Kitchen ~ See Pages 119 & 121*

### Egg Roll/Won Ton Wrappers

| | C | F | Cb |
|---|---|---|---|
| Egg/Spring Roll (1), 0.8 oz | 65 | 0 | 15 |
| Won Ton Wrapper (1), 0.3 oz | 20 | 0 | 4 |

---

## Quick Guide    C   F   Cb

**Fruit Pies:** *Average All Brands, 9"*
**Apple; Blueberry; Cherry:**

| | C | F | Cb |
|---|---|---|---|
| Small Serving, | | | |
| ⅛ pie, 4.8 oz | 350 | 16 | 49 |
| Medium Serving, | | | |
| ⅙ pie, 6.5 oz | 465 | 22 | 65 |
| Large Serving | | | |
| ¼ pie, 9.5 oz | 700 | 33 | 98 |
| Whole Pie (9"), 38 oz | 2800 | 131 | 392 |

**Other Pies:** *Per Serving, ⅙ of 8" Pie*

| | C | F | Cb |
|---|---|---|---|
| Chocolate Cream Pie | 345 | 22 | 38 |
| Custard: Egg | 220 | 12 | 22 |
| Coconut | 330 | 18 | 35 |
| Lemon Meringue | 305 | 10 | 53 |
| Peach | 260 | 12 | 39 |
| Pecan | 440 | 23 | 57 |
| Pumpkin Pie | 315 | 14 | 41 |

## Dessert/Fruit Pies ~ Brands

| | C | F | Cb |
|---|---|---|---|
| **Hostess:** | | | |
| Cherry Pie, 4.5 oz | 480 | 20 | 69 |
| Lemon Pie, 4.5 oz | 490 | 22 | 69 |
| **Marie Callender's:** | | | |
| Almond Glazed Cherry, ⅒ pie, 4.3 oz | 370 | 17 | 53 |
| Banana Cream, ⅑ pie, 4.2 oz | 310 | 17 | 37 |
| Peach, w/ Crmy Glaze, ⅒ pie, 4.2 oz | 360 | 16 | 50 |
| **Mrs Smith's:** | | | |
| **Original Flaky Crust:** *Per ⅛ Pie, 4.6 oz* | | | |
| Apple | 340 | 17 | 45 |
| Cherry | 350 | 17 | 47 |
| Peach | 340 | 19 | 41 |
| Pumpkin | 300 | 13 | 42 |
| Sweet Potato | 330 | 13 | 48 |
| Very Berry | 340 | 17 | 44 |
| **Sara Lee:** | | | |
| **Creme Pies:** | | | |
| Chocolate, ⅕ pie, 3.9 oz | 450 | 27 | 50 |
| Coconut, ⅙ pie, 4.5 oz | 370 | 20 | 44 |
| Key Lime, ⅕ pie | 410 | 17 | 60 |
| Lemon Meringue, ⅕ pie, 4.6 oz | 390 | 13 | 64 |
| **Oven Fresh Pies:** *Per 9" Pie, 4.6 oz Slice* | | | |
| Apple | 340 | 16 | 43 |
| Cherry | 340 | 17 | 44 |
| Peach | 320 | 15 | 42 |
| **Seasonal:** Pumpkin, 4.6 oz | 270 | 10 | 41 |
| Sthrn Sweet Potato, 4.6 oz | 280 | 9 | 46 |
| **Tastykake:** Apple | 270 | 11 | 41 |
| Lemon | 300 | 14 | 44 |

## Croissants    C   F   Cb

**Average all Brands**

| | C | F | Cb |
|---|---|---|---|
| **Plain/Butter/Cheese:** Mini, 1 oz | 115 | 6 | 13 |
| Small, 1.5 oz | 170 | 9 | 19 |
| Medium, 2 oz | 230 | 12 | 26 |
| Large, 2.5 oz | 290 | 15 | 32 |
| **Sweet Croissants:** | | | |
| Almond Filled, 3 oz | 330 | 18 | 39 |
| Chocolate Filled, 3 oz | 360 | 19 | 43 |
| **Dunkin' Donuts,** Plain Croissant | 330 | 17 | 37 |
| **Sara Lee:** | | | |
| French Style: Original, 1.8 oz | 185 | 9 | 21 |
| Mini, 1 oz | 230 | 11 | 26 |

**Croissant Sandwiches** ~ *See Page 165*

## Pastry & Pie Crust

| | C | F | Cb |
|---|---|---|---|
| **Pie Crust,** Baked, 9" diameter shell: | | | |
| 1 Pie Shell, 6.5 oz | 970 | 64 | 87 |
| 2-crust Pie, 9", 11.3 oz | 1660 | 109 | 150 |
| **Filo Pastry:** 4 sheets, 2.5 oz | 210 | 2.5 | 40 |
| *Athens,* Filo Dough, 5 sheets, 2 oz | 170 | 1 | 36 |
| **Puff:** | | | |
| *Pepperidge Farm:* ½ sheet | 480 | 30 | 48 |
| Bake & Fill Shell (1) | 180 | 11 | 18 |
| **Arrowhead Mills,** | | | |
| Graham Cracker Pie Crust, ⅛ of 9" | 110 | 5 | 14 |
| **Keebler:** | | | |
| **Ready Crust:** *Per ⅛ of 9" Crust* | | | |
| Chocolate | 100 | 4.5 | 14 |
| Graham: Regular | 100 | 5 | 14 |
| Reduced Fat | 100 | 3.5 | 15 |
| Shortbread Crust | 100 | 5 | 14 |
| **Marie Callenders,** | | | |
| Deep Dish Pie Crust, ⅛ pie, 1 oz | 140 | 10 | 11 |
| **Mrs Smith's,** | | | |
| Deep Dish, ⅛ pie, 1 oz | 130 | 7 | 14 |
| **Nabisco:** | | | |
| **Honey Maid,** | | | |
| Graham Cacker, ⅛ pie, 0.75 oz | 110 | 5 | 14 |
| **Nilla,** Pie Crust, | | | |
| ⅙ of 9", 1 oz | 140 | 8 | 18 |
| **Pillsbury,** | | | |
| **Rolled,** ⅛, 0.9 oz | 100 | 6 | 12 |
| **Trader Joe's,** Pie Crust, ⅛ pie, 1.2 oz | 190 | 13 | 17 |

## Pie Fillings ~ Canned

| | C | F | Cb |
|---|---|---|---|
| **Apple/Blueb./Cherry/Strawb.,** average: | | | |
| Sweetened: ⅓ cup, 3.2oz | 90 | 0 | 22 |
| 1 cup, 9.5 oz | 270 | 0 | 66 |
| 1 can, 21 oz | 600 | 0 | 150 |
| Light/Lite, ⅓ cup, 3.2 oz | 60 | 0 | 15 |
| Unsweetened, ⅓ cup, 3.2 oz | 35 | 0 | 8 |
| **Lemon Crm/Creme,** ⅓ cup, 3.2 oz | 130 | 1.5 | 28 |

**Pizzas ~ Ready To Eat**  **C**  **F**  **Cb**

*Figures Based On Pizza Hut*

## BBQ Lover's:
### Medium Size (12"):
**Hand Tossed/Classic Crust:**

| | C | F | Cb |
|---|---|---|---|
| ⅛ Pizza (1 slice) | 250 | 10 | 28 |
| ½ Pizza (4 slices) | 1000 | 40 | 112 |
| Whole Pizza (8 slices) | 2000 | 80 | 224 |

**Pan/Deep Dish:**

| | C | F | Cb |
|---|---|---|---|
| ⅛ Pizza (1 slice) | 290 | 13 | 31 |
| ½ Pizza (4 slices) | 1160 | 52 | 124 |
| Whole Pizza (8 slices) | 2320 | 104 | 248 |

**Thin 'N Crispy Crust:**

| | C | F | Cb |
|---|---|---|---|
| ⅛ Pizza (1 slice) | 240 | 11 | 25 |
| ½ Pizza (4 slices) | 960 | 44 | 100 |
| Whole Pizza (8 slices) | 1920 | 88 | 200 |

## Meat Lovers:
### Medium Size (12"):
**Hand Tossed/Classic:**

| | C | F | Cb |
|---|---|---|---|
| ⅛ Pizza (1 slice) | 280 | 15 | 25 |
| ½ Pizza (4 slices) | 1120 | 60 | 100 |
| Whole Pizza (8 slices) | 2240 | 120 | 200 |

**Pan/Deep Dish:**

| | C | F | Cb |
|---|---|---|---|
| ⅛ Pizza (1 slice) | 310 | 17 | 27 |
| ½ Pizza (4 slices) | 1240 | 68 | 108 |
| Whole Pizza (8 slices) | 2480 | 136 | 216 |

**Thin Crust:**

| | C | F | Cb |
|---|---|---|---|
| ⅛ Pizza (1 slice) | 270 | 15 | 22 |
| ½ Pizza (4 slices) | 1080 | 60 | 88 |
| Whole Pizza (8 slices) | 2160 | 120 | 176 |

## Pepperoni:
### Medium Size (12"):
**Hand Tossed/Classic Crust:**

| | C | F | Cb |
|---|---|---|---|
| ⅛ Pizza (1 slice) | 220 | 9 | 25 |
| ½ Pizza (4 slices) | 880 | 36 | 100 |
| Whole Pizza (8 slices) | 1760 | 72 | 200 |

**Pan/Deep Dish:**

| | C | F | Cb |
|---|---|---|---|
| ⅛ Pizza (1 slice) | 260 | 12 | 27 |
| ½ Pizza (4 slices) | 1040 | 48 | 108 |
| Whole Pizza (8 slices) | 2080 | 96 | 216 |

**Thin Crust:**

| | C | F | Cb |
|---|---|---|---|
| ⅛ Pizza (1 slice) | 210 | 10 | 21 |
| ½ Pizza (4 slices) | 840 | 40 | 84 |
| Whole Pizza (8 slices) | 1680 | 80 | 168 |

## Supreme:   C  F  Cb
### Medium Size (12")
**Hand Tossed:**

| | C | F | Cb |
|---|---|---|---|
| ⅛ Pizza (1 slice) | 240 | 10 | 26 |
| ½ Pizza (4 slices) | 960 | 40 | 104 |
| Whole Pizza (8 slices | 1920 | 80 | 208 |

**Pan/Deep Dish:**

| | C | F | Cb |
|---|---|---|---|
| ⅛ Pizza (1 slice) | 270 | 13 | 28 |
| ½ Pizza (4 slices) | 1080 | 52 | 112 |
| Whole Pizza (8 slices) | 2160 | 104 | 224 |

**Thin Crust:**

| | C | F | Cb |
|---|---|---|---|
| ⅛ Pizza (1 slice) | 220 | 10 | 23 |
| ½ Pizza (4 slices) | 880 | 40 | 92 |
| Whole Pizza (8 slices) | 1760 | 80 | 184 |

### Large (14"):
**Hand Tossed:**

| | C | F | Cb |
|---|---|---|---|
| **BBQ Lover's:** ⅛ Pizza (1 slice) | 340 | 15 | 39 |
| ½ Pizza (4 slices) | 1360 | 60 | 156 |
| **Cheese:** ⅛ Pizza (1 slice) | 290 | 11 | 34 |
| ½ Pizza (4 slices) | 1160 | 44 | 136 |
| **Meat Lover's:** ⅛ Pizza (1 slice) | 390 | 21 | 34 |
| ½ Pizza (4 slices) | 1560 | 84 | 136 |
| **Pepperoni:** ⅛ Pizza (1 slice) | 300 | 13 | 33 |
| ½ Pizza (4 slices) | 1200 | 52 | 132 |
| **Supreme:** ⅛ Pizza (1 slice) | 330 | 15 | 34 |
| ½ Pizza (4 slices) | 1320 | 60 | 136 |
| **Veggie Lover's:** ⅛ Pizza (1 slice) | 260 | 9 | 35 |
| ½ Pizza (4 slices) | 1040 | 36 | 140 |

### Individual Personal Pizzas (6"):
**Pan/Deep Dish:**

| | C | F | Cb |
|---|---|---|---|
| BBQ Lover's | 740 | 36 | 74 |
| Cheese | 600 | 25 | 69 |
| Pepperoni | 620 | 28 | 67 |
| Supreme | 690 | 34 | 70 |
| Veggie Lovers | 550 | 20 | 70 |

### Extra Large, Single Slices:
*Figures Based On Sbarro's*

| | C | F | Cb |
|---|---|---|---|
| **Pan:** Cheese | 590 | 25 | 69 |
| Meat Delight | 700 | 33 | 69 |
| Pepperoni | 650 | 31 | 69 |
| Supreme | 650 | 30 | 70 |

Updated Nutrition Data ~ www.CalorieKing.com
Persons with Diabetes ~ See Disclaimer (Page 22)

| Frozen Pizzas | C | F | Cb |
|---|---|---|---|
| **Amy's:** *Per ⅓ Pizza* | | | |
| Cheese Pizza | 290 | 12 | 33 |
| Mushroom & Olive | 260 | 10 | 33 |
| Pesto | 310 | 12 | 39 |
| Roasted Vegetable | 280 | 9 | 42 |
| Vegan, Roasted Vegetables, no Cheese | 260 | 4.5 | 50 |
| **California Pizza Kitchen:** | | | |
| **Crispy Thin Crust:** *Per ⅓ Pizza* | | | |
| Margherita | 320 | 16 | 31 |
| Sicilian Recipe | 360 | 18 | 30 |
| Signature Pepperoni | 350 | 19 | 29 |
| White | 320 | 17 | 30 |
| **Small Crispy Thin Crust:** *Per Whole Pizza* | | | |
| BBQ Recipe Chicken; Margh., av | 390 | 15 | 43 |
| Four Cheese | 400 | 18 | 40 |
| Hawaiian | 350 | 12 | 43 |
| Sicilian | 420 | 20 | |
| **Hand Tossed Style:** *Per ⅓ Pizza* | | | |
| BBQ Recipe Chicken, with Bacon | 360 | 9 | 50 |
| Californian Style White | 310 | 7 | 49 |
| The Works | 350 | 11 | 48 |
| **Celeste:** | | | |
| **Pizza For One:** Original, 1 pizza | 320 | 14 | 42 |
| Deluxe | 340 | 15 | 41 |
| Four Cheese | 330 | 15 | 38 |
| Pepperoni | 340 | 13 | 43 |
| Sausage & Pepperoni | 380 | 19 | 41 |
| Zesty Four Cheese | 350 | 16 | 43 |
| **DiGiorno:** *Per Slice, Unless Indicated* | | | |
| **Cheese Stuffed Crust:** | | | |
| Bacon Cheeseburger, ⅙ pizza, 4.5 oz | 310 | 13 | 34 |
| Five Cheese, ⅕ Pizza, 5.3 oz | 380 | 16 | 40 |
| Pepperoni, ⅕ pizza, 5.3 oz | 380 | 16 | 40 |
| Three Meat, ⅙ pizza 4.8 oz | 340 | 16 | 34 |
| Supreme, ⅙ pizza, 5 oz | 350 | 16 | 34 |
| **Classic Thin Crust**, Supreme, ⅕ pizza, 5 oz | 310 | 14 | 32 |
| **Garlic Bread:** *Per ⅙ Pizza* | | | |
| Pepperoni, 5 oz | 380 | 17 | 40 |
| Supreme, 4.3 oz | 300 | 12 | 36 |

| DiGiorno (Cont): | C | F | Cb |
|---|---|---|---|
| **Original Rising Crust:** *Per ⅙ Pizza* | | | |
| Four Cheese, 4.7 oz | 310 | 10 | 39 |
| Italian Sausage, 5 oz | 350 | 14 | 39 |
| Spicy Chicken Supreme, 5.3 oz | 300 | 9 | 40 |
| **Small Pizzas:** *Per ½ Pizza* | | | |
| Cheese Stuffed Crust: | | | |
| Four Cheese, 4.2 oz | 320 | 15 | 34 |
| Pepperoni, 4.2 oz | 330 | 16 | 34 |
| Three Meat, 4.6 oz | 360 | 18 | 34 |
| Traditional Crust: | | | |
| Pepperoni, 4.6 oz | 380 | 18 | 42 |
| Three Meat, 4.7 oz | 360 | 16 | 40 |
| **Freschetta:** | | | |
| **Brick Oven:** *Per ⅓ Pizza Unless Indicated* | | | |
| 5 Italian Cheese, ¼ Pizza, 5.2 oz | 380 | 18 | 40 |
| Chicken Club, ¼ Pizza, 5.5 oz | 360 | 15 | 41 |
| Pepp. & Italian Style Cheese, 4.6 oz | 340 | 17 | 33 |
| Rstd Portab. M'shrms & Spin., 4.6 oz | 270 | 10 | 34 |
| Three Meat Medley, 4.6 oz | 350 | 18 | 33 |
| Zesty Italian Supreme, 4.6 oz | 310 | 15 | 33 |
| **Naturally Rising:** *Per ⅙ of Large Pizza Unless Indicated* | | | |
| 4 Cheese Medley, ⅕ Pizza, 5 oz | 380 | 14 | 47 |
| Canada Style Bacon P'apple, 4.5 oz | 290 | 9 | 40 |
| Classic Supreme, 5 oz | 360 | 15 | 41 |
| Ssg & Pepperoni, 4.9 oz | 370 | 16 | 40 |
| Signat. Pepperoni, 4.5 oz | 340 | 13 | 40 |
| **Jeno's:** *Per Pizza* | | | |
| **Crispy 'N Tasty:** | | | |
| Cheese, 5 oz | 320 | 14 | 37 |
| Pepperoni, 5 oz | 350 | 18 | 36 |
| **Kashi:** | | | |
| **Thin Crust:** *Per ⅓ Pizza* | | | |
| Margherita, 4 oz | 260 | 9 | 29 |
| Mediterranean, 4.2 oz | 290 | 9 | 37 |
| Mushroom Trio & Spinach, 4 oz | 250 | 9 | 28 |
| **Kroger:** | | | |
| **3 Minute Microwave:** *Per 8 oz Pizza* | | | |
| 3-Meat | 500 | 17 | 64 |
| Cheese | 490 | 16 | 66 |
| Combination | 520 | 20 | 64 |
| Pepperoni | 530 | 20 | 65 |
| Supreme | 490 | 18 | 63 |
| **French Bread,** Pepperoni, 5 oz | 380 | 17 | 42 |

### Frozen Pizzas (Cont) **C** **F** **Cb**

**Lean Cuisine:**

**Simple Favorites,**

| | C | F | Cb |
|---|---|---|---|
| French Bread Cheese Pizza (1) | 340 | 6 | 53 |

**Red Baron:**

**Brick Oven:** *Per ¼ Pizza*

| | C | F | Cb |
|---|---|---|---|
| Cheese Trio, 4.4 oz | 320 | 14 | 36 |
| Meat Trio, Pepperoni, 4.6 oz | 340 | 16 | 36 |
| Sausage Supreme, 4.7 oz | 320 | 14 | 37 |

**Classic Crust:** *Per ¼ Pizza*

| | C | F | Cb |
|---|---|---|---|
| 4 Cheese, 5.2 oz | 370 | 16 | 41 |
| Sausage & Pepp., 5.3 oz | 390 | 18 | 42 |
| Supreme, 4.7 oz | 310 | 14 | 34 |

**Deep Dish Minis:**

| | C | F | Cb |
|---|---|---|---|
| Cheese, 4 pieces, 5.4 oz | 420 | 20 | 46 |
| Pepperoni, 4 pieces, 5.4oz | 470 | 25 | 46 |

**Rising Crust:**

| | C | F | Cb |
|---|---|---|---|
| Cheese; Pepperoni, average, 4.8 oz | 335 | 12 | 44 |
| Sausage & Pepperoni, 5 oz | 360 | 14 | 45 |

**Thin & Crispy Crust:** *Per ⅓ Pizza*

| | C | F | Cb |
|---|---|---|---|
| 5 Cheese, 5 oz | 360 | 16 | 40 |
| Pepperoni, 5.3 oz | 400 | 19 | 40 |

**Singles:** *Per Pizza*

**Deep Dish:**

| | C | F | Cb |
|---|---|---|---|
| Hawaiian Style, 5.3 oz | 350 | 13 | 47 |
| Meat-Trio, 5.6 oz | 400 | 17 | 47 |
| Sausage, 5.8 oz | 420 | 19 | 48 |

**French Bread:**

| | C | F | Cb |
|---|---|---|---|
| 5 Cheese & Garlic (1) | 430 | 23 | 41 |
| Pepperoni (1) | 370 | 15 | 44 |

**Safeway Select:**

**Pizzeria Crust:**

| | C | F | Cb |
|---|---|---|---|
| Cheese Trio, ¼ pizza | 340 | 15 | 34 |
| Fajita Chicken Ole, ⅕ pizza | 250 | 10 | 29 |
| Pepperoni & Sausage, ⅕pizza | 320 | 17 | 30 |

**Self Rising:** *Per ⅙ Pizza*

| | C | F | Cb |
|---|---|---|---|
| Four Cheese | 300 | 9 | 41 |
| Pepperoni | 350 | 14 | 41 |
| Sausage & Pepperoni | 340 | 13 | 41 |

**Smart Ones** *(Weight Watchers):*

**Classic Favorites,** Thin Crust,

| | C | F | Cb |
|---|---|---|---|
| Cheese Pizza, 6 oz | 290 | 6 | 42 |

**Smart Anytime,** Brick Oven Style,

| | C | F | Cb |
|---|---|---|---|
| Pepperoni Pizza, 6 oz | 430 | 13 | 57 |

**Stouffer's:** **C** **F** **Cb**

**French Bread Pizzas:**

**Two Per Box:**

| | C | F | Cb |
|---|---|---|---|
| Deluxe, 1 piece, 6 .2 oz | 430 | 21 | 44 |
| Sausage & Pepperoni, 1 piece, 6.3 oz | 460 | 24 | 43 |

**Nine Per Box:**

| | C | F | Cb |
|---|---|---|---|
| Cheese, 1 piece, 5.9 oz | 380 | 16 | 43 |
| Pepperoni, 1 piece, 5.7 oz | 430 | 21 | 44 |

**Tombstone:**

**Original:** *Per ¼ Pizza*

| | C | F | Cb |
|---|---|---|---|
| Canadian Style Bacon | 320 | 12 | 37 |
| Extra Cheese | 350 | 15 | 36 |
| Pepperoni | 390 | 20 | 37 |
| Pepperoni & Sausage | 360 | 17 | 37 |

**Thin Crust:** *Per ¼ Pizza*

| | C | F | Cb |
|---|---|---|---|
| Three Cheese | 310 | 15 | 28 |
| Pepperoni; Sausage, average | 315 | 16 | 28 |

| | C | F | Cb |
|---|---|---|---|
| **Brick Oven Style:** Cheese, ⅓ pizza | 350 | 15 | 37 |
| Pepperoni; Supreme, av., ¼ pizza | 315 | 16 | 29 |

**Tony's:**

**Pizzeria Style Crust:** *Per ⅓ Pizza*

| | C | F | Cb |
|---|---|---|---|
| Cheese, 4.8 oz | 330 | 13 | 42 |
| Pepperoni, 4.7 oz | 330 | 14 | 41 |
| Supreme, 5.3 oz | 350 | 15 | 42 |

**Singles:**

| | C | F | Cb |
|---|---|---|---|
| Deluxe (1), 8.7 oz | 470 | 18 | 66 |
| Pepperoni (1), 8.7 oz | 490 | 20 | 66 |

**Totino's:**

**Crisp Crust Party Pizza:** *Per ½ Pizza*

| | C | F | Cb |
|---|---|---|---|
| Cheese | 320 | 15 | 35 |
| Combination | 360 | 19 | 36 |
| Hamburger | 350 | 18 | 36 |
| Pepperoni | 360 | 19 | 35 |

**Pizza Rolls:**

| | C | F | Cb |
|---|---|---|---|
| Cheese (6), 3 oz | 210 | 8 | 28 |
| Pepperoni (6), 3 oz | 220 | 9 | 26 |

**Trader Joe's:**

| | C | F | Cb |
|---|---|---|---|
| 3 Cheese, ⅓ pizza | 310 | 9 | 42 |
| Parlanno, ¼ pizza | 340 | 16 | 34 |
| Pizza 4 Formaggi, ⅓ pizza | 310 | 9 | 42 |
| Spinach, ⅓ pizza | 300 | 12 | 38 |

## Quick Guide   C   F   Cb

### Chicken
From 3lb ready-to-cook chicken

| | C | F | Cb |
|---|---|---|---|
| **Breast/Wing Quarter:** | | | |
| **Roasted:** With skin | 300 | 15 | 0 |
| Without skin | 185 | 5 | 0 |
| **Fried,** batter dipped | 530 | 30 | 17 |
| **Leg Quarter:** | | | |
| **Thigh & Drumstick:** | | | |
| **Roasted:** With skin | 270 | 16 | 0 |
| Without skin | 185 | 8 | 0 |
| **Fried,** batter dipped | 435 | 25 | 15 |

KFC ~ *See Fast-Foods Section*

### Per 4 oz Edible Portion

**Average of Light Meat:** *Per 4 oz Without Bone*

| | C | F | Cb |
|---|---|---|---|
| Roasted: With skin | 250 | 12 | 0 |
| Without skin | 175 | 4.5 | 0 |
| Stewed: With skin | 230 | 12 | 0 |
| Without skin | 180 | 4.5 | 0 |
| Fried: Batter-dipped, with skin, 4 oz | 315 | 17 | 11 |
| Flour-coated, with skin, 4 oz | 280 | 14 | 2 |

**Average of Dark Meat:** *Per 4 oz Without Bone*

| | C | F | Cb |
|---|---|---|---|
| Roasted: With skin | 290 | 18 | 0 |
| Without skin | 235 | 11 | 0 |
| Stewed: With skin | 265 | 12 | 0 |
| Without skin | 220 | 10 | 0 |
| Fried: Batter-dipped, with skin, 4 oz | 340 | 21 | 11 |
| Flour-coated, with skin, 4 oz | 325 | 19 | 5 |

## Chicken Parts

**Broilers or Fryers:** *Edible Weights (no bone)*

**Breast:** *Per ½ Breast*

| | C | F | Cb |
|---|---|---|---|
| Raw: With skin, 5 oz | 250 | 14 | 0 |
| Without skin, 4.25 oz | 140 | 3 | 0 |
| Roasted: With skin, 3.5 oz | 195 | 8 | 0 |
| Without skin, 3 oz | 140 | 3 | 0 |
| Stewed: With skin, 4 oz | 200 | 8 | 0 |
| Without skin, 3.3 oz | 145 | 3 | 0 |
| Fried: Batter-dipped, w/ skin, 5 oz | 365 | 19 | 13 |
| Flour-coated, with skin, 3.5 oz | 220 | 9 | 2 |

**Drumstick:** *Per Drumstick*

| | C | F | Cb |
|---|---|---|---|
| Roasted: With skin, 2 oz | 115 | 6 | 0 |
| Without skin, 1.5 oz | 75 | 2.5 | 0 |
| Stewed: With skin, 2 oz | 115 | 6 | 0 |
| Without skin, 1.5 oz | 80 | 3 | 0 |
| Fried: Batter-dipped, w/ skin, 2.5 oz | 195 | 11 | 6 |
| Flour-coated, with skin, 1.8 oz | 120 | 7 | 1 |

## Chicken Parts (Cont)   C   F   Cb

**Broilers or Fryers (Cont):** *Edible Weights (no bone)*

**Thigh Portion:**

| | C | F | Cb |
|---|---|---|---|
| Raw: With skin, 3.3 oz (4¼ oz with bone) | 200 | 14 | 0 |
| Without skin, 2.4 oz | 80 | 3 | 0 |
| Roasted: With skin, 2.3 oz | 155 | 10 | 0 |
| Without skin, 2 oz | 110 | 6 | 0 |
| Stewed: With skin, 2.5 oz | 160 | 10 | 0 |
| Without skin, 2 oz | 105 | 5 | 0 |
| Fried: Batter-dipped, with skin 3 oz | 240 | 14 | 8 |
| Flour-coated, with skin, 2.3 oz | 165 | 9 | 2 |

**Wing:** *Per Wing, Bone In*
Raw Weight, 3.2 oz

| | C | F | Cb |
|---|---|---|---|
| Raw: With skin | 110 | 8 | 0 |
| Without skin | 35 | 1 | 0 |
| Roasted: With skin | 100 | 7 | 0 |
| Without skin | 45 | 2 | 0 |
| Fried: Batter-dipped, with skin | 160 | 11 | 5 |
| Flour-coated, with skin | 105 | 7 | 1 |
| Stewed, with skin, 4 oz | 100 | 7 | 0 |

**Buffalo Wings** ~ *See Fast-Foods Section*

| | C | F | Cb |
|---|---|---|---|
| **Neck:** Simmered, with skin | 95 | 7 | 0 |
| Without skin | 30 | 2 | 0 |

**Skin Only:** *Skin from ½ Chicken*

| | C | F | Cb |
|---|---|---|---|
| Raw skin, 3 oz | 275 | 26 | 0 |
| Roasted skin, 2 oz | 255 | 23 | 0 |
| Stewed skin, 2.5 oz | 260 | 24 | 0 |
| Fried, flour-coated, 2 oz | 280 | 24 | 5 |
| Fried, batter-dipped, 6.8 oz | 750 | 55 | 44 |

**Roasters:** *Average of Light & Dark Meat*

| | C | F | Cb |
|---|---|---|---|
| Roasted: With skin, 4 oz | 250 | 15 | 0 |
| Without skin, 4 oz | 190 | 8 | 0 |
| Light Meat, without skin, roasted | 175 | 5 | 0 |
| Dark Meat, without skin, roasted | 200 | 10 | 0 |

**Stewing Chicken:** *Per 4 oz, average of Light & Dark Meat*

| | C | F | Cb |
|---|---|---|---|
| Stewed: With skin | 325 | 22 | 0 |
| Without skin | 270 | 14 | 0 |
| Light Meat, without skin | 240 | 9 | 0 |
| Dark Meat, without skin | 290 | 17 | 0 |

**Capon Chicken:**

| | C | F | Cb |
|---|---|---|---|
| Roasted: With skin, 4 oz | 260 | 13 | 0 |
| ½ Chicken, with skin, 22.5 oz | 1460 | 74 | 0 |

**Chicken Offal & Stuffing:**

| | C | F | Cb |
|---|---|---|---|
| **Giblets:** Simmered, 1 cup | 230 | 7 | 0.5 |
| Fried, flour-coated, 1 cup | 400 | 20 | 6 |
| **Gizzard,** simmered, 1 cup | 210 | 4 | 0 |
| **Heart,** simmered, 1 cup | 270 | 12 | 0.2 |
| **Liver:** Raw, 4 oz | 130 | 5.5 | 0 |
| Simmered, 1 cup | 215 | 8.5 | 1 |
| **Liver Pate,** Fresh, 1 Tbsp, 0.5 oz | 30 | 2 | 1 |
| **Stuffing,** average, ½ cup | 180 | 9 | 22 |

## Chicken Products    **C** **F** **Cb**

**Bumble Bee:**
**Chicken In Water:** *Per 2 oz Drained*

| | C | F | Cb |
|---|---|---|---|
| Premium White | 70 | 1.5 | 0 |
| Premium Breast | 70 | 1 | 1 |

**Foster Farms:**

| | C | F | Cb |
|---|---|---|---|
| Chicken Breast Strips, grilled, 3 oz | 100 | 2 | 1 |
| Wings: Chipotle, 3 wings, 3 oz | 190 | 13 | 4 |
| Honey BBQ Glazed, 3 wings, 3 oz | 190 | 11 | 7 |
| Hot 'n' Spicy, 3 wings, 3 oz | 190 | 14 | 1 |

**Tyson:**
**Anytizers**, Frozen:
**Wings:**

| | C | F | Cb |
|---|---|---|---|
| Hot Wings, Buffalo Style (3) | 190 | 13 | 1 |
| Honey BBQ Seasoned (3) | 190 | 12 | 8 |

**Wyngz, Boneless:**

| | C | F | Cb |
|---|---|---|---|
| Buffalo Style, 3 pieces, 3 oz | 150 | 7 | 8 |
| Sweet Garlic Glazed, 3 pcs, 2.8 oz | 130 | 5 | 10 |

## Duck, Goose, Quail

**Duck:** Roasted,

| | C | F | Cb |
|---|---|---|---|
| With skin, 3 oz | 290 | 24 | 0 |
| Without skin, 3 oz | 170 | 10 | 0 |
| ½ duck, with skin, 13.5 oz | 1290 | 108 | 0 |
| **Goose:** Roasted with skin, 3 oz | 260 | 19 | 0 |
| Without skin, 3 oz | 200 | 11 | 0 |
| **Pheasant,** cooked, 3 oz | 210 | 10 | 0 |
| **Quail,** cooked, 1 whole, 6 oz | 385 | 24 | 0 |

## Turkey

**Fryer-Roasters:** *Per 3 oz Serving*
**Roasted:**

| | C | F | Cb |
|---|---|---|---|
| Light Meat: With skin | 140 | 4 | 0 |
| Without skin | 120 | 1 | 0 |
| Dark Meat: With skin | 155 | 6 | 0 |
| Without skin | 140 | 4 | 0 |

**½ of Whole Turkey:** (Approx. 3.3 lbs raw weight without neck and giblets; 1.8 lbs cooked weight)

| | C | F | Cb |
|---|---|---|---|
| **Roasted:** With skin | 1650 | 74 | 0 |
| Without skin | 1125 | 31 | 0 |

**Ground Turkey,** raw: (4 oz raw wt. = 3 oz ckd wt.)

| | C | F | Cb |
|---|---|---|---|
| 85% lean, regular, 4 oz | 170 | 10 | 0 |
| 93% lean: Average, 4 oz | 160 | 8 | 0 |
| *Jennie-O,* 4 oz | 170 | 8 | 0 |
| *Trader Joe's,* 4 oz | 150 | 8 | 0 |
| 94% lean, | | | |
| *Foster Farms,* 4 oz | 150 | 7 | 0 |
| Breast, no skin, 4 oz | 115 | 1 | 0 |
| Patties: Small, 3 oz | 130 | 7 | 0 |
| Medium, 4 oz | 170 | 7 | 0 |

## Turkey Parts    **C** **F** **Cb**

**Roasted, Edible Weights, without bone:**
**Breast,** (½), (from 17.3 oz raw weight with bone):

| | C | F | Cb |
|---|---|---|---|
| With skin, 12 oz (no bone) | 525 | 11 | 0 |
| Without skin, 10.8 oz | 415 | 2 | 0 |
| **Back (½):** With skin, 4.5 oz | 265 | 13 | 0 |
| Without skin, 3.5 oz | 165 | 6 | 0 |

**Leg (Thigh & Drumstick):**
(from 1 lb raw weight with bone)

| | C | F | Cb |
|---|---|---|---|
| With skin, 8.5 oz (without bone) | 410 | 13 | 0 |
| Without skin, 7.8 oz | 355 | 8.5 | 0 |

**Wing:** (From 7.3 oz raw weight)

| | C | F | Cb |
|---|---|---|---|
| With skin, 3 oz (without bone) | 185 | 9 | 0 |
| Without skin, 2 oz (with bone) | 100 | 2 | 0 |
| **Neck:** Simmered, 1 neck, 9 oz (with bone) | 275 | 11 | 0 |
| **Giblets,** simmered, 1 cup, 5 oz | 240 | 7 | 3 |

## Young Hens (Roasted)

**Light Meat:**

| | C | F | Cb |
|---|---|---|---|
| With skin, 3 oz | 175 | 8 | 0 |
| Without skin, 3 oz | 135 | 3 | 0 |
| **Dark Meat:** With skin, 3 oz | 200 | 11 | 0 |
| Without skin, 3 oz | 165 | 7 | 0 |

**Young Toms ~** *Similar to Young Hens*

## Turkey Products

**Foster Farms:** *Cooked & Frozen*
Meatballs, cooked:

| | C | F | Cb |
|---|---|---|---|
| Homestyle (3) | 160 | 9 | 3 |
| Italian Style (3) | 160 | 8 | 5 |

**Hormel,** Canned Turkey Breast,

| | C | F | Cb |
|---|---|---|---|
| in water, 2 oz | 50 | 1 | 0 |

**Jennie-O:**

| | C | F | Cb |
|---|---|---|---|
| Bacon, 1 slice, 0.5 oz | 30 | 2.5 | 0 |
| Bratwurst, lean, 1 link, 3.85 oz | 170 | 10 | 2 |
| Burgers, uncooked, All Natural, White Meat, 5.3 oz | 200 | 10 | 0 |
| Meatballs, Fully Cooked: Italian, 3 oz | 180 | 13 | 2 |
| Home Style, 3 oz | 180 | 13 | 3 |
| **Spam,** Oven Roasted Turkey, 2 oz | 80 | 4 | 2 |

**Trader Joe's,**

| | C | F | Cb |
|---|---|---|---|
| Italian Turkey Meatloaf, 3 oz | 140 | 8 | 5 |

**Valley Fresh,** 100% Natural,
Canned Prem. White Turkey Breast,

| | C | F | Cb |
|---|---|---|---|
| in water, 2 oz | 45 | 1 | 0 |

## White Rice   **C** **F** **Cb**

**Raw:**

| | C | F | Cb |
|---|---|---|---|
| Glutinous, 1 cup, 6.5 oz | 685 | 1 | 151 |
| Long Grain, 1 cup, 6.5 oz | 675 | 1 | 148 |
| Short Grain, 1 cup, 7 oz | 715 | 1 | 158 |
| Wild Rice, 1 cup, 5.5 oz | 570 | 2 | 120 |

**Cooked Rice:** *Boiled/Steamed*
**Short/Medium Grain:**

| | C | F | Cb |
|---|---|---|---|
| ½ cup, 3.3 oz | 140 | 0 | 30 |
| 1 cup (½ Pint), 7.2 oz | 265 | 0.5 | 59 |
| 2 cups (1 Pint), 13 oz | 480 | 1 | 106 |
| **Long Grain:** ½ cup, 2.8 oz | 100 | 0 | 22 |
| 1 cup, 5.5 oz | 205 | 0.5 | 44 |
| **Glutinous/Sticky,** 1 cup, 6 oz | 170 | 0.5 | 37 |
| **Parboiled,** ½ cup, 3 oz | 105 | 0.5 | 22 |

**Precooked/Instant:**

| | C | F | Cb |
|---|---|---|---|
| Dry, ½ cup, 3.5 oz | 380 | 1 | 82 |
| Cooked, ½ cup, 3 oz | 95 | 0.5 | 21 |

**Wild Rice,**

| | C | F | Cb |
|---|---|---|---|
| Cooked, 1 cup, 5.8 oz | 165 | 0.5 | 35 |

## Brown Rice

*Average of Short or Long Grain*

| | C | F | Cb |
|---|---|---|---|
| **Raw/Dry:** ½ cup, 3.3 oz | 340 | 2.5 | 71 |
| 1 cup, 6.5 oz | 685 | 5.5 | 143 |
| **Cooked:** ½ cup, 3.5 oz | 110 | 1 | 22 |
| 1 cup, 7 oz | 220 | 2 | 46 |

## Rice Dishes   **C** **F** **Cb**

**Chinese Fried Rice:**

| | C | F | Cb |
|---|---|---|---|
| ½ cup, 2.5 oz | 140 | 4.5 | 21 |
| 1 cup, (½ Pint), 5 oz | 280 | 9 | 42 |
| 2 cups, (1 Pint), 10 oz | 565 | 18 | 84 |

**Mexican Style Rice:**

| | C | F | Cb |
|---|---|---|---|
| Taco John's, Cilantro Lime, 6 oz | 220 | 3 | 39 |
| Taco Time, Mexi, 3.5 oz | 80 | 0.5 | 17 |

*Rice-A-Roni ~ See Page 119*

| | C | F | Cb |
|---|---|---|---|
| **Rice with Raisins/Pinenuts,** 1 cup | 400 | 11 | 60 |
| **Rice Pilaf:** Restaurant, 1 cup | 275 | 7.5 | 46 |
| O'Charley's, A La Carte, 1 order | 220 | 6 | 36 |

**Rice Pudding,**

| | C | F | Cb |
|---|---|---|---|
| Kozy Shack, Original, 1 pudding cup | 130 | 2.5 | 24 |
| **Risotto,** 1 cup | 420 | 12 | 70 |
| **Saffron Rice,** 4 oz | 175 | 7 | 25 |
| **Spanish Rice:** 1 cup, 5 oz | 390 | 9 | 72 |
| El Pollo Loco, Small, 4.5 oz | 170 | 2.5 | 33 |
| Taco Cababa, 3.6 oz | 120 | 0.5 | 25 |
| **Sticky Rice,** 1 cup, 5 oz | 155 | 0.5 | 34 |
| **Sushi Rice:** 1 Tbsp | 25 | 0 | 5 |
| 1 cup, 5.2 oz | 390 | 0 | 77 |

**Other Packaged Rice Products:**
*Uncle Ben's / Zatarain's ~ See Page 121*

---

# CalorieKing.com Recipes

*See the CalorieKing website for a salubrious selection of healthy recipes – all analyzed for calories, fat, protein, carbohydrate, fiber and sodium.*

**Choose from:**
- *Starters/Appetizers*
- *Salads*
- *Entrees: Meat, Fish and Chicken*
- *Vegetarian*
- *Desserts*
- *Cakes, Cookies*
- *Drinks*

*www.CalorieKing.com/recipes*

## HEALTHY RECIPE TIPS

- **Use non-fat milk** in place of whole or 2% milk
- **Use low-fat yogurt** in place of sour cream
- **Skim fat** from surface of soups and casseroles after cooling
- **Add extra vegetables** to soups and hot entreés
- **Cakes/cookies/muffins:** Replace most or all the fat/oil with applesauce and/or prune puree (Example, *Sunsweet Lighter Bake*)
- **Drinks:** Replace sugar with no-calorie sweeteners such as *Equal, Stevia, Splenda and Sweet 'N Low*

## Deli Salads

|  | C | F | Cb |
|---|---|---|---|
| *Average All Outlets* | | | |
| Antipasto Salad, ½ cup | 135 | 8 | 13 |
| 3-Bean Salad, ½ cup | 90 | 4.5 | 12 |
| Bulgur Salad, ½ cup | 70 | 2 | 12 |
| Caesar Salad, Classic, 1 cup | 200 | 14 | 15 |
| Side Salad, without Dressing | 25 | 0 | 6 |
| Carrot Raisin: With Dressing, ½ cup | 135 | 12 | 6 |
| Without Dressing, ½ cup | 20 | 0 | 5 |
| Chef's Salad: Regular, w/o Dressing | 620 | 37 | 8 |
| With 2 oz Thousand Island Drssng | 860 | 61 | 8 |
| Chicken Salad, ½ cup/scoop, 4 oz | 280 | 21 | 2 |
| Coleslaw: Traditional, ½ cup | 150 | 8 | 18 |
| W/ Low Cal Dressing, ½ c. | 50 | 2 | 8 |
| Corn, Mexican, ½ cup | 240 | 12 | 33 |
| Cucumber: Non-Oil Dressing, ½ cup | 60 | 0 | 14 |
| With Oil Dressing, ½ cup | 140 | 12 | 8 |
| Eggplant Salad, ½ cup | 75 | 5 | 7 |
| Fettucini, with veges, ½ cup | 135 | 6 | 16 |
| Garden Salad, without Dressing, 1 cup | 10 | 0 | 2 |
| Greek Salad, 1 cup | 105 | 8 | 7 |
| Greek Vegetables, 1 cup | 110 | 8 | 6 |
| Lobster Salad, ½ cup, 4 oz | 250 | 21 | 11 |
| Macaroni Salad, ½ cup, 5 oz | 360 | 26 | 26 |
| Nicoise, 1 cup | 450 | 32 | 18 |
| Pasta Salad, ½ cup | 200 | 11 | 19 |
| Potato Salad: Dijon, 3 oz | 120 | 7 | 13 |
| With Mayonnaise, ½ cup, 4 oz | 215 | 15 | 17 |
| Lowfat, ½ cup | 110 | 1.5 | 21 |
| Rice Salad, ½ cup | 150 | 10 | 13 |
| Saffron Rice, 4 oz | 175 | 7 | 25 |
| Spinach Salad, 1 cup | 180 | 13 | 13 |
| Tabouli, ½ cup | 125 | 7 | 13 |
| Three Bean Salad, ½ cup | 90 | 4.5 | 12 |
| Tomato & Mozzarella, ½ cup | 180 | 14 | 10 |
| Tortellini, with Basil Pesto, ½ cup | 150 | 9 | 15 |
| Waldorf, with Mayo, ½ cup | 110 | 7 | 12 |

**Signature Salads:** *Per 6 oz Serving*
(Supplied to Deli's and Institutions)

|  | C | F | Cb |
|---|---|---|---|
| Antipasto Salad | 510 | 50 | 4 |
| Artichoke Salad, marinated | 400 | 41 | 8 |
| California Medley | 120 | 7 | 15 |
| Cheese Agnolotti | 250 | 8 | 23 |
| Chicken Salad | 420 | 33 | 11 |
| Crabmeat Flavored | 450 | 38 | 20 |
| Egg Salad | 300 | 23 | 14 |
| Fresh Button Mushroom | 190 | 16 | 6 |

| Signature Salads (Cont): *Per 6 oz* | C | F | Cb |
|---|---|---|---|
| Fresh Button Mushroom | 190 | 16 | 6 |
| Ham Salad | 400 | 32 | 14 |
| Prima Pasta Salad | 360 | 30 | 18 |
| Seafood Pasta Del Mar | 170 | 10 | 21 |
| Seafood, Crab & Shrimp | 420 | 34 | 20 |
| Shrimp Salad | 360 | 32 | 8 |
| Tuna Salad | 450 | 36 | 14 |

*~ Also See Fast-Foods & Restaurants Section*

## Fresh Salad Packs

*Pre-Packaged (Supermarkets):*
**Dole:**

| *Kits: Per 3.5 oz, With Dressing* | C | F | Cb |
|---|---|---|---|
| Caesar | 150 | 12 | 8 |
| Chopped: Chipotle & Cheddar | 120 | 8 | 10 |
| Sesame Asian | 160 | 16 | 13 |
| Southwest | 140 | 10 | 10 |
| **Salad Blends:** *Without Dressing* | | | |
| American; Mediterranean, 3 oz | 15 | 0 | 3 |
| Arugula; Baby Spinach, average, 3 oz | 20 | 0.5 | 3 |

**Fresh Express:**

| *Complete Salad Kits: Per 3½ oz, Prepared* | | | |
|---|---|---|---|
| Asian | 120 | 5 | 17 |
| Caesar: Regular | 150 | 12 | 7 |
| Lite | 90 | 6 | 7 |
| Supreme | 160 | 14 | 6 |
| Pear Gorgonzola | 130 | 6 | 17 |
| **Gourmet Cafe:** *Per Package* | | | |
| Chopped Santa Fe | 290 | 19 | 18 |
| Tuscan | 330 | 28 | 9 |

**Ready Pac:**

| **Bowl Salads:** *Per Container, with Dressing* | | | |
|---|---|---|---|
| Apple Bleu Pecan, 4.5 oz | 230 | 17 | 15 |
| Asian Style Chkn, 6.2 oz | 210 | 11 | 14 |
| Cranb. Walnut, 4.5 oz | 220 | 9 | 26 |
| **Dinner Solutions:** *With Dressing* | | | |
| Chef, 3.5 oz | 160 | 11 | 7 |
| Southwestern, 3.5 oz | 130 | 9 | 7 |
| **Gourmet:** *Per Container, with Dressing* | | | |
| Baby Kale Apple Harvest, 8 oz | 390 | 23 | 42 |
| Turkey Cobb with Bacon, 11.5 oz | 460 | 32 | 24 |

## Salad Toppings

|  | C | F | Cb |
|---|---|---|---|
| Bac'n Pieces, McCormick, 1Tbsp, 0.3 oz | 30 | 1 | 2 |
| Bacon Bits (Hormel), 1Tbsp | 25 | 1 | 0 |
| Bac-Os, Bits (Betty Crocker), 1 Tbsp | 30 | 1 | 2 |
| Chow Mein Noodles, dry, ½ cup | 120 | 7 | 13 |
| Croutons, 2 Tbsp, 0.3 oz | 40 | 1 | 7 |
| Salad Toppins, McCormick, 4 tsp | 35 | 1.5 | 3 |
| Sunflower Seeds, 1 Tbsp, 0.3 oz | 45 | 4 | 1.5 |
| Toasted Sliced Almonds, 2 T., 0.5 oz | 85 | 7 | 3 |

### Quick Guide    C  F  Cb

**Salad Dressings**
Average All Brands: *Per 2 Tbsp, Approx 1 fl.oz*

| Balsamic Vinaigrette: | C | F | Cb |
|---|---|---|---|
| Regular | 90 | 9 | 3 |
| Light, 2 Tbsp | 45 | 4 | 2 |
| Fat Free, 2 Tbsp | 25 | 0 | 6 |
| **Blue Cheese:** Regular, 2 Tbsp | 145 | 15 | 1.5 |
| Regular, ¼ cup, 2 oz | 280 | 30 | 3 |
| Light, 2 Tbsp | 30 | 1 | 4 |
| **Caesar:** Regular, 2 Tbsp | 165 | 17 | 1 |
| Regular, ¼ cup, 2 oz | 310 | 34 | 2 |
| Light, 2 Tbsp | 35 | 1.5 | 5.5 |
| **Coleslaw:** Regular, 2 Tbsp | 125 | 11 | 8 |
| Regular, ¼ cup, 2 oz | 245 | 21 | 15 |
| Light, 2 Tbsp | 110 | 7 | 14 |
| **French:** Regular | 145 | 14 | 5 |
| Regular, ¼ cup, 2 oz | 260 | 25 | 9 |
| Light, 2 Tbsp | 65 | 4 | 9 |
| Fat/Oil-Free, 2 Tbsp | 40 | 0 | 10 |
| **Italian:** Regular, 2 Tbsp | 85 | 8.5 | 3 |
| Regular, ¼ cup, 2 oz | 165 | 16 | 6 |
| Light, 2 Tbsp | 55 | 5.5 | 2 |
| Fat/Oil-Free, 2 Tbas | 15 | 0 | 2.5 |
| **Ranch:** Regular, 2 Tbsp | 145 | 16 | 2 |
| Regular, ¼ cup, 2 oz | 290 | 30 | 4 |
| Light, 2 Tbsp | 60 | 4 | 6.5 |
| Fat-Free, 2 Tbsp | 35 | 0.5 | 8 |
| **Thousand Island:** Reg., 2 T. | 115 | 11 | 4.5 |
| Regular, ¼ cup, 2 oz | 210 | 20 | 9 |
| Light, 2 Tbsp | 60 | 3.5 | 7 |
| Fat-Free, 2 Tbsp | 40 | 0.5 | 10 |

### Brands ~ Salad Dressings

| **Annie's Naturals:** *Per 2 Tbsp* | C | F | Cb |
|---|---|---|---|
| Organic: Goddess Dressing | 120 | 12 | 2 |
| Green Garlic | 80 | 8 | 2 |
| Papaya Poppy Seed | 90 | 8 | 5 |
| Thousand Island | 90 | 8 | 5 |
| Vinaigrettes: | | | |
| Red Wine & Olive Oil | 140 | 15 | 0 |
| Sesame Ginger | 90 | 8 | 4 |
| Shitake & Sesame | 120 | 13 | 1 |
| **Bernstein's:** *Per 2 Tbsp* | | | |
| Creamy Caesar | 120 | 13 | 1 |
| Herb Garden French | 130 | 12 | 6 |
| Italian | 110 | 12 | 1 |
| Restaurant Recipe Italian | 120 | 12 | 1 |
| Sweet Herb Italian | 130 | 11 | 8 |
| Fat-Free, Cheese & Garlic Italian | 10 | 0 | 2 |
| Light Fantastic: Cheese Fantastico | 25 | 1.5 | 3 |
| Roasted Garlic Balsamic | 45 | 3.5 | 3 |
| **Best Foods:** *Per 1 Tbsp Unless Indicated* | | | |
| Dijonnaise, 1 tsp | 5 | 0 | 1 |
| Mayonnaise: Real | 90 | 10 | 0 |
| Light | 35 | 3.5 | 1 |
| Low-Fat | 15 | 1 | 2 |
| Canola | 40 | 4 | 1 |
| Olive Oil | 60 | 6 | 1 |
| Mayonesa, Lemom-Lime | 90 | 10 | 0 |
| **Cardini's:** *Per 2 Tbsp* | | | |
| Aged Parmesan Ranch | 150 | 16 | 1 |
| Caesar: Original | 160 | 17 | 1 |
| Fat-Free Caesar | 40 | 0 | 9 |
| Light Caesar | 80 | 7 | 5 |
| Honey Mustard | 120 | 11 | 6 |
| Roasted Asian Sesame | 120 | 10 | 6 |
| Vinaigrette, Balsamic: | | | |
| Regular | 100 | 8 | 5 |
| Lite | 50 | 3 | 5 |
| **Great Value** *(Walmart): Per 2 Tbsp* | | | |
| Caesar | 120 | 12 | 2 |
| **Ranch:** Bacon | 140 | 14 | 1 |
| Buttermilk | 110 | 11 | 2 |
| Chipotle | 120 | 13 | 2 |
| Classic | 130 | 14 | 1 |
| Zesty Italian | 70 | 6 | 3 |
| **Hidden Valley:** *Per 2 Tbsp* | | | |
| **Ranch Originals:** Regular | 140 | 14 | 2 |
| Light Original | 80 | 7 | 3 |
| Bacon; Spicy, average | 145 | 15 | 2 |
| Buttermilk | 130 | 14 | 2 |

Enjoy a healthy salad but don't drown it in high-fat salad dressings.
Use 'light' dressings to halve the fat and calories.

### Brands ~ Salad Dressings (Cont)

**Hidden Valley (Cont):**

|  | C | F | Cb |
|---|---|---|---|
| **Farmhouse Originals,** | | | |
| Dijon Mustard Vinaigrette | 100 | 9 | 4 |
| Homestyle Italian | 100 | 10 | 3 |
| Southwest Chipotle | 100 | 10 | 2 |

**Kraft:** *Per 2 Tbsp*

| **Regular Dressings:** | | | |
|---|---|---|---|
| Caesar Vinaigrette, with Parmesan | 70 | 6 | 3 |
| Catalina | 90 | 6 | 9 |
| Classic Caesar | 120 | 12 | 2 |
| Creamy Ranch | 110 | 11 | 2 |
| Creamy Italian | 100 | 10 | 2 |
| Greek Vinaigrette | 110 | 11 | 2 |
| Roka Blue Cheese | 120 | 13 | 1 |
| Sweet Honey Catalina | 100 | 8 | 8 |
| Thousand Island | 130 | 12 | 4 |
| Tuscan House, Italian | 130 | 13 | 3 |
| **Fat Free:** Catalina; Classic Ranch | 50 | 0 | 11 |
| French Style | 45 | 0 | 11 |
| Italian | 15 | 0 | 3 |
| Thousand Island | 45 | 0 | 10 |
| **Lite:** Asian Toasted Sesame | 50 | 2.5 | 7 |
| Balsamic Vinaigrette | 30 | 1 | 4 |
| Creamy Caesar | 35 | 2 | 4 |
| Zesty Italian | 25 | 1.5 | 3 |
| **Seven Seas:** | | | |
| Green Goddess | 130 | 13 | 2 |
| Viva Italian Anything | 50 | 4.5 | 1 |
| Reduced Fat: Viva Italian | 45 | 4 | 2 |
| Red Wine Vinaigrette | 45 | 4 | 3 |

**Marie's:** *Per 2 Tbsp*

| Blue Cheese, Premium Super | 160 | 17 | 1 |
|---|---|---|---|
| Caesar | 170 | 19 | 1 |
| Ranch: Buttermilk | 150 | 16 | 1 |
| Jalapeno Ranch | 160 | 17 | 1 |
| **Classics:** | | | |
| Chunky Blue Cheese | 160 | 17 | 0 |
| Coleslaw | 140 | 13 | 7 |
| Creamy Italian Garlic | 170 | 19 | 1 |
| Creamy Ranch | 170 | 19 | 1 |
| Thousand Island | 150 | 15 | 4 |
| **Specialty:** Honey Dijon | 130 | 12 | 5 |
| Poppy Seed | 150 | 13 | 8 |

**Marzetti's:**

|  | C | F | Cb |
|---|---|---|---|
| **Organic:** Blue Cheese | 130 | 14 | 1 |
| Caesar | 140 | 15 | 1 |
| Parmesan Ranch | 130 | 14 | 2 |
| Chunky Blue Cheese | 150 | 15 | 1 |
| Classic Ranch | 160 | 17 | 1 |
| Honey Dijon | 130 | 12 | 6 |

**Newman's Own:** *Per 2 Tbsp*

| **Regular:** Balsamic Vinaigrette | 90 | 9 | 3 |
|---|---|---|---|
| Creamy Caesar | 170 | 18 | 1 |
| Family Recipe Italian | 130 | 13 | 1 |
| Olive Oil & Vinegar | 150 | 16 | 1 |
| Parmesan & Rstd Garlic | 110 | 11 | 2 |
| Ranch | 150 | 16 | 2 |
| **Lite:** Italian | 60 | 6 | 1 |
| Raspberry & Walnut | 70 | 5 | 7 |
| **Organic:** | | | |
| Light Balsamic Vinaigrette | 45 | 4 | 4 |
| Tuscan Italian | 100 | 11 | 2 |

**Wish-Bone:** *Per 2 Tbsp*

| **Creamy:** Chunky Blue Cheese | 150 | 14 | 1 |
|---|---|---|---|
| Caesar | 180 | 18 | 1 |
| Deluxe French | 120 | 11 | 5 |
| Italian | 110 | 10 | 4 |
| Ranch | 130 | 13 | 2 |
| Russian | 110 | 6 | 14 |
| Sweet 'n Spicy French | 140 | 12 | 7 |
| Thousand Island | 130 | 12 | 5 |
| **Light:** Blue Cheese | 70 | 6 | 2 |
| Creamy Caesar | 70 | 6 | 2 |
| Honey Dijon | 70 | 5 | 6 |
| Italian | 35 | 2.5 | 3 |
| Parmesan Peppercorn Ranch | 60 | 5 | 2 |
| Ranch | 70 | 5 | 4 |
| Thousand Island | 60 | 5 | 4 |
| Vinaigrette: Balsamic & Basil | 50 | 4 | 3 |
| Asian with Sesame & Ginger | 70 | 5 | 5 |
| Raspberry Walnut | 70 | 4 | 7 |
| **Fat-Free:** | | | |
| Chunky Blue Cheese | 30 | 0 | 7 |
| Ranch | 30 | 0 | 6 |
| **Oil & Vinegar:** | | | |
| Balsamic Vinaigrette | 60 | 5 | 3 |
| House Italian | 110 | 10 | 3 |
| Red Wine Vinaigrette | 70 | 5 | 6 |
| Robusto Italian | 80 | 7 | 4 |

## Gravy

| | C | F | Cb |
|---|---|---|---|
| **Homemade Gravy,** average: | | | |
| Thin, little fat, | | | |
| 2 Tbsp, 1 oz | 20 | 1 | 3 |
| Thick: 2 Tbsp, 1.3 oz | 50 | 2 | 9 |
| ¼ cup, 2.5 oz | 100 | 4 | 18 |
| **McCormick:** | | | |
| Brown, 1 Tbsp | 25 | 0.5 | 3 |
| Turkey, 1 Tbsp | 20 | 0.5 | 4 |

## Gravy-In-Jars

| | C | F | Cb |
|---|---|---|---|
| **Boston Market,** | | | |
| Classic Beef, ¼ cup, 2 oz | 30 | 1 | 4 |
| **Campbell's,** Slow Roast, | | | |
| Beef/Chicken/Turkey, ¼ cup, 2 oz | 25 | 1 | 3 |
| *Heinz: Per ¼ Cup, 2 oz* | | | |
| Homestyle: Classic Chicken | 30 | 2 | 3 |
| Savory Beef | 30 | 1 | 4 |
| Sausage | 45 | 1.5 | 6 |
| Other varieties, average | 20 | 0.5 | 3 |
| Fat-Free, all varieties | 20 | 0 | 4 |
| **Safeway,** all varieties, ¼ cup, 2 oz | 20 | 0.5 | 4 |

## Tomato Products

| | C | F | Cb |
|---|---|---|---|
| **Whole/Chopped/Crushed/Diced:** | | | |
| Regular: 1 cup, 8.5 oz | 50 | 0 | 10 |
| In Aspic, ½ cup | 50 | 0 | 12 |
| With Green Chili, 1 c., 8.5 oz | 60 | 0 | 16 |
| Stewed, ½ cup, 1.7 oz | 40 | 1.5 | 7 |
| Wedges in Tomato Juice, 1 cup | 70 | 0.5 | 18 |
| Salsa, average, 2 Tbsp, 1 oz | 25 | 0 | 6 |
| **Tomato Ketchup:** | | | |
| Regular: 1 Tbsp, 0.5 oz | 15 | 0 | 4 |
| Single Serve, 1 packet | 10 | 0 | 3 |
| *Heinz,* Simply Heinz | | | |
| 1 Tbsp, 0.5 oz | 15 | 0 | 4 |
| **Tomato Paste:** | | | |
| Regular: 2 Tbsp, 1 oz | 25 | 0 | 6 |
| ¾ cup, 6 oz | 140 | 1 | 32 |
| **Tomato Puree,** ½ cup, 4.5 oz | 50 | 0 | 10 |
| **Tomato Sauce:** | | | |
| Regular, ½ cup, 4.4 oz | 50 | 0 | 11 |
| Spanish Style, ½ cup, 4.3 oz | 40 | 0 | 9 |
| With Mushr., ½ cup, 4.3 oz | 45 | 0 | 10 |
| With Onions, ½ cup, 4.3 oz | 50 | 0 | 12 |
| **Tomato Seasoning,** 3 tsp | 20 | 0 | 4 |
| **Sundried Tomatoes:** | | | |
| Natural, 5-6 pieces, 0.4 oz | 20 | 0 | 5 |
| In Oil, drained, 6 pieces, 0.5 oz | 40 | 2.5 | 4 |

## Sauces ~ Brands

| | C | F | Cb |
|---|---|---|---|
| **A-1:** | | | |
| **Marinades:** *Per Tbspn, ½ oz* | | | |
| Chicago Steakhouse | 20 | 1 | 3 |
| Classic | 15 | 0 | 4 |
| New Orleans Cajun | 25 | 0 | 5 |
| New York Steakhouse | 20 | 0 | 5 |
| **Steak Sauce:** Original | 15 | 0 | 3 |
| Bold & Spicy | 20 | 0 | 4 |
| Cracked Peppercorn | 15 | 0 | 0 |
| Thick & Hearty | 25 | 0 | 6 |
| **Barilla:** | | | |
| **Pasta Sauces:** *Per ½ Cup* | | | |
| Marinara; Tom. & Basil, av. | 70 | 1 | 15 |
| Mushroom | 80 | 2.5 | 12 |
| Rstd Garlic; Traditional, av. | 70 | 1 | 14 |
| Spicy Marinara | 60 | 0.5 | 13 |
| Sweet Peppers; Three Cheese, av. | 70 | 1 | 13 |
| Tuscan Herb | 70 | 0.5 | 14 |
| **Bertolli:** | | | |
| **Alfredo Sauces:** *Per ¼ Cup* | | | |
| Alfredo; Four Cheese Rosa | 110 | 10 | 3 |
| Garlic | 100 | 10 | 2 |
| Mushroom | 80 | 7 | 2 |
| **Gold Label:** | | | |
| Asiago Cheese with Artichokes | 110 | 6 | 10 |
| Balsamic Vinegar w/ Caramel Onions | 90 | 2.5 | 11 |
| Porcini Mushrooms with Truffle Oil | 100 | 5 | 9 |
| **Traditional:** *Per ½ Cup* | | | |
| Five Cheese | 90 | 3.5 | 14 |
| Italian Sausage | 90 | 3 | 14 |
| Olive Oil & Garlic | 80 | 3 | 14 |
| **Vineyard,** Marinara; Portobello Mshrm | 80 | 25 | 13 |
| *Best Foods/Hellmann's,* | | | |
| Tartar Sauce, 2 Tbsp | 80 | 7 | 4 |
| **Buitoni:** | | | |
| **Pasta Sauces:** | | | |
| Alfredo: Regular, ¼ cup | 140 | 12 | 4 |
| Light, ¼ cup | 90 | 6 | 4 |
| Marinara: Regular ½ cup | 70 | 3 | 10 |
| With Roasted Garlic, ½ cup | 60 | 1 | 10 |
| Pesto: With Basil, ¼ cup | 270 | 26 | 4 |
| Reduced Fat, ¼ cup | 230 | 17 | 8 |
| *Bull's-Eye: Per 2 Tbsp* | | | |
| BBQ Sauce: Origianl | 50 | 0 | 12 |
| Hickory Smoke | 60 | 0 | 15 |
| Regional, average all varieties | 50 | 0 | 11 |
| **Catelli:** *Per ½ Cup* | | | |
| **Pasta,** Garden Select Six Vegetable: | | | |
| Country Mushroom | 70 | 1.5 | 11 |
| Diced Tomato & Basil | 70 | 1 | 12 |
| **Meat Sauce** | 80 | 2.5 | 11 |
| **Pizza Sauce,** Tomato & Basil | 60 | 1.5 | 11 |

## Sauces ~ Brands (Cont)

| | C | F | Cb |
|---|---|---|---|
| **Cento:** *Per ½ Cup* | | | |
| **Clam,** Red, 4.3 oz | 60 | 2 | 6 |
| **San Marzano Pasta:** | | | |
| Arrabbiata, 4.3 oz | 70 | 3.5 | 6.5 |
| Marinara, 4.3 oz | 60 | 3.5 | 6 |
| Vodka, 4.3 oz | 75 | 3.5 | 6 |
| **Classico:** | | | |
| **Alfredo:** *Per ¼ Cup* | | | |
| Creamy | 60 | 4.5 | 3 |
| Roasted Red Pepper | 60 | 4 | 4 |
| **Pesto:** *Per ¼ Cup* | | | |
| Basil Pesto | 240 | 24 | 5 |
| Sun-Dried Tomato Pesto | 100 | 6 | 9 |
| **Red Sauces:** *Per ½ Cup* | | | |
| Family Favorites: Meat | 60 | 1 | 10 |
| Parmesan & Romano | 70 | 2 | 10 |
| Traditional | 80 | 2.5 | 13 |
| Seasonal Selection: Bolognese | 60 | 1.5 | 10 |
| Creamy Spinach & Parmesan | 80 | 4 | 8 |
| Signature Recipes: | | | |
| Cabernet Marinara with Herbs | 60 | 1.5 | 10 |
| Caramelized Onion & Rstd Garlic | 70 | 1.5 | 12 |
| Traditional Pizza Sauce | 40 | 1 | 7 |
| Tomato Cream Collection: | | | |
| Creamy Tomato & Roasted Garlic | 35 | 1.5 | 5 |
| Four Cheese Tomato | 40 | 2 | 5 |
| Spicy tomato & Parmesan | 40 | 2 | 5 |
| Traditional Favorites, Sweet Basil | 70 | 1 | 13 |
| **Colgin,** Liquid Smoke, 1 tsp | 0 | 0 | 0 |
| **Contadina:** | | | |
| **Pizza Sauce:** *Per 2.2 oz* | | | |
| Flavored with Pepperoni | 35 | 1 | 5 |
| Original; Four Cheese | 30 | 0.5 | 6 |
| **Tomato Sauce,** average | 20 | 0.5 | 4 |
| **Crosse & Blackwell:** | | | |
| **Meat:** Ham Glaze, 1 Tbsp | 25 | 0 | 7 |
| Mint Meat Sauce, 1 tsp | 5 | 0 | 2 |
| **Seafood:** | | | |
| Cocktail, ¼ cup, 2.5 oz | 80 | 0 | 20 |
| Shrimp, ¼ cup, 2.5 oz | 80 | 0 | 21 |
| **Dave's Gourmet:** *Per ½ Cup* | | | |
| **Pasta Sauce:** | | | |
| Butternut Squash | 100 | 4 | 17 |
| Organic: Red Heirloom | 45 | 1.5 | 7 |
| Rstd Garlic & Sweet Basil | 70 | 4.5 | 8 |
| **Del Monte:** | | | |
| **Pasta Sauces:** *Per ½ Cup* | | | |
| Four Cheese; Traditional, av. | 60 | 1 | 12 |
| Mushroom | 50 | 1 | 11 |
| Average other varieties | 70 | 1 | 13 |
| Sloppy Joe Sauce, Orig., ¼ cup | 50 | 0 | 13 |

| | C | F | Cb |
|---|---|---|---|
| **Emeril's:** | | | |
| **Pasta Sauces:** *Per ½ Cup* | | | |
| Homestyle Marinara | 90 | 3 | 14 |
| Kicked Up Tomato | 80 | 3.5 | 11 |
| Roasted Gaaahlic | 80 | 3.5 | 12 |
| Roasted Red Pepper | 70 | 3.5 | 9 |
| Vodka Sauce | 110 | 7 | 12 |
| **Francesco Rinaldi:** *Per ½ Cup* | | | |
| **Hearty:** Super Mushroom | 110 | 4.5 | 17 |
| Three Cheese | 90 | 2 | 16 |
| **Traditional:** Original | 80 | 3 | 14 |
| Meat Flavored | 90 | 3.5 | 14 |
| Mushroom | 80 | 3 | 13 |
| **French's,** | | | |
| **Worcestershire Sce,** 1 Tbsp | 5 | 0 | 1 |
| **Heinz:** *Per 1 Tbsp* | | | |
| 57/Steak Sauce | 20 | 0 | 4 |
| Chili Sauce | 20 | 0 | 5 |
| Cocktail Sauce, Original, | | | |
| ¼ cup, 2.2 oz | 60 | 0 | 15 |
| Horseradish Sauce | 75 | 6 | 3 |
| Tomato Ketchup: Regular | 20 | 0 | 5 |
| Reduced Sugar | 5 | 0 | 1 |
| Worcestershire Sauce, 1 Tbsp | 5 | 0 | 1 |
| **House of Tsang:** *Per 1 Tbsp* | | | |
| Bangkok Peanut Sauce | 40 | 2 | 4 |
| Ginger Flavored Soy | 20 | 0 | 4 |
| General Tsao | 45 | 0.5 | 10 |
| Ginger Sriracha | 15 | 0 | 4 |
| Hibachi Grill, Sweet Ginger Sesame | 40 | 1 | 8 |
| Hoisin, 1 tsp | 15 | 0 | 4 |
| Oyster Flavored | 30 | 0 | 7 |
| Saigon Sizzle Stir-Fry | 45 | 2 | 7 |
| Sweet & Sour Stir-Fry | 35 | 0 | 9 |
| **Hunt's:** | | | |
| BBQ Sauce, Original, 2 Tbsp | 60 | 0 | 15 |
| Hickory & Brown Sugar BBQ Sce, 2 Tbsp | 70 | 0 | 18 |
| **Manwich,** Sloppy Joe Sauce, | | | |
| Original, ¼ cup, 2.3 oz | 35 | 0 | 7 |
| **Pasta Sauce:** *Per ½ Cup* | | | |
| Four Cheese | 60 | 1 | 10 |
| Garlic & Herb | 40 | 1 | 8 |
| Meat Flavor | 60 | 1 | 10 |
| Mushroom | 50 | 0.5 | 10 |
| Traditional | 60 | 1 | 11 |

### Brands (Cont)

| Kikkoman: | C | F | Cb |
|---|---|---|---|
| **Asian Authentic:** | | | |
| Black Bean Sauce, w/ Garlic, 2 Tbsp | 50 | 1 | 6 |
| Hoisin Sauce, 2 Tbsp | 80 | 0 | 19 |
| **Marinades:** Gourmet Teriyaki | 30 | 0 | 7 |
| Honey Mustard, 1 Tbsp | 30 | 0 | 6 |
| Roasted Garlic & Herbs | 20 | 0 | 4 |
| **Knorr:** | | | |
| **Classic Sauce:** *Per Whole Package* | | | |
| Bernaise, dry mix only | 100 | 0 | 20 |
| Hollandaise, dry mix only | 100 | 0 | 20 |
| **Kraft:** | | | |
| Barbecue Sauces, av., 2 Tbsp | 65 | 0 | 15 |
| **Specialty Sauce:** Cocktail, 2 Tbsp | 60 | 0.5 | 11 |
| Coleslaw Dressing, 1.2 oz | 110 | 8 | 9 |
| Horseradish, 1 oz | 100 | 9 | 4 |
| Sandwich Spread, 1 Tbsp | 35 | 2.5 | 3 |
| Tartar, Original, 1 Tbsp | 60 | 5 | 4 |
| **Las Palmas:** | | | |
| Green Enchilada Sauce, all varieties, 2 oz | 25 | 1.5 | 3 |
| Red Chili Sauce, 2 oz | 15 | 0.5 | 3 |
| **La Victoria,** | | | |
| Red/Green Enchilada Sauce, av., 2 oz | 15 | 0.5 | 3 |
| **Lawry's:** | | | |
| **30 Minute Marinade:** *Per Tbsp* | | | |
| Caribbean Jerk | 30 | 0 | 7 |
| Herb & Garlic; Lemon Pepper | 10 | 0 | 2 |
| Mesquite, w/ Lime Juice | 10 | 0 | 2 |
| Steak & Chop, w/ Garl. Pepp. | 5 | 0 | 0.5 |
| Sesame Ginger, w/ Mandarin | 30 | 0 | 7 |
| **Packet Seasonings:** *Dry* | | | |
| Fajitas; Taco, average, 2 tsp | 15 | 0 | 3 |
| Other varieties, average, 2 tsp | 20 | 0 | 4 |
| **Lea & Perrins:** | | | |
| Marinade In-A-Bag, av. all var., 0.5 oz | 15 | 0 | 4 |
| Marinade for Chicken, 1 Tbsp | 15 | 0 | 1 |
| Steak Sauce, Bold, 1 Tbsp | 20 | 0 | 5 |
| Worcestershire Sauce, Original 1 tsp, 5 ml | 5 | 0 | 1 |
| **McCormicks:** | | | |
| **Seafood Sauces:** *Per 2 Tbsp* | | | |
| Asian | 50 | 1.5 | 7 |
| Cajun Style | 15 | 0 | 3 |
| Lemon Butter Dill | 100 | 9 | 4 |
| Lemon Herb | 140 | 15 | 0.5 |
| Mediterranean; Santa Fe Style | 20 | 0 | 4 |
| Scampi | 160 | 17 | 2 |

| Mrs. Dash: | C | F | Cb |
|---|---|---|---|
| **Marinades:** *Per 1 Tbsp* | | | |
| Garlic Herb | 15 | 0 | 3 |
| Lemon Pepper | 10 | 0 | 2 |
| Lime Garlic | 15 | 0 | 3 |
| Sweet Teriyaki | 35 | 0 | 9 |
| **Newman's Own:** *Per ½ Cup* | | | |
| Five Cheese | 80 | 2 | 11 |
| Fra Diavolo | 80 | 3 | 10 |
| Marinara; Sockarooni | 70 | 1 | 12 |
| Roasted Garlic & Peppers | 70 | 1.5 | 11 |
| Tomato & Basil Bombolina | 80 | 2 | 13 |
| Vodka | 120 | 5 | 13 |
| **O Organics (Von's):** *Per ½ Cup* | | | |
| Marinara; Roasted Garlic, av. | 60 | 1.5 | 9 |
| Mushroom; Tomato Basil | 50 | 1.5 | 8 |
| **Old El Paso:** | | | |
| **Enchilada Sauce:** | | | |
| Green Chile, ¼ cup | 25 | 1.5 | 4 |
| Other varieties, ¼ cup | 20 | 0 | 4 |
| **Salsa,** Thick & Chunky, all var., 2 Tbsp | 10 | 0 | 2 |
| **Taco Sauce,** all varieties, 1 Tbsp | 5 | 0 | 1 |
| **Pace:** *Per 2 Tbsp* | | | |
| Picante Sauce | 10 | 0 | 3 |
| **Salsa:** Thick & Chunky, av. | 10 | 0 | 2 |
| Fire, Mango & Habanero | 10 | 0 | 2 |
| Restaurant Style, Peach Mango | 15 | 0 | 4 |
| **Prego:** *Per ½ Cup* | | | |
| Alfredo, average all varieties | 150 | 14 | 6 |
| **Classic Italian:** | | | |
| Flavored with Meat | 90 | 3 | 13 |
| Fresh Mushroom; Traditional | 70 | 1.5 | 13 |
| Italian Sausage & Garlic | 90 | 3 | 13 |
| Marinara | 80 | 3 | 10 |
| Roasted Garlic & Herb | 80 | 2 | 13 |
| Three Cheese | 70 | 1.5 | 12 |
| Tomato, Basil & Garlic | 80 | 2.5 | 12 |
| **Chunky Garden:** | | | |
| Combo | 70 | 1.5 | 12 |
| Mushroom Supreme | 80 | 2.5 | 13 |
| **Heart Smart:** Ricotta Parmesan | 90 | 2.5 | 13 |
| Other varieties | 70 | 1.5 | 13 |
| **Pizza Sauce,** Pizzeria Style | 70 | 2 | 12 |
| **Premier Japan,** Hoisin; Teriyaki, 1 Tbsp | 15 | 0 | 3 |
| **Progresso:** *Per ½ Cup* | | | |
| **Recipe Starters:** | | | |
| Creamy Roasted Garlic | 70 | 5 | 4 |
| Fire Roasted Tomato | 60 | 2 | 10 |
| Average other varieties | 90 | 7 | 5 |

## Brands (Cont)

**C  F  Cb**

**Ragu:**

**Cheesy:** *Per ¼ Cup*

| | C | F | Cb |
|---|---|---|---|
| Classic Alfredo | 90 | 8 | 2 |
| Creamy Mozzarella | 80 | 7 | 2 |
| Creamy Tomato | 90 | 8 | 4 |
| Double Cheddar | 100 | 9 | 3 |
| Four Cheese | 80 | 8 | 2 |
| Light Parmesan Alfredo | 60 | 4 | 2 |
| Roasted Garlic Parmesan | 100 | 9 | 3 |
| Six Cheese | 90 | 3 | 13 |

**Chunky:** *Per ½ Cup*

| | C | F | Cb |
|---|---|---|---|
| Roasted Garlic | 80 | 2.5 | 14 |
| Average other varieties | 90 | 2.5 | 14 |

**Old World Style:** *Per ½ Cup*

| | C | F | Cb |
|---|---|---|---|
| Flavored with Meat | 70 | 2.5 | 10 |
| Marinara | 80 | 2.5 | 11 |
| Traditional | 80 | 2 | 11 |
| Light, Tomato & Basil | 50 | 0 | 10 |

| | C | F | Cb |
|---|---|---|---|
| **Pizza:** Homemade Style, ¼ cup | 30 | 1 | 5 |
| Quick Sauce, Traditional, ¼ cup | 45 | 1.5 | 6 |

**Safeway Select:**

| | C | F | Cb |
|---|---|---|---|
| Salsa, all varieties, average, 2 Tbsp | 15 | 0 | 3 |

**Select Sauces:** *Per ½ Cup*

| | C | F | Cb |
|---|---|---|---|
| Arrabbiata | 110 | 8 | 10 |
| Artichoke Pesto | 60 | 2 | 9 |
| Four Cheese | 80 | 3.5 | 11 |
| Marinara | 60 | 2 | 10 |
| Spicy Red Bell Pepper | 50 | 1 | 9 |
| Sundried Tomato & Olive | 60 | 1.5 | 11 |
| Tomato Alfredo; Vodka | 130 | 10 | 9 |

| | C | F | Cb |
|---|---|---|---|
| **Taco Bell,** Creamy Jalapeno Sauce, 1 Tablespoon, 0.5 oz | 70 | 7 | 1 |

**Tony Roma's:**

| | C | F | Cb |
|---|---|---|---|
| Bold & Spicy BBQ Sauce, 2 Tbsp | 50 | 0 | 12 |
| Carolina Honeys BBQ Sauce, 2 Tablespoons | 70 | 0 | 18 |

**Trader Joe's:**

BBQ Sauce,

| | C | F | Cb |
|---|---|---|---|
| Kansas City Style, 2 Tbsp | 60 | 0 | 15 |
| Tomato Basil Marinara, ½ cup | 80 | 4.5 | 10 |

**Walnut Acres,**

| | C | F | Cb |
|---|---|---|---|
| Organic Pasta Sauces, average all var., ½ cup, 4.5 oz | 50 | 1 | 9 |

## Seasonings & Flavorings

| | C | F | Cb |
|---|---|---|---|
| **Auromatic Bitters** *(Angostua)*, 1 tsp | 15 | 0 | 4 |
| **Bacon Bits,** average, 1 Tbsp | 35 | 2 | 2 |
| **Bacon Chips** *(Durkee)*, 1 Tbsp | 30 | 1 | 2 |
| **Bac-Os** *(Betty Crocker)*, 1Tbsp | 30 | 1.5 | 2 |
| **Blends** *(Mrs Dash)*, 1 tsp | 0 | 0 | 0 |
| **Butter Buds,** 1 tsp | 5 | 0 | 2 |
| **Flavor Enhancer** *(Accent)*, 1 tsp | 0 | 0 | 0 |
| **Flavor Sprinkles** *(Molly McButter)*, Natural/Cheese, 1 tsp | 5 | 0 | 1 |
| **Garlic Bread Sprinkle,** 1 tsp | 8 | 0.5 | 1 |
| **Garlic Salt,** 1 tsp | 2 | 0 | 0 |
| **Italian Seasoning,** 1 tsp | 4 | 0 | 1 |
| **Lemon Pepper Seasoning,** 1 tsp | 7 | 0 | 1 |
| **Meat Tenderizer,** av., 1 tsp | 7 | 0 | 1 |
| **Salad Crunchies** *(McCormick)*, 1 tsp | 10 | 0.5 | 2 |
| **Salt,** Reg., Sea Salt, Lite Salt | 0 | 0 | 0 |
| **Seasoning** *(Old Bay)*, ¼ tsp | 0 | 0 | 0 |
| **Seasoning Mix** *(Vegit)*, ¼ tsp | 0 | 0 | 0 |
| **Seasoning Mixes,** av., ¼ pkg | 70 | 1 | 9 |
| **Taco Seasoning,** av., ¼ pkg | 30 | 0.5 | 4 |
| **Bragg's,** Liquid Aminos | 0 | 0 | 0 |
| **Old El Paso:** Chili Season. Mix, 1 Tbsp | 8 | 0.5 | 1.5 |
| Cheesy Taco Seasoning Mix, 1 Tbsp | 10 | 0.5 | 2 |
| Taco/Burrito Seasoning Mix, 2 tsp | 15 | 0 | 4 |
| Fajita Seasoning Mix, 1 tsp | 5 | 0 | 1.5 |

## Spices & Herbs

| | C | F | Cb |
|---|---|---|---|
| **Average all types,** 1 tsp | 5 | 0 | 1 |
| **All Purpose,** 1 tsp | 0 | 0 | 0 |
| **Allspice,** ground | 5 | 0 | 1 |
| **Chili Powder** | 8 | 0 | 1 |
| **Cinnamon,** ground | 6 | 0 | 2 |
| **Curry Powder** | 6 | 0 | 1 |
| **Garlic Powder** | 9 | 0 | 2 |
| **Nutmeg,** ground | 12 | 0 | 1 |
| **Onion Powder** | 7 | 0 | 2 |
| **Parsley,** dried | 4 | 0 | 1 |
| **Pepper,** average | 6 | 0 | 1 |
| **Saffron** | 2 | 0 | 0 |
| **Salt-Free Blends,** 1 tsp | 0 | 0 | 0 |
| **Tumeric,** ground | 8 | 0 | 1 |
| **Seeds:** Fenugreek | 12 | 1 | 2 |
| Mustard, Poppyseed | 15 | 1 | 1 |
| Other varieties, average | 7 | 0 | 1 |

## Home-Popped Popcorn    **C**  **F**  **Cb**

| | C | F | Cb |
|---|---|---|---|
| **Popping Corn Kernels,** | | | |
| 2 Tbsp, 1 oz | 110 | 1 | 26 |
| (makes approximately 5 cups) | | | |
| **Air-popped,** without oil: Plain, 1 oz | 110 | 1 | 22 |
| 1 cup, 0.2 oz | 20 | 0 | 5 |
| **Oil-popped:** Plain, 1 oz | 145 | 8 | 16 |
| 1 cup, 0.4 oz | 55 | 3 | 6 |
| **Popcorn Oil,** 1 Tbsp | 120 | 14 | 0 |

## Microwave Popcorn

*Average all Brands: Per 1 Cup Popped, Unless Indicated*

| | C | F | Cb |
|---|---|---|---|
| Butter: Regular, 1 cup | 35 | 2 | 4 |
| Light, 1 cup | 25 | 1 | 4 |
| **Act II Popcorn:** | | | |
| **Butter:** 1 cup | 25 | 1 | 4 |
| 4½ cups, 1 oz | 120 | 5 | 19 |
| **94% Fat-Free Butter:** | | | |
| 1 cup | 20 | 0.5 | 4 |
| 6½ cups, 1 oz | 130 | 2 | 27 |
| **Butter Lovers:** 1 cup | 25 | 1 | 4 |
| 4½ cups, 1 oz | 120 | 4 | 19 |
| **Xreme Butter:** 1 cup | 25 | 1 | 4 |
| 4½ cups | 120 | 4 | 19 |
| **BodyKey** *(Amway),* Slim Popcorn, | | | |
| Sea Salt, 1 bag | 110 | 7 | 10 |
| **Jolly Time:** | | | |
| **Blast O Butter,** 1 cup | 45 | 3 | 4 |
| **Light Butter,** 1 cup | 25 | 1 | 4 |
| **Xtra Butter:** 1 cup | 40 | 2.5 | 4 |
| 4 cups | 160 | 10 | 16 |
| **Newman's Own:** | | | |
| **Butter Flavor,** Microwave: | | | |
| Regular, 3½ cups | 130 | 5 | 18 |
| Light, 3½ cups | 120 | 4 | 19 |
| **Butter Boom,** 3½ cups | 130 | 5 | 18 |
| **Orville Redenbacher's:** | | | |
| **Family Favorites:** | | | |
| Butter: 4 cups | 170 | 12 | 17 |
| Light, 5½ cups | 120 | 5 | 19 |
| Movie Theater Butter, 4 cups | 160 | 9 | 19 |
| Ultimate Butter, 5 cups | 170 | 12 | 16 |
| **Natural,** Lime & Salt, 5 cups | 220 | 15 | 21 |
| **Sweet & Savory,** | | | |
| Cheddar Cheese, 4½ cups | 180 | 14 | 16 |
| **Pop Secret:** *Per Cup* | | | |
| 94% Fat-Free, Butter | 20 | 0 | 3 |
| Double Butter | 40 | 2.5 | 3 |

## Bagged Popcorn    **C**  **F**  **Cb**

*Average All Brands (Ready-to-Eat)*

| | C | F | Cb |
|---|---|---|---|
| **Regular/Plain:** ½ oz package | 80 | 5 | 8 |
| 1 oz package | 160 | 10 | 16 |
| 4 oz package | 640 | 40 | 64 |
| 2 oz Box (store/airport) | 320 | 16 | 32 |
| 3 oz Bag (9" high x 5" wide) | 480 | 24 | 48 |
| **Caramel Popcorn,** | | | |
| with nuts, 1 cup, 1.5 oz | 230 | 12 | 39 |

## Bagged Popcorn ~ Brands

| | C | F | Cb |
|---|---|---|---|
| **Boston's,** Lite, 3½ cups, 1 oz | 130 | 4.5 | 20 |
| **Cracker Jack:** Original, 1 cup, 2 oz | 240 | 4 | 46 |
| Chocolate & Caramel, 1 cup, 2 oz | 220 | 1 | 50 |
| **Crunch 'N Munch:** | | | |
| **Buttery Toffee:** ⅔ cup, 1 oz | 150 | 6 | 22 |
| 1 cup, 1.6 oz | 220 | 9 | 32 |
| **Caramel:** ⅔ cup, 1 oz | 160 | 8 | 20 |
| 1 cup, 1.6 oz | 230 | 12 | 29 |
| 12 oz box | 1745 | 87 | 218 |
| **Fiddle Faddle:** | | | |
| Average all varieties: 1 oz | 120 | 2 | 24 |
| 1 cup, 2 oz | 240 | 4 | 48 |
| 6 oz box | 720 | 12 | 144 |
| **Popcorn Indiana:** | | | |
| **Kettlecorn,** | | | |
| Original, 2 cups, 1 oz | 130 | 5 | 21 |
| **Popcorn:** | | | |
| Aged White Cheddar, 2.5 cups, 1 oz | 150 | 9 | 14 |
| Chicago Style, | | | |
| Caramel & Cheese, 1 cup, 1 oz | 140 | 6 | 20 |
| Movie Theater, 2 cups, 1 oz | 160 | 12 | 13 |
| Seasalt, 3.5 cups, 1 oz | 130 | 6 | 17 |
| **Poppycock:** | | | |
| Original/Pecan Delight, av: | | | |
| ½ cup, 1 oz | 155 | 8 | 20 |
| 1 cup, 2 oz | 310 | 16 | 40 |
| Cashew Lovers, ½ cup, 1 oz | 150 | 6 | 20 |
| Chocolate Lovers, ½ cup, 1.2 oz | 160 | 7 | 22 |

## Movie Theater Popcorn

| | C | F | Cb |
|---|---|---|---|
| **Small,** (7 cups): Plain | 385 | 21 | 44 |
| With Butter (3 pumps, 0.8 oz) | 570 | 42 | 44 |
| **Medium,** (15 cups): Plain | 825 | 45 | 94 |
| With Butter (4 pumps, 1 oz) | 1075 | 73 | 94 |
| **Large,** (20 cups): Plain | 1100 | 60 | 124 |
| With Butter (6 pumps, 1.5 oz) | 1485 | 102 | 124 |
| **Butter:** 1 Pump, 0.3 oz | 65 | 7 | 0 |
| 4 Pumps (2 Tbsp), 1 oz | 250 | 28 | 0 |

## Corn & Tortilla Chips  C  F  Cb

*Average All Brands*

**Corn Chips:**

| | C | F | Cb |
|---|---|---|---|
| Average all types: 1 oz | 150 | 8 | 18 |
| 8 oz bag | 1200 | 64 | 144 |
| *Fritos*, Original, 32 chips, 1 oz | 160 | 10 | 15 |

**Tortilla Chips:** Average, 1 oz | 140 | 7 | 18

(1 oz = approx. 12 chips or 13 strips)

| | C | F | Cb |
|---|---|---|---|
| *Doritos*: Original, 1 oz | 140 | 7 | 18 |
| Nacho Chse; Salsa Verde, av., 1 oz | 140 | 8 | 18 |
| *Popchips*: Chili Limon, 1 oz | 120 | 4 | 19 |
| Nacho Cheese, 1 oz | 130 | 5 | 18 |
| *Snyder's:* | | | |
| El Restaurante, all flavors, 1 oz | 150 | 8 | 17 |
| Yellow Corn/White, av., 1 oz | 135 | 5 | 21 |
| *Tostitos:* | | | |
| Average all flav., 1 oz | 145 | 7 | 19 |
| Baked! Scoops, 1 oz | 120 | 3 | 22 |
| *Utz:* Multigrain, 1 oz | 150 | 8 | 16 |
| Baked, 1 oz | 120 | 2 | 23 |
| Other flavors, 1 oz | 140 | 8 | 18 |

## Potato Chips/Crisps

*Average All Brands*

**Regular:**

| | C | F | Cb |
|---|---|---|---|
| Plain or flavored, (4 chips) | 30 | 2 | 3 |
| 1 oz package (20 chips) | 150 | 10 | 15 |
| 4 oz quantity | 600 | 40 | 60 |
| 14 oz package | 2100 | 140 | 210 |

## Chips/Crisps ~ Brands

| | C | F | Cb |
|---|---|---|---|
| **Lay's** *(Fritolay):* | | | |
| Air Pops, av. all flavors, 1 oz | 125 | 4 | 21 |
| Regular; Wavy, av. all flavors, 1 oz | 160 | 10 | 15 |
| Kettle Cooked, 1 oz | 135 | 6 | 19 |
| **Pringles:** | | | |
| All Flavors, 1 oz | 150 | 9 | 15 |
| Large can, 6 oz | 900 | 54 | 90 |
| Reduced Fat, all flavors, 1 oz | 140 | 7 | 17 |
| Fat Free, all flavors, 15 crisps, 1 oz | 70 | 0 | 15 |
| Multi Grain, av. all flavors, 1 oz | 140 | 8 | 17 |
| Snack Stacks, all flav., 1 tub | 110 | 7 | 11 |
| Cheez Ummms, all flavors, 1 oz | 150 | 9 | 15 |
| **Ruffles:** Regular, av. all flavors, 1 oz | 160 | 11 | 15 |
| Baked!, average all flavors, 1 oz | 120 | 3.5 | 21 |
| **Simply7,** Hummus/Lentil Chips, | | | |
| average all flavors, 1 oz | 135 | 5 | 19 |
| **Sun Chips,** Original, 16 crisps, 1 oz | 140 | 6 | 18 |

## Pretzels  C  F  Cb

*Average All Brands*

**Hard-Baked Pretzels:** *Each*

| | C | F | Cb |
|---|---|---|---|
| 1 oz quantity | 110 | 1 | 23 |
| Sticks, thin, 2¼" (9/oz) | 12 | 0 | 3 |
| Twists, thin, ¼" thick, (5/oz) | 25 | 0 | 5 |
| Dutch (2¾"x 2⅝"), 0.5 oz | 55 | 1 | 11 |
| *Snyders*, Sourdough, 0.8oz | 100 | 0 | 22 |

**Soft Pretzel Twists,** average: *Each*

| | C | F | Cb |
|---|---|---|---|
| Plain: Small, 2 oz | 210 | 2 | 43 |
| Medium, 4 oz | 390 | 3.5 | 80 |
| Large, 5 oz | 485 | 4.5 | 100 |
| Big Cheese, 1.8 oz | 130 | 3 | 22 |
| New York Street Vendors, 7 oz | 660 | 6 | 135 |
| *Trader Joe's*, Peanut Butter filled, 1 oz | 140 | 8 | 14 |
| *Snyder's:* Milk Chocolate Dips, 1 oz | 140 | 6 | 19 |
| White Creme Dips, 1 oz | 130 | 6 | 19 |

## Pretzels ~ Brands

| | C | F | Cb |
|---|---|---|---|
| **Flipz:** Milk Choc, 8 pieces, 1 oz | 130 | 5 | 20 |
| White Fudge, 7 pcs, 1 oz | 130 | 5 | 20 |
| **Rold Gold** *(Frito-Lay):* | | | |
| Braided Twists, | | | |
| Honey Wheat (8), 1 oz | 110 | 1 | 24 |
| Pretzel, Sourdough (1) | 90 | 1 | 19 |
| Pretzel Dippers, 1 pkg | 230 | 12 | 29 |
| Pretzel Thins, 1 oz | 120 | 2 | 23 |
| Rods/Tiny Twists, av., 1 oz | 110 | 1 | 23 |
| Sticks, 1 oz | 100 | 0 | 23 |
| **Snyder's of Hanover:** | | | |
| Gluten Free Pretzel Sticks (30) | 110 | 1.5 | 25 |
| Homestyle (4), 1 oz | 120 | 1 | 25 |
| Pieces, Bacon Cheddar , 1 oz | 140 | 7 | 17 |
| Rods (3), 1 oz | 120 | 1 | 24 |
| Sticks (28), 1 oz | 110 | 1 | 23 |
| Thins (11), 1 oz | 110 | 0 | 23 |
| **SuperPretzel:** | | | |
| **Soft:** Original (1), 2.3 oz | 160 | 1 | 34 |
| Sweet Cinnamon (1), | | | |
| with topping, 2.5 oz | 200 | 2 | 42 |
| Bites (5), 1.9 oz | 140 | 0.5 | 32 |
| Softstix, av. all flavors, (2), 1.8 oz | 125 | 3 | 22 |
| **Utz:** Sourdough, Hard (1) | 90 | 0 | 18 |
| Cinnamon, 1 oz | 120 | 1.5 | 24 |

| Snacks | C | F | Cb |
|---|---|---|---|
| Note: Actual weight of packaged snacks is usually 5-10% more than label Net Wt. For accuracy, weigh snack and allow extra calories, fat and carbs for any extra weight. | | | |
| **Apple Chips** *(Seneca)*, av., 1 oz | **140** | 7 | 20 |
| **Bagel Crisps** *(N.Y. Style)*, 6 crisps, 1 oz | **130** | 6 | 17 |
| **Baguette Chips** *(Pillsbury)*, av., (21) | **130** | 5 | 20 |
| **Banana Chips** *(T.Joe's)*, 13 chips, 1 oz | **160** | 11 | 13 |
| **Beef Jerky** *(Jack Link's)*, av., 1 oz | **80** | 1 | 4 |
| **Beef Sticks:** *(Slim Jim)*, Orig., 2 oz | **150** | 3 | 10 |
|   *Jack Links*, Original, 1.5 oz | **160** | 13 | 2 |
| **BodyKey** *(Amway)*: | | | |
|   Mixed Nuts & Pumpkin Seeds, 1 bag | **200** | 16 | 8 |
|   Whole Grain Tortilla Chips, 1 bag | **210** | 11 | 24 |
| **Bugles,** Original; Nacho Cheese, 1 oz | **160** | 9 | 18 |
| **Cheese Balls** *(Utz)*, 1 oz serving | **150** | 9 | 16 |
| **Cheese Nips,** 1.3 oz package | **170** | 7 | 22 |
| **Cheese Puffs,** average, 1 oz | **160** | 10 | 15 |
| **Cheese Twists,** 1 oz | **140** | 8 | 15 |
| **Cheerios,** Snack Mix, | | | |
|   average, ⅔ cup, 1 oz | **120** | 3 | 21 |
| **Cheetos:** | | | |
|   Crunchy: Av. all flavors, 1 oz | **155** | 11 | 13 |
|     4 oz package | **640** | 40 | 60 |
|   Baked!; Fantastix, | | | |
|     all varieties, av., 1 oz | **130** | 5 | 19 |
|   Simply Puffs, | | | |
|     White Cheddar, 1 oz | **150** | 9 | 16 |
| **Cheez-It Crackers** *(Sunshine)*: | | | |
|   Original, 1.3 oz package | **180** | 9 | 20 |
|   Original Big (13), 1 oz | **150** | 8 | 17 |
|   Colby, 0.8 oz pouch | **110** | 6 | 12 |
|   Mozzarella (25), 1 oz | **150** | 7 | 19 |
|   Reduced Fat: Original, 1 oz | **130** | 4.5 | 20 |
|     White Cheddar, 1 oz | **130** | 4 | 22 |
| **Chester's:** Fries, Flamin' Hot, 1 pkg | **140** | 8 | 16 |
|   Puffcorn, Cheese, 1 oz | **160** | 11 | 14 |
| **Chex Mix,** *(General Mills)*, | | | |
|   Traditional, 1 oz | **120** | 3.5 | 21 |
| **Chips Ahoy!,** Choc Chip Cookies: | | | |
|   1.4 oz Single Serve Pack | **190** | 9 | 27 |
|   Minis: Go-Pak!, 1 package, 3.5 oz | **525** | 25 | 70 |
|     Snak Sak, 1 package, 8 oz | **1050** | 49 | 147 |
| **Chicharrones** ~ *See Pork Skins* | | | |
| **Churros** *(Rubio's)*, 9", 1.6 oz | **170** | 8 | 22 |
| **Combos:** | | | |
|   Crackers, av. all flavors, ⅓ cup, 1 oz | **140** | 6 | 18 |
| **Cool Cuts,** Carrot & Ranch, 2.3 oz | **70** | 5 | 5 |
| **Corn Chips** ~ *See Page 149* | | | |
| **Corn Nuts:** Av all flav., 1 oz | **130** | 4.5 | 20 |
|   1.7 oz bag | **210** | 8 | 34 |
| **Corn Puffs/Twists,** (32 approx), 1 oz | **160** | 11 | 15 |

| Snacks (Cont) | C | F | Cb |
|---|---|---|---|
| **Dunkin Stix** *(Dolly Madison)*, (3) | **490** | 25 | 63 |
| **Edamame,** | | | |
|   *Seapointe,* Dry Roasted, 1 oz | **130** | 4 | 10 |
| **Fritos:** Corn Chips, all varieties, av., 1oz | **150** | 10 | 15 |
|   Flavor Twists, Honey BBQ, 1 oz | **150** | 9 | 16 |
| **Funyuns,** Onion Flavored, 1 oz | **140** | 7 | 18 |
| **Goldfish,** av. all flavors 1 oz | **140** | 5 | 20 |
| **Gold-n-Chees** *(Lance)*: | | | |
|   Snack Mix, 1 oz | **150** | 8 | 17 |
|   Tube, 1 oz | **130** | 6 | 18 |
| **Gripz,** *(Sunshine)*, Mighty Tiny, 0.9 oz | **120** | 6 | 15 |
| **Hot Peanuts** *(Munchies)*, 1.7 oz | **310** | 25 | 10 |
| **Lance:** | | | |
|   Cracker Creations, Granola, av. all ,(2) | **190** | 9 | 24 |
|   Sandwich Crackers, av. all, 6 crackers | **200** | 9 | 25 |
| **Munchies** *(Frito-Lay)*, | | | |
|   Snack Mix, all flavors, 1 oz | **140** | 7 | 18 |
| **Munchos,** all flavors, 16 pieces, 1 oz | **160** | 10 | 16 |
| **Newtons:** | | | |
|   Single Serve: 2 oz pkg | **200** | 4 | 40 |
|   Fat-Free, 2 oz package | **200** | 0 | 46 |
| **Nutter Butter,** Sandwich Cookies: | | | |
|   Singles, 1.9 oz pkg | **250** | 10 | 37 |
|   Bites, Go-Pak, 3.5 oz | **490** | 21 | 74 |
| **Onion Rings** *(T.G.I. Friday)*, 1 oz | **140** | 7 | 16 |
| **Oreo Cookies,** all Creme Fillings: | | | |
|   Double Stuf (2), 1 oz | **140** | 7 | 21 |
|   Mini Bite Size: | | | |
|     1.3 oz pkg | **170** | 7 | 25 |
|     Go-Pak, 3.5 oz | **455** | 21 | 74 |
| **Oreo Cakesters,** soft, 2 oz | **250** | 12 | 36 |
| **Oriental Mix Rice Snacks,** 1 oz | **125** | 3.5 | 21 |
| **Peanut Butter Nuggets,** (10), 1 oz | **140** | 6 | 15 |
| **Pepitas,** dried or roasted, | | | |
|   ¼ cup, 1 oz | **155** | 14 | 3 |
| **Pirate's Booty:** | | | |
|   Aged White Cheddar, 4 oz bag | **520** | 20 | 76 |
|   Fruity Booty, 4 oz bag | **520** | 20 | 68 |
| **Pita Chips,** (9), average, 1 oz | **130** | 4 | 18 |
| **Plaintain Chips,** | | | |
|   *Goya*, 34 chips, 1 oz | **150** | 8 | 19 |
| **PopCorners,** Butter/Kettle, 1 oz | **125** | 3.5 | 20 |
| **Popcorn** ~ *See Page 148* | | | |
| **Pork Cracklins,** 1 oz | **160** | 12 | 0 |
| **Pork Skins/Rinds:** 1 oz | **160** | 10 | 0 |
|   *Baken-ets*, Traditional, 0.5 oz | **80** | 5 | 0 |
|   *Mission*, Chiccarones, 4 oz package | **640** | 40 | 0 |
| **Potato Chips** ~ *See Page 149* | | | |
| **Potato Skins** *(TGI Friday)*, | | | |
|   all flavors, 16 chips, 1 oz | **140** | 8 | 15 |
| **Puffed Wheat,** | | | |
|   *Sabritones*, Chili & Lime, 1 oz | **150** | 10 | 13 |
| **Pretzels** ~ *See Page 149* | | | |

## Snacks (Cont)

| | C | F | Cb |
|---|---|---|---|
| **Puffed Wheat,** | | | |
| Sabritones, Chili & Lime, 1 oz | 150 | 10 | 13 |
| **Pretzels** ~ See Page 149Rice Cakes: | | | |
| Lundberg, (1), average, 0.7 oz | 75 | 0.5 | 16 |
| Quaker: Plain, lightly salted, 0.3 oz | 35 | 0 | 7 |
| Chocolate (1), 0.5 oz | 60 | 1 | 12 |
| **Rice Chips:** | | | |
| Lundberg, average, 1 oz | 140 | 7 | 18 |
| Quaker, Popped White Cheddar & Herb, | | | |
| 16 chips, 1 oz | 130 | 5 | 19 |
| **Sandwich Crackers:** | | | |
| Austin, Cheese Crackers: | | | |
| With Cheddar, 1.4 oz | 190 | 10 | 23 |
| With Peanut Butter, 1.3 oz | 190 | 10 | 23 |
| PB & J Flavored, 1.4 oz | 190 | 8 | 26 |
| Lance: | | | |
| Nip Chee, 6 pieces | 190 | 9 | 24 |
| Toasty, 6 pieces | 180 | 8 | 21 |
| Toast Chee, 6 pieces | 210 | 10 | 25 |
| Ritz Bits: | | | |
| Cheese: 1.5 oz package | 220 | 12 | 25 |
| Go-Pak: 13 crackers, 1 oz | 150 | 8 | 16 |
| 3.5 oz Pak | 520 | 29 | 58 |
| P'nut Butter: 1.3 oz pkg | 170 | 10 | 20 |
| Big Bag, 3 oz | 450 | 25 | 50 |
| **Sesame Sticks,** | | | |
| SunRidge Farm, 1 oz | 170 | 12 | 14 |
| **Smart Puffs,** | | | |
| Pirates Booty, 1 oz | 140 | 7 | 16 |
| **Snack Mix,** | | | |
| Quaker, Baked Cheddar, 1 package | 230 | 8 | 34 |
| **Soy Crisps,** average, 1 oz | 120 | 3 | 17 |
| **Soy Nuts,** Dry Roasted, ¼ cup, 1 oz | 130 | 6 | 9 |
| Choc-coated, 1 oz | 140 | 7 | 13 |
| **Sun Chips,** | | | |
| Fritolay, average, 1 oz | 140 | 6 | 19 |
| **Takis:** Fajitas, 1 oz | 140 | 7 | 17 |
| 4 oz package | 560 | 28 | 68 |
| **Tings,** | | | |
| Robert's, 2 oz bag | 300 | 16 | 36 |
| **Toasted Chips** (Ritz), av. all, 1 oz | 130 | 5.5 | 20 |
| **Tortilla Chips/Tostitos** ~ Page 149 | | | |
| **Trail Mix** (Nuts/Seeds/Dried Fruit): | | | |
| Regular, 3 Tbsp, 1 oz | 140 | 9 | 13 |
| Tropical, 3 Tbsp, 1 oz | 130 | 7 | 16 |
| **Turkey Jerky:** Teriyaki, 1 oz | 80 | 1 | 8 |
| Trader Joe's, Original, 1 oz | 60 | 0.5 | 6 |
| **Veggie Crisps,** | | | |
| Snyder's, 1 oz | 140 | 7 | 18 |
| **Wheat Thins** (Nabisco), av. all, 1 oz | 135 | 5 | 19 |
| **Yogurt Pretzels,** 1.5 oz | 190 | 8 | 28 |
| **Yogurt Raisins,** | | | |
| Sun-Maid, 1 oz | 120 | 4.5 | 20 |

## Fruit Snacks

| | C | F | Cb |
|---|---|---|---|
| **Betty Crocker:** Fruit Gushers, 0.9 oz | 90 | 1 | 20 |
| Fruit by the Foot, 1 roll, 0.8 oz | 80 | 1 | 17 |
| Fruit Roll Ups, 1 roll, 0.5 oz | 50 | 1 | 12 |
| Fruit Flavored Shapes, | | | |
| all varieties, 0.9 oz | 80 | 0 | 19 |
| **Sunkist:** Fruit Snacks, 1 pouch | 80 | 0 | 19 |
| Fruit Smoothie Blitz, 1.3 oz | 140 | 1 | 32 |

## Vending Machines

| | C | F | Cb |
|---|---|---|---|
| **Bugles,** Nacho Cheese, 1 oz | 160 | 9 | 18 |
| **Cheese Balls** (Utz), 1 oz | 150 | 9 | 16 |
| **Cheetos,** Crunchy, 1 oz | 150 | 10 | 13 |
| **Cheeze-It,** Snack Mix, 1.5 oz | 195 | 6.5 | 30 |
| **Chex Mix,** Cheddar, 1 oz | 120 | 3.5 | 22 |
| **Chester's,** Flamin' Hot Fries, 1 oz | 140 | 8 | 16 |
| **Choc Chip Cookies:** | | | |
| Chips Ahoy, 1.4 oz | 190 | 9 | 27 |
| Famous Amos, (4), 1 oz | 150 | 8 | 18 |
| Grandma's, (2), 2.5 oz | 340 | 28 | 55 |
| **Chocolate Bars:** | | | |
| Hershey's, Milk Choc.,1.6 oz | 210 | 13 | 26 |
| Kit Kat, 1.5 oz | 210 | 11 | 27 |
| Snickers, 1.9 oz bar | 250 | 12 | 33 |
| **Donut,** plain cake, 1.4 oz | 160 | 9 | 18 |
| **Doritos,** av. all flavors, 1 oz | 145 | 8 | 18 |
| **Fritos,** Corn Chips, Orig., 1.8 oz | 280 | 17 | 26 |
| **Fruit Pie,** | | | |
| Hostess, 4.5 oz | 480 | 20 | 68 |
| **Granola/Cereal Bars,** av., 1 oz | 140 | 3 | 26 |
| **M & M's:** | | | |
| Milk Chocolate, 1.7 oz | 240 | 10 | 34 |
| Peanuts, 1.8 oz | 250 | 13 | 30 |
| **Oreo Cookies,** 2 oz | 270 | 11 | 41 |
| **Peanut Butter Cups,** | | | |
| Reese's, 1.5 oz | 210 | 13 | 24 |
| **Popcorn,** plain, 1 oz | 160 | 10 | 16 |
| **Pop Chips,** 0.8 oz | 100 | 3 | 16 |
| **Pork Skins,** 1.5 oz | 240 | 15 | 0 |
| **Potato Chips:** 1 oz | 150 | 10 | 15 |
| Baked! (Ruffles), Orig.,1 oz | 160 | 10 | 15 |
| **Potato Skins** (TGI Friday's), | | | |
| all flavors, 1 oz | 140 | 8 | 15 |
| **Pretzels** (Snyder's), Old Time, 1 oz | 120 | 1 | 24 |
| **Raisins,** 0.5 oz package | 45 | 0 | 11 |
| **Rice Krispies Treat** | 90 | 2 | 17 |
| **Skittles,** 2 oz | 230 | 2.5 | 52 |
| **Starburst,** Fruit Chews, Orig., 1.4 oz | 160 | 3.5 | 33 |
| **Tortilla Chips,** 1 oz | 140 | 7 | 18 |

## Homemade & Restaurant

| Restaurant & Take-Out:<br>*Average All Preparations: Per 8 fl.oz* | **C** | **F** | **Cb** |
|---|---|---|---|
| Bean Medley | 200 | 3 | 34 |
| Beef Consomme | 30 | 0 | 2 |
| Borscht, with Sour Cream | 130 | 8 | 14 |
| Bouillabaisse | 400 | 15 | 10 |
| Chicken & Corn | 290 | 14 | 20 |
| Chicken & Wild Rice | 80 | 4 | 9 |
| Chicken Consomme | 50 | 0 | 2 |
| Chicken Curry | 180 | 8 | 18 |
| Chicken Jambalaya | 160 | 7 | 8 |
| Chicken Noodle | 80 | 2 | 12 |
| With Chicken | 160 | 4 | 12 |
| Chicken Soup | 80 | 2 | 6 |
| Chili with Beans | 250 | 12 | 25 |
| Clam Chowder | 240 | 15 | 17 |
| Corn & Crab | 120 | 3 | 18 |
| Corn Chowder | 150 | 8 | 16 |
| Cream of Broccoli | 200 | 12 | 20 |
| Cream of Potato | 150 | 6.5 | 17 |
| Cream of Mushroom | 200 | 13 | 15 |
| Fish Chowder | 220 | 15 | 6 |
| French Onion | 420 | 15 | 25 |
| Gazpacho | 50 | 0 | 5 |
| Lentil Soup | 250 | 9 | 28 |
| Lobster Bisque | 320 | 15 | 10 |
| Matzo Ball, with 1 large ball | 180 | 7 | 24 |
| Minestrone | 125 | 2.5 | 20 |
| Mulligatawny | 300 | 15 | 8 |
| Pea & Ham | 240 | 10 | 25 |
| Potato & Bacon | 170 | 7 | 19 |
| Pumpkin, Creamy | 210 | 10 | 26 |
| Shark Fin Soup | 100 | 4 | 8 |
| Spicy Shrimp Soup, 1 bowl | 160 | 7 | 10 |
| Split Pea Soup | 180 | 2.5 | 30 |
| Vegetable (Fat Free) | 75 | 0 | 18 |
| Vegetable Beef | 80 | 2 | 10 |
| Vichyssoise | 200 | 9 | 15 |
| Watercress | 90 | 4 | 13 |

**Other Soups ~** *See International & Fast-Foods Sections (Arby's, Au Bon Pain, Boston Market, Dunkin' Donuts, Denny's, Schlotzsky's, Sizzler, Souplantation, Sweet Tomatoes, Zoup!)*
**Homemade Soups:** *Calculate calories, fat and carbohydrates from recipe ingredients.*

## Bouillon Cubes & Powders

| Bouillon Cubes: *Average all types* | **C** | **F** | **Cb** |
|---|---|---|---|
| Regular, 1 cube | 5 | 0 | 1 |
| Extra Large, 1 cube | 20 | 1 | 1 |
| **Powders**, average, 1 tsp | 10 | 0 | 1 |
| **Herb-Ox:**<br>Instant Broth & Seasoning, | | | |
| Beef, 1 envelope, 0.14 oz | 5 | 0 | 1 |
| Chicken, 1 envelope, 0.14 oz | 5 | 0 | 1 |

## Soup ~ Brands

**Amy's:**
**Heat & Serve (Organic):** *Per 1 Cup, Unless Indicated*

| | **C** | **F** | **Cb** |
|---|---|---|---|
| Alphabet | 80 | 0 | 16 |
| Chunky Vegetable | 60 | 0 | 13 |
| Cream of M'shrm, ¾ cup | 150 | 9 | 13 |
| Curried Lentil | 230 | 8 | 30 |
| Fire Roasted Sthwestern Veggie | 140 | 3 | 21 |
| Lentil | 180 | 5 | 25 |
| Lentil Vegetable | 160 | 4 | 24 |
| Rustic Italian Vegetable | 140 | 6 | 18 |
| Split Pea | 100 | 0 | 19 |
| Thai Coconut | 140 | 10 | 9 |
| Tuscan Bean & Rice | 160 | 4.5 | 25 |

**Andersen's:** *Per 1 Cup*

| | | | |
|---|---|---|---|
| Split Pea | 130 | 0 | 24 |
| Split Pea flavored with Bacon | 140 | 1 | 23 |

**Bertoli:** *Per ½ Package, 12 oz*
**Meal Soups:** 

| | | | |
|---|---|---|---|
| Chicken Minestrone | 370 | 18 | 32 |
| Roasted Chicken & Rotini Pasta | 290 | 12 | 28 |
| Ricotta & Lobster Ravioli,<br>in Seafood Bisque | 380 | 16 | 41 |
| Tomato Florentine<br>& Tortellini with Chicken | 410 | 19 | 36 |
| Tuscan-Style Beef & Vegetables | 360 | 20 | 26 |

**Campbell's:**
**Chunky:** *Per 8 fl.oz Cup*

| | | | |
|---|---|---|---|
| Baked Potato w/ Ched. & Bacon Bits | 190 | 9 | 23 |
| BBQ Seasoned Pork | 160 | 1 | 28 |
| Beef Burrito | 190 | 9 | 21 |
| Beer–n–Cheese, with Beef & Bacon | 190 | 9 | 21 |
| Chicken Corn Chowder | 190 | 10 | 20 |
| Classic Chicken Noodle | 110 | 3 | 14 |
| Healthy Request: | | | |
| Beef w/ Country Veggies | 110 | 1.5 | 17 |
| Chicken Corn Chowder | 140 | 3 | 22 |
| Chicken Noodle | 100 | 1 | 16 |
| New England Clam Chowder | 130 | 3 | 20 |
| Split Pea & Ham, Smoke Flavor | 160 | 2.5 | 22 |
| Mushroom Swiss Burger | 160 | 7 | 17 |
| Sausage & Pepper Rigatoni | 190 | 8 | 22 |

### Campbell's (Cont):
#### Chunky (Cont):

| | C | F | Cb |
|---|---|---|---|
| Hearty: Beef Noodle | 120 | 2 | 17 |
| Italian Style Wedding, with M'balls & Spinach | 120 | 3 | 15 |
| Wicked Thai Style Chicken, with Rice & Vegetables | 160 | 6 | 21 |

#### Condensed Soup: Per ½ Cup, 4 fl.oz

| | C | F | Cb |
|---|---|---|---|
| Bean with Bacon | 160 | 3 | 26 |
| Beef with Veggies & Barley | 80 | 1 | 15 |
| Chicken Noodle | 60 | 2 | 8 |
| Cream of Broccoli | 90 | 5 | 9 |
| Cream of Celery/Mushroom | 100 | 7 | 9 |
| Cream of Potato | 90 | 2 | 16 |
| Homestyle Chicken Noodle | 70 | 2 | 10 |
| Old Fashioned Tomato Rice | 130 | 1.5 | 26 |
| Split Pea w/ Ham & Bacon | 180 | 2 | 29 |
| Tomato | 90 | 0 | 20 |

#### Go Soups: Per 8 fl.oz Cup

| | C | F | Cb |
|---|---|---|---|
| Chicken & Quinoa with Chilies | 150 | 2.5 | 20 |
| Coconut Curry w/ Chicken & Shitaki Mushrooms | 150 | 5 | 17 |
| Creamy Red Pepper with Smoked Gouda | 220 | 15 | 15 |
| Golden Lentil w/ Madras Curry | 140 | 6 | 18 |
| Moroccan Style Chicken & Chickpeas | 180 | 2.5 | 26 |
| Spicy Chorizo, Chkn & Black Beans | 230 | 8 | 29 |

#### Gourmet Bisques: Per 8 fl.oz Cup

| | C | F | Cb |
|---|---|---|---|
| Golden Butternut Squash | 110 | 2 | 21 |
| Sweet Potato Tomatillo | 160 | 8 | 19 |
| Thai Tomato Coconut | 170 | 5 | 27 |
| Tomato Rstd Garlic Bacon | 210 | 8 | 31 |

#### Homestyle: Per 8 fl.oz Cup

| | C | F | Cb |
|---|---|---|---|
| Butternut Squash Bisque | 110 | 3 | 19 |
| Chicken Noodle | 90 | 2.5 | 10 |
| Creamy Chicken & Herb Dumplings | 160 | 9 | 14 |
| Creamy Gouda Bisque with Chicken | 190 | 11 | 16 |
| Harvest Tomato with Basil | 110 | 1 | 23 |
| Italian-Style Wedding | 120 | 3.5 | 15 |
| Maryland-Style Crab Soup | 80 | 0.5 | 14 |
| Mexican-Style Chkn Tortilla | 130 | 2 | 20 |
| Minestrone | 100 | 1 | 18 |
| New England Clam Chwdr | 170 | 10 | 15 |
| Potato Broccoli Cheese | 170 | 10 | 16 |
| Southwest-Style White Chkn Chili | 130 | 2.5 | 20 |
| Zesty Tomato Bisque | 110 | 2 | 19 |
| Light: Chicken Noodle | 70 | 1 | 9 |
| New England Clam Chowder | 120 | 4 | 15 |
| Italian-Style Wedding | 80 | 1.5 | 11 |
| Southwestern-Style Vegetable | 50 | 0 | 10 |

### Campbell's (Cont):
#### Slow Kettle Style: Per 8 fl.oz

| | C | F | Cb |
|---|---|---|---|
| Braised Beef Stew | 150 | 3 | 19 |
| Portobello Mushroom & Madeira Bisque | 240 | 18 | 16 |
| Southwest Style Chicken Chili with Black Beans | 190 | 2 | 28 |
| Tomato & Sweet Basil Bisque | 290 | 16 | 33 |
| Tuscan Style Chicken & White Bean | 140 | 2.5 | 17 |

### Health Valley Organics:
#### Creamed: Per 8 fl.oz Cup

| | C | F | Cb |
|---|---|---|---|
| Cream of Chicken | 110 | 3 | 15 |
| Cream of Celery | 100 | 2 | 17 |
| Cream of Mushroom | 90 | 2 | 14 |

#### Fat Free, 40% Less Sodium: Per 8 fl.oz Cup

| | C | F | Cb |
|---|---|---|---|
| Black Bean Vegetable | 110 | 0 | 25 |
| Corn & Vegetable | 100 | 0 | 22 |
| Lentil & Carrot | 110 | 0 | 24 |
| Split Pea & Carrots | 120 | 0 | 26 |
| Tomato Vegetable | 70 | 0 | 17 |

### Healthy Choice:
#### Canned: Per Cup

| | C | F | Cb |
|---|---|---|---|
| Bean & Ham, 8.8 oz | 180 | 2.5 | 28 |
| Chicken & Dumplings, 8.9 oz | 150 | 3 | 22 |
| Chicken Tortilla, 8.4 oz | 140 | 1.5 | 23 |
| Chicken with Rice, 8.4 oz | 110 | 2 | 17 |
| Country Vegetable, 8.7 oz | 100 | 0 | 19 |
| New England Clam Chowder | 110 | 1.5 | 20 |
| Split Pea & Ham, 8.4 oz | 160 | 2.5 | 27 |
| Tomato Basil, 8.8 oz | 100 | 0 | 22 |

#### Microwaveable Bowls: Per Cup

| | C | F | Cb |
|---|---|---|---|
| Beef Pot Roast, 8.6 oz | 110 | 1.5 | 17 |
| Chicken Tortilla, 8.6 oz | 140 | 1.5 | 23 |
| Chicken with Rice, 8.5 oz | 90 | 2 | 13 |
| Country Vegetable, 8.6 oz | 100 | 0 | 20 |
| Hearty Vegetable Barley, 8.8 oz | 140 | 1 | 30 |

### Imagine:
#### Broths, Organic: Per Cup

| | C | F | Cb |
|---|---|---|---|
| Beef Flavor | 20 | 1 | 2 |
| Free Range Chicken | 20 | 0.5 | 2 |
| Vegetable | 20 | 0 | 4 |
| Vegetarian, No-Chicken | 15 | 0 | 2 |

#### Chunky Style, Organic: Per Cup

| | C | F | Cb |
|---|---|---|---|
| Chicken & Dumplings | 130 | 4.5 | 18 |
| Cream of Mushroom | 100 | 3.5 | 15 |
| Ital. Vegetables & Beans | 120 | 1.5 | 24 |

Continued Nex Page...

## Imagine (Cont):

| | | C | F | Cb |
|---|---|---|---|---|
| **Creamy:** *Per 8 fl.oz Cup* | | | | |
| Acorn Squash & Mango | | 70 | 1 | 15 |
| Portobello Mushroom | | 70 | 2.5 | 12 |
| Potato Leek | | 80 | 2.5 | 13 |
| Sweet Pea | | 80 | 1.5 | 14 |
| Tomato Basil | | 110 | 2 | 21 |
| **Kettle Cuisine:** *Per 8 oz* | | | | |
| Angus Steak Chili with Beans | | 250 | 7 | 20 |
| Aztec Chili with Ancient Grains | | 170 | 2 | 29 |
| Broccoli Cheddar | | 320 | 24 | 15 |
| Caribbean Jerk Chicken | | 220 | 5 | 31 |
| Carrot Ginger | | 110 | 4 | 18 |
| Chicken Tortilla | | 120 | 3 | 15 |
| Chipotle Sweet Potato | | 140 | 7 | 20 |
| Cream of Crab | | 290 | 22 | 15 |
| Lobster Bisque | | 270 | 18 | 18 |
| Manhattan Clam Chowder | | 120 | 3 | 16 |
| North Atlantic Haddock Chowder | | 260 | 17 | 14 |
| **Knorr:** | | | | |
| **Cubes:** *Per ½ Cube, 1 Cup, Prepared* | | | | |
| Beef; Chicken, average | | 15 | 1.5 | 1 |
| Vegetable | | 20 | 1 | 1 |
| **Homestyle Stock:** *Per 1 Tsp* | | | | |
| Beef | | 10 | 1 | 0 |
| Chicken | | 10 | 2 | 0 |
| **Lipton:** | | | | |
| **Cup-a-Soup:** *Per Envelope* | | | | |
| Chicken Noodle, Original | | 50 | 1 | 8 |
| Cream of Chicken | | 60 | 1.5 | 12 |
| **Recipe Secrets:** *Per 1 Tbsp Dry Mix* | | | | |
| Onion | | 20 | 0 | 4 |
| Onion Mushroom | | 25 | 0 | 7 |
| Savory Herb with Garlic | | 25 | 0 | 6 |
| **Manischewitz:** | | | | |
| **Canned:** *Per 1 cup* | | | | |
| Broth: Beef | | 15 | 0.5 | 1 |
| Turkey | | 20 | 1 | 1 |
| Vegetable | | 5 | 0 | 1 |
| Chicken Consomme, Clear | | 30 | 0 | 4 |
| Chicken Noodle | | 180 | 2 | 20 |
| **Glass Jar:** *Per 1 Cup* | | | | |
| Matzo Ball | | 120 | 5 | 15 |
| Reduced Sodium | | 130 | 6 | 16 |
| Matzo Ball in Broth | | 180 | 8 | 23 |
| Reduced Sodium | | 180 | 8 | 21 |
| **Maruchan:** | | | | |
| **Instant Lunch**, | | | | |
| average all flavors, 1 pkg | | 290 | 12 | 38 |
| **Ramen**, all flavors, 1 pkg, 3 oz | | 380 | 14 | 52 |

## Nissin:

| | C | F | Cb |
|---|---|---|---|
| **Souper Meal:** *Per ½ of 4.3 oz Ctn* | | | |
| Chicken Flavor, with Vege Medley | 280 | 13 | 37 |
| Picante Shrimp Flavor, Hot & Spicy | 290 | 13 | 37 |
| **Top Ramen**, all flavors, 3 oz pkg | 380 | 14 | 53 |
| **Pacific Foods:** | | | |
| **Condensed:** | | | |
| Cream of Chicken, ½ cup | 90 | 3.5 | 10 |
| Cream of Mushroom, ½ cup | 100 | 2.5 | 18 |
| **Hearty Organic:** *Per 1 Cup* | | | |
| Butternut Squash Bisque | 110 | 3.5 | 18 |
| Cashew Carrot Ginger Bisque | 130 | 5 | 20 |
| Spicy Black Bean & Kale | 120 | 0 | 24 |
| Split Pea & Uncured Ham | 160 | 2.5 | 26 |
| Vegetable Quinoa | 90 | 2 | 18 |
| **Progresso:** | | | |
| **Broths:** Beef, 1 cup | 20 | 0 | 3 |
| Chicken, 1 cup | 20 | 0 | 1 |
| **Heart Healthy:** *Per Cup* | | | |
| Creamy Tomato with Basil | 120 | 3 | 22 |
| Creole Style Chkn Gumbo | 110 | 2 | 18 |
| Homestyle Vegetable Beef | 120 | 2 | 19 |
| Savory Garden Vegetable | 90 | 0 | 21 |
| S'West Style Black Bean & Vegetable | 110 | 2 | 21 |
| **Rich & Hearty:** *Per 1 Cup* | | | |
| Chkn & Hm'style Noodles | 110 | 3 | 14 |
| Chicken Corn Chowder | 200 | 9 | 23 |
| New Engl. Clam Chowder | 180 | 8 | 22 |
| Savory Beef Barley Vegetables | 110 | 2 | 16 |
| **Traditional:** *Per ½ Can, 1 Cup* | | | |
| Chickarina with Meatballs | 130 | 5 | 14 |
| Chicken & Sausage Gumbo | 120 | 3.5 | 17 |
| Creamy Tomato w/ Bacon & Cheese | 150 | 5 | 21 |
| **Vegetable Classic:** *Per 1 Cup* | | | |
| French Onion | 50 | 1 | 9 |
| Garden Vegetable | 90 | 0 | 20 |
| Minestrone | 100 | 2 | 20 |
| Tomato Basil | 150 | 3 | 29 |
| **Light:** *Per 1 cup* | | | |
| Beef Pot Roast | 80 | 2 | 10 |
| Chicken Pot Pie Style | 100 | 3 | 16 |
| Creamy Potato w/ Bacon & Cheese | 100 | 3 | 18 |
| Italian Style Vegetable | 70 | 0 | 16 |

| Safeway *(Vons)*: | C | F | Cb |
|---|---|---|---|
| **Signature Soups:** *Per Cup* | | | |
| Broccoli & Cheesy Cheddar | 250 | 18 | 12 |
| Chunky Chicken Noodle | 160 | 5 | 14 |
| Fiesta Chicken Tortilla | 110 | 2 | 15 |
| Italian-Style Wedding | 120 | 4 | 14 |
| Pacific Coast Clam Chowder | 320 | 20 | 27 |
| Tuscan Tomato & Basil Bisque | 290 | 22 | 20 |
| **Swanson:** | | | |
| **Broth:** *Per 8 fl.oz Cup* | | | |
| Beef | 15 | 0 | 1 |
| Chicken | 10 | 0.5 | 1 |
| Organic Chicken | 15 | 0.5 | 1 |
| Vegetable | 15 | 0 | 3 |
| **Flavor Boost:** *Per Pouch* | | | |
| Beef | 10 | 0 | 2 |
| Chicken | 35 | 2 | 3 |
| Vegetable | 20 | 0 | 4 |
| **Tabatchnick:** | | | |
| **Frozen:** | | | |
| **Dairy:** *Per 7.5 oz Pouch* | | | |
| Corn Chowder | 130 | 4.5 | 21 |
| Cream of Mushroom | 100 | 5 | 11 |
| **Gluten Free:** *Per 7.5 oz Pouch* | | | |
| Southwest Bean | 220 | 5 | 36 |
| Split Pea | 140 | 0 | 34 |
| Vegetarian Chili | 180 | 3.5 | 28 |
| **Low Sodium:** *Per 7.5oz Pouch* | | | |
| Barley & Mushroom | 80 | 1 | 17 |
| Split Pea | 140 | 0 | 34 |
| Vegetable | 90 | 1.5 | 17 |
| **Meat:** *Per 7.5 oz Pouch* | | | |
| Frenchman's Onion | 60 | 1.5 | 11 |
| Wilderness Wild Rice | 90 | 0.5 | 19 |
| **Parve:** *Per 7.5 oz Pouch* | | | |
| Black Bean | 220 | 2.5 | 38 |
| Minestrone | 110 | 1.5 | 20 |
| **Shelf Stable:** *Per ⅔ Cup, 5.3 fl.oz* | | | |
| **Broth:** Classic Chicken | 5 | 0 | 0 |
| Other Chicken Flavors | 10 | 0 | 1 |
| Gourmet Beef | 5 | 0 | 0 |
| **Soup:** Creamy Tomato | 70 | 2 | 14 |
| Rstd Red Pepper & Tomato | 70 | 2.5 | 13 |
| **Thai Kitchen:** | | | |
| **Rice Noodle Soup Bowls:** *Per Bowl* | | | |
| Hot & Sour | 250 | 4 | 51 |
| Lemongrass & Chili | 250 | 3.5 | 52 |
| Roasted Garlic | 250 | 3 | 52 |
| Spring Onion | 260 | 4.5 | 50 |
| Thai Ginger | 260 | 3 | 52 |

| Trader Joe's: | C | F | Cb |
|---|---|---|---|
| **28 fl.oz Cans:** *Per Cup* | | | |
| Chunky, Low Fat: | | | |
| Lentil with Vegetables | 140 | 3 | 21 |
| Minestrone | 110 | 2.5 | 19 |
| **14.5 oz Cans:** *Per 1 Cup* | | | |
| Organic: Black Bean | 140 | 1.5 | 26 |
| Lentil Vegetable | 160 | 4 | 24 |
| Split Pea | 100 | 0 | 19 |
| **10.75 oz Can,** | | | |
| Low Sodium, Minestrone | 200 | 4 | 37 |
| **15 oz Can,** | | | |
| Low Fat, Chicken Noodle, 1 cup | 90 | 1 | 14 |
| **32 fl oz. Cartons:** *Per 1 Cup* | | | |
| Butternut Squash | 90 | 2 | 16 |
| Carrot & Ginger | 80 | 1 | 17 |
| Creamy Corn & Rstd Pepper | 110 | 2 | 23 |
| Latin Style Black Bean | 70 | 1 | 12 |
| Sweet Potato Bisque | 130 | 1 | 28 |
| Organic: Butternut Squash | 70 | 0 | 17 |
| Tomato & Rstd Red Pepper | 100 | 3.5 | 15 |
| Low Sodium, Creamy Tomato | 90 | 3.5 | 15 |
| **17.6 fl.oz Cartons:** *Per Cup* | | | |
| Beef, Barley with Veggies | 100 | 0.5 | 16 |
| Chicken Noodle with Veggies | 100 | 1 | 16 |
| **Whole Foods:** *Per Cup* | | | |
| **365 Organic:** | | | |
| Chicken Noodle | 100 | 1.5 | 12 |
| Lentil | 70 | 0 | 15 |
| Minestrone | 140 | 1.5 | 23 |
| Southwestern Black Bean | 120 | 1 | 23 |
| Tomato Basil | 90 | 2 | 16 |
| **Wolfgang Puck:** *Per Cup* | | | |
| **Organic:** | | | |
| Butternut Squash | 140 | 11 | 10 |
| Chicken & Dumplings | 140 | 7 | 14 |
| Classic Minestrone | 120 | 2.5 | 20 |
| Corn Chowder | 210 | 13 | 20 |
| Free Range Chicken with Rice | 110 | 4 | 15 |
| New Engl. Clam Chowder | 150 | 7 | 18 |
| Signature Tortilla | 160 | 3.5 | 27 |
| Thick Hearty Lentil & Vegetable | 160 | 1 | 29 |
| Thick Hearty Garden Vegetable | 130 | 5 | 19 |
| Tomato with Basil | 150 | 6 | 21 |

| **Soybean Products** | **C** | **F** | **Cb** |
|---|---|---|---|
| Cheeses (Soy) ~ *See Page 78* | | | |
| **Miso Soy Bean Paste:** | | | |
| *Cold Mountain:* Light Yellow, 1 tsp | 10 | 0 | 1 |
| Mellow Red, 1 tsp | 15 | 0 | 3 |
| Red, 1 tsp | 10 | 0 | 1 |
| **Miso Soup (dry mix):** | | | |
| 1 Tbsp., dry mix | 35 | 1 | 5 |
| 1 cup, prepared | 35 | 1 | 5 |
| **Natto:** ½ cup, 3 oz | 160 | 7 | 14 |
| **Okara (Tofu fiber residue),** ½ c., 2 oz | 47 | 1 | 8 |
| **Tempeh:** 1 piece, 3 oz | 180 | 8 | 12 |
| Fried, 3 oz | 250 | 14 | 14 |
| **Seitan** *(Westsoy)*, Strips, 3 oz | 120 | 2 | 4 |
| **Soybean Protein** *(TVP)*, 1 oz | 95 | 0 | 8 |
| **Soy Bean Paste,** 1 tsp | 10 | 0 | 2 |
| Soy Beans ~ *See Page 160* | | | |
| Soy Drinks ~ *See Page 49* | | | |

### Tofu ~ Brands

| | **C** | **F** | **Cb** |
|---|---|---|---|
| **Azumaya Tofu:** | | | |
| Extra Firm; Firm, av., 3 oz | 70 | 4 | 2 |
| Soft (Silken), 3.2 oz | 45 | 2 | 1 |
| **House Foods:** *Per 3 oz* | | | |
| **Premium Tofu:** Extra Firm | 80 | 4.5 | 2 |
| Firm | 70 | 4 | 2 |
| Medium Firm | 60 | 3.5 | 2 |
| Soft (Silken) | 60 | 3 | 2 |
| **Organic Tofu:** Firm | 70 | 4 | 2 |
| Extra Firm | 70 | 3.5 | 2 |
| **Ethnic:** Tokusen Kinugoshi, Extra Soft | 80 | 4 | 3 |
| Sukui; Soon (Extra Soft) | 45 | 2 | 2 |
| Yaki Tofu (Broiled) | 90 | 5 | 2 |
| **Mori-Nu Tofu:** | | | |
| **Morinaga Silken:** | | | |
| Soft, 3 oz, 1" slice | 45 | 2.5 | 2 |
| Firm, 3 oz, 1" slice | 50 | 2.5 | 2 |
| Extra Firm, 3 oz, 1" slice | 45 | 1.5 | 2 |
| Organic, Silken 3 oz, 1" slice | 50 | 2.5 | 2 |
| Lite, Firm, 3 oz, 1" slice | 30 | 1 | 1 |
| **Nasoya:** Extra Firm, 3 oz | 80 | 4 | 3 |
| Firm, 3 oz | 70 | 3.5 | 2 |
| Silken, 3.2 oz | 45 | 2 | 1 |
| Soft, 2.8 oz | 60 | 3 | 1 |
| **Tofuplus:** | | | |
| Extra Firm, 3 oz | 80 | 4 | 2 |
| Firm, 3 oz | 70 | 3 | 2 |
| Sprouted, Super Firm, 3 oz | 100 | 5 | 3 |

| **Supplements** | **C** | **F** | **Cb** |
|---|---|---|---|
| **Aloe Vera Juice,** undiluted, 2 fl.oz | 5 | 0 | 1 |
| **Brewer's Yeast:** Tablets, 2 tabs | 4 | 0 | 0.5 |
| Flakes, 1 heaping Tbsp, 0.3 oz | 30 | 0.5 | 4 |
| Powder, 1 heaping Tbsp, 0.5 oz | 50 | 0.5 | 6 |
| **Calcium Chews:** *CVS,* 1 chew | 20 | 0 | 3 |
| *Trader Joe's,* Chocolate,1 chew | 20 | 1 | 3 |
| **Cod Liver Oil,** 1 Tbsp | 125 | 13 | 0 |
| *Fiber Choice,* 2 tabs | 15 | 0 | 4 |
| **Fiber,** | | | |
| *Fibersure,* 1 heaping tsp | 25 | 0 | 6 |
| **Fish Oil Capsules,** (1), av. | 10 | 1 | 0 |
| **Flax Oil:** | | | |
| Capsules (2) | 10 | 1 | 0 |
| *Barlean's,* softgels (3) | 110 | 11 | 0 |
| **Garlic Tablets/Capsules,** each | 3 | 0 | 0 |
| **Glowelle:** | | | |
| Beauty Drink, 8 fl.oz | 100 | 0 | 24 |
| Powder Stick (1) | 50 | 0 | 12 |
| **Lecithin Granules,** 1 Tbsp | 55 | 4 | 0.5 |
| **Metamucil,** Powder: | | | |
| Orange (Smooth Texture), 1 rounded Tbsp | 45 | 0 | 12 |
| Sugar-Free, 1 rounded tsp | 20 | 0 | 5 |
| Pink Lemonade, Sugar-Free, 1 rounded tsp | 20 | 0 | 5 |
| **Fiber Wafers,** (2) | 120 | 5 | 17 |
| **Capsules:** | | | |
| Heart & Digestive (6) | 10 | 0 | 3 |
| Strong Bones (5) | 10 | 0 | 3 |
| **Protein,** Powders, av., 1 oz | 100 | 0.5 | 0 |
| **Seaweed:** Dried, 1 oz | 85 | 0.5 | 22 |
| Soaked, drained, 1 oz | 15 | 0.5 | 3 |
| **Spirulina,** 1 tablet | 2 | 0 | 0.5 |
| **Vitamins/Minerals:** Tabs/Caps (1) | 2 | 0 | 0 |
| Vitamin E Capsules, each | 5 | 0.5 | 0 |
| **Viactiv Chews,** Choc. (1) | 20 | 0.5 | 4 |

### Cough & Pharmaceutical

| | **C** | **F** | **Cb** |
|---|---|---|---|
| **Antacids:** Av., 1 tablet | 4 | 0 | 1 |
| Liquid, 1 Tbsp | 6 | 0 | 1 |
| Antacid Sodium Counts ~ *See Page 280* | | | |
| **Cough/Cold Syrups:** | | | |
| Regular: With sugar, 1 Tbsp | 35 | 0 | 9 |
| With alcohol, 1 Tbsp | 46 | 0 | 9 |
| *Diabetic Tussin,* Sugar Free, 1 T. | 0 | 0 | 0 |
| Cough Drops/Lozenges ~ *See Page 75* | | | |
| *Sudafed,* Syrup 1 tsp | 14 | 0 | 3 |
| *Tylenol,* Liquid: Child, 1 tsp | 17 | 0 | 4 |
| Extra Strength, 1 tsp | 11 | 0 | 3 |

## Sugar

**C  F  Cb**

**White Sugar, granulated:**

| | C | F | Cb |
|---|---|---|---|
| 1 level teaspoon, 4g | 15 | 0 | 4 |
| 1 heaping teaspoon, 6g | 25 | 0 | 6 |
| 1 Tablespoon, 12g | 50 | 0 | 12 |
| 1 ounce, 1 oz | 110 | 0 | 28 |
| 1 cup, 7 oz | 775 | 0 | 200 |
| 1 lb (16 oz) | 1760 | 0 | 454 |
| Single Portion Packages: | | | |
| 1 stick | 15 | 0 | 4 |
| 1 packet | 15 | 0 | 4 |
| 1 cube | 10 | 0 | 2.5 |
| **Brown Sugar:** 1 Tbsp | 50 | 0 | 13 |
| 1 ounce, 1 oz | 110 | 0 | 28 |
| 1 cup, not packed, 5 oz | 550 | 0 | 140 |
| 1 cup, packed, 7.8 oz | 835 | 0 | 216 |
| **Powdered Sugar:** | | | |
| Sifted, 1 cup, 3.5 oz | 390 | 0 | 100 |
| Unsifted, 1 cup, 4¼ oz | 470 | 0 | 120 |
| **Coconut Palm Sugar**, 1 tsp, 4g | 15 | 0 | 4 |
| **Dextrose**, 1 tsp | 12 | 0 | 3 |
| **Fructose**, powder, 1 tsp | 12 | 0 | 3 |
| **Glucose Powder**, 1 oz | 110 | 0 | 27 |
| **Glucose Tablets**, (1) | 20 | 0 | 5 |
| **Palm Sugar**, 3 Tbsp | 45 | 0 | 11 |
| **Piloncillo**, (Brown Sugar), 3oz | 325 | 0 | 81 |
| **Turbinado Sugar**, 2 Tbsp, 1 oz | 110 | 0 | 27 |

## Sugar Substitutes

| | C | F | Cb |
|---|---|---|---|
| **Agave**, 1 Tbsp, 0.7 oz | 60 | 0 | 16 |
| **DiabetiSweet**, 1 teaspoon | 9 | 0 | 4.5 |
| *Note: Carb figure includes 4.5 g sugar alcohol* | | | |
| **Domino**, Light, ½ tsp | 5 | 0 | 2 |
| **Equal:** Tablet (2) | 0 | 0 | 0 |
| Granular, 1 tsp | 0 | 0 | 0 |
| Packet (1) | 0 | 0 | 0 |
| **Next,** 1 packet | 0 | 0 | 0 |
| **Nectresse**, 1 packet | 0 | 0 | 0 |
| **NutraSweet**, 1 tsp | 0 | 0 | 0 |
| **Splenda**, Granulated No Calorie Sweetener: | | | |
| 1 tsp | 0 | 0 | 0 |
| 1 cup | 95 | 0 | 24 |
| Packets, all flavors | 0 | 0 | 0 |
| Sugar Blend, Orig/Brown, ½ cup | 385 | 0 | 96 |
| **Stevia**, single serving | 0 | 0 | 0 |
| **Sugar Twin**, 1 packet | 0 | 0 | 0 |
| **Sweet 'N Low**, 1 packet | 0 | 0 | 0 |
| **Truvia**, 1 packet | 0 | 0 | 0 |
| **Walgreens**, Wal-Sweet, 1 packet | 0 | 0 | 0 |
| **Whey Low**, 1 tsp | 4 | 0 | 1 |

## Syrups, Molasses, Agave

**Syrups· Plain:** *Average All Brands (Corn/Rice/Maple/Pancake/Sundae/Waffle) Includes Aunt Jemima, Cary's, Karo, Hershey's, Hungry Jack, IHOP, Log Cabin, Mrs Butterworth's*

| **Regular/Dark/Light Color:** | C | F | Cb |
|---|---|---|---|
| 1 Tbsp, 0.5 fl.oz | 55 | 0 | 14 |
| ¼ cup (4 Tbsp) | 220 | 0 | 55 |
| Single Portion, 1.5 oz pkg | 170 | 0 | 42 |
| **Lite**, 1Tbsp, 1 oz | 25 | 0 | 6 |
| **Sugar-Free:** 2 Tbsp, 1 oz | 18 | 0 | 5 |
| Maple Grove, Cozy Cottage, 2 Tbsp | 10 | 0 | 3 |
| IHOP, 4 Tbsp, 2 oz | 20 | 0 | 7 |
| **Fruit Syrups,** (IHOP), ¼ cup, 2 oz | 200 | 0 | 52 |
| **Honey Cream Syrup**, ¼ cup, 2 oz | 220 | 0 | 55 |
| **Molasses:** Dark/Light: 1 T, 0.7 oz | 60 | 0 | 15 |
| 1 cup, 12 oz | 975 | 0.5 | 252 |
| **Blackstrap**, 1 Tbsp, 0.8 oz | 47 | 0 | 13 |
| **Agave Nectar**, av. all flavors, 1 Tablespoon, 0.8 oz | 60 | 0 | 15 |

## Flavored Syrups/Ice Cream Toppings

| **Hershey's:** Per 2 Tbsp | | | |
|---|---|---|---|
| Average all flavors | 105 | 0 | 26 |
| Lite | 45 | 0 | 12 |
| **Smuckers:** Per 2 Tbsp | | | |
| **Magic Shell**, average all flavors | 220 | 17 | 16 |
| **Spoonables:** Reg., average all flavors | 115 | 1 | 28 |
| Sugar Free: Caramel; Chocolate | 90 | 0 | 24 |
| Strawberry | 25 | 0 | 9 |
| *Note: Carb figures include 9g-17g sugar alcohol* | | | |
| **Sundae Syrups:** Regular, av. all flavors | 105 | 0 | 25 |
| Sugar Free, average all flavors | 90 | 0 | 24 |
| *Note: Carb figures includes 15g sugar alcohol* | | | |

## Honey, Jam, Preserves

*Average all Brands*

| **Honey:** 1 tsp, 0.3 oz | 22 | 0 | 5.5 |
|---|---|---|---|
| 1 Tbsp, 0.8 oz | 65 | 0 | 17 |
| 1 ounce, 1 oz | 85 | 0 | 23 |
| 1 cup, 12 oz | 1030 | 0 | 269 |
| Single Portion, 0.5 oz package | 45 | 0 | 11 |
| **Jams/Jellies/Marmalade/Preserves:** | | | |
| Regular: 1 tsp, 0.3 oz | 20 | 0 | 5 |
| 1 Tbsp, 0.8 oz | 55 | 0 | 14 |
| 1 ounce, 1 oz | 80 | 0 | 20 |
| Single Portion, 0.5 oz pkg | 40 | 0 | 11 |
| **Apple/Fruit Butters**, 1 T., 0.6 oz | 20 | 0 | 6 |
| **Fruit Spreads:** Regular, 1 tsp | 15 | 0 | 4 |
| Low Sugar, 1 tsp | 8 | 0 | 2 |
| **Jelly:** Regular, average, 1 tsp | 18 | 0 | 4.5 |
| Imitation, Low Calorie, 1 tsp | 4 | 0 | 1 |

| Vegetables | C | F | Cb |
|---|---|---|---|
| **Alfalfa Sprouts**, ½ cup, 0.5 oz | 5 | 0 | 0.5 |
| **Artichokes**, Globe/French: | | | |
| 1 medium, 4.5 oz | 60 | 0 | 13 |
| 1 large, 5.7 oz | 75 | 0 | 17 |
| **Artichoke Heart**, plain, 2 pieces | 15 | 0 | 3 |
| **Asparagus**, raw/frozen: | | | |
| Cuts & Tips, ½ cup, 4.3 oz | 20 | 0 | 3 |
| Spears, 3 medium | 10 | 0 | 2 |
| **Bamboo Shoots**, cooked, ½ cup, 2 oz | 7 | 0 | 1 |
| **Beans**, Green/Snap/String: | | | |
| 10 beans (4" long), 2 oz | 20 | 0 | 4 |
| Pieces, ½ cup, 3 oz | 30 | 0 | 7 |
| Dried Beans (Kidney, Brown, Lima, Navy, Pinto, White): | | | |
| Raw: 2 Tbsp, 1 oz | 95 | 0.5 | 18 |
| 1 cup, 7 oz | 665 | 3 | 126 |
| Cooked: 1 oz | 35 | 0 | 7 |
| ½ cup, 3 oz | 105 | 0 | 21 |
| **Bean Sprouts**, average, ½ cup, 2 oz | 15 | 0 | 3.5 |
| **Beets (Beetroot)**: | | | |
| Raw, 1 beet (2" diam.), 4 oz | 35 | 0 | 8 |
| Cooked, 1 cup, slices, 3 oz | 35 | 0 | 8 |
| **Canned** ~ See Page 161 | | | |
| **Beet Greens**, cooked, ½ cup, 2.5 oz | 20 | 0 | 4 |
| **Bell Pepper** ~ See Peppers | | | |
| **Bitter Melon/Gourd**, 1 cup, 1.5 oz | 15 | 0 | 1.5 |
| **Blackeye Peas**, cooked, ½ cup, 3 oz | 100 | 0.5 | 18 |
| **Bok Choy (Chinese Chard)**, | | | |
| cooked, 3 oz | 10 | 0 | 1.5 |
| **Breadfruit**, ¼ small fruit, 3 oz | 100 | 0 | 26 |
| **Broadbeans (Fava Beans):** | | | |
| Green, raw, (in pod): 4 pods | | | |
| (3.5 oz with shells, 1.2 oz beans) | 30 | 0 | 6 |
| 1 cup beans, without shell, 4.5 oz | 110 | 1 | 22 |
| Mature Seeds: Raw, 1 cup, 5.3 oz | 510 | 2.5 | 87 |
| Cooked, ½ cup, 3 oz | 95 | 0 | 17 |
| **Broccoflower**, ⅕ head, 3.5 oz | 35 | 0 | 7 |
| **Broccoli**: Raw, chopped,1 cup, 3 oz | 30 | 0 | 6 |
| 3 Florets, 2.5 oz | 25 | 0 | 5 |
| 1 Spear (5" long), 1.oz | 10 | 0 | 2 |
| 1 Whole: Medium, 14 oz | 135 | 1.5 | 26 |
| Large, 21 oz | 205 | 2 | 40 |
| 1 Head (no stalk), 11 oz | 105 | 1 | 21 |
| 1 Stalk, small (5" long), 5.3 oz | 50 | 0.5 | 10 |
| **Brocco Sprouts**, ½ cup, 1 oz | 15 | 0 | 2 |
| **Brussels Sprouts:** Cooked, ½ cup, 2.8 oz | 30 | 0.5 | 6 |
| 2 Sprouts, 1.5 oz | 15 | 0 | 3 |
| **Butterbeans**, cooked, ½ cup, 3 oz | 90 | 0 | 16 |
| **Cabbage**, average other flavors: | | | |
| Raw: 1 leaf, large, 1 oz | 5 | 0 | 2 |
| Shredded, 1 cup, 2.5 oz | 15 | 0 | 4 |
| ½ large head (7" diam), 22 oz | 150 | 1 | 35 |
| Cooked, shredded, ½ cup, 2.5 oz | 15 | 0.5 | 3.5 |

| Vegetables (Cont) | C | F | Cb |
|---|---|---|---|
| **Cactus Leaf (Nopales):** | | | |
| 1 leaf, 4.5 oz | 20 | 0 | 4 |
| 1 cup (slices), 3 oz | 15 | 0 | 3 |
| **Carrots**, regular thick variety: | | | |
| 1 small, 4 oz | 45 | 0 | 11 |
| 1 medium, 6 oz | 70 | 0 | 16 |
| 1 large, 8 oz | 95 | 0 | 22 |
| Chopped, 1 cup, 4.5 oz | 50 | 0 | 12 |
| Grated, 1 cup, 4 oz | 45 | 0 | 11 |
| Slices, 1 cup, 4.5 oz | 50 | 0 | 12 |
| Sticks (4"), 4-5, 1.5 oz | 20 | 0 | 4 |
| Long thin variety, 1 medium, 2.2 oz | 25 | 0 | 6 |
| Baby: Snack size, 3 medium, 1 oz | 10 | 0 | 2.5 |
| Snack Pack, 3 oz | 30 | 0 | 7 |
| **Cassava**, raw, 1 cup, 2.5 oz | 330 | 0.5 | 78 |
| **Cauliflower**: raw: Pieces, 1 cup, 3.5 oz | 25 | 0 | 5 |
| ½ medium head, 10 oz | 70 | 0 | 15 |
| Cooked, 3 florets, 2 oz | 10 | 0 | 2 |
| **Celeriac**, ½ cup, raw, 2.8 oz | 35 | 0 | 7 |
| **Celery**: 1 large stalk, 11", 2.2 oz | 10 | 0 | 2 |
| 4 Strips, thin sticks, 0.5 oz | 5 | 0 | 1 |
| Chopped, 1 cup, 3.5 oz | 15 | 0 | 3 |
| **Chard (Swiss)**, ½ cup, cooked, 3 oz | 20 | 0 | 3.5 |
| **Chayote Squash:** 1 medium, 7 oz | 40 | 0 | 9 |
| Pieces, 1 cup, 4.5 oz | 25 | 0 | 6 |
| **Chickpeas**, (Garbanzo Beans): | | | |
| Dry, 1 cup, 7 oz | 730 | 12 | 121 |
| Cooked, 1 cup, 5.8 oz | 270 | 4 | 45 |
| **Chicory Greens**, 1 cup, 1 oz | 7 | 0 | 1.5 |
| **Chili Peppers** ~ See Peppers | | | |
| **Chinese Long Bean**, slices, 1 cup, 3.2 oz | 45 | 0 | 8 |
| **Chives**, chopped, 1 Tbsp | 1 | 0 | 0 |
| **Choy Sum**, 3 oz | 15 | 0 | 3 |
| **Cilantro**, (Coriander), 1 cup | 5 | 0 | 0.5 |
| **Collards**, cooked, ½ cup, 3 oz | 25 | 0 | 5 |
| **Corn**, Yellow/White: | | | |
| Raw: Kernels, ½ cup, 3 oz | 80 | 0.5 | 19 |
| Ear (5"x 1¾"), 5.5 oz | 155 | 1 | 37 |
| Cooked: Kernels, ½ cup, 3 oz | 77 | 0.5 | 18 |
| Cob, small, 2.3 oz | 60 | 0.5 | 14 |
| Ear, large, 5.5 oz | 120 | 1 | 28 |
| **Courgette** ~ See Zucchini | | | |
| **Cowpeas** ~ See Blackeye Peas | | | |
| **Cress**, garden, raw, 1 cup, 1.8 oz | 15 | 0 | 3 |
| **Cucumber**, average other flavors: | | | |
| Slices, ½ cup, 2 oz | 10 | 0 | 2 |
| Green, 1 medium (9"), 11 oz | 45 | 0 | 11 |
| Persian, 1 medium (8"), 6 oz | 25 | 0 | 5 |
| **Daikon Radish**, ½ cup, slices, 2 oz | 9 | 0 | 2 |
| **Dandelion Greens**, raw, ½ cup, 1 oz | 10 | 0 | 2.5 |
| **Edamame**, (Immature green soybeans): | | | |
| Shelled, ½ cup, 2.6 oz | 110 | 5 | 8 |
| With shells, 10 pods, 1.3 oz | 30 | 1 | 3 |

## Vegetables (Cont)

| | C | F | Cb |
|---|---|---|---|
| **Eggplant**, raw: 4 oz | 30 | 0 | 7 |
| ½ cup, 1" pieces, 1.5 oz | 10 | 0 | 2 |
| 1 slice, fried, 1 oz | 75 | 4 | 10 |
| **Endive**, Belgian/French: Raw, | | | |
| 1 medium head (6"), 2.5 oz | 12 | 0 | 3 |
| **Fennel**, 1 cup, sliced, 3 oz | 25 | 0 | 7 |
| **Gai Choy Cabbage**, cooked, 1 cup, 6 oz | 20 | 0 | 3 |
| **Gai Lan**, (Chinese Kale), cooked, 1 cup | 35 | 0.5 | 7 |
| **Garbanzo Beans** ~ See Chick Peas | | | |
| **Garlic**, 1 clove | 4 | 0 | 1 |
| **Ginger**: ¼ cup slices, 1 oz | 20 | 0 | 5 |
| Crystallized (sugared), 7 pieces, 1.5 oz | 130 | 0 | 35 |
| **Horseradish**, raw, 1 pod, 0.5 oz | 5 | 0 | 1 |
| **Jerusalem Artichoke**, raw, ½ cup | 55 | 0 | 13 |
| **Jicama**, raw, sliced, ½ cup, 2.3 oz | 25 | 0 | 6 |
| **Kale**, 1 cup, chopped, 2.5 oz | 35 | 0.5 | 7 |
| **Kohlrabi**, cooked, ½ cup, 1.8 oz | 17 | 0 | 5 |
| **Leek**, cooked, 1 whole, 4.5 oz | 40 | 0 | 9 |
| **Lentils**, green/brown: Dry, 1 oz | 100 | 0.5 | 17 |
| 1 cup, 6.8 oz | 675 | 3 | 115 |
| Cooked, ½ cup, 3.5 oz | 115 | 0.5 | 20 |
| **Lettuce**: 1 cup, chopped/shredded, 2 oz | 7 | 0 | 1 |
| Butterhead, 2 leaves, 0.5 oz | 2 | 0 | 0.5 |
| Cos/Romaine, shredded, 1 cup | 10 | 0 | 2 |
| Iceberg: 1 outer leaf, 0.5 oz | 2 | 0 | 0.5 |
| 1 medium head, 16 oz | 75 | 1 | 16 |
| **Lima Beans**, baby, cooked, ½ cup, 3 oz | 105 | 0 | 20 |
| **Lotus Root**, cooked, 10 slices, 3 oz | 60 | 0 | 14 |
| **Mung Bean Sprouts**, ½ cup, 2 oz | 15 | 0 | 3 |
| **Mushrooms**, average all varieties: | | | |
| Raw, diced/siced, 1 cup, 3 oz | 20 | 0 | 3 |
| Pieces, 1 cup, 1.3 oz | 8 | 0 | 1 |
| Fried/Sauteed, 6 oz | 220 | 16 | 10 |
| Grilled, pieces, ½ cup, 2.5 oz | 20 | 0.5 | 4 |
| Shitake, dried, 1 oz package | 90 | 0 | 22 |
| **Mustard Greens**, raw, ½ cup, 1 oz | 7 | 0 | 2 |
| **Okra:** Raw, 8 pods, 4 oz | 30 | 0 | 7 |
| Cooked, ½ cup, 2.8 oz | 20 | 0 | 4 |
| **Onions**, Raw: 1 small, 2.5 oz | 30 | 0 | 7 |
| 1 medium, 4 oz | 50 | 0 | 11 |
| 1 large, 5.5 oz | 65 | 0 | 15 |
| 1 jumbo, 16 oz | 190 | 0.5 | 46 |
| Chopped: ½ cup, 3 oz | 35 | 0 | 8 |
| 1 Tbsp, 0.4 oz | 5 | 0 | 1 |
| Slices: 1 cup, 4 oz | 50 | 0 | 12 |
| 1 medium slice (⅛"), 0.5 oz | 5 | 0 | 1 |
| 1 large slice (¼"), 1.3 oz | 15 | 0 | 4 |
| Flakes, dried ¼ cup, 0.5 oz | 50 | 0 | 12 |
| Rings, breaded & fried, 2 rings | 80 | 5 | 9 |
| Scallions, ½ cup, 2 oz | 15 | 0 | 3 |
| Spring, chopped, ½ cup, 2 oz | 15 | 0 | 3 |

## Vegetables (Cont)

| | C | F | Cb |
|---|---|---|---|
| **Parsley**, chopped, ½ cup, 1 oz | 10 | 0 | 2 |
| **Parsnip**: 1 medium, 4 oz | 85 | 0 | 20 |
| Cooked, slices, ½ cup, 2.8 oz | 55 | 0 | 13 |
| **Peas**: Green, raw, ¼ cup, 1.5 oz | 30 | 0 | 5 |
| With pods, 0.5 lb | 70 | 0 | 13 |
| Snow Peas, 10 pods, 1.2 oz | 15 | 0 | 3 |
| Split: Dry, hulled, 1 oz | 100 | 0.5 | 17 |
| Cooked, 1 cup, 7 oz | 230 | 1 | 42 |
| **Peppers:** | | | |
| Sweet, 1 medium, 4.2 oz | 30 | 0 | 7 |
| Bell: 1 medium, 4.2 oz | 30 | 0 | 7 |
| raw, chopped, ½ cup, 2.5 oz | 20 | 0 | 5 |
| 2 rings (5" diam. x ¼" thick) | 3 | 0 | 1 |
| Chili: Green/Red, 1.5 oz | 20 | 0 | 5 |
| Habanero, 1 only, 0.3 oz | 10 | 0 | 2 |
| **Pigeon Peas**, cooked, ½ cup, 3 oz | 95 | 1 | 17 |
| **Pimientos**, 3 medium, 3.5 oz | 25 | 0 | 5 |
| **Poi**, ½ cup, 4.2 oz | 135 | 0 | 33 |
| **Potatoes:** | | | |
| Raw (with skin): | | | |
| 1 baby, 2 oz | 45 | 0 | 10 |
| 1 small, 6 oz | 135 | 0 | 30 |
| 1 medium, 8 oz | 180 | 0 | 40 |
| 1 large, 12 oz | 270 | 0 | 60 |
| 1 extra large, 16 oz | 360 | 0 | 80 |
| Baked, (no added fat), large, 10 oz (raw wt): | | | |
| Plain: With skin, 7 oz (cooked wt) | 185 | 0 | 42 |
| W/o skin, 5.5 oz (cooked wt) | 145 | 0 | 34 |
| With Skin/Toppings: | | | |
| With 2 tsp fat | 270 | 8 | 58 |
| With Grated Cheese, 1 oz | 370 | 9 | 58 |
| With Plain Yogurt, 2 Tbsp | 260 | 1 | 60 |
| With Sour Crm & Chives, 2 Tbsp | 320 | 6 | 60 |
| Mashed: | | | |
| With milk plus fat, ½ cup, 4 oz | 120 | 4.5 | 18 |
| KFC Style without gravy, 4 oz | 90 | 3 | 15 |
| Loaded (fat/cream/cheese/bacon): | | | |
| Side serving, 6 oz | 180 | 9 | 22 |
| Large serving, 12 oz | 360 | 18 | 44 |
| Potato Skins, baked w/ cheese topping, | | | |
| ½ whole, 4 oz | 240 | 13 | 22 |
| French Fries: Small serving, 2.6 oz | 250 | 13 | 30 |
| Medium serving, 4 oz | 380 | 20 | 47 |
| Frozen, uncooked, 18 fries, 4 oz | 165 | 5.5 | 28 |
| Oven-heated, 18 fries, 4 oz | 165 | 5.5 | 28 |
| Take-Out, 1 cup, 5 oz | 440 | 25 | 60 |
| Au Gratin, ½ cup, 4.3 oz | 160 | 9 | 14 |
| Pancakes, 2 small, 2 oz | 120 | 6.5 | 12 |
| Puffs, fried, 4 puffs, 1 oz | 55 | 2.5 | 8 |
| Scalloped, 8.5 oz | 220 | 9 | 26 |

## Vegetables (Cont)

| | C | F | Cb |
|---|---|---|---|
| **Pumpkin:** | | | |
| Raw, 1" cubes, 1 cup, 4 oz | 30 | 0 | 7 |
| Cooked: | | | |
| Baked, without fat, 4 oz | 90 | 7 | 9 |
| Mashed: 1 scoop, 2 oz | 10 | 0 | 2 |
| ½ cup, 4.3 oz | 25 | 0 | 6 |
| Pumpkin Flowers, 1 cup, 1.2 oz | 5 | 0 | 1 |
| **Purslane:** Cooked, ½ cup, 2 oz | 10 | 0 | 2 |
| Raw, 1" cubes, 1 cup, 1.5 oz | 5 | 0 | 1.5 |
| **Radicchio:** 2 leaves, 0.5 oz | 5 | 0 | 1 |
| Shredded, 1 cup, 1.5 oz | 20 | 0 | 4 |
| **Radishes:** 1 small | 0 | 0 | 0 |
| 10 medium/5 large, 1.6 oz | 5 | 0 | 1 |
| Slices, ½ cup, 2 oz | 10 | 0 | 2 |
| **Rhubarb**, raw, ½ cup, 2 oz | 15 | 0 | 3 |
| **Rutabaga**, cubes, cooked, ½ cup, 3 oz | 30 | 0 | 7 |
| **Salsify**, cooked, slices, ½ cup, 2.5 oz | 50 | 0 | 11 |
| **Sauerkraut**, ½ cup, 2.5 oz | 15 | 0 | 3 |
| **Seaweed:** Dried, 1 oz | 5 | 0 | 2 |
| Soaked, drained, 1 oz | 15 | 0 | 4 |
| Nori/Laver, dried, 6 sheets, 0.5 oz | 35 | 0 | 5 |
| **Shallots**, chopped, 1 Tbsp, 0.5 oz | 5 | 0 | 1 |
| **Sorrel**, raw, ½ cup, 4 oz | 20 | 0 | 4 |
| **Soybeans:** Dry, ½ cup, 3.3 oz | 390 | 18 | 28 |
| Mature, dry, 1 oz | 120 | 5.5 | 8 |
| Cooked, ½ cup, 3 oz | 150 | 7.5 | 8 |
| **Soy Products/Tofu/Tempeh** ~ *See Page 156* | | | |
| **Spinach:** Cooked, ½ cup, 3 oz | 20 | 0 | 4 |
| Creamed, average, ½ cup, 4.5 oz | 190 | 15 | 8 |
| Raw: 3 leaves, 1 cup, 1 oz | 7 | 0 | 1 |
| 1 Bunch, 12 oz | 80 | 1.5 | 12 |
| **Squash:** | | | |
| Summer: Raw, ½ cup, 2.5 oz | 10 | 0 | 2 |
| Cooked, slices, ½ cup, 3 oz | 15 | 0 | 3 |
| Winter, cooked: | | | |
| Acorn: Cubes, ½ cup, 3.5 oz | 35 | 0 | 9 |
| ½ medium (10 oz raw weight) | 115 | 0 | 30 |
| Butternut: Cubes, ½ cup, 3.5 oz | 40 | 0 | 10 |
| ¼ medium (9 oz raw weight) | 115 | 0 | 30 |
| Spaghetti, ½ cup, 1.8 oz | 15 | 0 | 3 |
| **Succotash**, cooked, ½ cup, 3.3 oz | 110 | 1 | 23 |
| **Sweetcorn** ~ *See Corn* | | | |
| **Sweet Potatoes:** | | | |
| Cooked with skin (w/o fat), | | | |
| 1 medium, 4 oz | 105 | 0 | 24 |
| Without skin, mashed, ½ cup, 5.5 oz | 125 | 0 | 29 |
| Fries (Alexia, Julienne syle), | | | |
| approximately 12 pieces, 3 oz | 140 | 5 | 24 |

## Vegetables (Cont)

| | C | F | Cb |
|---|---|---|---|
| **Swiss Chard**, cooked, chopped, 1 c., 6 oz | 35 | 0 | 7 |
| **Taro**, cooked, ½ cup, 2.3 oz | 95 | 0 | 23 |
| **Tomatoes:** 1 small (2¼" diam.), 3 oz | 15 | 0 | 3 |
| 1 medium (2¾" diameter), 5 oz | 25 | 0 | 5 |
| 1 large (3½" diameter), 8 oz | 40 | 0.5 | 9 |
| 1 extra lge (4" diam.), 12 oz | 60 | 0.5 | 14 |
| Chopped, 1 cup, 6.5 oz | 35 | 0.5 | 7 |
| **Tomatillo:** 1 medium, 1.2 oz | 10 | 0 | 2 |
| 1lb quantity for recipe | 135 | 4.5 | 27 |
| **Turnip:** Cooked, ½ cup, 2.8 oz | 15 | 0 | 4 |
| Greens, cooked, ½ cup, 2.5 oz | 15 | 0 | 3 |
| **Water Chestnuts:** 5-6 nuts, 1 oz | 56 | 0.5 | 13 |
| Raw, slices, ½ cup, 2.3 oz | 60 | 0 | 15 |
| Canned, 1 oz | 15 | 0 | 3 |
| **Watercress**, 10 sprigs, 1 oz | 3 | 0 | 0.5 |
| **Yams:** Cooked, steamed, ½ cup, 2.5 oz | 80 | 0 | 19 |
| Baked: | | | |
| 1 medium (6") 8 oz | 265 | 0.5 | 63 |
| 1 large (9") 12 oz | 400 | 0.5 | 94 |
| **Yardlong Bean**, 1 pod, 0.5 oz | 5 | 0 | 1 |
| **Yucca Root**, raw, ½ cup, 3.5 oz | 165 | 0 | 39 |
| **Zucchini:** Raw, 1 medium, 7 oz | 30 | 0.5 | 7 |
| 1 large, 12 oz | 60 | 1 | 12 |
| Cooked, slices, | | | |
| ½ cup, 3 oz | 15 | 0 | 4 |

## Frozen Vegetables

| | C | F | Cb |
|---|---|---|---|
| **Birds Eye:** | | | |
| **Mixtures & Blends:** | | | |
| Broccoli, Cauliflower & Carrots, 3 oz | 35 | 0 | 5.5 |
| Stir-Fry: Broccoli, 3.4 oz | 35 | 0 | 6 |
| Crisp Bean, 5.5 oz | 60 | 0 | 11 |
| Sugar Snap, 3.4 oz | 40 | 0 | 7.5 |
| **Pure & Simple:** | | | |
| Baby: Broccoli Florets, 1 cup, 3 oz | 35 | 0.5 | 5 |
| Gold & White Corn, ⅔ cup, 3.2 oz | 105 | 1 | 22 |
| Sweet Peas, ⅔ cup, 3 oz | 80 | 0 | 14 |
| **Recipe Ready:** | | | |
| Chopped Green Peppers & Onions, 2.8 oz | 25 | 0 | 5 |
| Southwest Blend, 3.3 oz | 80 | 0.5 | 15 |
| **Sauced & Seasoned:** *Per 1 Cup* | | | |
| Green Beans & Spaetzle, | | | |
| in Bavarian Sauce | 95 | 4.5 | 10 |
| Pasta & Veggies in Creamy Cheese Sauce | 125 | 3 | 20 |
| **Steamfresh:** | | | |
| Pure & Simple Blends: | | | |
| Baby Broccoli Blend, 1 cup | 65 | 1.5 | 8 |
| Baby Potato Blend, ¾ cup | 50 | 0 | 10 |
| Brocc. & Cauliflower, 1 cup, 3.4 oz | 30 | 0.5 | 4.5 |

## Frozen Vegetables (Cont)  C F Cb

**Green Giant:**
**Create A Meal Stir Fry:** *Unprepared*

| | C | F | Cb |
|---|---|---|---|
| Lo Mein, 1.6 cups | 130 | 1 | 27 |
| Sweet & Sour, 1.3 cups | 140 | 0 | 34 |
| Szechuan, 1.3 cups | 70 | 1 | 14 |
| Teriyaki, 1.3 cups | 60 | 0 | 14 |

**Just for One:**

| | | | |
|---|---|---|---|
| Broccoli & Cheese Sauce, 4.3 oz | 40 | 1 | 7 |
| Caulifl. & Cheese Sauce, 4.3 oz | 40 | 1 | 8 |

**Seasoned Steamers:** *Per ¾ Cup, Frozen*

| | | | |
|---|---|---|---|
| Honey Dijon Carrots, 3 oz | 60 | 2 | 10 |
| Mediterranean Blend, 3 oz | 80 | 3 | 11 |

**Valley Fresh Steamers:**
Prepared, with Cheese Sauce:

| | | | |
|---|---|---|---|
| Broccoli, ⅔ cup, 4 oz | 60 | 2.5 | 7 |
| Broccoli, Cauliflower & Carrots, ⅔ cup, 4.3 oz | 60 | 2.5 | 8 |
| Garden Vegetable Medley, 3.5 oz | 60 | 0.5 | 12 |

Prepared, Without Sauce:

| | | | |
|---|---|---|---|
| Broccoli Cuts, ½ cup | 15 | 0 | 3 |
| Mixed Vegetables, ½ cup | 50 | 0 | 12 |
| Sweet Peas, ½ cup | 50 | 0 | 12 |

**Ore-Ida:** *Per 3 oz Unless Indicated*
**Fries:**

| | | | |
|---|---|---|---|
| Classic: Golden Crinkles | 120 | 4.5 | 19 |
| Golden | 130 | 3.5 | 21 |
| Steak | 110 | 3 | 19 |
| Extra Crispy Easy, Golden Crinkles | 170 | 6 | 25 |
| Extra Crispy: Fast Food Fries | 150 | 6 | 24 |
| Golden Crinkles | 160 | 7 | 22 |
| Seasoned Crinkles | 150 | 6 | 22 |
| Tater Tots | 170 | 9 | 20 |

Premium:

| | | | |
|---|---|---|---|
| Country Style French | 130 | 4.5 | 20 |
| Crispers | 230 | 14 | 23 |
| Golden Twirls | 150 | 6 | 23 |
| Texas Crispers | 150 | 7 | 20 |

| | | | |
|---|---|---|---|
| **Grillers:** Golden Thick Cut Potatoes | 130 | 5 | 19 |
| Seasoned Thick Cut Potatoes | 140 | 5 | 21 |
| **Hash Browns:** Golden Patties (1) | 140 | 8 | 15 |
| Potatoes O'Brien | 60 | 0 | 13 |
| Shredded Hash Browns Pattie (1) | 70 | 0 | 16 |
| **Onion:** Chopped, 3 oz | 20 | 0 | 5 |
| Gourmet Rings, 2.7 oz | 185 | 9 | 24 |
| Onion Ringers, 3 oz | 180 | 10 | 21 |

**Simply:** Cracked Pepper & Sea Salt,

| | | | |
|---|---|---|---|
| Country Style French Fries | 130 | 4.5 | 22 |
| Homestyle Wedges, all varieties | 120 | 3.5 | 20 |
| **Steam n' Mash,** Cut Russet, 3.5 oz | 70 | 0 | 16 |
| **Tater Tots:** Regular | 160 | 8 | 20 |
| Crispy Crowns | 170 | 10 | 19 |

## Canned/Bottled  C F Cb

*Solids & Liquid*

**Artichoke Hearts:**

| | C | F | Cb |
|---|---|---|---|
| *Fancifoods:* Plain, 1 oz (1) | 8 | 0 | 1 |
| Marinated, ¼ bottle, 1 oz | 25 | 1.5 | 2 |
| **Asparagus:** Drained, 3 spears | 10 | 0 | 1.5 |
| Pieces, ½ cup, 4.3 oz | 25 | 0.5 | 3 |
| **Bamboo Shoots,** 1 cup, 4.5 oz | 25 | 0 | 4 |
| **Bean Salad,** ½ cup, 4.4 oz | 90 | 0 | 20 |
| **Beans:** Baked, ½ cup, 4.5 oz | 120 | 0.5 | 27 |
| Butter, ½ cup, 4.5 oz | 90 | 0 | 16 |
| Green, ½ cup, 2.5 oz | 15 | 0 | 3 |
| Italian, ½ cup, 4.5 oz | 30 | 0 | 6 |
| Kidney, ½ cup 3.5 oz | 105 | 0.5 | 19 |
| Lima, ½ cup, 4.5 oz | 80 | 0 | 15 |
| Pinto, ½ cup, 4.5 oz | 105 | 1 | 18 |
| **Beets:** Sliced, ½ cup, 3 oz | 25 | 0 | 6 |
| Crinkle/Pickled, ½ cup | 80 | 0 | 20 |
| **Carrots:** Sliced, ½ cup, 2.5 oz | 20 | 0 | 4 |
| *Del Monte,* Honey Glazed, ½ cup | 75 | 0 | 18 |
| **Corn:** Kernels, ½ cup, 4.5 oz | 80 | 0.5 | 18 |
| Creamed style, ½ cup, 4.5 oz | 90 | 0.5 | 23 |
| **Garbanzo/Chick Peas,** ½ c, 4.2 oz | 145 | 1.5 | 27 |
| **Hearts of Palm,** (1), 1.2 oz | 7 | 0 | 1 |
| **Mushrooms:** ½ cup, 2.5 oz | 20 | 0 | 4 |
| In Butter Sauce, 2 oz | 20 | 1 | 2 |
| **Onions:** Cocktail (1) | 0 | 0 | 0 |
| Pickled, 1 medium, 0.5 oz | 10 | 0 | 2 |
| **Peas,** ½ cup, 3 oz | 60 | 0.5 | 10 |
| **Peppers:** Hot Chili, Jalapeno (1), 1 oz | 5 | 0 | 1 |
| Red/Green, 1 oz | 5 | 0 | 1 |
| Sweet, undrained, 2.5 oz | 13 | 0 | 3 |
| Jalapeno, with liquid, ½ cup chopped | 20 | 0.5 | 3 |
| Fried, drained, 2 Tbsp, 1 oz | 60 | 5 | 3 |
| **Salsa,** average all varieties, 2 Tbsp | 10 | 0 | 2 |
| **Sauerkraut,** drained, 1 cup, 5 oz | 25 | 0 | 6 |
| **Spinach,** ½ cup, 3.5 oz | 25 | 0.5 | 3.5 |
| **Succotash:** Cream Style, ½ cup | 100 | 0.5 | 23 |
| W/ whole kernels, undrained, ½ cup | 80 | 0.5 | 18 |
| **Sweetcorn** ~ *See Corn* | | | |
| **Sweet Potato,** ½ cup, 3.5 oz | 90 | 0 | 24 |
| **Tomatoes,** Sundried: Nat., 5–6 pieces | 20 | 0 | 5 |
| In Oil, drained, 6 pieces, 0.5 oz | 40 | 2.5 | 4 |
| **Tomato Products** ~ *See Page 144* | | | |
| **Vegetables,** mixed, ½ cup, 4 oz | 45 | 0 | 8 |
| **Yams:** In Light Syrup, ½ cup, 4 oz | 105 | 0 | 25 |
| Candied, ½ cup, 5 oz | 170 | 0 | 46 |
| **Zucchini,** in Tomato Sauce, ½ cup, 4 oz | 30 | 0 | 8 |

## Quick Guide

| | C | F | Cb |
|---|---|---|---|
| **Yogurt:** *Average All Brands: Per 8 oz Container* | | | |
| **Plain Yogurt:** Whole | 140 | 8 | 10 |
| Low-Fat | 145 | 3.5 | 16 |
| Fat-Free | 125 | 0.5 | 17 |
| **Fruit Flavored:** Whole | 225 | 8 | 32 |
| Low-Fat | 230 | 3 | 43 |
| Fat-Free, regular | 215 | 0.5 | 43 |
| Fat-Free, no sugar added | 80 | 0 | 15 |
| **Yogurt Parfait/Deli Cups:** | | | |
| **With Fruit Pieces:** (⅔ Yogurt + ⅓ Fruit) | | | |
| Small, 8 oz cup | 140 | 3 | 20 |
| Large, 12 oz cup | 210 | 4.5 | 30 |
| **With Fruit + Granola:** | | | |
| Small, 8 oz cup (+ 0.75 oz Granola) | 235 | 7 | 30 |
| Large, 12 oz cup (+ 1.3 oz Granola) | 400 | 13 | 58 |

## Yogurt ~ Brands

| | C | F | Cb |
|---|---|---|---|
| **Activia:** *Per 4 oz Unless Indicated* | | | |
| Fiber/Fruit flavors, average | 115 | 2 | 21 |
| Light flavors, fat free, all flav. | 60 | 0 | 10 |
| Greek: Av. all flavors, 5.3 oz | 130 | 0 | 20 |
| Light, Fruit Flavors | 80 | 0 | 8 |
| **Alpina:** | | | |
| **Greek**, Strained, av., 5.3 oz | 125 | 0 | 19 |
| **Artisan Granolas:** *Per 6 oz* | | | |
| Plain | 170 | 2.5 | 22 |
| Black Cherry | 220 | 2.5 | 36 |
| Pineapple | 230 | 4.5 | 38 |
| Other Fruit Flavors, av. | 210 | 4.5 | 29 |
| **Bon Yurt:** *Per 5.3 oz Container* | | | |
| Cookies & Cream | 180 | 3.5 | 33 |
| Other fruit flavors, av. | 150 | 1.5 | 28 |
| **Cafe Selections**, av. 5.3oz | 120 | 1 | 18 |
| **Amande:** | | | |
| **Almond Milk Yogurt:** Plain, 8 oz | 170 | 9 | 19 |
| Fruit Flavors, 6 oz | 150 | 6 | 23 |
| Vanilla, 8 oz | 220 | 8 | 26 |
| **Axelrod:** | | | |
| **32 oz Containers:** | | | |
| Low Fat, Plain, 8 oz | 140 | 2.5 | 18 |
| Nonfat, Plain, 8 oz | 140 | 0 | 21 |
| **6 oz Containers:** | | | |
| Low Fat, Fruit flavors, average | 180 | 1.5 | 36 |
| Nonfat, Fruit flavors, average | 90 | 0 | 17 |
| **Brown Cow:** *Per 6 oz Container* | | | |
| **Cream Top:** | | | |
| Fruit On The Bottom: | | | |
| Apricot Mango | 170 | 6 | 23 |
| Cherry-Vanilla; Strawb. | 180 | 6 | 28 |
| Chocolate | 190 | 6 | 28 |

| **Brown Cow (Cont):** | C | F | Cb |
|---|---|---|---|
| **Cream Top:** | | | |
| Smooth & Creamy: Plain | 130 | 7 | 9 |
| Coffee; Vanilla | 160 | 7 | 19 |
| Maple | 170 | 7 | 22 |
| **Greek:** *Per 5.3 oz Containers* | | | |
| Fruit On The Bottom, Fruit Flav., av. | 125 | 0 | 19 |
| Smooth & Creamy, Plain, nonfat | 80 | 0 | 6 |
| **Cabot:** *Per 8 oz Serving* | | | |
| **32 oz Containers, Greek Style:** | | | |
| Plain | 310 | 22 | 12 |
| Lowfat (2%): Plain | 180 | 5 | 12 |
| Strawberry; Vanilla Bean | 240 | 4 | 34 |
| **Chobani:** *Per 5.3 oz Containers* | | | |
| **Blended:** Plain | 130 | 6 | 7 |
| Coconut | 150 | 4.5 | 16 |
| Fruit Flavors, average | 145 | 3 | 17 |
| Vanilla | 120 | 0 | 16 |
| **Flip:** Almond Coco Loco | 240 | 10 | 26 |
| Key Lime Crumble | 200 | 6 | 26 |
| Nutty for 'Nana | 200 | 8 | 20 |
| **Fruit On The Bottom:** | | | |
| 2% Fat, Fruit Flavors, av. | 140 | 3 | 18 |
| Fat Free, Fruit Flavors, av. | 125 | 0 | 20 |
| **Simply 100**, av. all flavors | 100 | 0 | 15 |
| **Dannon:** | | | |
| **Activia ~** *See Activia* | | | |
| **All Natural:** | | | |
| Plain: Regular, 8 oz | 150 | 8 | 11 |
| Lowfat, 6 oz | 100 | 2.5 | 12 |
| Nonfat, 6 oz | 80 | 0 | 12 |
| **Classic:** Coffee, 6 oz | 160 | 2.5 | 26 |
| Vanilla, 6 oz | 150 | 2.5 | 25 |
| **Creamy**, Fruit Flavors, average, 4 oz | 95 | 0.5 | 18 |
| **Danimals:** Nonfat, Strawberry, 4 oz | 80 | 0 | 16 |
| Greek, all flavors, 4 oz | 110 | 1.5 | 15 |
| Squeezables, all flavors, 1 Pouch, 4 oz | 100 | 1.5 | 18 |
| **Fruit On The Bottom,** | | | |
| av. all flavors, 6 oz | 150 | 1.5 | 29 |
| **Light & Fit:** | | | |
| 50-Calorie Packs, av. all flavors, 4 oz | 50 | 0 | 9 |
| Regular: 6 oz Cup, average all flavors | 80 | 0 | 14 |
| Quarts Cont., av. all flavors, 8 oz | 105 | 0 | 19 |
| Greek, av. all flavors, 5.3 oz cup | 80 | 0 | 9 |
| Carb & Sugar Control, 4- Pack, | | | |
| all flavors, 4 oz cup | 45 | 1.5 | 3 |
| **Oikos:** *Per Single, 5.3 oz Container, Unless Indicated* | | | |
| Chocolate On Top: Raspberry Truffle | 150 | 4 | 18 |
| Chocolate Covered Strawberry | 210 | 4.5 | 32 |
| Traditional Fruit flavors | 160 | 4.5 | 19 |
| Triple Zero, all flavors | 120 | 0 | 15 |
| Non-Fat Yogurt: Plain | 80 | 0 | 6 |
| Fruit On Bottom, average all flav. | 125 | 0 | 20 |

## Yogurt Brands (Cont)

**C** **F** **Cb**

**Ehrmann Mixim:** *Per 5.3 oz Cup*
**Fat Free Greek Yogurt with:**

| | C | F | Cb |
|---|---|---|---|
| Blackb. & Pomegranate, w/ Granola & Dr. Fruit | 160 | 3 | 22 |
| Blueb. & Choc Chip Cookies | 150 | 1.5 | 23 |
| Cherry & Dark Chocolate Curls | 160 | 0 | 31 |
| Mango, P'apple, Coconut & Almonds | 150 | 3 | 21 |
| Raspbery & Dark/White Chocolate | 160 | 3 | 23 |
| Other varieties | 150 | 1.5 | 23 |

**Fage:**

| | C | F | Cb |
|---|---|---|---|
| **Fruyo Greek:** Reg., av. all flav., 6 oz | 195 | 7 | 20 |
| Fat free, av. all flavors, 6 oz | 140 | 0 | 21 |
| **Total Classic:** Plain, Single Serve, 7 oz | 190 | 10 | 8 |
| Split Cup, Fruit Flavors, 5.3 oz | 170 | 6 | 17 |
| **Total 2%:** | | | |
| Plain, Single Serve, 7 oz | 150 | 4 | 8 |
| Split Cup, Fruit Flavors, 5.3 oz | 140 | 2.5 | 17 |
| **Total 0%:** Plain, 6 oz | 100 | 0 | 7 |
| Split Cup, Fruit Flavors, 5.3 oz | 120 | 0 | 17 |

**Horizon Organic:** *Per 8 oz Cup*
**Cream On Top:**

| | C | F | Cb |
|---|---|---|---|
| Whole Milk: Plain | 170 | 8 | 16 |
| Vanilla | 230 | 6 | 33 |
| **Fat-Free:** Plain | 110 | 0 | 17 |
| Vanilla | 190 | 0 | 35 |
| **Tuberz,** all flavors, 1 tube | 60 | 0.5 | 11 |

**Kemps:**
**Greek Style:**

| | C | F | Cb |
|---|---|---|---|
| Fat Free: Vanilla, 5.3 oz | 140 | 0 | 22 |
| Average Fruit Flavors, 5.3 oz | 130 | 0 | 18 |
| Snack Mousse, all flavors, 4.8 oz | 190 | 2.5 | 31 |
| **Light,** 80 Calories, av. all flav., 6 oz | 80 | 0 | 16 |

**La Yogurt:** *Per 6 oz Container*

| | C | F | Cb |
|---|---|---|---|
| **Low Fat:** Original, average all flavors | 155 | 1.5 | 29 |
| Rich & Creamy, average all flavors | 180 | 1.5 | 35 |
| **Sabor Latino,** Low Fat, av. all flavors | 185 | 1.5 | 37 |

**LALA:**

| | C | F | Cb |
|---|---|---|---|
| **32 oz Tubs,** Plain, 8 oz | 130 | 2.5 | 17 |
| **Single Serve:** | | | |
| Fruit Flavors, av., 6 oz | 150 | 1.5 | 30 |
| Pina Colada, 6 oz | 160 | 2 | 30 |

**Liberté:**
**Méditerranée:**

| | C | F | Cb |
|---|---|---|---|
| Average Fruit flavors, 6 oz | 250 | 12 | 29 |
| Average other flavors | 265 | 12 | 31 |

**Lucerne:** *Per 6 oz Container*

| | C | F | Cb |
|---|---|---|---|
| **Low-Fat,** average all flavors | 170 | 2 | 32 |
| **Fat-Free:** Plain | 80 | 0 | 13 |
| Light Fat-Free, fruit, 6 oz | 90 | 0 | 17 |

**Mountain High:** *Per 8 oz*
**32 oz Containers:**

| | C | F | Cb |
|---|---|---|---|
| Original Style: Plain | 170 | 6 | 19 |
| Vanilla | 200 | 6 | 28 |
| Lowfat: Plain | 140 | 2.5 | 18 |
| Honey; Vanilla | 185 | 2.5 | 30 |
| Fat-Free: Plain | 120 | 0 | 18 |
| Vanilla | 160 | 0 | 30 |

**Nancy's:** *Per 8 oz Container Unless Indicated*
**Natural:**

| | C | F | Cb |
|---|---|---|---|
| Whole Milk: Honey Yogurt, Plain | 180 | 8 | 17 |
| With Fruit on Top, av. | 230 | 5 | 41 |
| Lowfat: Lemon; Van., av. | 145 | 3 | 16 |
| Average other flavors | 175 | 2.5 | 28 |

**Organic:**

| | C | F | Cb |
|---|---|---|---|
| Low Fat, Plain | 140 | 3 | 16 |
| Nonfat: Fruit-On-Top, av. | 150 | 0 | 28 |
| Maple; Vanilla, 6 oz | 120 | 0 | 21 |

**Oikos ~** *see Dannon*

| | C | F | Cb |
|---|---|---|---|
| **O Organics,** Blended Low-Fat, av. | 160 | 2.5 | 26 |
| **Publix:** | | | |
| Fat Free, Light, average all flavors, 6 oz | 110 | 0 | 19 |
| Premium Greek, av. all flavors, 5.3 oz | 130 | 0 | 18 |
| **Schnucks,** Light (Nonfat), av. all flavors, 6 oz | 110 | 0 | 20 |

**Silk** *(Dairy Free):*
**Fruity & Creamy:**

| | C | F | Cb |
|---|---|---|---|
| Black Cherry, 5.3 oz | 140 | 3.5 | 21 |
| Blueberry, 5.3 oz | 140 | 3.5 | 22 |
| Peach Mango; Strawb.; Van., 5.3 oz | 135 | 3.5 | 20 |

**So Delicious:**
**Cultured Almond Milk:**

| | C | F | Cb |
|---|---|---|---|
| Chocolate, 6 oz | 150 | 6 | 24 |
| Vanilla, 6 oz | 120 | 5 | 18 |
| **Cultured Coconut Milk:** | | | |
| Plain, unsweetened, 4 oz | 50 | 4 | 6 |
| Blueberry, 4 oz | 140 | 6 | 24 |
| Greek: Plain, 6 oz | 130 | 5 | 22 |
| Vanilla, 6 oz | 140 | 4.5 | 27 |

**Stonyfield Organic:**
**Fruit On Bottom:** *Per 6 oz Container*

| | C | F | Cb |
|---|---|---|---|
| Fat Free: Chocolate Underground | 170 | 0 | 36 |
| Fruit flavors, average | 115 | 0 | 22 |

**Greek:** *Per 5.3 oz Containers*

| | C | F | Cb |
|---|---|---|---|
| Plain | 80 | 0 | 6 |
| Chocolate | 140 | 0 | 23 |
| Average Fruit Flavors | 120 | 0 | 19 |
| **Oh My Yog,** average all flavors, 6 oz | 180 | 5 | 28 |

**Smooth & Creamy (32 oz Ctn):** *Per 8 oz Serving*

| | C | F | Cb |
|---|---|---|---|
| Fat Free: Plain | 100 | 0 | 16 |
| French Vanilla | 170 | 0 | 33 |
| Low Fat: Plain | 120 | 2 | 15 |
| French Vanilla | 170 | 2 | 29 |
| Strawberry; Banilla, average | 195 | 2 | 36 |

## Yogurt Brands (Cont)

| | C | F | Cb |
|---|---|---|---|
| **Trader Joes:** | | | |
| **French Village:** *Per 32 oz Containers* | | | |
| **Non-Fat:** Plain, 8 oz | 120 | 0 | 17 |
| Vanilla, 8 oz | 180 | 0 | 34 |
| Cream Line, Plain, 8 oz | 170 | 10 | 12 |
| 6 oz Container, av. all flav. | 130 | 0 | 26 |
| **Greek Style:** Plain, 8 oz | 260 | 18 | 14 |
| Apricot Mango; Honey, av., 8 oz | 300 | 15 | 28 |
| Low-Fat: With Almonds/Granola: | | | |
| Pomegranate, 4.6 oz | 140 | 2.5 | 27 |
| Vanilla, 4.6 oz | 160 | 7 | 20 |
| **Squishers**, Org., low fat, 1 tube, 2 oz | 60 | 1 | 10 |
| **Voskos**, Greek, Non-Fat, Van., 8 oz | 200 | 0 | 30 |
| **Wallaby Organic**, Blended, | | | |
| Low-Fat, Fruit Flavors, average, 6 oz | 140 | 2.5 | 24 |
| **Wegmans:** *Per 6 oz Container* | | | |
| **Blended Lowfat**, Fruit Flavors | 170 | 1.5 | 33 |
| **Fruit On The Bottom, Lowfat:** | | | |
| Strawberry | 180 | 2 | 35 |
| Average other Fruit Flavors | 165 | 2 | 31 |
| **Greek**, Non-Fat: Plain | 90 | 0 | 8 |
| Fruit flavors, average | 140 | 0 | 20 |
| Vanilla Flavored | 120 | 0 | 15 |
| **Whole Foods (365):** | | | |
| Non-Fat: Plain, 6 oz | 90 | 0 | 13 |
| Fruit flavors, av., 6 oz | 145 | 0 | 30 |
| Greek, non-fat, 5.3 oz | 150 | 0 | 25 |
| **Whole Soy**, Plain, 6 oz | 150 | 4.5 | 19 |
| Av. other flavors, 6 oz | 170 | 3.5 | 33 |
| **YoCrunch:** | | | |
| **YoCrunch**, Vanilla, Lowfat, | | | |
| w/ Nestle Crunch/Snickers pcs, 6 oz | 180 | 4 | 31 |
| **Yopa Greek:** | | | |
| Fruit Parfaits, with Granola, 4 oz | 110 | 0.5 | 24 |
| Light Plus: Strawberry, | | | |
| with Dble Dark Choc. pcs, 5.3 oz | 150 | 2.5 | 12 |
| Nonfat: Blueberry, with | | | |
| 9 Whole Grain Granola, 5.3 oz | 180 | 2 | 28 |
| Vanilla & Almonds, 5.3 oz | 190 | 8 | 20 |
| **Yoplait:** | | | |
| **Original**, 25% less sugar: | | | |
| Caramel, 6 oz | 140 | 2.5 | 23 |
| Other flavors, 6 oz | 150 | 2 | 25 |
| **Light:** Fruit flavors, 6 oz | 90 | 0 | 16 |
| Thick & Creamy, 6 oz | 100 | 0 | 21 |
| **Lactose Free**, all flavors, 6 oz | 170 | 1.5 | 33 |
| **GoGurt:** All flavors, | | | |
| 1 tube, 2.3 oz | 60 | 0.5 | 12 |
| Simply GoGurt, 1 tube, 2.3 oz | 60 | 0.5 | 12 |
| Twisted 1 tube, 2.3 oz | 60 | 0.5 | 12 |

## Yogurt Brands (Cont)

| | C | F | Cb |
|---|---|---|---|
| **Yoplait (Cont):** | | | |
| **Greek:** *Per 5.3 oz Carton* | | | |
| 100 Calorie Flav., av. | 100 | 0 | 12 |
| 2% Fat, all flavors | 150 | 3 | 20 |
| Fruit Flavors (fat-free) av. | 140 | 0 | 21 |
| **Plenti**, all flavors, 5.5 oz | 140 | 1.5 | 21 |
| **Thick & Creamy**, av., 6 oz | 180 | 2.5 | 31 |
| **Trix**, all flavors, av., 4 oz cup | 100 | 0.5 | 20 |
| **Whips!:** Choc. flav., 4 oz | 160 | 4 | 25 |
| Fruit flavors, 4 oz cup | 140 | 2.5 | 25 |
| Greek 100, all flav., 4 oz | 100 | 0 | 15 |
| **Yoplait Kids:** All flavors, 3 oz cup | 70 | 1 | 12 |
| 4 oz Cups, all flavors | 100 | 0.5 | 20 |

### Yogurt Drinks & Probiotics

| | C | F | Cb |
|---|---|---|---|
| **Cacique,** Yonique, | | | |
| av. other flavors, 7 fl.oz | 200 | 1.5 | 35 |
| **Dannon:** | | | |
| **Activia**, av. all flavors, 7 fl oz | 165 | 3 | 27 |
| **DanActive**, fruit flavors, 3.1 fl.oz | 70 | 1 | 14 |
| **Danimals Smoothies:** | | | |
| Av. all flavors, 3.1 fl.oz | 60 | 0.5 | 11 |
| Max, av. all flavors, 7 fl.oz | 120 | 1.5 | 23 |
| **Dan-o-nino**, all flav., 3.1 fl.oz | 70 | 0.5 | 15 |
| **Light & Fit**, Protein Shake, 10 fl.oz | 140 | 0 | 23 |
| **Glen Oaks**, av. all flavors, 8 fl.oz | 150 | 3 | 33 |
| **Good Belly:** *Per 2.7 fl.oz Bottle* | | | |
| **Probiotics:** BigShot, all flav. | 60 | 1 | 11 |
| Plus, average all flavors | 50 | 0 | 12 |
| Straightshot, Plain | 30 | 0 | 6 |
| **Kemps**, Smoothie To Go, | | | |
| average all flavors, 4 fl.oz | 105 | 1 | 18 |
| **LaLa:** | | | |
| **Lalacult:** 5-pack, 1 bottle | 35 | 0 | 9 |
| **Proactive:** Prune, 6.3 oz bottle | 180 | 3 | 36 |
| Average other flavors, 6.3 oz bottle | 155 | 3.5 | 30 |
| **Yogurt Smoothies**, all flav. 7 fl.oz | 175 | 4.5 | 29 |
| **Lifeway Kefir:** | | | |
| Original, 8 fl.oz | 150 | 8 | 12 |
| Lowfat: Plain, 8 fl.oz | 110 | 2 | 12 |
| Chocolate Truffle, 8 fl.oz | 160 | 2 | 25 |
| Other flavors, 8 fl.oz | 140 | 2 | 20 |
| **Stonyfield Organic:** | | | |
| **Smoothies**, av. all flav., 10 oz | 230 | 3 | 40 |
| **Yobaby**, av. all flavors, 6 oz | 185 | 7 | 24 |
| **Yakult:** Reg., 2.7 fl.oz bottle | 50 | 0 | 12 |
| Light, 2.7 fl.oz | 30 | 0 | 6 |
| **Yoplait,** Yogurt & Juice, av., 8 fl.oz | 115 | 0 | 21 |

## Cafeteria-Style Foods  C  F  Cb

*Average All Preparations:*

| | C | F | Cb |
|---|---|---|---|
| **Beef Stroganoff**, 5 oz | 195 | 13 | 7 |
| **Beef Stroganoff**, with 4 oz noodles | 350 | 14 | 36 |
| **Chicken Lasagna**, 1 piece | 300 | 11 | 32 |
| **Chicken Chop Suey**, with 4 oz rice | 245 | 4 | 37 |
| **Deep Dish Burrito**, 7 oz | 265 | 13 | 20 |
| **Ground Beef Casserole**, 2 scps, 6 oz | 245 | 13 | 17 |
| **Italian Meat Sce**, for Spaghetti, 5 oz | 150 | 9 | 9 |
| with 5 oz Spaghetti | 350 | 10 | 49 |
| **Lasagna**, 1 piece | 275 | 11 | 25 |
| **Meatloaf**, 3 oz | 205 | 13 | 4 |
| **Ranch Beans**, 2 scoops, 6 oz | 350 | 11 | 45 |
| **Red Beans & Rice**, 7 oz | 280 | 9 | 37 |
| **Scalloped Potato/Ham**, 2 scoops, 6 oz | 160 | 6 | 20 |
| **Stuffed Shells in Sauce**, (1) | 105 | 3 | 17 |
| **Swedish Meatballs**, (3) | 205 | 12 | 9 |
| **Sweet & Sour Pork/Rice**, 9 oz | 240 | 3 | 40 |
| **Swiss Steak**, w/ Mushroom Gravy, 6 oz | 280 | 11 | 4 |
| **Tator Tot Casserole**, 2 scoops, 6 oz | 260 | 15 | 20 |
| **Tenderloin Tips/Mshrm Gravy:** 5 oz | 210 | 13 | 3 |
| With 5 oz noodles | 395 | 15 | 38 |
| **Tuna Noodle Casserole**, 2 scoops, 6 oz | 180 | 6 | 17 |
| **Turkey Tetrazzini**, 2 scoops, 6 oz | 195 | 7 | 17 |
| **Vegetable Lasagna**, 1 piece | 250 | 13 | 21 |

## Croissants

| | C | F | Cb |
|---|---|---|---|
| **Unfilled,** medium 1.5 oz | 180 | 10 | 21 |
| **Filled:** With Ham (2 oz), garnish | 280 | 14 | 24 |
| With Ham (2 oz), Cheese (2 oz) | 470 | 30 | 20 |
| With Chick (2 oz) Cheese (2 oz) | 470 | 30 | 20 |
| With Turkey/Ham/Cheese (2 oz ea.) | 580 | 36 | 20 |
| *Au Bon Pain:* Ham & Cheese | 390 | 21 | 35 |
| Spinach & Cheese | 290 | 17 | 28 |

7-Eleven ~ See Page 236

## Bagels

| | C | F | Cb |
|---|---|---|---|
| **Plain:** Large, 4 oz (without filling) | 320 | 2 | 65 |
| With 2 oz Cream Cheese | 500 | 27 | 54 |
| With 2 oz Lox (Smoked Salmon) | 400 | 4 | 65 |

**Also see Bagels Section ~** *Page 54*
**Fast-Foods Restaurants ~** *Page 175*
Au Bon Pain ~ *Page 179*
Bruegger's ~ *Page 185*
Einstein Bros Bagels ~ *Page 199*

## Sandwiches  C  F  Cb

*No Spreads Unless Indicated:*
*Includes 2 Slices Bread ~ 3 oz*

| | C | F | Cb |
|---|---|---|---|
| **BLT**, (5 strips Bacon, 2 Tbsp Mayo) | 600 | 40 | 46 |
| **Breaded Chicken & Garnish** | 540 | 28 | 46 |
| **Chicken Salad**, with Mayo., 5 oz | 580 | 30 | 49 |
| **Chopped Liver, Egg Mayonnaise** | 630 | 25 | 44 |
| **Corned Beef with Mustard**, 5 oz | 560 | 28 | 44 |
| **Egg Salad**, with Mayonnaise | 570 | 29 | 49 |
| **Egg Salad Club**, with Bacon & Mayo, | 780 | 53 | 49 |
| **Grilled Cheese**, (3 oz) | 540 | 30 | 44 |
| **Ham**, (4 oz), Cheese (4 oz), & Mayo. | 910 | 56 | 44 |
| **Lobster Salad**, (4 oz), w/ Mayo. | 530 | 25 | 45 |
| **Overstuffed Tuna Salad**, (7 oz) | 870 | 39 | 75 |
| **Philly Cheese Steak Sandwich** | 550 | 23 | 42 |
| **Reuben**, (6 oz Beef/Pastrami, | | | |
| 2 oz Cheese, 2 Tbsp Dressing) | 920 | 60 | 28 |
| **Roast Beef**, (4 oz), with Mustard | 460 | 12 | 45 |
| **Roast Pork**, (4 oz), with Apple Sauce | 500 | 16 | 55 |
| **Shrimp Salad Club**, w/ Bacon & Mayo | 800 | 57 | 48 |
| **Sloppy Joe with Sauce**, (7 oz) | 600 | 30 | 45 |
| **Steak Sandwich**, (5 oz cooked) | 680 | 32 | 41 |
| **Triple Cheese Melt**, (4 oz) | 720 | 45 | 46 |
| **Tuna Salad**, (5 oz), with Mayonnaise | 610 | 30 | 49 |
| **Turkey Breast**, (5 oz), w/ Mayo. | 460 | 18 | 44 |
| **Turkey Breast**, (5 oz,) with Mustard | 360 | 7 | 44 |
| **Turkey Club**, with Bacon & Mayo. | 830 | 38 | 31 |
| **Vegetarian**, with Avocado & Cheese | 820 | 49 | 72 |

7-Eleven ~ *Page 236*
Schlotzsky's ~ *Page 237*
Subway ~ *Page 245*

## Wraps & Roll-Ups

*Average All Types*
**Meat/Chicken/Fish/Veggie:**

| | C | F | Cb |
|---|---|---|---|
| Small, approximately 9 oz | 500 | 25 | 48 |
| Regular, approximately 15 oz | 830 | 40 | 80 |
| Large, approximately 22 oz | 1400 | 70 | 134 |

**Fast-Foods Restaurants ~** *Page 175*
Au Bon Pain ~ *Page 179*
Sonic Drive-In ~ *Page 241*
Subway ~ *Page 245*
WAWA ~ *Page 254*

Updated Nutrition Data ~ www.CalorieKing.com
Persons with Diabetes ~ See Disclaimer (Page 22)

# Eating Out – Fair ◆ Carnival

## Fair & Carnival Foods  | C | E | CP |

**Barbeque Chicken/Meats:**

| | C | E | CP |
|---|---|---|---|
| **Chicken**, ½ chicken, 15 oz | 740 | 24 | 34 |
| **Grilled Chicken Pita**, with dressing | 680 | 19 | 82 |
| **Teriyaki Chicken**, on stick, w/ dress. | 250 | 6 | 4 |
| **Pork Ribs**, 18 oz | 1360 | 68 | 21 |
| **Turkey Leg:** Regular, 19 oz | 1135 | 54 | 0 |
| Caveman (2lb Turkey Leg, with 1lb Bacon) | 2360 | 177 | 3 |
| **Bacon:** Fried, on-a-stick, with syrup | 230 | 16 | 5 |
| Choc-covered Bacon, 4.5 oz dish | 640 | 43 | 30 |
| **Beef Stew over Rice**, 2 cups | 440 | 14 | 61 |
| **Butter Balls**, deep fried, 4 Balls | 460 | 38 | 24 |
| **Cheese Curds**, Breaded & fried, Culver's, 6.7 oz | 670 | 38 | 54 |
| **Corn Dogs:** Regular, 4 oz | 250 | 14 | 23 |
| Jumbo, 6 oz | 375 | 21 | 36 |
| Pretzel-Wrapped Dog | 300 | 16 | 30 |
| Papa Pup, on-a-stick | 400 | 24 | 32 |
| Pronto Pup, on-a-stick | 170 | 9 | 16 |
| **Corn On The Cob**, 8"(1), 16 oz | 200 | 1 | 42 |

**Finger Foods:**

| | C | E | CP |
|---|---|---|---|
| **Artichoke**, fried, 9 pieces | 250 | 14 | 24 |
| **Chicken Nuggets**, (6) | 340 | 17 | 26 |
| **Chicken Strips**, (4), 4.5 oz | 445 | 21 | 33 |
| **Onion Rings**, 3 rings | 310 | 13 | 40 |
| **Onion Flower** | 1320 | 72 | 140 |
| **Shrimp**, Fried, 10-12 pieces, 5 oz | 555 | 30 | 36 |
| **Spam**, deep-fried in batter, 2 pieces | 330 | 24 | 18 |

**Gator:**

| | C | E | CP |
|---|---|---|---|
| **Big Gator**, Nuggets/Hushpuppies | 550 | 31 | 54 |
| **Stick Gator**, 1 sausage | 250 | 20 | 4 |

**Greek:**

| | C | E | CP |
|---|---|---|---|
| **Baklava**, 2" square | 245 | 13 | 32 |
| **Falafel**, 11.6 oz | 660 | 27 | 85 |
| **Greek Salad**, 14 oz | 520 | 48 | 17 |
| **Gyro**, 7.5", 12 oz | 680 | 40 | 55 |
| **Spanakopita**, 8 oz | 200 | 7.5 | 23 |

**Hamburgers:**

| | C | E | CP |
|---|---|---|---|
| **⅓ Pound Burger**, 7.5 oz | 670 | 41 | 26 |
| **Cheeseburger**, 6 oz | 550 | 36 | 25 |

**Hot Dogs:** *With Bun*

| | C | E | CP |
|---|---|---|---|
| **Regular:** No extras | 215 | 14 | 28 |
| With Chili, 6 oz | 450 | 32 | 32 |
| With Chili & Cheese, 7.3 oz | 500 | 36 | 31 |
| **⅓ Pound Hot Dog** | 550 | 41 | 31 |
| **Foot Long Hot Dog** | 470 | 26 | 41 |
| **Jumbo**, Bratwurst/Kielbasa, average | 800 | 60 | 28 |

## Fair & Carnival Foods (Cont)

**Mexican:**

| | C | F | Cb |
|---|---|---|---|
| **Burrito**, with Bean/Beef, 17 oz | 1100 | 41 | 104 |
| **Carne Asada**, 14.5 oz | 820 | 44 | 58 |
| **Cheese Quesadilla**, 1.8 oz | 480 | 27 | 40 |
| **Chicken Taco**, 3.3 oz | 210 | 12 | 16 |
| **Fish Taco**, 5 oz | 270 | 13 | 31 |
| **Jalapeno Pepper**, choc-covered (3) | 270 | 15 | 31 |
| **Nachos with Cheese**, 9" plate | 860 | 59 | 70 |
| **Tamale**, 3.5 oz | 180 | 8 | 21 |
| **Taquito**, 5 oz | 370 | 17 | 43 |

**Pizza:**

| | C | F | Cb |
|---|---|---|---|
| **Pizza Bread**, Pepperoni, ½ loaf, 12 oz | 1115 | 32 | 151 |
| **Pizza on-a-stick**, 1 piece | 535 | 28 | 55 |
| **Personal Pizza:** *Per 7"* | | | |
| Cheese | 670 | 24 | 80 |
| Pepperoni | 795 | 35 | 80 |
| Ham & Pineapple | 800 | 31 | 87 |

**Potatoes & Fries:**

| | C | F | Cb |
|---|---|---|---|
| **Australian Battered Potatoes** | 1290 | 66 | 155 |
| **Baked Potato**, 14 oz | 435 | 0.5 | 100 |
| **Fries:** French, 7 oz | 560 | 24 | 79 |
| Cheese Fries, 10 oz | 645 | 38 | 62 |
| Chili Fries, 10 oz | 700 | 36 | 83 |
| Curly Fries, 7 oz | 620 | 30 | 78 |
| Jamaican Jerk Fries, 7 oz | 640 | 34 | 77 |
| **Sweet Potato**, baked, 14 oz | 405 | 0.5 | 97 |
| **Tornado**, on-a-stick | 210 | 15 | 18 |

**Salads/Sides:**

| | C | F | Cb |
|---|---|---|---|
| **Chili**, 1 cup | 280 | 11 | 24 |
| **Cole Slaw**, 5 oz | 350 | 21 | 37 |
| **Pickle**, whole (6") | 30 | 0 | 8 |
| **Potato Salad**, 5 oz | 290 | 15 | 35 |

**Sandwiches:** *7½" Roll*

| | C | F | Cb |
|---|---|---|---|
| **Ham**, 11 oz | 645 | 39 | 47 |
| **Hot Pastrami**, 9 oz | 760 | 17 | 62 |
| **Roast Beef**, 11 oz | 620 | 36 | 46 |
| **Philadelphia Cheese Steak**, 13 oz | 680 | 36 | 49 |
| **Turkey**, 11 oz | 665 | 24 | 65 |

**Drinks:**

| | C | F | Cb |
|---|---|---|---|
| **Icee**, 16 fl.oz | 235 | 0 | 59 |
| **Shakes**, average, 16 fl.oz | 690 | 33 | 85 |
| **Slushies:** Horchata, 16 fl.oz | 280 | 8 | 50 |
| Lemonade, 18 fl.oz | 210 | 0 | 52 |
| Orange Julius, 20 fl.oz | 490 | 10 | 96 |
| Strawberry Julius, 20 fl.oz | 430 | 0 | 98 |
| **Soft Frozen Lemonade**, 12 fl.oz | 300 | 0 | 78 |
| **Smoothies**, Berry Flavors, 16 fl.oz | 350 | 1 | 80 |

## Fair & Carnival Foods (Cont)

| Cakes, Pastries: | C | F | Cb |
|---|---|---|---|
| **Funnel Cake,** Plain (1) | 760 | 44 | 80 |
| **Toppings:** | | | |
| Apple Cinnamon, 2 oz | 85 | 3 | 16 |
| Cinnamon & Sugar, 2 tsp | 40 | 0 | 10 |
| Strawberry & Cream, 2 oz | 70 | 0 | 16 |
| **Cheesecake on-a-stick,** 6 oz | 655 | 47 | 56 |
| **Churro,** (1), 9", 1.6 oz | 170 | 8 | 22 |
| **Cream Puff,** 4.3 oz | 500 | 43 | 22 |
| **Fried Twinkie,** (1) | 420 | 34 | 45 |
| **Puff-on-a-Stick,** (4), 8.6 oz | 995 | 86 | 44 |
| **Strawberry Crepe,** 4.3 oz | 280 | 14 | 36 |
| **Twinkie Dog,** (Sundae) | 500 | 14 | 89 |
| **Candied Apple,** 7 oz | 330 | 0 | 80 |
| **Cookies:** | | | |
| **Sweet Martha,** (1), 0.8 oz | 90 | 4 | 14 |
| **Deep Fried: Oreos,** tray (5) | 890 | 48 | 108 |
| Cookie Dough on stick, 3 pieces | 670 | 32 | 89 |
| **Cotton Candy:** | | | |
| Small, 1 oz | 110 | 0 | 27 |
| Large, 2.3 oz | 250 | 0 | 62 |
| Family Size, 5.5 oz | 610 | 0 | 151 |
| **Dirt Dessert,** 1 cup, 9.3 oz | 405 | 12 | 69 |
| **Donuts,** Jumbo Twist, (1), 7.5 oz | 905 | 49 | 109 |
| **Fried Dough/FryBread:** | | | |
| **Plain:** 7", 3.7 oz | 390 | 19 | 47 |
| 9", 4¾ oz | 510 | 25 | 61 |
| **Toppings:** Cinnamon Sugar, 2 tsp | 40 | 0 | 10 |
| Butterscotch; Caramel, 2 Tbsp | 115 | 0 | 29 |
| Hot Fudge, average, 2 Tbsp | 110 | 4 | 22 |
| Cheese Powder, 2 tsp | 70 | 3 | 2 |
| Honey, 1 Tbsp, 0.8 oz | 65 | 0 | 17 |
| **Fudge,** 1.5 oz | 200 | 11 | 25 |
| **Ice Cream & Frozen Treats:** | | | |
| **Deep-fried Klondike Bar,** w/ syrup | 430 | 16 | 18 |
| **Dippin' Dots Ice Cream,** 6 oz cup | 380 | 20 | 46 |
| **Frozen Banana,** choc. coated, 5 oz | 240 | 4 | 53 |
| **Frozen Yogurt,** in sugar cone, 14 oz | 475 | 2 | 94 |
| **Ice Cream:** Small, sugar cone, 10 oz | 775 | 42 | 83 |
| Large, sugar cone, 14 oz | 935 | 54 | 96 |
| **Sherbet,** 8 oz | 270 | 4 | 59 |
| **Snow Cone,** with 3 oz syrup | 270 | 0 | 68 |
| **Strawberry,** Choc. Dipped, 1 piece | 125 | 7 | 15 |
| **Popcorn:** | | | |
| **Plain:** Small, 3 oz | 450 | 24 | 48 |
| Large, 6 oz | 900 | 48 | 96 |
| **Kettle Corn:** Small, 5 oz | 600 | 15 | 110 |
| Large, 10 oz | 1200 | 30 | 220 |
| **Pretzels,** Soft, 4.5 oz | 340 | 2 | 70 |
| **S'more,** on stick | 275 | 16 | 27 |

## Stadium Foods

| | C | F | Cb |
|---|---|---|---|
| **Burgers:** | | | |
| **Bacon Burger,** 8.3 oz | 470 | 25 | 34 |
| **Cheeseburger,** 8.3 oz | 450 | 23 | 33 |
| **Hamburger,** 7.8 oz | 400 | 19 | 33 |
| **French Fries,** 6.4 oz | 470 | 34 | 39 |
| **Fruit Cup,** 6 oz | 80 | 0 | 20 |
| **Hot Dogs:** | | | |
| **Chili Dog,** 7.7 oz | 520 | 29 | 45 |
| **Hot Dog,** 6.4 oz | 465 | 21 | 50 |
| **Jumbo Dog,** 6 oz | 440 | 25 | 38 |
| **Kraut Dog with Sauerkraut** , 7.8 oz | 490 | 27 | 41 |
| **Individual Pan Pizza (6"):** *Per Pizza* | | | |
| **BBQ Chicken** | 630 | 24 | 71 |
| **Cheese** | 630 | 27 | 71 |
| **Pepperoni** | 660 | 30 | 70 |
| **Nachos,** 40 chips, with 4 oz cheese | 1100 | 59 | 132 |
| **Sandwiches:** | | | |
| **Chicken:** With Bacon, 8.3 oz | 530 | 31 | 41 |
| With Cheese, 8.3 oz | 510 | 29 | 40 |
| Without Cheese, 7.7 oz | 460 | 25 | 40 |
| **Polish Sausage Sandwich,** 7 oz | 565 | 33 | 46 |
| **Snacks:** | | | |
| **Brownie,** 2.5" x 4.5" | 360 | 18 | 44 |
| **Cheese Sauce,** 1.3 oz | 100 | 8 | 4 |
| ***Cheetos,*** 2.8 oz package | 440 | 28 | 42 |
| **Chocolate Chip Cookie,** 2.3 oz | 280 | 12 | 40 |
| **Churro,** (1), 10", 2 oz | 210 | 10 | 26 |
| ***Doritos,*** Nacho, 2.8 oz package | 390 | 20 | 48 |
| **King Size Candy:** | | | |
| *Butterfinger,* 3.8 oz | 480 | 18 | 75 |
| *Nestle Crunch,* 2.8 oz | 390 | 21 | 85 |
| ***Lay's,*** Chips, 2.8 oz package | 440 | 28 | 42 |
| **Peanuts,** in shell, 8 oz | 930 | 80 | 24 |
| **Popcorn:** Small (9 cup size) | 575 | 35 | 56 |
| Large (15 cup size) | 950 | 58 | 93 |
| **Pretzel,** Soft, Reg., 5.5 oz | 490 | 3.5 | 101 |
| **Red Vines,** 5 oz box | 500 | 0 | 117 |
| **Snow Cone:** With 3 oz syrup | 270 | 0 | 68 |
| With 6 oz syrup | 540 | 0 | 136 |
| **Beverages:** | | | |
| **Orange Juice,** 12 fl.oz | 180 | 0 | 2 |
| **Beer:** | | | |
| *Heineken,* 16 fl.oz | 200 | 0 | 16 |
| *Miller:* Draft, 16 fl.oz | 195 | 0 | 17 |
| Lite, 16 fl.oz | 125 | 16 | 4 |
| *Jack Daniels,* Punch, 12 fl.oz | 235 | 0 | 34 |
| **Wine,** White, 9 fl.oz | 190 | 0 | 6 |
| **Soda,** (with ½ ice), average: | | | |
| 20 fl.oz | 160 | 0 | 40 |
| 32 fl.oz | 260 | 0 | 65 |
| ***Starbuck's,*** Coffee, Frappuccino, 9.5 fl.oz | 200 | 3 | 37 |

# Restaurant & International Foods

## Asian & Chinese Dishes

| | C | F | Cb |
|---|---|---|---|
| **Appetizers:** | | | |
| **Crab Cake**, 2.3 oz | 125 | 10 | 1 |
| **Dumplings:** *Per Dumpling* | | | |
| Pork: Steamed | 80 | 4.5 | 5 |
| Fried | 90 | 6 | 5 |
| Vegetable, steamed | 35 | 1 | 5 |
| **Egg Rolls,** Mini, 3 rolls | 100 | 3 | 11 |
| **Spring Roll:** | | | |
| Small, 1.5 oz | 85 | 4 | 9 |
| Medium, 3 oz | 170 | 8 | 17 |
| Large, 5 oz | 290 | 15 | 29 |
| **Wonton,** 1 only | 75 | 4 | 5 |
| **Soup:** Egg Flower, bowl 12 oz | 90 | 2 | 16 |
| Hot & Sour Soup, bowl 12 oz | 110 | 3.5 | 14 |
| **Rice:** Plain, 1 cup, 6.5 oz | 320 | 2 | 66 |
| 2 Cups, 13 oz | 640 | 4 | 132 |
| Fried: 1 cup, 5 oz | 365 | 11 | 55 |
| Large dish, 16 oz | 950 | 28 | 67 |
| **Noodles,** Chinese Egg, cooked, 1 cup | 200 | 4 | 37 |
| **Entrees & Mains:** *Per Serving* | | | |
| **Almond Chicken**, 6 oz | 270 | 10 | 21 |
| **BBQ Pork**, 5.5oz | 440 | 23 | 15 |
| **Beef in Black Bean Sauce**, 8.5 oz | 390 | 17 | 17 |
| **Broccoli Beef**, 6 oz | 370 | 21 | 13 |
| **Chicken & Broccoli**, 5.5 oz | 160 | 8 | 10 |
| **Chicken Skewers**, 3 oz | 210 | 9 | 18 |
| **Chop Suey:** | | | |
| Chicken, 5 oz | 140 | 9 | 2 |
| Pork, 5 oz | 170 | 12 | 3 |
| **Chow Mein**, Beef/Chicken, 8 oz | 390 | 12 | 59 |
| **Crab Puff/Rangoon**, 1 dumpling | 190 | 11 | 13 |
| **Crispy Fried Chicken**, 8 oz | 485 | 33 | 12 |
| **Egg Drop Soup:** With Noodles, 1 cup | 110 | 3 | 16 |
| Without Noodles, 1 cup | 60 | 3 | 4 |
| **Egg Foo Yung with Sauce**, 1 cup | 270 | 15 | 16 |
| **Kung Pao Chicken**, 5.5 oz | 240 | 15 | 12 |
| **Lemon Chicken**, 5 oz | 525 | 21 | 57 |
| **Lo Mein**, stir-fried, 8 oz | 705 | 42 | 49 |
| **Omelet**, Chicken/Shrimp, 16 oz | 990 | 82 | 10 |
| **Orange Chicken**, 5.5 oz | 500 | 27 | 42 |
| **Steamed Whole Fish,** | | | |
| ½ Sockeye Salmon | 646 | 36 | 23 |
| **Sweet & Sour:** | | | |
| Fish, 20 oz | 1160 | 58 | 106 |
| Pork, 5.5 oz | 400 | 23 | 35 |
| **Vegetable Combo**, with oil, 6 oz | 367 | 5 | 66 |
| **Vegetables**, Steamed, without oil, 6 oz | 135 | 1 | 29 |
| **Sauces:** Mandarin Sauce 1.5 oz | 70 | 0 | 17 |
| Potsticker Sauce, 1.5 oz | 35 | 0 | 8 |
| **Bubble Tea**, average, 12 fl oz | 280 | 0.5 | 68 |
| **Fortune Cookie**, each | 32 | 0.5 | 7 |

## Cajun & Creole

| | C | F | Cb |
|---|---|---|---|
| **Alligator**, cooked, 4 oz | 160 | 2 | 0 |
| **Baked Herb Chicken**, 1 serving | 850 | 53 | 2 |
| **Bouillabaisse** | 400 | 15 | 10 |
| **Cajun Fried Turkey**, 1 serving | 630 | 25 | 0 |
| **Cocktail Sauce**, 2 Tbsp | 30 | 0 | 6 |
| **Couche-Couche**, ½ cup | 80 | 0 | 17 |
| **Crawfish Bisque**, 1 serving | 500 | 10 | 10 |
| **Crawfish**, cooked, 2 oz | 45 | 0.5 | 0 |
| **Creole Jambalaya,** | | | |
| 1 serving | 550 | 30 | 15 |
| **Frog Legs**, steamed (2) | 45 | 0 | 0 |
| **Guinea Fowl**, flesh, 4 oz, cooked | 160 | 4 | 0 |
| **Hogshead Cheese**, ¼ cup | 80 | 5.5 | 0 |
| **Jambalaya**, Shrimp & Crabmeat | 520 | 14 | 12 |
| **Red Beans & Rice**, 1 serving | 400 | 17 | 52 |
| **Roasted Quail**, with Bacon, on Toast | 550 | 25 | 15 |
| **Remoulade Sauce**, 2 Tbsp, 1 oz | 110 | 11 | 2 |
| **Shrimp Creole**, 1 serving | 450 | 20 | 10 |
| **Stuffed Smothered Steak,** | | | |
| with 1 cup Rice | 890 | 50 | 50 |
| **Turtle**, cooked, 3 oz | 120 | 3 | 0 |

## Canadian

| | C | F | Cb |
|---|---|---|---|
| **Bagels,** Montreal-Style: | | | |
| Plain, 100g/3.5 oz | 300 | 2 | 60 |
| Poppyseed, 100g/3.5 oz | 310 | 4 | 58 |
| Sesame, 100g/3.5 oz | 320 | 6 | 56 |
| **Bannock:** Plain 33g/1.2 oz | 120 | 3 | 20 |
| With currants/raisins, 85g/3 oz | 215 | 9 | 32 |
| **Meals:** | | | |
| **Baked Beans in Maple Syrup,** | | | |
| 1 cup, 250g/8.8 oz | 320 | 1 | 62 |
| **Donnairs** (*Pizza Delight*): | | | |
| Famous, regular, 250g/8.8 oz | 510 | 21 | 60 |
| Super, regular, 310g/11 oz | 685 | 34 | 62 |
| **Poutine:** | | | |
| *A&W*, 330g/12 oz | 610 | 33 | 58 |
| *Boston Pizza*, regular, 400g/14 oz | 610 | 30 | 67 |
| *Burger King*, Classic, 330g/11.6 oz | 680 | 36 | 72 |
| *Harvey's*, 240g/8.5 oz | 730 | 41 | 63 |
| *McDonald's*, 1 serving | 510 | 29 | 44 |
| *Swiss Chalet,* | | | |
| Chalet -Style, 340g/12 oz | 150 | 12 | 195 |
| **Shish Taouk:** | | | |
| Chicken: 1 skewer, 200g/7 oz | 270 | 25 | 9 |
| Wrap, 455g/16 oz | 1150 | 12 | 195 |
| **Tassot:** | | | |
| Beef, 283g/10 oz | 430 | 28 | 12 |
| Goat, 100g/3.5 oz | 360 | 36 | 9 |
| **Toutiere**, 170g/6oz | 600 | 42 | 35 |

### Canadian (Cont) | C | F | Cb

**Pastries:**

**Beaver Tails:**

| | C | F | Cb |
|---|---|---|---|
| Cheese & Garlic, 80g/2.8 oz | 390 | 30 | 28 |
| Cinnamon & Sugar, 80g/2.8 oz | 315 | 13 | 30 |
| **Butter Tart**, mini, 1 tart | 120 | 3 | 16 |
| **May West,** | | | |
| Original, 54g/1.9 oz | 240 | 11 | 34 |
| **Nanaimo Bar**, 56g/2 oz | 270 | 16 | 30 |
| **Snacks:** Maple Syrup Taffy, 40g/1.4 oz | 130 | 0 | 33 |
| Potato Chips: Dill Pickle Flav., 40g | 160 | 10 | 15 |
| Ketchup Flavor, 50g/1.8 oz | 260 | 16 | 26 |

### French Foods

| | C | F | Cb |
|---|---|---|---|
| **Blanquette d' Agneau,** (Lamb Stew) | 800 | 30 | 17 |
| **Brioche**, 1 cake | 280 | 14 | 34 |
| **Bouillabaisse** | 400 | 15 | 10 |
| **Coq au Vin,** leg/thigh | 700 | 28 | 31 |
| **Coquilles St. Jacques** | 320 | 13 | 36 |
| **Crème Brulée,** 1 serving | 460 | 40 | 21 |
| **Baguette,** 3 slices, 2.2 oz | 150 | 1 | 35 |
| **Creme Caramel,** (Caramel Custard) | 260 | 10 | 38 |
| **Crepe Suzette,** 1x6" crepe with sauce | 220 | 10 | 13 |
| **Duck a l'Orange,** ¼ duck, 22 oz | 970 | 44 | 19 |
| **Escargot,** (Snails), in garlic butter (6) | 200 | 10 | 4 |
| **Frog Legs,** fried, 4 medium pairs | 400 | 20 | 10 |
| **Lamb Noisettes,** fried, 2 chops | 500 | 40 | 1 |
| **Potage Creme Crecy,** (Carrot Soup) | 360 | 18 | 14 |
| **Salade Nicoise,** (Tuna/Olives/Vegs) | 450 | 13 | 14 |
| **Veal Cordon Bleu,** (Veal/Ham) | 650 | 25 | 18 |
| **Vichyssoise,** (Potato /Leek Soup), 1 c. | 200 | 9 | 15 |
| **Baguette & French Stick ~** *Page 54* | | | |

### German

| | C | F | Cb |
|---|---|---|---|
| **Beef:** Goulash with Veggies | 520 | 20 | 46 |
| Weiner Schnitzel, 1 medium | 750 | 35 | 38 |
| **Chicken:** Fried, Viennese-style | 530 | 20 | 28 |
| Livers with Apple/Onion, 6 oz | 460 | 28 | 10 |
| **Herring,** pickled: Rollmops, 4 oz | 260 | 16 | 3 |
| With Sour Cream, 4 oz | 310 | 20 | 3 |
| **Pork,** Sauerbraten (Pot Roast) | 650 | 35 | 15 |
| **Sausage:** Bratwurst, grilled, 6 oz | 450 | 37 | 2 |
| Hot Sausage Curry | 300 | 7 | 6 |
| **Cakes:** | | | |
| **Black Forest**, 1 slice | 380 | 16 | 30 |
| **Bavarian Bread Dumpling**, 3 small | 330 | 10 | 28 |
| **Kugelhupf Cake**, 1 large slice, 4 oz | 400 | 23 | 40 |
| **Torte:** Linzer (Almond/Raspb. Jam) | 430 | 18 | 58 |
| Sacher (Chocolate/Apricot Jam) | 260 | 12 | 23 |

### Greek | C | F | Cb

| | C | F | Cb |
|---|---|---|---|
| **Baklava Pastry:** Small | 240 | 13 | 32 |
| Large, 3.8 oz | 400 | 21 | 45 |
| **Calamari,** deep fried, 1 cup | 300 | 13 | 17 |
| **Chicken Kebob Plate** | 345 | 13 | 8 |
| **Dolmades,** 2 rolls, 6 oz | 200 | 5 | 13 |
| **Galactobureko,** 1 only | | | |
| (Filo, Custard, Pastry in Syrup) | 360 | 15 | 48 |
| **Greek Chicken Salad** | 400 | 18 | 9 |
| **Gyros:** 6" Pita, 8 oz | 475 | 32 | 35 |
| 7½" Pita, 12 oz | 680 | 40 | 55 |
| **Hummus & Pita,** 4 oz | 260 | 12 | 30 |
| **Kataifi,** (Filo, Nut, Pastry in Syrup) | 350 | 11 | 56 |
| **Moussaka:** Small serving, 8 oz | 350 | 22 | 22 |
| Large serving, 16 oz | 700 | 44 | 44 |
| **Soup,** Avgolemono (Egg & Lemon | | | |
| with Chicken & Rice), 1 cup | 85 | 6 | 5 |
| **Souvlaki,** (Lamb), each, 2 oz | 120 | 6 | 1 |
| **Stuffed Tomatoes,** (2) | 250 | 12 | 17 |
| **Taramosalata,** 1 T., 0.5 oz | 40 | 3 | 2 |
| **Tyropita,** (Filo/Egg/Cheese Pastry) | 350 | 26 | 31 |

### Hawaiian

| | C | F | Cb |
|---|---|---|---|
| **Ahi Tuna,** grilled w/o fat, 6 oz fillet | 220 | 2 | 0 |
| **Chicken Long Rice,** 1 cup, 7 oz | 240 | 14 | 12 |
| **Gyoza,** 1 only | 55 | 2 | 6 |
| **Haupia,** (Coconut Pudd.), 1 pce, (4"x 2½") | 120 | 6 | 17 |
| **Hawaiian Sweet Bread,** ½" slice, 2 oz | 180 | 4.5 | 29 |
| **Kalua:** Chicken, 4 oz | 280 | 16 | 0 |
| Pork, 4 oz | 350 | 24 | 0 |
| **Kim Chee,** (pickled cabbage), ½ cup, 4 oz | 20 | 0 | 5 |
| **Kulolo,** (Taro Pudding), 1 slice | 125 | 5 | 19 |
| **Lau Lau:** | | | |
| Chicken (1), 7 oz | 280 | 21 | 3 |
| Pork (1), 7 oz | 320 | 26 | 5 |
| **Loco Moco,** (rice/burger/egg/gravy) | 650 | 27 | 63 |
| **Lomi Salmon,** ¼ cup, 4 oz | 20 | 1 | 2 |
| **Malasadas,** (Donut), 2 oz | 240 | 13 | 26 |
| **Manapua,** (Char Siu Pork Bun), 2.3 oz | 180 | 8 | 25 |
| **Poi** ,(mashed cooked taro), 1 cup, 8.5 oz | 270 | 0.5 | 65 |
| **Poke,** average all types, 3 oz | 90 | 1 | 0 |
| **Portuguese Sausage,** 2 oz | 180 | 15 | 2 |
| **Potato Salad,** ½ cup, 5 oz | 170 | 10 | 17 |
| **Shave Ice,** *(Matsumoto)*, all flavors: | | | |
| With Ice Cream, 1 large | 300 | 4 | 64 |
| With Beans, 1 large | 290 | 0 | 72 |
| **Spam Musubi:** | | | |
| With Regular Spam | 265 | 11 | 34 |
| (4 oz rice+1.3 oz Spam/7-Eleven Hawaii) | | | |
| Homemade, w/ Lite Spam (50% less fat) | 220 | 5 | 34 |
| **Taro Pancake Mix,** ⅓ cup (makes 2) | 140 | 2 | 26 |

## Hawaiian (Cont)    C   F   Cb

**Plate Lunches:**

| | C | F | Cb |
|---|---|---|---|
| **Chicken Katsu**, (9 oz:) With Rice | 1110 | 48 | 108 |
| + Macaroni Salad, ¾ cup | 1360 | 68 | 123 |
| or Tossed Salad + 2Tbsp Fr. Dress. | 1240 | 61 | 111 |
| **Hamburger**, (5 oz): With Rice | 710 | 24 | 81 |
| Gravy + Macaroni Salad | 1135 | 49 | 112 |
| **Mahi Mahi**, (7 oz): With Rice | 650 | 12 | 90 |
| + Macaroni Salad + Tartar Sce | 1150 | 58 | 109 |
| or Macaroni Salad, w/o Tartar ce | 935 | 34 | 108 |
| or Tossed Salad + 3 Tbsp Fr. Dress. | 815 | 27 | 96 |
| or Tossed Salad, without dressing | 670 | 12 | 93 |
| **Teri Beef, (5 oz):** With 2 scoops Rice | 790 | 23 | 94 |
| + Macaroni Salad, ¾ cup | 1095 | 47 | 113 |
| or Tossed Salad, without dressing | 800 | 23 | 95 |

## Indian & Pakistani

*Per Serving, Meat dishes allow 4 oz meat/serving*

| | C | F | Cb |
|---|---|---|---|
| **Aloo Samosa**, each | 155 | 12 | 12 |
| **Alu Gosht Kari**, (Meat/Potato Curry) | 600 | 40 | 23 |
| **Chicken Korma** | 500 | 35 | 6 |
| **Chicken Pilaf** | 700 | 53 | 50 |
| **Chicken Tikka** | 260 | 16 | 2 |
| **Chicken Vindaloo** | 400 | 20 | 8 |
| **Chapati/Roti**, 7" diameter, 1 piece | 60 | 0.5 | 11 |
| **Dahl**, (Lentil Puree): | | | |
| 1 cup, without oil | 230 | 1 | 37 |
| 1 Tbsp Tadka (oil topping) | 120 | 13 | 0 |
| **Dhakla**, (Lentil Dish), 1" square, 1 oz | 105 | 5 | 13 |
| **Dhansak**, ½ cup | 105 | 3.5 | 11 |
| **Gosht Kari** | 460 | 25 | 17 |
| **Lamb Pilaf** | 520 | 35 | 40 |
| **Lassi**, (Sweet or Mango), 1 cup, 8 oz | 160 | 4 | 24 |
| **Masala Gosht**, (Beef/Tomato/Gravy) | 400 | 25 | 18 |
| **Mulligatawney Soup** | 300 | 15 | 8 |
| **Murgh Tikka**, 1 cup | 300 | 4 | 7 |
| **Naan Flatbread**, 2 oz | 160 | 3.5 | 29 |
| **Pappadum**, 1 large/2 small | 50 | 3 | 5 |
| **Pesrattu**, (Lentil Crepe), 9", 2.6 oz | 130 | 5 | 15 |
| **Pork Vindaloo Curry**, without Rice | 620 | 47 | 3 |
| **Rajmah**, 1 cup | 225 | 5 | 35 |
| **Rogan Josh**, | | | |
| without Rice/Potatoes | 500 | 30 | 3 |
| **Shahi Korma**, (Braised Lamb) | 430 | 28 | 3 |
| **Tandoori Chicken:** | | | |
| Breast | 260 | 13 | 5 |
| Leg/Thigh portion | 300 | 17 | 6 |

## Italian Dishes    C   F   Cb

**Entrees:**

| | C | F | Cb |
|---|---|---|---|
| **Baked Ziti:** Small | 370 | 27 | 32 |
| Regular | 575 | 42 | 49 |
| **Breadstick**, 2 oz piece | 120 | 2.5 | 25 |
| **Broccoli Fettucine Alfredo**, regular | 815 | 23 | 125 |
| **Bruschetta**, 2 slices | 380 | 17 | 53 |
| **Calzones**, av. all varieties | 840 | 34 | 101 |
| **Cannelloni**, 1 tube, 6 oz | 280 | 15 | 18 |
| **Cheese Breadstick**, 2.4 oz piece | 180 | 8 | 20 |
| **Cheese Ravioli**, with sauce | 495 | 17 | 65 |
| **Chicken Alfredo** | 775 | 29 | 82 |
| **Chicken Parmigiana**, 11 oz | 520 | 22 | 16 |
| **Chicken Scallopine**, dinner | 1110 | 71 | 68 |
| **Eggplant Parmigiana** | 900 | 39 | 78 |
| **Fettucine Alfredo:** Lunch, 9 oz | 885 | 65 | 63 |
| Dinner, 15 oz | 1475 | 108 | 104 |
| **Linquine & Seafood**, dinner | 1130 | 71 | 79 |
| **Manicotti Formaggio** | 800 | 38 | 57 |
| **Meat Lasagne:** | | | |
| Small, 10 oz | 440 | 23 | 39 |
| Large, 16 oz | 700 | 36 | 60 |
| **Meat Ravioli** | 725 | 22 | 102 |
| **Minestrone Soup**, 1 bowl | 110 | 2 | 18 |
| **Penne Rustica:** Lunch | 1300 | 71 | 76 |
| Dinner | 1540 | 80 | 101 |
| **Ravioli**, over-stuffed, average | 990 | 67 | 57 |
| **Panini Sandwich:** | | | |
| Chicken, 16 oz | 900 | 38 | 81 |
| Meats, average, 18 oz | 940 | 39 | 81 |
| Vegetarian, 15 oz | 750 | 31 | 83 |

**Pizza, Ready-To-Eat** ~ *See Page 135*

**Spaghetti & Meatballs:**

| | C | F | Cb |
|---|---|---|---|
| With Tomato Sauce: Kids | 500 | 20 | 58 |
| Medium/Lunch | 1080 | 63 | 89 |
| Large/Dinner | 1430 | 81 | 119 |
| With Meat Sauce: Kids | 550 | 25 | 56 |
| Medium/Lunch | 1300 | 79 | 84 |
| Large/Dinner | 1700 | 103 | 110 |
| **Veal Marsala**, dinner | 1320 | 66 | 132 |
| **Veal Parmigiana**, dinner | 1270 | 65 | 116 |
| **Vegetable Primavera** | 610 | 8 | 116 |

**Salad,**

| | C | F | Cb |
|---|---|---|---|
| **Caprese ,** 11 oz | 445 | 34 | 10 |

**Desserts:**

| | C | F | Cb |
|---|---|---|---|
| **Gelato:** Vanilla (Milk Base), ½ cup | 200 | 15 | 18 |
| Choc. Hazelnut (Milk), ½ cup | 370 | 29 | 26 |
| Water Base, ½ cup | 100 | 0 | 25 |
| **Lemon Ice,** | 180 | 0 | 45 |
| **Tiramisu**, 1 piece, 5 oz | 400 | 29 | 30 |

**Further listings** ~ *See Fast-Foods Section*

## Japanese | **C** **F** **Cb**

| | C | F | Cb |
|---|---|---|---|
| **Sashimi:** (Sliced Raw Seafood/Beef) | | | |
| Ika (Squid), 4 oz | 105 | 2 | 0 |
| Hamachi (Yellowtail), 4 oz | 165 | 6 | 0 |
| Maguro (Yellowfin Tuna), 4 oz | 120 | 1 | 0 |
| Niku (Beef), 5 oz | 200 | 10 | 0 |
| Saba (Mackerel), 4 oz | 160 | 7 | 0 |
| Suzuki (Sea Bass), 4 oz | 110 | 0.5 | 0 |
| Tako (Octopus), 4 oz | 95 | 1 | 0 |
| **Sushi Rice:** Cooked, 1 Tbsp | 25 | 0 | 5 |
| 1 cup, 5.3 oz | 380 | 3 | 82 |
| **Sushi (Maki) Rolls:** *Per Piece* | | | |
| Average all types (California Rolls; Cream Cheese with Crab; Eel; Salmon; Shrimp; Tuna; Yellowtail; Vegetable) | | | |
| Small (1.2" diam. x 1.2" high), 0.8 oz | 25 | 0.5 | 3.5 |
| Medium (1¾" diam. x 1¾" high), 1.6 oz | 50 | 1 | 7 |
| Large (2¼" diam. x ⅞" high), 2 oz | 60 | 1.5 | 9 |
| **Sushi Packs:** *Per Pack* | | | |
| Average all types: 6 large pieces | 370 | 5 | 55 |
| 9 medium pieces | 360 | 6 | 60 |
| 12 small pieces | 265 | 3 | 45 |
| Futomaki (thick roll), 6 pieces | 380 | 5 | 72 |
| Hand Roll (Cone), 4 oz | 120 | 2 | 18 |
| Inari (rice filled soybean pocket), 4 pces | 420 | 9 | 73 |
| **Sushi-Nigiri,** (fish on rice), average all varieties, 1 piece | 70 | 0.5 | 12 |
| **Sushi Plate,** Assorted: 6 pieces | 420 | 3 | 36 |
| Combination (Sushi & Sushi Rolls) 2 Sushi + 6 small & 3 medium rolls | 400 | 7 | 72 |
| **Dipping Sauces:** Average, 2 Tbsp | 30 | 0 | 7 |
| Ginger Vinegar Dressing, 2 Tbsp | 20 | 0 | 5 |
| **Edamame:** (young green soybeans): | | | |
| Boiled beans (no pods), 4 oz | 160 | 7 | 12 |
| Steamed (in pods), 4 oz | 60 | 3 | 5 |
| **Katsu-don,** Pork with Rice | 1100 | 39 | 141 |
| **Miso Soup,** with Tofu pieces, 1 cup | 85 | 3 | 11 |
| **Sake Wine,** (16% alcohol), 3 fl.oz | 115 | 0 | 7 |
| **Seaweed Salad,** 1.5 oz | 20 | 2 | 0 |
| **Sukiyaki,** (Beef/Tofu/Veggies), 8 oz | 400 | 24 | 32 |
| **Tempura:** | | | |
| 3 large shrimp & veggies | 320 | 18 | 25 |
| 1 shrimp only | 60 | 4 | 3 |
| **Teppan Yaki,** (Steak, Seafood & Veggies), 10 oz serving | 470 | 30 | 15 |
| **Teriyaki:** Beef, 4 oz | 350 | 25 | 4 |
| Chicken, 4 oz | 260 | 9 | 7 |
| Salmon, medium, 6 oz | 270 | 8 | 3 |
| **Yakatori,** 1 skewer, 2.5 oz | 140 | 5 | 1 |

## Kosher/Deli Foods | **C** **F** **Cb**

| | C | F | Cb |
|---|---|---|---|
| **Bagel/Bialy,** 1 small, 2 oz | 160 | 2 | 32 |
| **Beiglach,** (Cheese Knish) | 350 | 17 | 35 |
| **Blintzes:** Average, 1 only | 120 | 1 | 25 |
| With Sour Cream & Preserves | 370 | 10 | 30 |
| **Borscht,** (Without Sour Cream): 1 cup | 85 | 3 | 14 |
| Diet/Reduced Calorie, 1 cup | 30 | 1 | 7 |
| **Cabbage Roll,** (meat/rice), 5 oz | 170 | 6 | 21 |
| **Chicken Broth:** 1 cup | 80 | 8 | 0 |
| With vegetables | 100 | 8 | 5 |
| With noodles | 150 | 9 | 16 |
| Lowfat, plain, 1 cup | 25 | 1 | 0 |
| **Cholent,** 1 medium serving, 1 cup | 350 | 16 | 48 |
| **Chopped Liver:** 1 serving, 3 oz | 110 | 6 | 5 |
| With Egg Salad, ¼ cup | 100 | 7 | 3 |
| **Farfel,** dry, ½ cup | 90 | 0.5 | 21 |
| **Gefilte Fish Balls:** | | | |
| Regular, 2 oz | 55 | 2 | 4 |
| With Jelled Broth | 80 | 2 | 6 |
| Cocktail size, 1 oz | 30 | 1 | 2 |
| Sweet: Medium, 2 oz | 65 | 2 | 4 |
| With Jelled Broth | 95 | 2 | 9 |
| **Hallah,** (Yeast Bread), 1 slice, 1 oz | 85 | 2 | 14 |
| **Herring:** Smoked, 2 oz | 120 | 8 | 0 |
| In Sour Cream, 2 oz | 150 | 10 | 0 |
| **Kasha,** cooked, ½ cup | 100 | 0.5 | 20 |
| **Kipfel,** (Vanilla/Almdond Cookie), 1 pce | 60 | 2 | 7 |
| **Knaidlach ~** *See Matzo Balls* | | | |
| **Knish:** Kasha/Potato, 1 only | 130 | 4 | 22 |
| Cheese, 1 only | 350 | 17 | 35 |
| **Kreplach,** beef, 1 piece | 40 | 1 | 6 |
| **Kugel,** potato/noodle, 1 serving | 300 | 20 | 25 |
| **Latkes,** (Potato Pancake): 2 oz | 200 | 11 | 22 |
| 3 Latkes w/ Sour Cran Apple Sauce | 750 | 25 | 95 |
| **Lochshen:** Plain, 1 cup | 130 | 2 | 26 |
| Pudding, 1 cup | 380 | 13 | 48 |
| **Lox,** (Smoked Salmon), 2 oz | 65 | 2 | 0 |
| **Mandelbrot,** (Almond Bread), 1 slice, ¼" thick | 45 | 2 | 5 |
| **Matzo,** 1 oz board | 110 | 0.5 | 21 |
| **Matzo Balls:** 2 small, or 1 large, 2" | 90 | 3 | 12 |
| Extra large ball, 3" | 180 | 6 | 24 |
| **Matzo Ball Soup:** | | | |
| Cup w/ 2 small or 1 large ball | 150 | 5 | 27 |
| Bowl w/ Chkn & Noodles | 325 | 13 | 34 |
| *Jerry's Deli,* large bowl | 560 | 17 | 56 |
| **NY Cheesecake,** 4 oz | 350 | 24 | 26 |
| **Pierogi,** potato/cheese, 1 piece | 90 | 4 | 11 |
| **Reuben S'wich,** w/ ½ lb Corned Beef | 920 | 60 | 28 |
| **Schmaltz,** (Rend'd Chicken Fat), 1 T. | 90 | 10 | 0 |

# Restaurant & International Foods

## Korean Food

| | C | F | Cb |
|---|---|---|---|
| **Bibimbab**, (Veg. & Beef on Rice), 1 cup | 565 | 15 | 89 |
| **Bulgogi**, (Barbeque Beef), 3.5 oz | 325 | 12 | 15 |
| **Galbi (Short Ribs)**, 16 oz | 975 | 61 | 16 |
| **Gujeolpan**, (Pancake with Meat & Vegetables), 1 cup with 1 pancake | 340 | 11 | 39 |
| **Japchae**, (Noodle w/ Veggies & Meat), 1¼ cups | 365 | 19 | 34 |
| **Sides:** | | | |
| **Kimchee**, (Cabbage Relish), ½ cup | 30 | 0 | 6 |
| **Namool**, (Assorted Vegetables), 1 cup | 125 | 6.5 | 9 |
| **Soups:** Per Serving | | | |
| **Muguk**, (Radish & Chive Soup), 6 oz | 105 | 7 | 6 |
| **Samgyetang**, (Ginseng Chkn Soup): | | | |
| Without Chicken Skin, 1 cup | 520 | 11 | 60 |
| With Chicken Skin, 1 cup | 725 | 35 | 60 |
| **Yuk Gae Jang**, (Spicy Beef Soup), 1¼ cups | 180 | 13 | 5 |

## Lebanese/Middle East

| | C | F | Cb |
|---|---|---|---|
| **Baba Ghannouj**, 2 Tbsp, 1 oz | 70 | 6 | 2 |
| **Baklava**, (Pastry, Nuts, Syrup), 1 pastry, 13/4 oz | 245 | 18 | 18 |
| **Cabbage Rolls**, (Cabb. Leaf, Meat, Rice), 1 roll, 3 oz, | 100 | 3 | 12 |
| **Cous Cous**, (Semolina, Milk, Fruit, Nuts), 1 cup | 400 | 21 | 43 |
| **Falafel**, (Chick Pea Fritter), Fried, 1 medium, 1 oz | 60 | 4 | 4 |
| **Hummus**, ¼ cup, 2.2 oz | 105 | 3 | 5 |
| **Fried Kibbi**, (Wheat, Meat Pinenuts), 1 piece, 3 oz | 180 | 8 | 15 |
| **Kafta**, (Ground Lamb, Ssge on Skewer), 1 skewer, 1.5 oz | 85 | 5 | 2 |
| **Kibbeh Naye**, (raw Lamb, Bulgur & Spice) 1 cup, 9 oz | 450 | 18 | 28 |
| **Lebanese Omelet**, 1 serving, 4 oz (Egg, Spinach, Pinenuts, Onion) | 200 | 12 | 13 |
| **Pilaf**, (Rice, Onion, Raisins, Apr., Spice) 1 cup | 400 | 11 | 60 |
| **Shawourma**, (Spit-Roast Beef), 4 oz serving | 280 | 15 | 2 |
| **Shish Kabob**, 1 stick, 2.5 oz | 130 | 7 | 2 |
| **Spinach Pie**, 1 piece, 3.5 oz | 290 | 21 | 20 |
| **Sweet Almond Sanbusak**, (Pastry, Almonds, Spices), 1 piece | 200 | 15 | 11 |
| **Tabouli**, 1 serving, 4 oz | 125 | 7 | 13 |
| **Tahini Sauce**, average, 1 Tbsp | 90 | 8 | 2 |

## Mexican

| | C | F | Cb |
|---|---|---|---|
| **Burritos** (Taco Bell): Bean | 370 | 10 | 56 |
| Supreme Beef | 420 | 16 | 53 |
| **Chili**, plain, ¼ cup | 90 | 6 | 8 |
| **Chili con Carne:** With Beans, 1 cup | 310 | 17 | 15 |
| Without Beans, 1 cup | 370 | 28 | 10 |
| **Chimichangas**, Beef, 5 oz | 400 | 19 | 43 |
| **Chorizo Sausage**, 2 oz | 265 | 23 | 0 |
| **Churro**, (1), 1.5 oz | 150 | 8 | 18 |
| **Corn Chips**, ½ cup, 1 oz | 160 | 10 | 17 |
| **Enchilada**, average | 330 | 10 | 49 |
| **Fajitas**, Chicken | 200 | 7 | 20 |
| **Guacamole**, average, 2 Tbsp, 1 oz | 45 | 4 | 2 |
| **Horchata:** (Don Jose), 1 cup, 8 fl.oz | 140 | 4 | 25 |
| Cacique, 1 pint bottle, 16 fl.oz | 320 | 7 | 62 |
| **Margarita**, with 1.5 oz Tequila | 160 | 0 | 6 |
| **Masa**, (Pre-mixed for Tamales), 1 oz | 80 | 5 | 9 |
| **Menudo:** | | | |
| With Hominy, 1 cup | 240 | 9 | 19 |
| Without Hominy, 1 cup | 170 | 9 | 2 |
| **Nachos:** With cheese, peppers, 1 portion, 6-8 nachos, 7 oz | 600 | 33 | 60 |
| With cheese, beans, beef, peppers, 1 portion, 6-8 nachos, 9 oz | 570 | 31 | 56 |
| Del Taco: Regular, 4 oz | 300 | 19 | 30 |
| Macho Nachos, 17 oz | 1000 | 56 | 94 |
| Taco Bell, BellGrande®, 10.8 oz | 780 | 40 | 84 |
| **Nopal Cactus Salad**, 1 cup | 130 | 9 | 11 |
| **Papas Fritas**, (1), 6 oz | 325 | 18 | 40 |
| **Piloncillo**, (Brown Sugar): | | | |
| 1 Tbsp, 0.5 oz | 50 | 0 | 13 |
| Cone, small, 3", 3 oz | 325 | 0 | 81 |
| **Quesadilla**, Cheese | 490 | 28 | 39 |
| **Queso Fresco**, ¼ cup | 80 | 4.5 | 8 |
| **Refried Beans**, ¾ cup, 6 oz | 160 | 3 | 26 |
| **Rice Pudding**, (Arroz Con Leche), 4 oz | 140 | 3 | 24 |
| **Soup**, Black Bean, 1 bowl | 200 | 3 | 34 |
| **Tacos** (Taco Bell): | | | |
| Crunchy: Regular | 170 | 10 | 12 |
| Supreme | 200 | 12 | 15 |
| Soft: Crispy Potato | 270 | 13 | 31 |
| Grilled Steak | 250 | 14 | 19 |
| Taco Salad with Salsa | 840 | 52 | 85 |
| **Taco Sauce**, average, ¼ cup | 15 | 0 | 3 |
| **Taco Shell**, regular | 50 | 2 | 8 |
| **Tamales**, Beef/Chicken, av. 4.5 oz | 250 | 11 | 27 |
| **Taquitos**, Beef & Cheese, 4.5 oz | 330 | 15 | 36 |
| **Tostada** (Taco Bell) | 250 | 10 | 29 |
| **Tortilla**, Corn, 6" diameter | 70 | 1 | 14 |
| **Tortilla Chips**, 1 oz | 150 | 8 | 18 |
| **Soup**, Black Bean, 1 bowl | 200 | 3 | 34 |

*Extra Food Listings ~ See Fast Food Section*
*(Examples: Del Taco, Taco Bell, Taco Cabana, Taco Time)*

## Mexican (Cont)

| | C | F | Cb |
|---|---|---|---|

**Breads:**
| | C | F | Cb |
|---|---|---|---|
| **Bolillos**, 1 roll, 3.5 oz | 240 | 4 | 42 |
| **Mexican Cornbread**, 4" square | 210 | 11 | 19 |
| **Pan de Leche**, 1 roll, 1.3 oz | 110 | 2.5 | 20 |
| **Telera**, 2 oz | 150 | 1.5 | 19 |

**Cakes, Cookies, Pastries Pan Dulce:**
| | C | F | Cb |
|---|---|---|---|
| **Banderilla**, 1 piece | 140 | 10 | 8 |
| **Bigotes**, 7" | 570 | 22 | 44 |
| **Capirotada**, (Bread Pudding), 10 oz | 810 | 38 | 107 |
| **Cinnamon Cookies**, 2 | 125 | 8 | 13 |
| **Concha**, av. all varieties: | | | |
|   Small (3" diameter), 2.5 oz | 250 | 8 | 38 |
|   Medium (4" diameter), 3.5 oz | 350 | 11 | 53 |
|   Large (5" diameter), 5.5 oz | 550 | 18 | 84 |
| **Cream Puff**, with Custard, 4.3 oz | 255 | 14 | 25 |
| **Cuernos**, (Horns), 3 oz | 340 | 17 | 41 |
| **Donut**, large, 4", 3.5 oz | 440 | 21 | 58 |
| **Elotes**, 3.5 oz | 450 | 24 | 51 |
| **Empanadas**, average all varieties: | | | |
|   Medium, 3 oz | 300 | 14 | 42 |
|   Large, 4 oz | 400 | 19 | 56 |
| **Fiesta Cookie**, (1), 2.3 oz | 280 | 8 | 47 |
| **Galletas Mixtas:** | | | |
|   Small, 1 oz | 100 | 2.5 | 16 |
|   Medium, 2 oz | 200 | 5 | 32 |
|   Large, 3 oz | 300 | 7.5 | 48 |
| **Guayaba**, 3.3 oz | 360 | 14 | 53 |
| **Jelly Roll**, (1), 3.3 oz | 240 | 4 | 46 |
| **Mantecadites**, 4.5 oz | 670 | 42 | 64 |
| **Mini Cupcake**, (1),1.8 oz | 180 | 8 | 25 |
| **Muffins/Nino Enbuelto**, large, 6 oz | 465 | 11 | 48 |
| **Nuez**, 3.3 oz | 380 | 17 | 52 |
| **Ojo de Buey**, 4 oz | 360 | 15 | 55 |
| **Orejas**, 1 medium, 3 oz | 310 | 15 | 38 |
| **Pan Dulce**, 1 bun | 330 | 10 | 45 |
| **Panquecitos**, 2.5 oz | 260 | 11 | 36 |
| **Piedras**, 4 oz | 470 | 15 | 76 |
| **Polvorones:** Small, 1.5 oz | 180 | 9 | 24 |
|   1 large, 3 oz | 370 | 18 | 48 |
| **Pound Cakes**, mini, 3.5 oz | 380 | 16 | 52 |
| **Puerquitos**, 3.5 oz | 350 | 12 | 55 |
| **Rebanadas**, 3.5 oz | 390 | 18 | 51 |
| **Roles De Canela**, (Cinn. Roll), 4.5 oz | 490 | 15 | 81 |
| **Roscas**, 1 piece, 2.8 oz | 360 | 18 | 44 |
| **Semitas** (*Bimbo*), 1 piece, 2.2 oz | 210 | 6 | 33 |
| **Sopapillas**, (flaky pastry puffs): 1 piece | 100 | 7 | 10 |
|   With Honey & Cream | 200 | 14 | 18 |
| **Strawberry Crema Roll**, 2.5 oz slice | 240 | 5 | 45 |

**Extra Food Listings** ~ *See CalorieKing.com*

## Polish

| | C | F | Cb |
|---|---|---|---|
| **Cabbage Rolls**, w/ Sour Cream, 2 small | 220 | 10 | 30 |
| **Chicken Casserole**, w/ Mshrms, 1 cup | 520 | 27 | 5 |
| **Kielbasa**, (Sausages, Onions, fried), | | | |
|   2 large | 350 | 28 | 2 |
| **Meatballs**, | | | |
|   in sour cream, 3 x 1½" balls | 300 | 16 | 11 |
| **Pierogi**, Fruit/Vegetables, 3" ball | 80 | 2 | 15 |
| **Pork Goulash**, (Pork/Vegetable Stew) | 550 | 21 | 38 |
| **Pot Roast**, with Vegetables | 630 | 21 | 28 |

## Soul Foods

| | C | F | Cb |
|---|---|---|---|
| **Breakfast Sausage**, fried, 2 patties | 250 | 17 | 0 |
| **Brunswick Stew**, 1 cup, 8.5 oz | 320 | 14 | 19 |
| **Cornbread**, homemade, 3 oz | 200 | 7.5 | 28 |
| **Fatback**, 0.5 oz | 110 | 11 | 0 |
| **Ham Hock**, pickled, 3 oz | 200 | 12 | 0 |
| **Hog Maw,** 1 oz | 70 | 4.5 | 0 |
| **Hominy**, cooked, ¾ cup | 110 | 0.5 | 25 |
| **Hush Puppies**, 5 pieces | 260 | 12 | 35 |
| **Kale**, cooked, ½ cup | 20 | 0.5 | 4 |
| **Opossum**, roasted, without bone, 3 oz | 190 | 9 | 0 |
| **Oxtail**, cooked, without bone, 2 oz | 85 | 4.5 | 0 |
| **Pig's Ear**, ¼ ear | 50 | 3 | 0 |
| **Pig's Foot**, ½ foot | 70 | 4.5 | 0 |
| **Pig's Tail**, ⅓ tail | 115 | 10 | 0 |
| **Poke Salad**, cooked, ½ cup | 16 | 0.5 | 3 |
| **Pork Brains,** braised, 3 oz | 115 | 8 | 0 |
| **Pork Chitterlings**, simmered, 3 oz | 260 | 25 | 0 |
| **Pork Cracklings**, 0.5 oz | 80 | 6 | 0 |
| **Pork Neck Bones**, cooked, no bone, 2 oz | 100 | 4.5 | 0 |
| **Pork Skin**, 1 cup | 70 | 4.5 | 0 |
| **Pork Tongue**, ⅓ tongue | 75 | 5.5 | 0 |
| **Sousemeat**, 1 oz | 60 | 4.5 | 0 |
| **Succotash**, ½ cup | 80 | 1 | 17 |
| **Sweet Potato Pie**, ⅛ of 9" pie | 250 | 12 | 34 |
| **Tripe**, 2 oz | 55 | 2 | 0 |
| **Vienna Sausage:** | | | |
|   2 small, 1 oz | 90 | 8 | 1 |
|   1 small, 0.5 oz | 45 | 4 | 0.5 |

OLD McDONALDS FARM
128  FOR PEOPLE WHO WANT BETTER

**Brooklyn**

# Restaurant & International Foods

## Spanish

| | C | F | Cb |
|---|---|---|---|
| **Arroz Abanda,** (Fish with Rice) | 340 | 8 | 31 |
| **Arroz Con Pollo,** (Rice/Chkn Salad) | 500 | 23 | 50 |
| **Clams Marinara,** 8 clams | 330 | 16 | 22 |
| **Cochifrito,** (Lamb with Lemon/Garlic) | 650 | 25 | 5 |
| **Cochinillo Asado,** | | | |
| (Rst Suckling Pig), 2 slices | 300 | 15 | 3 |
| **Cocido Madrileno,** | | | |
| (Madrid-Style Boiled Dinner) | 450 | 27 | 18 |
| **Flan de Leche,** (Caramel Custard) | 325 | 9 | 52 |
| **Fritadera de Ternera,** (Sauteed Veal) | 450 | 27 | 2 |
| **Gazpacho,** 1 bowl | 60 | 0 | 15 |
| **Mole Poblano,** ½ cup | 205 | 14 | 16 |
| **Paella a la Valenciana,** | | | |
| (Chicken & Shellfish Rice) | 900 | 42 | 70 |
| **Pollo a la Espanola,** (Chicken) | 475 | 30 | 4 |
| **Ternera al Jerez,** (Veal with Sherry) | 660 | 29 | 6 |
| **Zarzuela,** (Fish & Shellfish Medley) | 530 | 27 | 40 |

## Thai Foods

| | C | F | Cb |
|---|---|---|---|
| **Appetizers:** Satay Pork, 1 oz | 100 | 4 | 2 |
| Spring Roll, 1.3 oz | 110 | 6 | 13 |
| **Soups,** Tom Yam (Hot & Sour): | | | |
| Spicy Shrimp/Seafood: | | | |
| 1 cup | 100 | 4 | 6 |
| 1 bowl | 160 | 7 | 10 |
| Vegetarian, 1 cup | 50 | 0 | 11 |
| **Curries:** Chicken with Ginger, 1 cup | 390 | 34 | 4 |
| Thick Red Curry with Beef, 1 cup | 600 | 50 | 7 |
| Thai Chicken Curry, 1 cup | 340 | 23 | 4 |
| Massaman Curry, 1 cup | 680 | 57 | 8 |
| Green Curry with Pork, 1 cup | 480 | 44 | 5 |
| **Pad Thai,** large serving, 18 oz | 990 | 38 | 125 |
| **Fish:** Steamed with Spicy Thai Sce | 450 | 8 | 46 |
| Crispy Fried, 5 oz | 290 | 15 | 9 |
| **Spicy Chicken,** stir-fry | 450 | 22 | 14 |
| **Spicy Garlic Tofu,** stir-fry | 340 | 18 | 18 |
| **Sticky Thai Rice:** Plain 1 cup, 6 oz | 170 | 0.5 | 36 |
| With Coconut & Sesame Seeds, 1 cup | 880 | 28 | 120 |
| **Stir-fried Rice Noodles,** 1 cup 5.5 oz | 270 | 9 | 40 |
| **Stir-fried Vegetables,** 1 cup | 100 | 3 | 18 |
| **Salads:** Green Papaya Salad | 160 | 0 | 40 |
| Spicy Prawn, 9 shrimp | 170 | 3 | 15 |
| Thai Beef Salad, 1 serving | 260 | 9 | 15 |
| Thai Chicken, 1 serving | 330 | 9 | 17 |
| Thai Noodle, 1 serving | 410 | 13 | 45 |
| **Satay Chicken & Peanut Sauce,** | | | |
| 1 satay stick | 390 | 24 | 20 |
| **Sauce,** Peanut Satay, | | | |
| ½ cup, 4 oz | 160 | 10 | 13 |

## Vietnamese

| | C | F | Cb |
|---|---|---|---|
| **Banh Cuon,** (Steam Rice w/ Pork), 1 roll | 105 | 7 | 8 |
| **Bo Nuong,** (Beef Satay), 2 sticks | 265 | 9 | 4 |
| **Bo Xao Dau Phong,** | | | |
| (Ginger Beef with Onion, Fish Sce) | 750 | 30 | 10 |
| **Ca Chien Gung,** (Whole Snapper/Ginger) | 600 | 16 | 6 |
| **Canh Chay,** (Vegetable/Tofu Soup) | 80 | 3 | 13 |
| **Cari Chicken,** 1 cup | 475 | 29 | 16 |
| **Cari Chicken,** with Rice Noodle, | | | |
| 1 cup curry & 1 cup noodles | 660 | 29 | 60 |
| **Cari Chicken,** with Steamed Rice, | | | |
| 1 cup curry & 1 cup rice | 650 | 29 | 55 |
| **Cuu Xao Lan,** (Curried Lamb and | | | |
| Veggies in Coconut) | 900 | 40 | 80 |
| **Ga Chien,** (Crisp Chick + Plum Sauce) | 900 | 40 | 105 |
| **Ga Nuong,** (Chicken Satay + Sauce) | 240 | 10 | 4 |
| **Ga Xao Rau,** (Marinated Chicken | | | |
| Braised with Vegetables) | 800 | 26 | 100 |
| **Gio Lua,** (Lean Pork Pie), ⅛ of pie | 245 | 12 | 0 |
| **Goi Cuon,** (Cold Spring Rolls), 1 roll | 60 | 1 | 7 |
| **Rau Cai Xao Chay,** (Stir Fried Veggies) | 400 | 15 | 65 |
| **Thit Bo Vien,** (Beef Balls), 6 balls | 225 | 14 | 2 |
| **Thit Heo Goi Baup Cai,** | | | |
| (Spicy Cabb. Rolls with Pork), 1 roll | 200 | 7 | 11 |
| ***Soup:*** *Per Bowl, ½ Cup* | | | |
| Bun Bo Hue, (Hot & Spicy Soup): | | | |
| Without Pork Feet | 340 | 9 | 35 |
| With Pork Feet | 830 | 45 | 35 |
| Chicken & Rice Noodle Soup | 400 | 3 | 55 |
| Pho Bo, (Beef Noodle Soup) | 410 | 7 | 59 |
| Pho Ga, (Chicken Noodle Soup) | 460 | 6 | 58 |
| Pho Tai, (Rare Beef & Noodle Soup) | 440 | 7 | 73 |
| **Salad,** Goi Du Du, | | | |
| (Green Papaya), ½ cup | 155 | 3 | 29 |
| **Sauce,** Nuoc Cham (Hot Sauce) | 5 | 0 | 1 |

## Gourmet & Miscellaneous

| | C | F | Cb |
|---|---|---|---|
| **Ants Eggs/Larvae,** 1 Tbsp | 20 | 0 | 0 |
| **Ants,** chocolate coated, 3 Tbsp | 140 | 7 | 2 |
| **Bee Maggots,** canned, 3 Tbsp | 65 | 2 | 0 |
| **Caviar,** black/red, 1 Tbsp | 40 | 3 | 0 |
| **Caterpillars,** canned, 2 oz | 60 | 2 | 0 |
| **Frog Legs,** fried, 1 pair (large) | 125 | 7 | 0 |
| **Haggis,** boiled, 4 oz | 350 | 24 | 22 |
| **Locusts,** roasted, 1 oz | 35 | 1 | 0 |
| **Silkworms,** raw, 1 oz | 60 | 2 | 0 |
| **Snails in garlic butter,** 6 large | 200 | 10 | 4 |
| **Snake,** roasted, 4 oz | 160 | 6 | 0 |

# Fast - Foods & *Restaurants*

©2016 Allan Borushek

*Nutritional data is based on U.S. outlets*

**For More Restaurants &
Full Nutritional Data
~ See CalorieKing.com**

# Fast - Foods & Restaurants

## A&W® (Aug '15)

| | C | F | Cb |
|---|---|---|---|
| **Burgers:** | | | |
| Hamburger | 340 | 16 | 39 |
| Cheeseburger | 440 | 25 | 41 |
| Double Cheeseburger | 455 | 26 | 40 |
| Original: Bacon Cheeseburger | 440 | 25 | 41 |
| Bacon Double Cheeseburger | 645 | 41 | 42 |
| Papa Burger | 550 | 33 | 43 |
| **Sandwiches:** | | | |
| Crispy Chicken | 440 | 18 | 51 |
| Grilled Chicken | 400 | 15 | 40 |
| **Chicken Tenders,** breaded, 3 pcs | 260 | 9 | 5 |
| **Corn Dog Nuggets:** 5 pieces | 180 | 8 | 20 |
| 10 pieces | 350 | 17 | 40 |
| **Hot Dogs:** Plain | 310 | 19 | 23 |
| Coney Chili Dog | 340 | 20 | 26 |
| Coney Chili Cheese Dog | 380 | 23 | 28 |
| **Fries/Sides:** | | | |
| **Cheese Curds,** 5 oz | 570 | 40 | 27 |
| **Chili Cheese Fries,** 7 oz | 410 | 17 | 52 |
| **French Fries:** Small/Kids, 2.5 oz | 200 | 8 | 28 |
| Regular, 4 oz | 310 | 13 | 45 |
| Large, 5.5 oz | 430 | 17 | 61 |
| **Onion Rings,** 7-9 rings | 350 | 16 | 45 |
| Large, 5.5 oz | 480 | 27 | 62 |
| **Dipping Sauces:** BBQ, 1 oz | 40 | 0 | 10 |
| Honey Mustard, 1 oz | 100 | 6 | 12 |
| Ranch, 1 oz | 160 | 17 | 2 |
| **Regional Favorites:** California Recipe Only | | | |
| BBQ Bacon Crunch Cheeseburger | 565 | 34 | 49 |
| Deluxe Double Cheeseburger | 560 | 34 | 43 |
| Fish Sandwich | 575 | 29 | 58 |
| Mozza Burger Double | 570 | 34 | 41 |
| **Sweets & Treats:** | | | |
| **Polar Swirl:** M&M; Oreo, av. | 700 | 25 | 107 |
| Reese's | 740 | 31 | 97 |
| **Sundaes:** Chocolate | 320 | 8 | 53 |
| Caramel; Hot Fudge, av. | 345 | 10 | 56 |
| **Soft Serve Cone,** Vanilla, 5.5 oz | 260 | 7 | 41 |
| **Floats:** | | | |
| **A&W Root Beer:** Medium, 20 oz | 350 | 5 | 77 |
| Large, 32 oz | 640 | 10 | 136 |
| Diet, Medium, 20 oz | 170 | 5 | 30 |
| **Freeze,** A&W Root Beer, 16 oz | 370 | 8 | 68 |
| **Milkshakes:** Strawb., Small, 16 oz | 670 | 29 | 90 |
| Chocolate; Vanilla, average: | | | |
| Small, 16 fl.oz | 710 | 30 | 98 |
| Medium, 20 oz | 890 | 38 | 123 |
| **Smoothies:** Pineapple Banana, 16 oz | 400 | 6 | 85 |
| Strawberry, 16 oz | 360 | 6 | 70 |
| Strawberry Banana, 16 oz | 390 | 6 | 78 |

## Applebee's® (Aug '15)

| | C | F | Cb |
|---|---|---|---|
| **Appetizers:** As Served | | | |
| Chicken Quesadillas | 970 | 58 | 61 |
| **Pub Plates:** | | | |
| Boneless Wings w/out Dressing | 810 | 42 | 62 |
| +Bleu Cheese Dresssing | 240 | 25 | 1 |
| + Buttermilk Ranch Dressing | 210 | 22 | 1 |
| **Sharables:** | | | |
| Brew Pub Pretzels | | | |
| & Beer Cheese Dip | 1120 | 49 | 143 |
| Mozzarella Sticks | 910 | 50 | 79 |
| Pot Stickers | 650 | 32 | 75 |
| Spinach & Artichoke Dip | 980 | 60 | 89 |
| Sriracha Shrimp | 720 | 46 | 58 |
| Sweet Chili Brisket Sliders | 1220 | 54 | 145 |
| Sweet Potato Fries & Dip | 1070 | 64 | 118 |
| **Burgers:** Without Sides | | | |
| The American Standard | 1030 | 71 | 48 |
| Classic Burger: No cheese or bacon | 780 | 40 | 44 |
| + American or Swiss, average | 155 | 13 | 1 |
| + Cheddar; Monterey Jack, av. | 95 | 8 | 1 |
| + Bacon | 100 | 8 | 1 |
| Cowboy Burger | 1280 | 73 | 101 |
| Mushroom Swiss | 1090 | 78 | 47 |
| Quesadilla Burger | 1440 | 108 | 46 |
| Sweet Asian Pineapple | 1030 | 67 | 56 |
| **Chicken:** Includes Standard Sides | | | |
| Chicken Tenders, Basket | 1120 | 63 | 99 |
| Fiesta Lime Chicken | 1430 | 85 | 104 |
| **Pasta & Seafood:** As Served | | | |
| Shrimp Scampi Linguine | 980 | 50 | 96 |
| Three-Cheese Chicken Penne | 1010 | 45 | 98 |
| **Seafood:** As Served | | | |
| Blackened Tilapia | 450 | 17 | 45 |
| Double Crunch Shrimp | 1350 | 64 | 156 |
| Hand-Battered Fish & Chips | 1540 | 96 | 118 |
| New England Fish & Chips | 1970 | 136 | 134 |
| **Sizzling Entrees:** Includes Sides | | | |
| Bourbon Street Chicken & Shrimp | 620 | 28 | 42 |
| Bourbon Street Steak, 9 oz | 740 | 43 | 39 |
| Skillet Fajitas with Rice: | | | |
| Chicken | 1300 | 47 | 146 |
| Shrimp | 1190 | 45 | 146 |
| Steak | 1380 | 51 | 153 |

*Continued Next Page...*

## Applebees® cont... (Aug '15)

| Steaks & Toppers: *Without Sides* | C | F | Cb |
|---|---|---|---|
| House Sirloin, 9 oz | 330 | 17 | 2 |
| New York Strip, 12 oz | 480 | 25 | 1 |
| Ribeye, 12 oz | 500 | 28 | 1 |
| Shrimp 'N Parmesan Sirloin | 560 | 34 | 5 |
| Steak Combos: With Fried Shrimp | 720 | 35 | 50 |
| With Grilled Shrimp | 360 | 17 | 3 |
| With Honey BBQ Chicken | 620 | 19 | 40 |
| **Toppers:** Grilled Onions | 45 | 2.5 | 5 |
| Sauteed Garlic Mushrooms | 130 | 13 | 3 |
| Shrimp 'N Parmesan | 230 | 17 | 4 |

| *Have it All: Includes Sides* | | | |
|---|---|---|---|
| Cedar Grilled Lemon Chicken | 570 | 25 | 46 |
| Napa Chicken & Portobellos | 500 | 16 | 38 |
| Savory Cedar Salmon | 540 | 32 | 24 |
| Shrimp & Broccoli Cavatappi | 520 | 22 | 49 |
| Steakhouse Bruschetta Sirloin | 520 | 28 | 28 |
| Thai Shrimp Salad | 390 | 19 | 32 |

| *Salads: Regular, With Dressing* | | | |
|---|---|---|---|
| Fiesta Chicken, Chopped | 900 | 45 | 85 |
| Fried Chicken | 1130 | 78 | 59 |
| Oriental Grilled Chicken | 1290 | 82 | 90 |
| Pecan Crusted Chicken | 1340 | 80 | 115 |

| *Sides: As Served* | | | |
|---|---|---|---|
| Baked Potato | 340 | 18 | 40 |
| BBQ Spiced Fries, side | 440 | 20 | 60 |
| Chili Cheese Fries, side | 630 | 33 | 65 |
| Classic Fries | 440 | 20 | 59 |
| Crunchy Onion Rings, side | 530 | 29 | 60 |
| Fried Shrimp | 430 | 20 | 48 |
| Garlic Mashed Potatoes | 250 | 14 | 29 |
| Garlic Mashed Potatoes, loaded | 470 | 32 | 31 |
| Grilled Shrimp | 160 | 11 | 2 |
| Loaded Baked Potato | 400 | 23 | 40 |

| *Soup:* | | | |
|---|---|---|---|
| Chicken Noodle Soup | 140 | 4 | 17 |
| Chicken Tortilla Soup | 220 | 9 | 23 |
| Chili | 410 | 24 | 18 |
| French Onion Soup | 370 | 23 | 24 |
| Tomato Basil Soup | 260 | 16 | 24 |

| *Desserts: As Served* | | | |
|---|---|---|---|
| Butter Pecan Blondie | 1180 | 62 | 139 |
| Shooters: Chocolate Mousse | 480 | 25 | 44 |
| Hot Fudge Sundae | 460 | 22 | 57 |
| Strawberry Cheesecake | 390 | 24 | 38 |
| Triple Choc. Meltdown | 980 | 52 | 125 |

## Arby's® (Aug '15)

| Sandwiches: | C | F | Cb |
|---|---|---|---|
| **Beef 'n Cheddar:** Classic | 450 | 20 | 45 |
| Mid | 560 | 27 | 45 |
| Reuben | 660 | 29 | 63 |
| **Roast Beef:** Classic | 360 | 14 | 35 |
| Mid | 460 | 21 | 35 |
| Max | 560 | 27 | 35 |
| **Chicken:** | | | |
| Chicken Bacon & Swiss, Crispy | 600 | 29 | 49 |
| Chicken Cordon Bleu , Crispy | 610 | 32 | 45 |
| Crispy Chicken | 500 | 25 | 47 |
| **Turkey:** | | | |
| Roast Turkey & Swiss | 700 | 28 | 77 |
| Roast Turkey, Ranch & Bacon | 800 | 35 | 76 |
| **Wraps:** | | | |
| Roast Turkey & Swiss | 520 | 27 | 38 |
| Roast Turkey, Ranch & Bacon | 620 | 34 | 38 |

| *Chicken:* | | | |
|---|---|---|---|
| **Chicken Tenders,** 3 tenders | 350 | 17 | 25 |
| **Chicken Tenders,** 5 tenders | 590 | 28 | 42 |

| *Optional/Regional Menu:* | | | |
|---|---|---|---|
| **Homestyle Fries:** Kids | 240 | 11 | 33 |
| Small | 360 | 17 | 49 |
| Medium | 480 | 22 | 66 |
| Large | 610 | 28 | 82 |
| **Melts:** Arby's | 340 | 13 | 37 |
| Ham & Swiss | 300 | 9 | 35 |

| *Kids Meals:* | | | |
|---|---|---|---|
| Curly Fries, 2.75 oz | 240 | 13 | 28 |
| Jr Roast Beef Sandwich | 210 | 8 | 22 |
| Jr Turkey & Cheese Sandwich | 220 | 6 | 23 |
| Prime Cut Chkn Tenders, (2), 3 oz | 230 | 11 | 17 |

| *Fries:* | | | |
|---|---|---|---|
| **Curly Fries:** Small, 4.5 oz | 400 | 22 | 47 |
| Medium, 6 oz | 540 | 29 | 62 |
| Large, 7 oz | 630 | 35 | 74 |

| *Snack 'N Save:* | | | |
|---|---|---|---|
| **Jalapeno Bites:** 5 bites | 280 | 16 | 31 |
| 8 bites | 460 | 25 | 49 |
| **Mozzarella Sticks:** 4 sticks | 420 | 21 | 35 |
| 6 sticks | 620 | 32 | 52 |
| **Potato Cakes:** 3 cakes | 340 | 20 | 37 |
| 4 cakes | 460 | 27 | 50 |
| **Steakhouse Onion Rings,** 5 rings | 410 | 20 | 51 |
| **Turnovers:** Apple with Icing | 430 | 18 | 64 |
| Cherry Turnover with Icing | 390 | 13 | 64 |

*Continued Next Page...*

# Fast - Foods & *Restaurants*

## Arby's® cont... (Aug '15)

*Market Fresh Salads:* Without Dressing

| | C | F | Cb |
|---|---|---|---|
| **Farmhouse:** | | | |
| Crispy Chicken | 400 | 23 | 20 |
| Roast Turkey | 230 | 13 | 8 |
| **Dressings:** *Per 1.5 oz packet* | | | |
| Balsamic Vinaigrette | 130 | 12 | 5 |
| Buttermilk Ranch | 210 | 22 | 2 |
| Dijon Honey Mustard | 180 | 16 | 8 |
| *Breakfast: Per Serving* | | | |
| **Biscuits:** Bacon, Egg & Cheese | 470 | 27 | 35 |
| Ham, Egg & Cheese | 420 | 21 | 34 |
| Sausage, Egg & Cheese | 620 | 43 | 36 |
| **Croissants:** Bacon, Egg & Cheese | 400 | 26 | 25 |
| Ham, Egg & Cheese | 350 | 20 | 24 |
| Sausage, Egg & Cheese | 550 | 42 | 26 |
| **Sourdoughs:** | | | |
| Bacon, Egg & Cheese | 480 | 22 | 45 |
| Ham, Egg & Cheese | 430 | 16 | 44 |
| Sausage, Egg & Cheese | 630 | 38 | 46 |
| **Wraps:** Bacon, Egg & Cheese | 500 | 27 | 42 |
| Ham, Egg & Cheese | 410 | 20 | 41 |
| Sausage, Egg & Cheese | 630 | 41 | 43 |
| *Sauces:* Arby's, 0.5 oz | 15 | 0 | 3 |
| Bronco Berry, 1 oz | 60 | 0 | 15 |
| Cheddar Cheese, 1.5 oz | 50 | 3.5 | 4 |
| Horsey, 0.5 oz | 50 | 5 | 3 |
| Marinara, 1 oz | 25 | 0.5 | 3 |
| Spicy Three Pepper, 0.5 oz | 25 | 1 | 3 |
| Tangy BBQ, 1 oz | 45 | 0 | 11 |
| *Dipping Sauces:* Buffalo, 1 oz | 10 | 1 | 1 |
| Honey Mustard, 1 oz | 140 | 13 | 5 |
| Ranch, 1 oz | 100 | 11 | 1 |
| *Shakes: Per Regular Size* | | | |
| Chocolate, 22 oz | 570 | 15 | 99 |
| Vanilla, 22 oz | 470 | 15 | 75 |
| *Sodas: Without Ice* | | | |
| **Average all flavors:** | | | |
| Small, 16 fl.oz | 200 | 0 | 50 |
| Medium, 22 fl.oz | 280 | 0 | 70 |
| Large, 32 fl.oz | 400 | 0 | 100 |
| *Iced Tea,* no added sugar, 18 fl.oz | 5 | 0 | 1 |

## Atlanta Bread Co® (Aug '15)

*Signature Sandwiches:* As Per Menu Board Components

| | C | F | Cb |
|---|---|---|---|
| ABC Special on French Baguette | 720 | 30 | 62 |
| Chicken Salad | 630 | 34 | 45 |
| Curry Chicken Salad | 650 | 42 | 44 |
| Fresh Caprese | 570 | 29 | 51 |
| Roast Beef | 510 | 16 | 56 |
| Salmon Banh-Mi on Ciabatta | 420 | 9 | 52 |
| Tuna Salad | 620 | 39 | 40 |
| *Paninis:* Buffalo Chicken | 770 | 30 | 102 |
| Gourmet Grilled Cheese | 900 | 50 | 102 |
| Grilled Caprese | 570 | 29 | 51 |
| NY Hot Pastrami | 830 | 58 | 39 |
| Steakhouse | 620 | 29 | 49 |
| *Pasta:* Fettuccine Salmon | 440 | 20 | 27 |
| Penne Pomodora | 310 | 18 | 18 |
| *Pizza:* BBQ Chicken | 870 | 24 | 99 |
| Buffalo Chicken | 970 | 42 | 87 |
| Four Cheese | 940 | 41 | 85 |
| Margherita | 740 | 25 | 84 |
| Pepperoni | 690 | 23 | 86 |
| White | 840 | 37 | 99 |
| *Salads:* With Dressing | | | |
| Balsamic Bleu | 510 | 40 | 29 |
| Buffalo Chicken | 720 | 60 | 13 |
| Caesar | 540 | 47 | 20 |
| House Salad | 430 | 36 | 18 |
| Montamore Berry | 360 | 25 | 24 |
| Salsa Fresca Salmon | 510 | 30 | 32 |

*For Complete Menu & Data ~ see CalorieKing.com*

## Au Bon Pain® (Aug '15)

*Bagels: Per Bagel*

| | C | F | Cb |
|---|---|---|---|
| Asiago Cheese | 370 | 8 | 56 |
| Cinnamon Crisp | 410 | 7 | 77 |
| Everything | 300 | 2 | 58 |
| Honey 9 Grain | 310 | 2 | 63 |
| Jalapeno Double Cheddar | 320 | 8 | 52 |
| *Cream Cheese Spreads:* | | | |
| Garden Vegetable, 1.5 oz | 100 | 10 | 2 |
| Honey Pecan, 1.5oz | 150 | 12 | 7 |
| Lite Cream Cheese, 1.5 oz | 90 | 8 | 3 |

*Continued Next Page... ...*

## Au Bon Pain® cont... (Aug '15)

| Breakfast Sandwiches: | C | F | Cb |
|---|---|---|---|
| 2 Egg on a Bagel | 430 | 12 | 58 |
| With Bacon | 510 | 17 | 58 |
| With Cheese | 480 | 16 | 58 |
| Egg Whites & Cheddar | 210 | 7 | 22 |
| Smoked Salmon & Wasabi, | | | |
| on Onion Dill | 400 | 9 | 62 |

**Cafe Sandwiches:** *Per Whole Sandwich*

| | C | F | Cb |
|---|---|---|---|
| Black Angus Roast Beef & Cheddar | 510 | 18 | 53 |
| Black Forest Ham & Cheddar | 640 | 17 | 92 |
| Classic Chicken Salad | 440 | 11 | 59 |
| Grilled Chicken | 470 | 14 | 54 |
| Tuna Salad | 520 | 22 | 47 |
| Turkey & Swiss | 750 | 30 | 79 |

**Signature Sandwiches:** *Per Whole Sandwich*

| | C | F | Cb |
|---|---|---|---|
| Black Angus Roast Beef | | | |
| & Herb Cheese | 510 | 13 | 70 |
| Caprese | 550 | 27 | 53 |
| Chipotle Turkey & Avocado | 690 | 32 | 61 |
| Turkey Club | 620 | 24 | 53 |
| **Wraps:** Chicken Caesar | 600 | 32 | 50 |
| Thai Peanut Chicken | 530 | 17 | 72 |
| Veggie & Hummus | 660 | 37 | 64 |
| Waldorf Turkey | 670 | 32 | 63 |

**Harvest Rice Bowls:**

| | C | F | Cb |
|---|---|---|---|
| Roasted: Angus Steak Teriyaki | 610 | 14 | 91 |
| Mayan Chicken | 580 | 17 | 80 |

**Soups:** *Per Medium 12 oz Bowl*

| | C | F | Cb |
|---|---|---|---|
| Baked Stuffed Potato | 380 | 24 | 33 |
| Chicken Gumbo | 190 | 9 | 22 |
| Corn & Green Chili Bisque | 270 | 16 | 26 |
| Cream of Chicken & Wild Rice | 270 | 15 | 26 |
| French Onion | 110 | 5 | 15 |
| Italian Wedding | 170 | 8 | 16 |
| Lobster & Corn Bisque | 280 | 16 | 25 |
| Vegetarian Chili | 270 | 2.5 | 47 |
| Wild Mushroom Bisque | 190 | 9 | 23 |

**Specialty Soups:** *Per 12 fl.oz Bowl*

| | C | F | Cb |
|---|---|---|---|
| Beef & Vegetable Stew | 340 | 19 | 26 |
| Macaroni & Cheese | 880 | 43 | 92 |
| Turkey Chili | 340 | 9 | 44 |

## Au Bon Pain® cont... (Aug '15)

| Salads: *Without Dressing* | C | F | Cb |
|---|---|---|---|
| Chicken Caesar Asiago | 370 | 16 | 22 |
| Chicken Cobb, with Avocado | 460 | 27 | 16 |
| Farm Stand Steak | 360 | 17 | 21 |
| Harvest Turkey | 440 | 16 | 38 |
| Lobster & Corn | 350 | 15 | 26 |
| Southwest Chicken | 420 | 16 | 43 |
| Steak Caesar Asiago | 420 | 20 | 24 |

**Dressings:** Balsamic Vinaig., 2 oz

| | C | F | Cb |
|---|---|---|---|
| Balsamic Vinaig., 2 oz | 110 | 9 | 7 |
| Bleu Cheese, 2 oz | 310 | 33 | 2 |
| Caesar, 2 oz | 290 | 30 | 2 |
| Sesame Ginger, 2 oz | 230 | 20 | 12 |
| Thai Peanut, 2 oz | 160 | 8 | 20 |

**Bakery:** *Per Item*

| | C | F | Cb |
|---|---|---|---|
| Brownie Bites, 1.4 oz | 160 | 7 | 22 |
| **Cakes:** Red Velvet Cupcake, 3 oz | 400 | 22 | 46 |
| Pound Cakes: Iced Lemon, 4.5 oz | 470 | 21 | 66 |
| Marble, 4 oz | 450 | 24 | 54 |
| **Cookies:** English Toffee, 2.3 oz | 320 | 16 | 42 |
| Choc. Dipped Shortbread, 2.6 oz | 390 | 23 | 43 |
| **Croissants:** Almond, 4.1 oz | 500 | 31 | 48 |
| Apple & Cinnamon, 3.4 oz | 240 | 8 | 38 |
| Chocolate, 4 oz | 480 | 25 | 57 |
| Raspberry Cheese, 4 oz | 360 | 16 | 48 |
| Sweet Cheese, 3.9 oz | 430 | 23 | 48 |
| **Muffins:** Blueberry, 4.7 oz | 490 | 19 | 73 |
| Berry, Low-Fat, 4.5 oz | 290 | 3 | 61 |
| Carrot Walnut, 5 oz | 540 | 25 | 73 |
| Raisin Bran, 5.5oz | 420 | 11 | 78 |

**Beverages:** Caffe Latte, 16 fl.oz

| | C | F | Cb |
|---|---|---|---|
| Caffe Latte, 16 fl.oz | 140 | 7 | 12 |
| Caramel Macchiato, 16 fl.oz | 270 | 7 | 43 |
| Raspberry Iced Tea, 24 fl.oz | 180 | 0 | 50 |
| Strawberry Smoothie, 16 fl.oz | 290 | 0 | 68 |

*For Complete Nutritional Data ~ see CalorieKing.com*

## Auntie Anne's® (Aug '15)

| Pretzels: *With Butter* | C | F | Cb |
|---|---|---|---|
| Cinnamon Sugar | 470 | 12 | 84 |
| Jalapeno | 330 | 5 | 63 |
| Original | 340 | 5 | 65 |
| Original Stix, 6 sticks | 340 | 5 | 65 |
| Pepperoni | 480 | 16 | 65 |
| Sour Cream & Onion | 360 | 5 | 68 |
| Sweet Almond | 390 | 6 | 74 |

*Continued Next Page ...*

## Auntie Anne's® cont... (Aug '15)

### Dipping Sauces:

| | C | F | Cb |
|---|---|---|---|
| Caramel Dip, 1.5 oz | 130 | 3 | 23 |
| Cheese Dip; Hot Salsa Cheese, av., 1 oz | 95 | 8 | 3 |
| Light Cream Cheese, 1.3 oz | 80 | 6 | 1 |
| Marinara, 2 oz | 45 | 1 | 7 |
| Sweet Glaze, 1.4 oz | 130 | 0 | 32 |
| Sweet Mustard, 1.3 oz | 60 | 2 | 10 |

### Beverages: Per Serving

**Frozen Lemonade Mixer:** Per 16 fl.oz

| | C | F | Cb |
|---|---|---|---|
| Blue Raspberry; Strawberry, av. | 235 | 0 | 60 |

## Back Yard Burgers® (Aug '15)

### Burgers:

| | C | F | Cb |
|---|---|---|---|
| American Cheeseburger, ⅓ lb | 750 | 49 | 36 |
| Bacon Cheddar | 840 | 57 | 37 |
| Black Jack | 860 | 64 | 34 |
| Bleu Cheeseburger: ⅓ lb | 700 | 44 | 36 |
| Double ⅔ lb | 1140 | 78 | 36 |
| Cheddar Cheeseburger: ⅓ lb | 765 | 50 | 37 |
| Double ⅔ lb | 1265 | 89 | 38 |
| Classic Burger, ⅓ lb | 650 | 40 | 36 |
| Mushroom Swiss | 760 | 50 | 35 |
| Pepper Jack Cheesseburger, ⅓ lb | 740 | 49 | 36 |
| Swiss Cheeseburger: ⅓ lb | 760 | 49 | 36 |
| Double ⅔ lb | 1260 | 88 | 38 |

### Chicken:

| | C | F | Cb |
|---|---|---|---|
| **Sandwiches:** Blackened Chicken | 500 | 25 | 41 |
| Chicken Club | 670 | 43 | 38 |
| Grilled Chicken | 365 | 12 | 36 |
| Hawaiian Chicken | 415 | 12 | 48 |
| *Specialities:* Back Yard Dog | 320 | 18 | 29 |
| Chicken Tender Basket | 465 | 25 | 33 |
| Chili Cheese Dog | 635 | 45 | 32 |
| Loaded Smoked Sausage | 575 | 39 | 30 |
| Original Smoked Sausage | 450 | 28 | 32 |
| Veggie Burger | 410 | 15 | 57 |
| *Turkey Burgers:* Classic | 565 | 38 | 36 |
| Wild Turkey Wrap | 675 | 50 | 35 |

### Fries:

| | C | F | Cb |
|---|---|---|---|
| Seasoned, Regular, 6 oz | 510 | 36 | 45 |
| Sweet Potato, Regular, 5 oz | 555 | 43 | 43 |
| Waffle, 4.5 oz | 570 | 37 | 52 |

## Back Yard Burgers® cont... (Aug '15)

### Salads: Without Dressing

| | C | F | Cb |
|---|---|---|---|
| Chicken: Blackened | 590 | 38 | 22 |
| Grilled | 485 | 26 | 22 |
| Cranberry Pecan | 760 | 42 | 55 |
| With Blackened Chicken | 865 | 53 | 55 |
| *Sides:* Cole Slaw | 35 | 1.5 | 4.5 |
| Panko Onion rings, 4 oz | 295 | 14 | 37 |

### Dressings: Per Serving

| | C | F | Cb |
|---|---|---|---|
| Bleu Cheese | 220 | 24 | 1 |
| Gorgonzola Vinaigrette | 170 | 15 | 6 |
| Honey Mustard | 240 | 23 | 7 |
| Ranch, Homestyle | 150 | 15 | 2 |

### Desserts: Per Serving

| | C | F | Cb |
|---|---|---|---|
| Cobblers: Apple | 360 | 14 | 59 |
| Blackberry | 285 | 7.5 | 51 |
| Cherry | 345 | 12 | 59 |
| Pecan | 740 | 26 | 119 |

### Shakes: Per 12 fl.oz

| | C | F | Cb |
|---|---|---|---|
| Chocolate | 760 | 36 | 100 |
| Strawberry/Vanilla | 730 | 32 | 100 |

## Baja Fresh® (Aug '15)

### Burritos: With Standard Menu Board Components

| | C | F | Cb |
|---|---|---|---|
| **Baja:** | | | |
| With Carnitas | 830 | 45 | 67 |
| With Chicken | 790 | 38 | 65 |
| With Steak | 850 | 46 | 67 |
| **Bean & Cheese:** | | | |
| With Carnitas | 1010 | 42 | 98 |
| With Chicken | 970 | 35 | 96 |
| With Steak | 1030 | 43 | 97 |
| Vegetarian, without Meat | 840 | 33 | 96 |
| **Mexicano:** | | | |
| With Carnitas | 830 | 20 | 119 |
| With Chicken | 790 | 13 | 117 |
| With Steak | 860 | 21 | 118 |
| **Ultimo:** With Chicken | 880 | 38 | 84 |
| With Steak | 950 | 44 | 85 |
| **Vegetarian,** Grilled Veggie | 800 | 33 | 94 |

### Fajitas: As Served, Without Tortilla Chips

| | C | F | Cb |
|---|---|---|---|
| Chicken, with Corn Tortillas | 860 | 24 | 105 |
| Chicken, with Flour Tortillas | 1140 | 33 | 147 |

### Nachos: As Served

| | C | F | Cb |
|---|---|---|---|
| **Regular:** With Cheese | 945 | 54 | 82 |
| With Chicken | 1010 | 55 | 82 |
| With Steak | 1060 | 59 | 82 |

*Continued Next Page...*

Updated Nutrition Data ~ www.CalorieKing.com
Persons with Diabetes ~ See Disclaimer (Page 22)

## Baja Fresh® cont... (Aug '15)

*Quesadillas: With Grilled Flour Tortilla and Standard Menu Board Components*

| | C | F | Cb |
|---|---|---|---|
| With Cheese | 1200 | 78 | 84 |
| With Chicken | 1330 | 80 | 84 |
| With Steak | 1430 | 87 | 84 |
| Vegetarian | 1260 | 78 | 96 |

*Tacos: With Standard Menu Board Components*

| | C | F | Cb |
|---|---|---|---|
| **Americano, Soft Taco:** Carnitas | 250 | 12 | 21 |
| Chicken | 230 | 10 | 20 |
| **Crispy Wahoo** | 250 | 13 | 27 |
| **Grilled Wahoo,** with black beans | 180 | 1 | 30 |
| **Original Baja,** average all varieties | 215 | 6.5 | 28 |

*Salads: With Standard Menu Board Components Without Dressing*

| **Baja Ensalada:** | | | |
|---|---|---|---|
| With Carnitas | 370 | 18 | 20 |
| With Chicken | 310 | 7 | 18 |
| With Shrimp | 230 | 6 | 18 |
| With Steak | 450 | 18 | 18 |
| **Tostada:** | | | |
| With Carnitas | 1180 | 62 | 100 |
| With Chicken | 1140 | 55 | 98 |
| With Shrimp | 1120 | 55 | 99 |
| With Steak | 1230 | 63 | 98 |

*For Complete Nutritional Data ~ see CalorieKing.com*

## Baskin Robbins® (Aug '15)

| Cones: | C | F | Cb |
|---|---|---|---|
| Cake | 25 | 0 | 5 |
| Fresh-Baked Waffle | 130 | 3.5 | 24 |
| Sugar | 45 | 0.5 | 9 |

*Ice Creams: Per 4 oz Scoop*

| **Classic Flavors:** Cherries Jubilee | 220 | 11 | 26 |
|---|---|---|---|
| Chocolate | 240 | 14 | 26 |
| Jamoca Almond Fudge | 260 | 15 | 28 |
| Mint Chocolate Chip | 250 | 16 | 23 |
| Nutty Coconut | 290 | 19 | 24 |
| Old Fashioned Butter Pecan | 260 | 18 | 20 |
| Oreo Cookies 'n Cream | 260 | 15 | 28 |
| Peanut Butter 'n Chocolate | 300 | 20 | 25 |
| Pistachio Almond | 270 | 19 | 21 |
| Pralines 'n Cream | 270 | 14 | 32 |
| Rainbow Sherbet | 130 | 2 | 27 |
| Reese's P'nut Butter Cup | 300 | 17 | 32 |
| Vanilla | 240 | 16 | 21 |
| Very Berry Strawberry | 200 | 11 | 24 |
| World Class Chocolate | 260 | 16 | 25 |

## Baskin Robbins® cont... (Aug '15)

*Ice Creams (Cont): Per 4 oz Scoop*

| | C | F | Cb |
|---|---|---|---|
| **Seasonal Flavors:** Baseball Nut | 260 | 14 | 29 |
| Black Walnut | 260 | 18 | 20 |
| Chocolate Fudge | 250 | 15 | 27 |
| Creole Cream Cheese | 230 | 13 | 24 |
| Red Velvet | 250 | 14 | 28 |
| Strawberry Cheesecake | 250 | 13 | 29 |

*Grab-N-Go,*

| Brownie a la Mode, 2.77 oz slice | 260 | 13 | 36 |
|---|---|---|---|

*Soft Serve:*

| **Cups:** Vanilla: Kid's, 3 oz | 130 | 4.5 | 18 |
|---|---|---|---|
| Regular, 6 oz | 250 | 9 | 37 |
| Large, 9 oz | 380 | 14 | 55 |

*Parfaits: Per Regular 15 oz Size*

| M&M's | 820 | 31 | 124 |
|---|---|---|---|
| Oreo | 740 | 27 | 114 |
| Reese's | 990 | 63 | 86 |
| Snickers | 780 | 25 | 127 |
| Strawberry 'n Almonds | 600 | 27 | 76 |

*31 Below' Mix-In: Per 16 oz Medium Cup*

| Butterfinger | 840 | 32 | 127 |
|---|---|---|---|
| Choc. Chip Cookie Dough | 860 | 30 | 132 |
| Heath | 860 | 43 | 106 |
| Oreo | 750 | 28 | 110 |
| Reese's PB Cup | 830 | 40 | 100 |

*Sundaes:*

| Banana Royale | 620 | 28 | 87 |
|---|---|---|---|
| Brownie | 920 | 47 | 119 |
| Chocolate Chip Cookie Dough | 990 | 43 | 138 |
| Classic Banana | 1010 | 34 | 173 |
| Made with Snickers | 1010 | 42 | 146 |
| Two Scoop | 530 | 29 | 61 |
| Warm Brownie | 740 | 41 | 85 |

*Beverages:*

**Fruit Blast:** *Per Medium, 24 fl.oz*

| Mango | 500 | 1.5 | 123 |
|---|---|---|---|
| Strawberry Citrus | 350 | 0 | 87 |

**Milk Shakes:** *Per Medium, 24 fl.oz*

| Choc. with Choc. Ice Cream | 920 | 40 | 125 |
|---|---|---|---|
| Chocolate Chip | 880 | 43 | 106 |
| Mint Chocolate Chip | 880 | 44 | 106 |

**Smoothie:** *Per Medium, 24 fl.oz*

| Mango Banana | 630 | 2 | 150 |
|---|---|---|---|
| Strawberry Banana | 520 | 1 | 126 |
| Tropical Banana | 550 | 1.5 | 132 |

## Big Apple Bagels® (Aug '15)

*Bagels:*

| | C | F | Cb |
|---|---|---|---|
| **Regular flavors,** average all, 5 oz | 340 | 2 | 70 |
| **Choice Bagels:** *Per Bagel* | | | |
| Blueberry Cobbler | 390 | 8 | 70 |
| Cheddar Nacho | 350 | 6 | 60 |
| Cinnamon Bun | 400 | 8 | 70 |
| Cinnamon Danish | 395 | 8 | 72 |
| Quiche Lorraine | 355 | 8 | 54 |
| Strawberry White Chocolate | 365 | 4 | 72 |
| Swiss Melt | 370 | 8 | 58 |
| White Chocolate Swirl | 395 | 8 | 70 |
| *Cream Cheese: Per 2 Tbsp, 1 oz* | | | |
| Plain | 90 | 9 | 2 |
| Plain, Lite | 60 | 4.5 | 3 |
| Other varieties, average | 90 | 8 | 2 |
| Whipped: Classic Plain | 70 | 7 | 1 |
| Brown Sugar Cinnamon | 70 | 5 | 5 |
| Reduced-Fat Spring Veggie | 60 | 5 | 2 |
| *Overstuffed Sandwich,* | | | |
| Manhattan Club | 1120 | 40 | 120 |
| *Specialty Sandwiches:* | | | |
| All-American Duo | 750 | 28 | 78 |
| Big Apple Club | 795 | 37 | 75 |
| Chicken Caesar | 610 | 19 | 78 |
| Turkey Club | 780 | 34 | 75 |
| *Toasted Sandwiches:* | | | |
| Cafe Chicken Melt | 815 | 32 | 80 |
| Roast Beef Parmesan Grinder | 585 | 15 | 76 |
| Tuna Melt | 640 | 23 | 75 |
| *Breakfast,* | | | |
| Morning Classic | 485 | 11 | 73 |

*For Complete Nutritional Data ~ see CalorieKing.com*

## Biggby Coffee® (Aug '15)

*Hot Drinks:*

*Per Tall, 16 fl.oz, w/o Whipped Cream & Sugar Unless Indicated*

| | C | F | Cb |
|---|---|---|---|
| **Caffe au Lait:** | | | |
| With 2% Milk | 100 | 4 | 9 |
| With Non-Fat Milk | 65 | 0 | 9 |
| With Soy | 90 | 3 | 11 |
| **Caffe Latte:** With 2% Milk | 175 | 7.5 | 16 |
| With Non-Fat Milk | 115 | 0 | 16 |
| With Soy | 160 | 5 | 19 |
| **Cappuccino:** With 2% Milk | 105 | 4.5 | 10 |
| With Non-Fat Milk | 70 | 0 | 10 |
| With Soy | 95 | 3 | 11 |
| **Chai Latte:** With 2% Milk | 315 | 7.5 | 51 |
| With Non-Fat Milk | 255 | 0 | 51 |
| **Dark Hot Chocolate:** With 2% Milk | 275 | 7 | 39 |
| With Non-Fat Milk | 215 | 0 | 39 |

## Biggby Coffee® cont... (Aug '15)

*Cold Drinks: Per Tall, 16 fl.oz*

| | C | F | Cb |
|---|---|---|---|
| **Creme Freeze:** *With Whipped Cream* | | | |
| Banana Berry | 535 | 15 | 95 |
| Chocolate Chip, 2% Milk | 820 | 33 | 131 |
| Mango | 670 | 15 | 125 |
| **Freeze Specials,** | | | |
| Almond Blizzard Creme Freeze, | | | |
| 2% milk & Whipped Cream | 570 | 17 | 97 |

*For Complete Menu & Data ~ see CalorieKing.com*

## Blimpie® (Aug '15)

*Cold Deli Subs:*

*Per Regular, 6" White Sub, with Standard Menu Board Toppings*

| | C | F | Cb |
|---|---|---|---|
| Blimpie Best | 450 | 18 | 47 |
| BLT | 430 | 22 | 43 |
| Club | 410 | 13 | 49 |
| Ham & Swiss | 410 | 14 | 47 |
| Roast Beef & Provolone | 430 | 15 | 44 |
| Tuna without Cheese | 460 | 21 | 41 |
| Turkey & Provolone | 410 | 14 | 47 |
| *Wraps: Includes Dressing* | | | |
| Chicken Caesar | 590 | 26 | 56 |
| Southwestern | 490 | 18 | 57 |
| *Hot Deli Subs: Per 6" White Sub with Standard Menu Board Toppings* | | | |
| Meatball Parmigiana | 560 | 29 | 47 |
| Pastrami | 430 | 16 | 42 |
| VegiMax | 520 | 21 | 55 |
| *Salads: Regular, Without Dressing* | | | |
| Buffalo Chicken | 200 | 8 | 11 |
| Garden | 30 | 0 | 6 |
| Tuna | 270 | 19 | 6 |
| Ultimate Club | 270 | 14 | 11 |
| *Dressings & Sauces: Per 1.5oz* | | | |
| Creamy Caesar | 210 | 21 | 2 |
| Creamy Italian | 180 | 18 | 4 |
| *Soups: Per 8.6 oz Serving* | | | |
| Chicken Noodle | 130 | 4 | 18 |
| Cream of Broccoli with Cheese | 250 | 19 | 13 |
| Harvest Vegetable | 100 | 1 | 19 |
| New England Clam Chowder | 170 | 3 | 28 |
| Vegetable Beef | 80 | 2 | 13 |
| *Breakfast:* | | | |
| **Biscuits:** Bacon, Egg & Cheese | 440 | 25 | 37 |
| Sausage, Egg & Cheese | 520 | 33 | 37 |
| **Bluffin,** Egg & Cheese | 180 | 4 | 27 |
| **Burritos:** Ham, Egg & Cheese | 580 | 25 | 57 |
| Sausage, Egg & Cheese | 800 | 52 | 54 |
| **Sandwich,** Grilled Bacon | 520 | 26 | 43 |
| **Cinnamon Roll** | 540 | 24 | 72 |
| *Desserts:* Brownie | 230 | 10 | 28 |
| Cookie, Oatmeal Raisin | 160 | 8 | 23 |

## Bob Evans® (Aug '15)

| Starters: | C | F | Cb |
|---|---|---|---|
| Breaded Garlic Mushrooms | 620 | 35 | 64 |
| Country Fair Cheese Bites | 1220 | 95 | 44 |
| Fruit Plate w/ Low Fat Strawb Yog. | 340 | 2 | 95 |

**Burgers:** *Without Fries or Coleslaw*

| | C | F | Cb |
|---|---|---|---|
| **Big Farm Burgers:** Regular | 910 | 61 | 48 |
| Bacon Cheeseburger | 1090 | 76 | 50 |
| Favorite Burger | 1010 | 70 | 48 |
| Smokehouse Burger | 1380 | 98 | 66 |

**Sandwiches:** *Full Sandwich, without Sides*

| | C | F | Cb |
|---|---|---|---|
| Farm Favorite Chicken: Cripsy | 590 | 23 | 59 |
| Grilled | 500 | 18 | 48 |
| Farm-Grill Chicken Club: Crispy | 610 | 25 | 58 |
| Grilled | 520 | 19 | 47 |
| Pot Roast Sandwich Platter | 650 | 36 | 48 |
| Turkey Bacon Melt Platter | 560 | 26 | 48 |

**Dinners:** *Without Sides or Bread*

**Slow Roasted:**

| | C | F | Cb |
|---|---|---|---|
| Chicken-N-Noodles, Deep-Dish | 630 | 28 | 67 |
| Country Fried Steak, with Country Gravy | 830 | 50 | 72 |
| Meatloaf & Gravy, 1 slice | 500 | 31 | 23 |
| Pot Roast | 590 | 39 | 43 |

**Chicken:** *Without Sides or Bread*

| | C | F | Cb |
|---|---|---|---|
| Chicken Tender: Crispy, 4 tenders | 490 | 26 | 26 |
| Grilled, 4 tenders | 140 | 2.5 | 0 |
| Fried Chicken, 1 breast | 230 | 10 | 11 |
| Grilled Chicken, 1 breast | 150 | 3.5 | 0 |

**Seafood:** *Without Sides or Bread*

| | C | F | Cb |
|---|---|---|---|
| Grilled Salmon Fillet | 300 | 20 | 2 |
| Potato-Crusted Flounder | 240 | 12 | 13 |

**Farmhouse Sides:**

| | C | F | Cb |
|---|---|---|---|
| **Baked:** Russet Potato | 220 | 5 | 49 |
| Sweet Potato | 310 | 10 | 52 |
| Bread & Celery Dressing, 6 oz | 280 | 15 | 29 |
| Buttered Sweet Corn | 190 | 12 | 20 |
| Coleslaw, 3.5 oz | 210 | 14 | 19 |
| **Loaded:** Baked Potato | 420 | 16 | 52 |
| French Fries | 690 | 37 | 73 |
| Hash Browns | 400 | 26 | 28 |
| Home Fries | 390 | 23 | 33 |
| Macaroni & Cheese | 280 | 15 | 24 |
| Mashed Potatoes | 190 | 9 | 24 |
| *Gravy:* Beef, 2.3 oz | 20 | 2 | 3 |
| Chicken, 2 oz | 20 | 2 | 2 |
| Country, 3 oz | 50 | 2 | 8 |

## Bob Evans® cont... (Aug '15)

| Sauces: | C | F | Cb |
|---|---|---|---|
| Bob Evans Wildfire, 1 ramekin | 60 | 0 | 15 |
| Garlic Herb Butter, 0.3 oz | 10 | 1 | 1 |
| Honey Mustard, 1 pkt | 140 | 13 | 6 |
| Old Route 35, 2 Tbsp | 140 | 14 | 3 |
| Spicy Chipotle, 2 Tbsp | 180 | 19 | 1 |

**Soups:** *Per Bowl, with 2 Saltine Crackers*

| | C | F | Cb |
|---|---|---|---|
| Cheddar Baked Potato | 380 | 20 | 34 |
| Chicken-N-Noodles | 225 | 4 | 31 |
| Farm Festival Bean | 220 | 4.5 | 33 |
| Hearty Beef Vegetable | 220 | 4.5 | 34 |
| Tomato Basil | 390 | 17 | 48 |

**Salads:** *Full Size, Without Dressing or Bread*

| | C | F | Cb |
|---|---|---|---|
| Apple, Cranberry Spinach | 260 | 9 | 33 |
| Heritage Chef | 400 | 25 | 12 |
| Wildfire Grilled Chicken | 410 | 15 | 39 |

**Dressings:** *Per Ramekin*

| | C | F | Cb |
|---|---|---|---|
| Blue Cheese | 180 | 16 | 8 |
| Buttermilk Ranch | 130 | 13 | 1 |
| Sweet Italian | 160 | 15 | 7 |

**Breakfast:**

**Hotcakes:** *With Margarine & Syrup*

| | C | F | Cb |
|---|---|---|---|
| Cinnamon Hotcakes (4) | 1010 | 30 | 175 |
| Chocolate Chip (4) | 1030 | 32 | 178 |
| Multigrain (4) | 1030 | 18 | 203 |

**Omelets:** *With Hash Browns & Cinnamon Bread*

| | C | F | Cb |
|---|---|---|---|
| Border Scramble | 1440 | 82 | 123 |
| Farmer's Market | 1320 | 73 | 119 |
| Western | 1240 | 67 | 113 |

**Farm-Fresh Egg Combinations:** *Includes 2 Eggs, 3 Sausage Links, Grits & 2 Slices Cinnamon Bread*

| | C | F | Cb |
|---|---|---|---|
| Pot Roast Hash | 1150 | 64 | 99 |
| Sunrise | 920 | 45 | 107 |
| The Rise | 1300 | 78 | 107 |

**Sweet & Stacked Hotcakes:**

| | C | F | Cb |
|---|---|---|---|
| Cinnamon Supreme, w/-Bacon | 1170 | 42 | 178 |
| Dble Blueb. w/- sausage links | 1300 | 54 | 173 |

**Breakfast Sides:**

| | C | F | Cb |
|---|---|---|---|
| Golden-Brown Home Fries | 190 | 6 | 31 |
| Low-Fat Strawberry Yogurt | 90 | 1 | 17 |
| Seasonal Fresh Fruit Dish | 60 | 0 | 14 |
| *Dessert:* Coconut Cream Pie, 1 slice | 590 | 36 | 63 |
| French Silk Pie, 1 slice | 650 | 43 | 59 |
| Peanut Butter Brownie Bites (8) | 880 | 40 | 120 |

**183**

## Bojangles® (Aug '15)

### Biscuit:

| | C | F | Cb |
|---|---|---|---|
| Plain | 280 | 14 | 33 |
| Bacon, Egg & Cheese | 550 | 37 | 35 |
| Cajun Filet | 515 | 28 | 45 |
| Country Ham | 355 | 18 | 33 |
| Egg & Cheese | 515 | 34 | 35 |
| Gravy Biscuits | 390 | 20 | 43 |
| Sausage | 420 | 27 | 33 |
| Steak | 555 | 35 | 44 |

### Dinner:

| | | | |
|---|---|---|---|
| 2 Breast | 1380 | 80 | 77 |
| 1 Leg, 2 Thighs | 1470 | 95 | 86 |
| 3 Wing | 1090 | 67 | 83 |

### Sandwiches:

| | | | |
|---|---|---|---|
| Cajun Filet: Regular | 495 | 27 | 43 |
| Club | 640 | 39 | 44 |
| Grilled Chicken: Regular | 375 | 15 | 33 |
| Club | 520 | 27 | 34 |

### Fixins': *Per Individual Serve Unless Indicated*

| | | | |
|---|---|---|---|
| Bo-Tato Rounds | 230 | 14 | 24 |
| Cole Slaw | 255 | 20 | 18 |
| Dirty Rice | 165 | 6 | 24 |
| Macaroni & Cheese | 240 | 7 | 33 |
| Mashed Potatoes 'N Gravy | 150 | 6 | 21 |
| Seasoned Fries: Individual | 215 | 14 | 20 |
| Medium size | 300 | 20 | 27 |
| Picnic size | 530 | 35 | 49 |
| *Salads:* Chicken Supreme | 460 | 18 | 33 |
| Garden | 190 | 9 | 9 |
| Grilled Chicken | 305 | 11 | 11 |

### Sweets:

| | | | |
|---|---|---|---|
| Bo-Berry Biscuit (1) | 375 | 15 | 55 |
| Cinnamon Twist (1) | 270 | 12 | 36 |
| Sweet Potato Pie | 410 | 23 | 48 |

*For Complete Nutritional Data ~ see CalorieKing.com*

## Boston Market® (Aug '15)

### Sandwiches:

*Per Whole With Set Menu Board Toppings*

| | C | F | Cb |
|---|---|---|---|
| All-White Chicken Salad | 890 | 56 | 62 |
| Meatloaf Carver | 950 | 39 | 93 |
| Roasted Turkey Carver | 850 | 46 | 62 |
| Rotisserie Chicken Carver | 750 | 34 | 62 |

### Individual Meals: *Without Sides Or Bread*

| | | | |
|---|---|---|---|
| Meatloaf, regular, 7.6 oz | 510 | 29 | 26 |
| Rotisserie Chicken, half, 12 oz | 640 | 33 | 2 |
| St Louis Style BBQ Ribs, ½ rack | 1180 | 74 | 67 |

## Boston Market® cont... (Aug '15)

### Salads:

*Per Whole, With Dressing, Without Cornbread*

| | C | F | Cb |
|---|---|---|---|
| Chicken Caesar, 10.8 oz | 440 | 29 | 16 |
| Mediterranean, 13.4 | 550 | 39 | 14 |
| Southwest Santa Fe, 13.7 oz | 530 | 30 | 30 |

### Sides:

| | | | |
|---|---|---|---|
| Creamed Spinach, 6.3 oz | 250 | 20 | 11 |
| Fresh Steamed Vegetables, 4.8 oz | 70 | 4 | 7 |
| Fresh Vegetable Stuffing, 5.5 oz | 220 | 10 | 30 |
| Garlic Dill New Potatoes, 4.5 oz | 100 | 2 | 20 |
| Green Beans, 4.3 oz | 90 | 6 | 9 |
| Macaroni & Chse, 7.4 oz | 280 | 11 | 33 |
| Mashed Potatoes: Regular, 7.oz | 240 | 10 | 32 |
| Loaded, 7 oz | 310 | 16 | 31 |
| Sweet Corn | 120 | 2.5 | 25 |
| Sweet Potato Casserole, 7.4 oz | 430 | 12 | 79 |

### Soups:

| | | | |
|---|---|---|---|
| Chicken Noodle, 14 oz | 240 | 9 | 22 |
| Chicken Tortilla | 410 | 22 | 33 |

### Desserts:

| | | | |
|---|---|---|---|
| Apple Pie, 5.8 oz slice | 430 | 21 | 59 |
| Chocolate Brownie (1), 4.7 oz | 530 | 26 | 74 |
| Chocolate Cake, 1 Slice, 5 oz | 580 | 32 | 67 |

*For Complete Nutritional Data ~ see CalorieKing.com*

## Boston Pizza® Canada (Aug '15)

### Starters:

| | C | F | Cb |
|---|---|---|---|
| Oven Roasted Wings, 8.4 oz | 580 | 37 | 7 |
| Poutine, 14 oz | 610 | 30 | 67 |
| Spinach & Artichoke Dip, 13.7 oz | 660 | 35 | 65 |
| *Burgers:* Prime Rib with Bacon | 880 | 76 | 58 |
| Pepperoni & Bacon Pizzaburger | 1040 | 88 | 51 |
| Spicy Perogy Burger | 1200 | 107 | 64 |

### Gourmet Pastas: *Full Order, Without Garlic Toast*

| | | | |
|---|---|---|---|
| Boston's Lasagna | 790 | 23 | 107 |
| Montréal Smoked Meat Pasta | 890 | 16 | 142 |
| Spicy Sausage Arrabiata Penne | 1230 | 54 | 142 |

### Gourmet Pizza: *Per Individual Pizza*

**Classic Crust:**

| | | | |
|---|---|---|---|
| Boston Royal | 710 | 30 | 69 |
| Deluxe | 730 | 33 | 65 |
| Hawaiian | 660 | 24 | 72 |
| Pepperoni | 630 | 30 | 60 |

**Thin Crust:**

| | | | |
|---|---|---|---|
| Bacon Double Cheeseburger | 430 | 22 | 36 |
| The Meateor | 450 | 23 | 34 |

*Continued Next Page...*

# Fast - Foods & Restaurants

## Boston Pizza® Canada cont... (Aug '15)

**Sandwiches:** *Without Sides*

| | C | F | Cb |
|---|---|---|---|
| BBQ Pulled Pork | 1070 | 57 | 92 |
| Boston Brute | 800 | 24 | 108 |
| Buffalo Chicken | 920 | 35 | 119 |
| Chipotle Chicken Club | 710 | 35 | 57 |
| NY Striploin Steak Sandwich | 1060 | 51 | 95 |
| Smoked Meat | 910 | 59 | 40 |

**Salads:** *Full Order With Dressing*

| | C | F | Cb |
|---|---|---|---|
| Crispy Chicken Pecan | 1170 | 88 | 46 |
| Santa Fe | 710 | 51 | 64 |

**Desssert:**

| | C | F | Cb |
|---|---|---|---|
| NY Cheesecake | 600 | 32 | 76 |
| The Panookie, with ice cream | 880 | 38 | 133 |

*For Complete Nutritional Data ~ see CalorieKing.com*

## Braum's® ~ *see CalorieKing.com*

## Bruegger's® (Aug '15)

**Bagels:**

| | C | F | Cb |
|---|---|---|---|
| Chocolate Chip, 4 oz | 330 | 3.5 | 65 |
| Jalapeno Cheddar, 5.5 oz | 440 | 9 | 75 |
| Plain, 4.1 oz | 300 | 2 | 60 |
| Sesame; Whole Wheat, av., 4 oz | 310 | 3.5 | 61 |

**Breakfast Bagel S'wiches:** *With Standard Toppings*

| | C | F | Cb |
|---|---|---|---|
| Egg & Cheese | 430 | 18 | 63 |
| Egg White, Cheese & Bacon | 460 | 12 | 64 |
| Smoked Salmon | 460 | 10 | 66 |
| Spinach & Cheddar Omelet | 490 | 16 | 63 |
| Sriracha, Egg & Sausage | 660 | 31 | 64 |
| Western | 670 | 34 | 67 |

**Burgers:** *With Standard Toppings*

| | C | F | Cb |
|---|---|---|---|
| Bacon & Bleu Burger Melt | 770 | 53 | 35 |
| Barnyard Burger | 920 | 54 | 68 |
| Bistro Burger | 850 | 44 | 79 |

**Deli Sandwiches:** *With Standard Toppings*

| | C | F | Cb |
|---|---|---|---|
| BLT on Hearty White Bread | 720 | 42 | 62 |
| Chicken Breast on Plain Bagel | 550 | 6 | 81 |
| Garden Veggie on Plain Bagel | 360 | 2 | 72 |
| Ham On Honey Wheat Bread | 500 | 13 | 62 |

**Hot Paninis:** *On Ciabatta With Standard Toppings*

| | C | F | Cb |
|---|---|---|---|
| Four Cheese & Tomato | 570 | 26 | 59 |
| Harvest Turkey | 690 | 24 | 84 |
| Primo Pesto Chicken | 560 | 19 | 58 |
| Roast Beef Cheddar Melt | 630 | 26 | 72 |
| Turkey, Artichoke, Mozzarella | 520 | 14 | 61 |

**Signature & Classic Sandwiches:** *With Standard Toppings*

| | C | F | Cb |
|---|---|---|---|
| Herby Turkey on Sesame Bagel | 570 | 15 | 75 |
| Leon. da Veggie on Asiago Parm. Bagel | 490 | 14 | 70 |
| Thai Peanut Chicken on Plain Bagel | 580 | 11 | 91 |
| Turkey Chipotle Club on Wheat Bread | 400 | 17 | 36 |

## Bruegger's® cont... (Aug '15)

**Cafe Salads:** *Without Dressing*

| | C | F | Cb |
|---|---|---|---|
| Blue Apple, 7 oz | 300 | 14 | 20 |
| Chicken Almond, 11 oz | 260 | 14 | 8 |
| Chicken Caesar, 6 oz | 190 | 7 | 11 |

**Dressings:** *Balsamic Vinaig., 1 oz*

| | C | F | Cb |
|---|---|---|---|
| Balsamic Vinaig., 1 oz | 60 | 6 | 3 |
| Caesar, 1 oz | 80 | 7 | 2 |
| Ranch | 90 | 10 | 1 |

**Dessert Bars:**

| | C | F | Cb |
|---|---|---|---|
| Chocolate Chunk Brownie, 2.7 oz | 340 | 17 | 42 |
| Marshmallow Chew, 2.7 oz | 290 | 7 | 54 |
| Toffee Almond, 2.7 oz | 350 | 17 | 44 |

*For Complete Menu & Data ~ see CalorieKing.com*

## Burgerville® (Aug '15)

**Burgers:** *With Spread Unless Indicated*

| | C | F | Cb |
|---|---|---|---|
| Original Hamburger | 310 | 17 | 26 |
| Cheeseburger | 360 | 21 | 27 |
| Colossal Cheseburger | 550 | 29 | 41 |
| Double Colossal Cheeseburger with Mayo | 800 | 46 | 41 |
| Pepper Bacon Cheeseburger with Mayo | 670 | 41 | 37 |
| Tillamook Chseburger, with Mayo | 600 | 35 | 40 |
| Walla Walla Sweet Onion Chsebgr | 730 | 43 | 55 |

**Fish & Chips:** *With Lemon & Tartar Sce*

| | C | F | Cb |
|---|---|---|---|
| Hallibut, 3 pieces | 840 | 50 | 73 |
| Hallibut, 4 pieces | 940 | 54 | 80 |

**Sandwiches:** *With Spread*

| | C | F | Cb |
|---|---|---|---|
| Crispy Chicken | 590 | 29 | 58 |
| Deluxe Crispy Chicken | 750 | 41 | 60 |
| Hallibut Fish without fries | 460 | 27 | 38 |
| Turkey Club, all components | 610 | 38 | 38 |

**French Fries:** *Small, 2.8 oz*

| | C | F | Cb |
|---|---|---|---|
| Small, 2.8 oz | 220 | 11 | 28 |
| Regular, 5 oz | 400 | 19 | 50 |
| Large, 6.5 oz | 510 | 25 | 65 |

**Salads:** *Entree Size, Without Dressing*

| | C | F | Cb |
|---|---|---|---|
| Blue Cheese & Apple | 250 | 8 | 36 |
| Grilled Chicken Club | 360 | 19 | 7 |
| Wild Smoked Salmon & Hazelnuts | 410 | 30 | 11 |

**Breakfast:**

| | C | F | Cb |
|---|---|---|---|
| Bagel with Egg, Bacon & Cheese | 520 | 22 | 52 |
| Breakfast Platter, Bacon | 580 | 35 | 43 |
| Engl. Muffin w/- Egg Ham & Chse | 430 | 22 | 28 |
| Hash Browns (6) | 310 | 23 | 24 |

**Ice Cream Sundaes:** *Caramel*

| | C | F | Cb |
|---|---|---|---|
| Caramel | 420 | 20 | 56 |
| Hot Fudge | 440 | 22 | 53 |
| Triple Berry | 380 | 19 | 46 |

## Burger King® (Aug '15)

### Burgers and Sandwiches:

| | C | F | Cb |
|---|---|---|---|
| A.1. Mozzarella Bacon Cheeseburger | 800 | 48 | 42 |
| Bacon Cheeseburger | 290 | 13 | 27 |
| Big King Sandwich | 530 | 31 | 38 |
| Cheeseburger | 270 | 12 | 27 |
| Double Cheeseburger | 360 | 19 | 27 |
| Extra Long: BBQ Cheeseburger | 590 | 28 | 62 |
| Cheeseburger | 590 | 33 | 50 |
| Pulled Pork S'wich | 370 | 8 | 55 |
| Hamburger | 230 | 9 | 26 |
| Rodeo Burger | 310 | 13 | 38 |
| Veggie Burger | 390 | 16 | 44 |
| **Whopper Sandwich** | 650 | 37 | 50 |
| Bacon & Cheese Whopper | 770 | 48 | 47 |
| Double Whopper Sandwich | 880 | 55 | 50 |
| Triple Whopper Sandwich | 1160 | 75 | 50 |
| Whopper JR. Sandwich | 300 | 16 | 27 |

### Chicken & More:

| | C | F | Cb |
|---|---|---|---|
| Bacon & Chse Tendercrisp S'wich | 790 | 51 | 51 |
| BBQ Bacon Tendercrisp Sandwich | 640 | 32 | 59 |
| Big Fish Sandwich | 520 | 28 | 52 |
| Original Chicken S'wich | 640 | 36 | 53 |
| TenderGrill Chicken Sandwich | 450 | 19 | 41 |
| TenderCrisp Chicken Sandwich | 630 | 37 | 50 |
| **Chicken Fries**, 3.6 oz | 290 | 17 | 18 |
| **Chicken Nuggets:** 4 pieces | 190 | 11 | 13 |
| 6 pieces | 280 | 17 | 20 |
| 10 pieces | 470 | 29 | 34 |
| *Dipping Sauces:* BBQ | 40 | 0 | 11 |
| Buffalo | 80 | 8 | 2 |
| Chicken Fry | 140 | 13 | 6 |
| Ranch; Zesty Onion Ring, average | 145 | 15 | 2 |

### Sides:

| | C | F | Cb |
|---|---|---|---|
| **French Fries:** | | | |
| Small, 4.3 oz | 340 | 15 | 49 |
| Medium, 5.8 oz | 410 | 18 | 58 |
| Large, 7 oz | 500 | 22 | 72 |
| **Fresh Apple Slices,** 2 oz | 30 | 0 | 7 |
| **Onion Rings:** Small | 320 | 16 | 41 |
| Medium | 410 | 21 | 53 |
| **Satisfries,** small | 270 | 11 | 41 |

### Garden Fresh Salads: *With Dressing*

| | C | F | Cb |
|---|---|---|---|
| **Chicken Caesar:** | | | |
| With TenderCrisp Chicken | 650 | 43 | 39 |
| With TenderGrill Chicken | 450 | 27 | 20 |
| **Grilled Chicken,** Apple & Cranb. | 480 | 26 | 34 |

### Dressings: *Per 1.8 oz Packet*

| | C | F | Cb |
|---|---|---|---|
| **Ken's:** Apple Cider Vinaigrette | 210 | 18 | 10 |
| Avocado Ranch | 170 | 17 | 4 |
| Honey Mustard | 220 | 18 | 13 |

## Burger King® cont... (Aug '15)

### Breakfast:

| | C | F | Cb |
|---|---|---|---|
| **Biscuits:** Bacon, Egg & Cheese | 440 | 27 | 33 |
| Ham, Egg & Cheese | 430 | 23 | 35 |
| Sausage, Egg & Cheese | 540 | 36 | 34 |
| **Burritos:** | | | |
| Sausage Breakfast | 410 | 26 | 24 |
| Southwestern Breakfast | 600 | 38 | 43 |
| **Croissan'wich:** | | | |
| Bacon Egg & Chse | 370 | 21 | 31 |
| Egg & Cheese | 330 | 18 | 31 |
| Fully Loaded | 640 | 42 | 35 |
| Ham Egg & Cheese | 390 | 20 | 33 |
| **King Croissan'wich:** | | | |
| with Double Sausage | 630 | 45 | 32 |
| with Ham & Sausage | 600 | 39 | 35 |
| with Sausage & Bacon | 490 | 32 | 31 |
| **French Toast Sticks:** 5 pieces | 380 | 18 | 49 |
| with 1.5 oz Syrup | 500 | 18 | 70 |
| **Hash Browns:** Small, 3 oz | 250 | 16 | 24 |
| Medium, 6 oz | 500 | 33 | 48 |
| Large, 8 oz | 670 | 44 | 65 |
| **Muffin Sandwiches:** | | | |
| Sausage & Cheese | 380 | 23 | 27 |
| Ssg., Egg & Cheese | 430 | 26 | 28 |
| **Platters:** Pancakes & Sausage | 660 | 31 | 83 |
| Ultimate Breakfast | 1420 | 79 | 139 |
| **Oatmeal:** Fruit Topped Maple Flav. | 270 | 20 | 55 |
| Kids Oatmeal | 170 | 3 | 32 |

### Desserts:

| | C | F | Cb |
|---|---|---|---|
| **Cookies,** Chocolate Chip (2) | 320 | 16 | 48 |
| **Pies:** Dutch Apple Pie | 340 | 14 | 51 |
| Hershey's Sundae Pie | 310 | 19 | 32 |
| **Sundaes,** Choc./Caramel av. | 300 | 7 | 55 |
| **Vanilla Soft Serve,** in cone | 160 | 4 | 27 |

### Shakes:

| | C | F | Cb |
|---|---|---|---|
| **Chocolate/Oreos:** Small, 12 fl.oz | 580 | 17 | 97 |
| Medium, 16 fl.oz | 760 | 21 | 131 |
| Large, 20 fl.oz oz | 980 | 24 | 174 |
| **Strawberry,** Small, 12 fl.oz | 500 | 16 | 79 |
| **Vanilla,** Small, 12 fl.oz | 550 | 16 | 91 |
| **Smoothies,** average 16 oz | 320 | 0 | 75 |

### Beverages:

| | C | F | Cb |
|---|---|---|---|
| **Coca Cola Classic:** Small, 20 fl.oz | 190 | 0 | 51 |
| Medium, 30 fl.oz | 290 | 0 | 77 |
| **Frozen Coke,** 16 oz | 140 | 0 | 38 |
| **Frozen Lemonade,** 16 oz | 80 | 0 | 21 |
| **Orange Freeze,** 16 oz | 260 | 0 | 66 |
| **Iced Coffee,** 16 oz | 160 | 7 | 19 |
| **Iced Tea,** sweetened, 20 oz | 120 | 0 | 35 |

*For Complete Nutritional Data ~ see CalorieKing.com*

Updated Nutrition Data ~ www.CalorieKing.com
Persons with Diabetes ~ See Disclaimer (Page 22)

## Captain D's Seafood® (Aug '15)

*Fish: Without Sides*

| | C | F | Cb |
|---|---|---|---|
| Battered Dipped Fish, 1piece | 210 | 15 | 22 |
| Breaded Flounder, 1 piece | 235 | 14 | 12 |

*From The Grill: Without Sides*

| | | | |
|---|---|---|---|
| Grilled Salmon | 240 | 11 | 1 |
| Grilled Steak Tips, 1 kabob | 110 | 4 | 2 |
| Grilled Whitefish Fillet | 175 | 8 | 1 |
| Seasoned Tilapia, 1 pce | 225 | 9 | 0.5 |
| Shrimp Scampi, 1 serving | 655 | 35 | 64 |

*Other Favorites:*

| | | | |
|---|---|---|---|
| Cheese Sticks, 1order | 500 | 32 | 34 |
| Jalapeno Poppers, 1 order | 1160 | 75 | 102 |

*Seafood:*

| | | | |
|---|---|---|---|
| Butterfly Shrimp (6) | 330 | 24 | 22 |
| Popcon Shrimp | 485 | 27 | 48 |
| Stuffed Crab, 1 piece | 140 | 10 | 10 |

*Side Dishes:*

| | | | |
|---|---|---|---|
| Baked Potato (1) | 210 | 0 | 47 |
| Cole Slaw, 1 order | 180 | 12 | 15 |
| French Fries, 1 serving | 365 | 26 | 29 |
| Hushpuppy (1) | 80 | 4 | 9 |
| *Dessert,* Chocolate Cake, 1 order | 300 | 10 | 48 |

## Caribou Coffee® (Aug '15)

*Without Whipped Cream Unless Indicated*

*Hot Coffees: Per Medium*

| | C | F | Cb |
|---|---|---|---|
| **Classic:** Coffee Of The Day, 2% Milk | 90 | 3.5 | 9 |
| Espresso, 4 oz | 0 | 0 | 0 |
| Cappuccino, with 2% Milk | 110 | 4.5 | 10 |
| Latte, with 2% Milk | 180 | 7 | 17 |
| Macchiato, with 2% Milk | 20 | 1 | 1 |

*Hot Chocolate: Per Medium, With Whipped Cream*

| | | | |
|---|---|---|---|
| Milk Chocolate, 2% Milk | 600 | 36 | 50 |

*Specialty,* Mint Condition Mocha,

| | | | |
|---|---|---|---|
| Milk Choc., 2% Milk, medium | 470 | 20 | 65 |

*Cold Beverages: Per Medium*

**Blended:** *Without Whipped Cream*

Fruit & Yogurt Smoothies:

| | | | |
|---|---|---|---|
| Mango Orange Key Lime | 450 | 0 | 113 |
| Strawberry Banana | 380 | 0 | 88 |
| White Peach Berry | 330 | 0 | 80 |

Snowdrift, with Milk Chocolate:

| | | | |
|---|---|---|---|
| Cookies & Crm, with 2% Milk | 610 | 17 | 98 |
| Mint, with 2% Milk | 480 | 12 | 80 |

| **Classics:** Iced Americano | 5 | 0 | 0 |
|---|---|---|---|
| Iced Latte, with 2% Milk | 90 | 3.5 | 8 |
| Iced Mocha, Milk Choc, 2% Milk | 320 | 10 | 47 |

**Specialty, Coolers:** *With Whipped Cream*

| | | | |
|---|---|---|---|
| Caramel High Rise | 550 | 19 | 87 |
| Mint Condition, Milk Chocolate | 750 | 26 | 116 |
| Turtle Mocha, Milk Chocolate | 750 | 26 | 117 |

## Carl's Jr.® (Aug '15)

*California menu only. Please check instore for further nutritional information.*

*Charbroiled Burgers:*

| | C | F | Cb |
|---|---|---|---|
| Big Hamburger | 480 | 18 | 56 |
| Famous Star with Cheese | 670 | 37 | 57 |
| Kid's Hamburger | 270 | 10 | 33 |
| Super Star with Cheese | 930 | 56 | 59 |
| The Big Carl | 920 | 58 | 56 |
| Western Bacon Cheeseburger | 730 | 34 | 74 |
| ½ lb Thickburgers: Original $6 | 1050 | 72 | 62 |
| Guacamole Bacon | 1210 | 89 | 57 |
| Low-Carb | 670 | 56 | 9 |
| Western Bacon | 1090 | 69 | 74 |

*Chicken Sandwiches:*

| | | | |
|---|---|---|---|
| Bacon Swiss Crispy Chicken | 860 | 49 | 67 |
| Big Chicken Fillet | 760 | 41 | 65 |
| Charbroiled: BBQ Chicken | 390 | 7 | 50 |
| Chicken Club | 580 | 28 | 46 |
| Santa Fe Chicken | 560 | 27 | 46 |
| Teriyaki Chicken | 530 | 17 | 60 |
| Spicy Chicken Sandwich | 460 | 24 | 47 |

*Chicken Tenders,* hand breaded,

| | | | |
|---|---|---|---|
| 5 pieces, without Sauce | 440 | 21 | 21 |
| *Chicken Stars,* 6 pieces, w/o Sce | 260 | 16 | 18 |
| *Fish,* Beer Battered Cod Sandwich | 550 | 19 | 74 |

*Breakfast:*

| | | | |
|---|---|---|---|
| Bacon & Egg Burrito | 570 | 34 | 38 |
| Breakfast Burger | 800 | 43 | 68 |
| Grilled Pork Chop Biscuit | 400 | 19 | 36 |
| With Egg & Cheese | 530 | 30 | 38 |
| Hash Brown Nuggets: Small, 3.8 oz | 350 | 23 | 32 |
| Medium, 4.2 oz | 390 | 26 | 36 |
| Large, 6 oz | 560 | 37 | 52 |
| Loaded Breakfast Burrito | 790 | 50 | 53 |
| Sourdough Breakfast Sandwich | 450 | 23 | 40 |
| Steak & Egg Burrito | 650 | 36 | 44 |

*Fries:* CrissCut Fries, 5 oz

| | | | |
|---|---|---|---|
| | 450 | 29 | 42 |
| Natural Cut: Small, 3.5 oz | 300 | 15 | 39 |
| Medium, 6 oz | 430 | 21 | 55 |
| Large, 6.5oz | 460 | 22 | 59 |
| *Fried Zucchini,* 5 oz | 330 | 18 | 36 |
| *Onion Rings,* 4.5 oz | 530 | 28 | 61 |

*Salads: Without Dressing or Croutons*

| | | | |
|---|---|---|---|
| Chicken: Crispy | 350 | 16 | 29 |
| Original Grilled | 280 | 12 | 26 |
| Garden, Side | 110 | 4.5 | 14 |

*Dressings: Per 2 oz Package*

| | | | |
|---|---|---|---|
| Blue Cheese | 320 | 34 | 1 |
| House | 220 | 22 | 3 |
| Low-Fat Balsamic | 35 | 1.5 | 5 |

*Malts,* with Ice Cream:

| | | | |
|---|---|---|---|
| Oreo Cookie | 780 | 40 | 94 |
| Other flavors, average | 760 | 36 | 99 |

*Shakes,* with Ice Cream:

| | | | |
|---|---|---|---|
| Oreo Cookie | 710 | 39 | 79 |
| Vanilla; Choc.; Strawb. av. | 695 | 36 | 85 |

## Carvel® (Aug '15)

| *Carvelanche:* | C | F | Cb |
|---|---|---|---|
| **Average all flavors:** Small, 12 oz | 600 | 30 | 70 |
| Regular, 16 oz | 870 | 46 | 100 |
| Large, 24 oz | 1300 | 70 | 150 |
| *Classic Sundaes:* Per Small, 12 oz | | | |
| Caramel | 700 | 36 | 84 |
| Hot Fudge | 540 | 30 | 60 |
| Strawberry | 610 | 34 | 67 |
| *Sundae Dashers:* Per Regular, 16 oz | | | |
| Banana's Foster | 1020 | 31 | 176 |
| Fudge Brownie | 1170 | 60 | 147 |
| Mint Chocolate Chip | 1230 | 64 | 157 |
| Peanut Butter Cup | 1850 | 105 | 163 |
| Strawberry Shortcake | 730 | 38 | 91 |
| *Soft Serve:* | | | |
| **Chocolate/Vanilla, average:** | | | |
| Junior Cup, 4.5 oz | 260 | 14 | 28 |
| Small Cup, 7.5 oz | 430 | 24 | 47 |
| Medium Cup, 9.5 oz | 550 | 30 | 60 |
| *Thick Shakes:* Per 16 oz | | | |
| Chocolate | 650 | 27 | 93 |
| Strawberry | 600 | 31 | 70 |
| Vanilla | 660 | 31 | 86 |

## Checkers®

**Same Menu & Data as Rally's ~ See Page 231**

## Cheesecake Factory® (Aug '15)

| *Cheesecake:* Per Slice | C | F | Cb |
|---|---|---|---|
| Original | 830 | n/a | 62 |
| Godiva Chocolate | 1280 | n/a | 96 |
| Reese's P.B. Chocolate Cake | 1510 | n/a | 153 |
| White Chocolate Raspb. Truffle | 1170 | n/a | 87 |
| *Small Plates & Snacks:* Per Dish, As Served | | | |
| Crispy Crab Bites | 350 | n/a | 11 |
| Pretzel Crusted Chicken | 770 | n/a | 62 |
| Stuffed Mushrooms | 460 | n/a | 15 |
| *Glamburgers & Sandwiches:* Without Sides | | | |
| Bacon Bacon Chseburger | 1590 | n/a | 74 |
| Factory Burger | 860 | n/a | 81 |
| Grilled Turkey Burger | 1160 | n/a | 72 |
| *Specialties:* Per Dish, As Served | | | |
| Crispy Chicken Costoletta | 2590 | n/a | 103 |
| Famous Factory Meatloaf | 1630 | n/a | 117 |
| White Chicken Chili | 570 | n/a | 36 |
| *Salads:* As Served, Includes Dressing | | | |
| Herb-Crusted Salmon | 760 | n/a | 22 |
| Santa Fe Salad | 1820 | n/a | 99 |
| Sheila's Chicken & Avocado | 1890 | n/a | 140 |

*n/a = not available*
*For Complete Menu & Data ~ see CalorieKing.com*

## Charley's Grilled Subs® (Aug '15)

| *Subs:* Regular Size, Includes Standard Toppings, Without Sauce or Dressings Unless Indicated | C | F | Cb |
|---|---|---|---|
| Bacon 3 Cheese Steak | 720 | 31 | 56 |
| Chicken Buffalo, with Sauce | 610 | 18 | 60 |
| Chicken California | 690 | 28 | 52 |
| Chicken Teriyaki, with Sauce | 630 | 18 | 62 |
| Italian Deli Deluxe | 750 | 36 | 58 |
| Pepperoni Steak | 780 | 37 | 55 |
| Philly Cheesesteak | 640 | 24 | 58 |
| Philly Chicken | 590 | 17 | 58 |
| Turkey Cheddar Melt | 670 | 21 | 62 |
| Ultimate Club | 710 | 27 | 61 |
| *Salads:* Cheese or Dressings not included | | | |
| Grilled Chicken; Grilled Steak, average | 130 | 3 | 8 |
| *Fries:* Original | 400 | 22 | 46 |
| Cheese Gourmet | 550 | 31 | 62 |
| Ultimate Gourmet | 720 | 49 | 61 |
| *Breakfast:* | | | |
| Hashbrowns | 460 | 29 | 45 |
| **Omelet Platter:** | | | |
| Bacon, Egg & Cheese | 1010 | 63 | 74 |
| Sausage, Egg & Cheese | 1110 | 70 | 73 |
| Steak, Egg & Cheese | 1050 | 62 | 74 |
| **Sandwiches:** | | | |
| Bacon, Egg & Cheese | 490 | 26 | 36 |
| Sausage, Egg & Cheese | 590 | 33 | 36 |
| Steak, Egg & Cheese | 520 | 25 | 36 |
| Toast, 2 slices | 130 | 2 | 24 |

*For Complete Menu & Data ~ see CalorieKing.com*

## Chevys Fresh Mex® (Aug '15)

| *Burritos:* As Served | C | F | Cb |
|---|---|---|---|
| Fajita Carnitas | 1260 | 51 | 144 |
| Fajita Chicken | 1240 | 46 | 142 |
| Fajita Steak | 1300 | 54 | 142 |
| *Fresh Mex Combos:* As Served | | | |
| Chevys Super Cinco | 1920 | 100 | 171 |
| Mar Y Tierra Combo | 1230 | 54 | 108 |
| Taste of Chevys | 1480 | 68 | 155 |
| *Fresh Mex Innovations:* As Served | | | |
| **Enchiladas:** Chipotle Chicken | 1070 | 65 | 93 |
| Farmers' Market | 1130 | 72 | 101 |
| Shrimp & Crab | 1250 | 80 | 94 |
| *Tacos:* As Served | | | |
| **Mesquite Grilled:** Chicken | 980 | 28 | 123 |
| Steak | 1050 | 38 | 123 |
| Fish | 920 | 27 | 123 |
| *Grande Salads:* Without Dressing Unless Indicated | | | |
| Sizzling Fajita Chicken w/ dressing | 1220 | 90 | 51 |
| Santa Fe Chopped | 660 | 39 | 26 |
| Tostada Steak | 1560 | 100 | 91 |
| *Soup,* Tortilla, 1 bowl | 420 | 18 | 38 |
| *Tortilla,* El Machino, 6" | 140 | 4 | 22 |
| *Tortilla Chips* | 430 | 20 | 56 |

## Chick-fil-A® (Aug '15)

### Breakfast:

| | C | F | Cb |
|---|---|---|---|
| **Bagel,** Chicken, Egg & Cheese | 480 | 20 | 48 |
| **Biscuits:** Chicken | 440 | 20 | 48 |
| Bacon, Egg & Cheese | 450 | 23 | 44 |
| Sausage, Egg & Cheese | 670 | 44 | 44 |
| **Burritos:** Chicken | 440 | 19 | 43 |
| Sausage | 500 | 28 | 40 |
| **Chick-n-Minis,** 1 box, 3 pieces | 280 | 11 | 30 |
| **Cinnamon Cluster** | 430 | 17 | 63 |
| **Hash Browns,** 2.7 oz | 240 | 15 | 25 |
| **Oatmeal:** Multigrain w/ toppings | 290 | 11 | 50 |
| Without toppings | 140 | 2.5 | 28 |

### Chick-fil-A Sandwiches: *Without Sauce*

| | C | F | Cb |
|---|---|---|---|
| Chicken | 440 | 18 | 41 |
| Chicken Salad | 500 | 20 | 53 |
| Grilled Chicken | 320 | 5 | 40 |
| Grilled Chicken Club | 440 | 14 | 41 |

### Cool Wrap, Grilled Chicken,

| | C | F | Cb |
|---|---|---|---|
| without dressing | 340 | 13 | 30 |

### Chicken:

| | C | F | Cb |
|---|---|---|---|
| Chick-n-Strips, breaded, 4 count | 470 | 24 | 21 |
| Nuggets: Breaded, 8 count | 270 | 13 | 10 |
| 12 count | 400 | 19 | 15 |

### Salads: *Without Dressing or Toppings*

| | C | F | Cb |
|---|---|---|---|
| Asian | 330 | 13 | 24 |
| Cobb | 430 | 22 | 22 |
| Grilled Market | 200 | 5 | 17 |

### Condiments:

| | C | F | Cb |
|---|---|---|---|
| Charred Tom. Crispy Bell Peppers | 80 | 6 | 6 |
| Garlic & Butter Croutons, 0.5 oz | 70 | 3 | 9 |
| Harvest Nut Granola, salad portion | 60 | 3 | 8 |

### Dressings:

| | C | F | Cb |
|---|---|---|---|
| Buttermilk Ranch, 1.5 oz | 280 | 30 | 2 |
| Honey Mustard, fat-free | 100 | 0 | 23 |
| Light Italian, 1.5 oz | 25 | 1.5 | 3 |
| *Sauces:* BBQ | 45 | 0 | 10 |
| Buffalo, 0.8 oz | 10 | 0 | 1 |
| Buttermilk Ranch, 0.8 oz | 110 | 11 | 1 |
| Chick-fil-A, 1 oz | 140 | 13 | 6 |
| Honey Roasted BBQ, 0.5 oz | 60 | 5 | 3 |

### Sides:

| | C | F | Cb |
|---|---|---|---|
| Chicken Salad Cup, 6 oz | 360 | 24 | 7 |
| Cole Slaw, medium | 360 | 31 | 19 |
| Fruit Cup, w/ Blueberries, medium | 50 | 0 | 13 |
| Hearty Brst of Chicken Soup, med. | 140 | 2.5 | 18 |
| Side Salad | 80 | 4.5 | 6 |
| Waffle Potato Fries: Small | 310 | 16 | 37 |
| Medium | 400 | 21 | 48 |
| Large | 520 | 27 | 63 |
| *Dessert,* Chocolate Chunk Cookie | 330 | 14 | 45 |
| *Milkshakes:* Chocolate, large | 710 | 26 | 108 |
| Vanilla, large | 620 | 25 | 86 |

## Chili's® (Aug '15)

### For The Table: *As Served*

| | C | F | Cb |
|---|---|---|---|
| Bottomless Tostada Chips w/ Salsa | 910 | 45 | 113 |
| **Classic Nachos:** Beef, lge | 1590 | 103 | 60 |
| Chicken, large | 1420 | 88 | 61 |
| Southwest Eggrolls | 800 | 41 | 82 |
| Texas Cheese Fries, full order | 1710 | 119 | 85 |

### Triple Dipper: *As Served*

| | C | F | Cb |
|---|---|---|---|
| Big Mouth Bites w/ Ranch | 770 | 52 | 47 |
| Original Chicken Crispers | 570 | 37 | 31 |

### Burgers: *As Served, with Fries*

| | C | F | Cb |
|---|---|---|---|
| Classic Bacon | 1340 | 80 | 103 |
| Oldtimer, with Cheddar Cheese | 1180 | 65 | 101 |
| Southern Smokehouse Bacon | 1550 | 89 | 129 |

### Chicken: *As Served, with Set Sides*

| | C | F | Cb |
|---|---|---|---|
| Cajun Pasta with Grilled Chicken | 1290 | 61 | 115 |
| Chicken Crispers, Crispy w/out sce | 1140 | 51 | 123 |

### Fresh Mex: *As Served*

| | C | F | Cb |
|---|---|---|---|
| **Bowls:** Chipotle Chicken | 880 | 38 | 81 |
| Chipotle Shrimp | 790 | 35 | 86 |
| Chipotle Steak | 970 | 54 | 81 |
| Margarita Chicken | 870 | 25 | 108 |
| Margarita Shrimp | 770 | 22 | 112 |

### Enchiladas: *With Rice & Black Beans*

| | C | F | Cb |
|---|---|---|---|
| Beef | 1160 | 52 | 116 |
| Chicken, with Green Chile Sce | 1040 | 39 | 112 |
| Chicken, with Sour Cream Sce | 1140 | 50 | 111 |

### Top Shelf Tacos: *With Rice & Black Beans*

| | C | F | Cb |
|---|---|---|---|
| Grilled Fish | 1070 | 47 | 112 |
| Pork Carnitas | 1250 | 60 | 99 |
| Ranchero Chicken | 1080 | 45 | 104 |

### Fresh Tex Lighter Choices: *As Served*

| | C | F | Cb |
|---|---|---|---|
| Ancho Salmon | 600 | 27 | 43 |
| Grilled Chicken Salad | 430 | 23 | 23 |
| Mango Chile Chicken/Tilapia, av. | 520 | 18 | 57 |
| Margarita Grilled Chicken | 580 | 13 | 66 |

### Fresh Tex Ribs: *Full Rack, As Served*

| | C | F | Cb |
|---|---|---|---|
| Original BBQ | 1360 | 74 | 92 |
| Craft Beer BBQ | 1380 | 74 | 94 |
| *Sides:* Homestyle Fries | 390 | 17 | 55 |
| Loaded Mashed Potatoes | 380 | 23 | 32 |
| Southwest Mac 'n' Cheese | 490 | 30 | 38 |
| Spiced Panko Onion Rings | 400 | 19 | 48 |

### Salads: *Includes Dressing*

| | C | F | Cb |
|---|---|---|---|
| Boneless Buffalo Chicken | 1040 | 72 | 49 |
| Caribbean with Seared Shrimp | 620 | 26 | 84 |
| Quesadilla Explosion | 1430 | 96 | 83 |

### Sweet Stuff: *Per Slice*

| | C | F | Cb |
|---|---|---|---|
| Cheesecake | 750 | 47 | 69 |
| Molten Chocolate Cake | 1180 | 62 | 150 |

*For Complete Menu & Data ~ see CalorieKing.com*

# Fast - Foods & Restaurants

## Chipotle® (Aug '15)

| Tortillas: | C | F | Cb |
|---|---|---|---|
| Burrito Size Flour Tortillas (1) | 300 | 10 | 46 |
| Taco Size: Crispy Corn Tortilla (3) | 210 | 7.5 | 30 |
| Soft Corn Tortillas (Taco), (3) | 210 | 0 | 45 |
| Soft Flour Tortillas (Taco), (3) | 255 | 3 | 39 |
| *Meal Components:* | | | |
| Barbacoa, 4 oz | 165 | 7 | 2 |
| Black/Pinto Beans, average, 4 oz | 120 | 1 | 22 |
| Brown Rice, 4 oz | 200 | 7 | 32 |
| Carnitas, 4 oz | 210 | 12 | 0 |
| Cheese, 1 oz | 100 | 7.5 | 1 |
| Chicken, 4 oz | 180 | 7 | 0.5 |
| Fajita Vegetables, 2.5 oz | 20 | 0.5 | 4 |
| Guacamole, 3.5 oz | 230 | 22 | 8 |
| Lettuce, 1 oz | 5 | 0 | 0 |
| Sofritas, 4 oz | 145 | 10 | 9 |
| Steak, 4 oz | 190 | 6.5 | 2 |
| *Condiments:* | | | |
| **Salsa:** Chili Corn, 3.5 oz | 80 | 1.5 | 16 |
| Green Tomatillo, 2 oz | 15 | 0 | 4 |
| Red Tomatillo, 2 oz | 30 | 0 | 8 |
| Tomato, 3.5 oz | 20 | 0 | 5 |
| Sour Cream, 2 oz | 115 | 10 | 1 |
| *Extras,* Chips, serving, 4 oz | 570 | 27 | 73 |

## Chuck E. Cheese® (Aug '15)

| Appetizers: | C | F | Cb |
|---|---|---|---|
| Buffalo Wings, Traditional (1) | 125 | 9 | 1 |
| Cheesy Breadstick, with Marinara, and Light Ranch Dressing | 110 | 6 | 9 |
| *Oven Baked Sandwiches:* | | | |
| Ham & Cheese | 620 | 24 | 70 |
| Italian Sub | 910 | 53 | 75 |
| *Pizzas: Per Medium Slice* | | | |
| BBQ Chicken | 145 | 4 | 21 |
| Canadian Bacon & Pineapple | 160 | 4 | 22 |
| Cheese | 150 | 4 | 21 |
| Pepperoni | 180 | 7 | 21 |
| Super Combo | 180 | 7 | 22 |
| Veggie Combo | 160 | 5 | 22 |
| *Platters:* Sandwich, ½ Platter | 185 | 8 | 20 |
| Veggie, ⅛ Platter | 130 | 11 | 7 |
| *French Fries,* | | | |
| W/ Ketchup & Light Ranch, 8 oz | 645 | 33 | 83 |
| *Desserts:* Apple Dessert Pizza, 1 sl. | 105 | 1 | 21 |
| Chocolate Cake (8"), 1 slice | 290 | 13 | 41 |
| Cinnamon Stick, w/ Toppings (1) | 70 | 2 | 11 |

## Church's Chicken® (Aug '15)

| Chicken: Per Serving | C | F | Cb |
|---|---|---|---|
| **Original:** Breast, 1 piece | 200 | 11 | 3 |
| Leg, 1 piece | 110 | 6 | 3 |
| Thigh, 1 piece | 330 | 23 | 8 |
| Wing, 1 piece | 300 | 18 | 7 |
| **Spicy:** Breast, 1 piece | 320 | 20 | 12 |
| Leg, 1 piece | 180 | 11 | 8 |
| Thigh, 1 piece | 480 | 35 | 20 |
| Wing, 1 piece | 430 | 27 | 17 |
| **Tender Strips,** average, 1 piece | 130 | 6 | 6 |
| *Sides: Per Small Serving* | | | |
| Baked Macaroni & Cheese, 6.3 oz | 260 | 8 | 24 |
| Cajun Rice, 6 oz | 290 | 17 | 27 |
| Cole Slaw, 4.15 oz | 150 | 10 | 15 |
| French Fries, 1.6 oz | 140 | 6 | 19 |
| Honey Butter Biscuits (1), 2 oz | 240 | 15 | 28 |
| Mashed Potatoes & Gravy, 6 oz | 110 | 2 | 21 |
| Okra, 1.95 oz | 170 | 11 | 17 |
| Sweet Corn Nuggets (6), 3.5 oz | 240 | 7 | 40 |
| *Sauces: Per Packet* | | | |
| BBQ; Sweet & Sour, av. | 40 | 0 | 10 |
| Creamy Jalapeno | 125 | 13 | 2 |
| Honey Mustard | 140 | 13 | 4 |
| Ranch | 140 | 15 | 2 |

## Cici's Pizza® (Aug '15)

| Buffet & Large To Go Pizzas: Per Slice | C | F | Cb |
|---|---|---|---|
| Alfredo | 150 | 5 | 22 |
| BBQ Pork | 160 | 4.5 | 24 |
| Beef Topping | 190 | 7 | 24 |
| Buffalo Chicken | 160 | 5 | 22 |
| Cheese | 180 | 6 | 23 |
| Pepperoni & Jalapeno | 190 | 7 | 24 |
| Sausage | 180 | 7 | 24 |
| Spin. Alfredo; Zesty Ham & Chedd. | 155 | 5.5 | 22 |
| *Extras:* Oven Roasted Wings (5) | 190 | 12 | 1 |
| Hot/Mild Sauce | 25 | 1 | 3 |

## Cinnabon® (Aug '15)

| Baked Goods: | C | F | Cb |
|---|---|---|---|
| Caramel Pecanbon (1) | 1080 | 51 | 146 |
| Churro (1) | 280 | 11 | 39 |
| Cinnabon Bites (6) | 650 | 24 | 95 |
| Cinnabon Stix (5) | 400 | 21 | 46 |
| Classic Cinnabon (1) | 880 | 37 | 127 |
| Frosting Cup, 1.7 oz | 210 | 13 | 23 |
| *Strawberry Chillata,* 16 oz | 520 | 11 | 105 |

**190**

## Claim Jumper® (Aug '15)

*Appetizers:* As Served

| | C | F | Cb |
|---|---|---|---|
| Southwest Eggrolls | 1190 | 53 | 114 |
| Three Cheese Potatocakes (3) | 1075 | 71 | 80 |

*Burgers & Sandwiches:* Without Sides

| | | | |
|---|---|---|---|
| Grilled Cobb Sandwich | 1210 | 78 | 78 |
| Widow Maker Burger | 1370 | 87 | 84 |
| *Calzones:* Specialty | 1430 | 80 | 137 |
| Traditional | 1350 | 66 | 140 |

*Meals:*

**Favorites:** With Menu Set Sides & Toppings

| | | | |
|---|---|---|---|
| Country Fried Steak | 2030 | 107 | 189 |
| Giant Stuffed Chicken Baker | 990 | 34 | 118 |
| Meatloaf & Mashed Potatoes | 1300 | 75 | 117 |
| **Pasta:** Black Tie Pasta | 1535 | 84 | 126 |
| Parmesan Crusted Chicken | 975 | 47 | 83 |
| **Pizza:** Calif. Works, Classic Crust | 1295 | 64 | 127 |
| Steakhouse, Flatbread | 820 | 47 | 65 |

**Specialties:**

| | | | |
|---|---|---|---|
| BBQ Baby Back Pork Ribs, Full Rack | 1745 | 111 | 111 |
| Roasted Tri-Tip with Demi Glaze | 800 | 47 | 19 |
| **Seafood:** Atlantic Salmon, Blackened | 715 | 42 | 48 |
| Tilapia Bianca, with Shrimp, Artichoke Hearts & Sauce | 1165 | 80 | 56 |

*Entree Salads:* Without Dressing Or Bread

| | | | |
|---|---|---|---|
| Calif. Citrus Chkn, Charbroiled | 865 | 53 | 58 |
| Seared Ahi Spinach | 515 | 24 | 31 |

*Soups:* Per Bowl

| | | | |
|---|---|---|---|
| New England Clam Chowder | 525 | 45 | 23 |
| Potato Cheddar | 710 | 61 | 31 |
| *Sweets:* Choc. Motherlode Cake | 2770 | 144 | 340 |
| Italian Lemon Cake | 1240 | 62 | 158 |

## Coldstone Creamery® (Aug '15)

*Ice Creams:*

| | C | F | Cb |
|---|---|---|---|
| **Amaretto:** Like it | 330 | 20 | 33 |
| Love it | 530 | 31 | 53 |
| Gotta have it | 790 | 47 | 80 |
| **Chocolate:** Like it | 320 | 20 | 33 |
| Love it | 520 | 31 | 53 |
| Gotta have it | 780 | 48 | 79 |

**Hot Stone:**

| | | | |
|---|---|---|---|
| Brownie A La Cold Stone, 11 oz | 810 | 55 | 99 |
| Chocolate Lava Meltdown, 9 oz | 730 | 36 | 97 |
| Churro Caramel Crave, 8.6 oz | 700 | 33 | 98 |

*Sorbet:*

| | | | |
|---|---|---|---|
| **Strawberry Mango:** Like it | 220 | 0 | 55 |
| Love it | 350 | 0 | 87 |
| Gotta have it | 520 | 0.5 | 131 |

## Cosi® (Aug '15)

*Flatbread Pizza:* Individual

| | C | F | Cb |
|---|---|---|---|
| **Original Crust:** | | | |
| Chicken & Spinach | 940 | 37 | 102 |
| Margherita | 805 | 30 | 94 |
| Pepperoni | 855 | 33 | 92 |
| Sausage | 810 | 27 | 93 |
| Traditional Cheese | 715 | 21 | 92 |

*Melts:* Includes Set Menu Components

| | | | |
|---|---|---|---|
| Chicken TBM | 540 | 25 | 30 |
| Pesto Chicken | 460 | 21 | 28 |
| Steakhouse Gorgonzola | 690 | 44 | 44 |

*Bowls:* Includes Set Menu Components

| | | | |
|---|---|---|---|
| Adobo Chicken with Avocado | 515 | 19 | 63 |
| Korean BBQ Pork | 540 | 22 | 56 |
| Stuffed Portobello | 455 | 19 | 59 |

*Soup:* Per Regular

| | | | |
|---|---|---|---|
| Classic Clam Chowder | 310 | 20 | 25 |
| Tomato Basil | 400 | 31 | 20 |

*Salads:*

| | | | |
|---|---|---|---|
| Cobb, with Sherry Shallot Dressing | 740 | 56 | 20 |
| Greek, with Italian Vinaigrette | 535 | 47 | 20 |
| Signature, w/ Sherry Shallot Drsng | 615 | 45 | 40 |
| Steakhouse, with Blue Chse Drsng | 655 | 53 | 15 |

*Breakfast:* Includes Set Menu Components

| | | | |
|---|---|---|---|
| **Sandwiches:** Cosi Club Squagel | 560 | 21 | 64 |
| Sausage & Pepper Frittata | 780 | 42 | 65 |
| Western Croissant | 560 | 32 | 43 |
| **Pastries:** Banana Nut Muffin | 510 | 25 | 62 |
| Chocolate Biscotti | 280 | 13 | 38 |

## Cousins Subs® (Aug '15)

*Subs:*

| | C | F | Cb |
|---|---|---|---|
| BLT, with Mayo | 600 | 36 | 49 |
| Cheese Steak | 675 | 33 | 50 |
| Chicken Cheddar Deluxe, w/ Mayo | 680 | 37 | 52 |
| Club, with Mayo | 715 | 39 | 53 |
| Double Cheese Steak | 1085 | 58 | 50 |
| Ham & Provolone, wth Mayo | 675 | 39 | 51 |
| Italian Special, with Dressing | 895 | 56 | 51 |
| Philly Cheese Steak | 695 | 38 | 51 |
| Roast Beef & Cheddar, with Mayo | 705 | 35 | 51 |
| Tuna with Mayo | 690 | 40 | 51 |
| Turkey Breast w/ Mayo | 530 | 31 | 53 |

*Soup:* Per Regular

| | | | |
|---|---|---|---|
| Beef Steak with Noodle | 105 | 3.5 | 12 |
| Cheddar Cauliflower | 115 | 5 | 13 |
| Chicken Noodle | 115 | 3 | 16 |
| Cream of Broccoli | 165 | 10 | 13 |
| New England Clam Chowder | 150 | 2.5 | 25 |

*For Complete Nutritional Data ~ See CalorieKing.com*

*For Complete Nutritional Data ~ see CalorieKing.com*

## Culver's® (Aug '15)

*ButterBurgers:*

| | C | F | Cb |
|---|---|---|---|
| **Original:** Single | 390 | 19 | 39 |
| Double | 560 | 32 | 39 |
| Triple | 730 | 45 | 39 |
| Cheddar with Bacon, Single | 510 | 29 | 39 |
| Cheese: Single | 460 | 25 | 40 |
| Double | 700 | 44 | 41 |
| Culver's Bacon Deluxe: Single | 610 | 39 | 42 |
| Double | 850 | 58 | 43 |
| Culver's Deluxe: Single | 570 | 36 | 42 |
| Double | 810 | 55 | 43 |
| Mushroom & Swiss, Single | 490 | 27 | 40 |
| Sourdough Melt, Single | 460 | 26 | 36 |
| Corn Dog, Kids | 230 | 14 | 17 |
| Chicken Tenders, Breaded, 4 pcs | 540 | 24 | 42 |
| **Sandwiches:** Beef Pot Roast | 410 | 16 | 41 |
| Crispy Chicken | 460 | 16 | 57 |
| Crispy Southwest Chicken | 630 | 31 | 54 |
| Grilled Reuben Melt | 670 | 35 | 49 |
| North Atlantic Cod Filet | 600 | 33 | 48 |
| Pork Tenderloin | 630 | 27 | 73 |
| Shaved Prime Rib | 620 | 37 | 41 |

*Sides:*

| | | | |
|---|---|---|---|
| Chili Cheddar Fries | 670 | 31 | 78 |
| Crinkle Cut Fries, regular | 360 | 14 | 53 |
| Mashed Potatoes, w/ Gravy, reg. | 140 | 2 | 25 |
| Wisconsin Cheese Curds, 5.3 oz | 510 | 25 | 51 |

*Dinners: With Fries, Cole Slaw & Bread Roll*

| | | | |
|---|---|---|---|
| Butterfly Jumbo Shrimp, 6 pieces | 1090 | 55 | 130 |
| Fried Chicken, 1 breast, 1 wing | 890 | 38 | 61 |
| North Atlantic Cod, Fried, 2 pieces | 1480 | 100 | 107 |

*Soup:*

| | | | |
|---|---|---|---|
| Broccoli Cheese, 10.5 oz | 220 | 12 | 17 |
| Chicken Noodle, 10.5 oz | 110 | 2 | 14 |
| Potato with Bacon, 10.5 oz | 240 | 10 | 28 |

*Salads: Without Dressing*

| | | | |
|---|---|---|---|
| Chicken Cashew w/ Gr. Chicken | 460 | 24 | 19 |
| Cranberry Bacon Bleu, with Grilled Chicken | 360 | 13 | 18 |
| Garden Fresco w/ Gr. Chicken | 360 | 13 | 20 |
| Side Salad | 55 | 2 | 4 |

*Dressings:*

| | | | |
|---|---|---|---|
| Chunky Bleu Cheese, 1.8 oz | 310 | 33 | 2 |
| French Dressing, 1.8 oz | 190 | 13 | 19 |
| Ranch, 1.75 oz | 180 | 19 | 2 |
| Sesame Ginger, 2 oz | 70 | 0 | 16 |

## Culver's® cont... (Aug '15)

*Concrete Mixers: Per Regular*

| | C | F | Cb |
|---|---|---|---|
| Chocolate | 950 | 46 | 121 |
| Cookie Dough | 1010 | 56 | 113 |

*Sundaes: Per 2 Scoops*

| | | | |
|---|---|---|---|
| Banana Split | 1060 | 60 | 121 |
| Caramel Cashew | 1000 | 51 | 122 |
| Fudge Pecan | 1040 | 64 | 107 |
| Turtle | 1040 | 62 | 112 |

*Beverages:* Chocolate Malt, reg.

| | | | |
|---|---|---|---|
| Chocolate Malt, reg. | 880 | 39 | 120 |
| Chocolate Shake, regular | 820 | 38 | 108 |
| Strawberry Malt, regular | 770 | 38 | 96 |
| Strawberry Shake, regular | 730 | 38 | 86 |

## D'Angelo's® (Aug '15)

*Toasted & Hot Sandwiches: Per Medium Size, Menu Board Toppings Only, w/out Bread*

| | C | F | Cb |
|---|---|---|---|
| Classic Veggie | 350 | 23 | 16 |
| Italian Toasted | 840 | 69 | 14 |
| Meatball & Cheese | 770 | 59 | 25 |
| **Add Sandwich Bread:** *Per Medium Size* | | | |
| Classic Italian Sub | 310 | 3.5 | 58 |
| Multigrain Sub | 310 | 3.5 | 60 |
| Pokket | 160 | 0 | 34 |

*Wraps: Menu Board Toppings, Without Wraps*

| | | | |
|---|---|---|---|
| Buffalo Chicken, Whole | 520 | 36 | 17 |
| Chicken Caesar, Whole | 620 | 42 | 25 |
| **Add Wraps:** Wheat, 4 oz | 310 | 8 | 55 |
| Tortilla Wrap, 4 oz | 310 | 9 | 49 |

*Dressings:* Caesar, 1.5 oz

| | | | |
|---|---|---|---|
| Caesar, 1.5 oz | 200 | 21 | 3 |
| Greek, 1.5 oz | 210 | 24 | 1 |
| Ranch, 1.5 oz | 150 | 15 | 2 |

*Salads: Entree Size, without Bread*

| | | | |
|---|---|---|---|
| Caesar, with Dressing | 630 | 53 | 28 |
| Chicken Caesar, with Dressing | 770 | 55 | 30 |
| Chicken Cobb, w/o Dressing | 310 | 17 | 11 |
| Greek, w/o Dressing | 240 | 13 | 17 |

*Soup: Per Bowl*

| | | | |
|---|---|---|---|
| Extreme Broccoli & Cheddar | 370 | 28 | 18 |
| Hearty Beef Stew | 330 | 12 | 34 |
| Main Lobster Bisque | 540 | 43 | 24 |
| New England Clam Chowder | 480 | 27 | 46 |

*For Complete Menu & Data ~ see CalorieKing.com*

# Dairy Queen® (Aug '15)

*Burgers & Sandwiches:*

| | C | F | Cb |
|---|---|---|---|
| **Burgers:** | | | |
| Cheeseburger: Original | 380 | 19 | 34 |
| Double | 580 | 34 | 35 |
| **GrillBurgers:** | | | |
| ¼ lb Bacon Cheese | 620 | 36 | 41 |
| ½ lb Burger, with Cheese | 770 | 46 | 43 |
| ½ lb Flame Thrower | 950 | 66 | 39 |
| ¼ lb Mushroom Swiss | 560 | 33 | 39 |
| **Sandwiches:** Crispy Chicken | 610 | 30 | 50 |
| Grilled Chicken | 390 | 14 | 44 |
| *Baskets:* | | | |
| Chicken Strips: 4 pce w/ Ctry Gravy | 1020 | 52 | 101 |
| 6 piece | 1250 | 65 | 115 |
| **Hot Dogs:** Beef | 300 | 18 | 23 |
| Beef, Chili & Cheese | 390 | 25 | 25 |
| *Salads: Without Dressing* | | | |
| **Chicken BLT:** Crispy Chicken | 520 | 31 | 25 |
| Grilled Chicken | 380 | 19 | 11 |
| *Sides:* | | | |
| French Fries, regular, 5 oz | 380 | 17 | 54 |
| Onion Rings, 4 oz | 360 | 16 | 48 |
| *Desserts: Per Medium* | | | |
| **Blizzard Treats:** Banana Split | 590 | 16 | 100 |
| Butterfinger | 730 | 26 | 111 |
| Cookie Dough | 1030 | 41 | 151 |
| Heath | 860 | 38 | 119 |
| Oreo Cookies | 790 | 30 | 117 |
| Reese's Peanut Butter Cups | 750 | 32 | 103 |
| Strawberry Cheesecake | 690 | 25 | 100 |
| **DQ Blizzard Cakes (10"):** | | | |
| Oreo, ¹⁄₁₂ cake | 550 | 23 | 78 |
| Reese's P'nut Butter Cup, ¹⁄₁₂ cake | 580 | 27 | 77 |
| **DQ Dipped Cone,** Chocolate, med. | 470 | 22 | 61 |
| **DQ Sundaes:** *Per Medium, 8.3 oz* | | | |
| Caramel | 430 | 11 | 75 |
| Hot Fudge | 440 | 15 | 67 |
| Strawberry | 360 | 10 | 61 |
| *Malts: Per Medium* | | | |
| Caramel | 830 | 24 | 136 |
| Chocolate | 790 | 23 | 130 |
| Strawberry | 710 | 22 | 112 |
| *Moo Latte: Per Medium, With Whipped Topping* | | | |
| Cappuccino | 570 | 19 | 90 |
| French Vanilla | 630 | 19 | 106 |
| Mocha | 690 | 27 | 104 |

*For Complete Nutritional Data ~ see CalorieKing.com*

# Daphne's Greek Cafe® (Aug '15)

*Starters:*

| | C | F | Cb |
|---|---|---|---|
| Fire Feta & Warm Pita | 400 | 19 | 43 |
| Hummus & Warm Pita | 330 | 13 | 44 |
| *Pita Sandwiches: With Sides, Without Tzatsiki Sauce* | | | |
| Chicken | 480 | 16 | 43 |
| Crispy Shrimp | 450 | 19 | 51 |
| Falafel | 560 | 25 | 72 |
| Gyros | 730 | 47 | 52 |
| *Plates: Without Sides, Pita Bread or Tzatziki* | | | |
| **Mix & Match:** | | | |
| Crispy Shrimp | 150 | 8 | 9 |
| Falafel | 260 | 15 | 29 |
| Fresh-Carved Gyros | 420 | 37 | 9 |
| Grilled Chicken Kabob | 120 | 4 | 3 |
| Grilled Steak Kabob | 120 | 4 | 4 |
| *Classic Greek Salads: With Dressing, W/O Pita & Sce* | | | |
| Crispy Shrimp | 440 | 31 | 25 |
| Falafel | 540 | 37 | 45 |
| Grilled Chicken | 460 | 28 | 18 |
| *Dressings:* Greek | 120 | 12 | 4 |
| Gorgonzola | 170 | 16 | 4 |
| **Sides:** Fire Roasted Vegetables | 60 | 3 | 6 |
| French Fries | 320 | 16 | 40 |
| Moroccan Carrot-Walnut | 180 | 13 | 16 |
| Multigrain Pita Chips | 170 | 5 | 27 |
| Pita Bread | 240 | 5 | 39 |
| Seasoned Rice | 250 | 6 | 47 |
| Tabouli Salad | 220 | 15 | 20 |

# Davanni's® (Aug '15)

*Half Hoagies: Includes 6" White Bun and Standard Toppings*

| | C | F | Cb |
|---|---|---|---|
| Assorted | 490 | 30 | 39 |
| Cheese | 500 | 31 | 39 |
| Chicken & Bacon w/ Honey Mstrd | 505 | 22 | 46 |
| Chicken Parmigiana | 445 | 16 | 40 |
| Club | 495 | 27 | 40 |
| Pastrami | 470 | 27 | 40 |
| Roast Beef | 470 | 25 | 39 |
| Southwestern Chicken | 535 | 26 | 43 |
| Tuna Melt | 645 | 44 | 42 |
| Turkey Bacon Chipotle | 565 | 33 | 39 |
| Veggie | 445 | 24 | 43 |
| *Pasta: As Served, With Garlic Toast* | | | |
| Chicken Florentine, half portion | 570 | 23 | 56 |
| Lasagna, half portion | 625 | 43 | 37 |

*continued next page...*

## Davanni's® cont... (Aug '15)

### Pizzas: *Per Slice*

| | C | F | Cb |
|---|---|---|---|
| Five Meat: Thin Crust | 255 | 13 | 19 |
| Traditional Crust | 305 | 13 | 30 |
| Solo, Thin Crust | 655 | 36 | 44 |
| Veggie: Thin Crust | 220 | 10 | 19 |
| Traditional Crust | 275 | 10 | 30 |
| Works: Thin Crust | 265 | 14 | 19 |
| Traditional Crust | 315 | 15 | 30 |

## Del Taco® (Aug '15)

### Breakfast:

| | C | F | Cb |
|---|---|---|---|
| **Burritos:** Breakfast | 290 | 13 | 28 |
| ½ lb Sausage & Egg | 500 | 26 | 38 |
| ½ lb Steak & Egg | 460 | 20 | 40 |
| Egg & Cheese | 400 | 17 | 38 |
| **Hash Brown Sticks:** 5 pieces | 230 | 17 | 18 |
| 8 pieces | 360 | 27 | 28 |
| **Quesadilla,** Bacon & Egg | 410 | 22 | 32 |

### American Grill:

| | | | |
|---|---|---|---|
| **Burgers:** Cheeseburger | 430 | 22 | 40 |
| Double Del Cheeseburger | 720 | 48 | 40 |
| **Crinkle Cut Fries:** Kids, 3 oz | 160 | 10 | 17 |
| Regular, 4 oz | 210 | 13 | 22 |
| Medium, 6 oz | 320 | 19 | 34 |
| Macho, 8.8 oz | 470 | 28 | 49 |
| Chili Cheddar Fries, 10.5 oz | 570 | 34 | 41 |

### Burritos:

| | | | |
|---|---|---|---|
| Classic Grilled Chicken | 530 | 33 | 40 |
| Del Beef | 490 | 20 | 40 |
| Grilled Chicken Avocado | 840 | 36 | 90 |
| Macho Combo | 940 | 34 | 100 |
| *Nachos:* 4 oz | 300 | 19 | 30 |
| Macho Beef | 960 | 49 | 98 |
| Macho, Chicken; Steak, average | 940 | 53 | 101 |
| Salsa Verde | 430 | 6 | 77 |

### Quesadillas:

| | | | |
|---|---|---|---|
| Cheddar; Spicy Jack, average | 460 | 27 | 32 |
| Chicken Cheddar/Spicy Jack, av | 550 | 31 | 35 |

### Tacos:

| | | | |
|---|---|---|---|
| Al Carbon, Chkn; Steak, av., 3.5 oz | 150 | 4.5 | 19 |
| Beer Battered Fish , 5.1 oz | 280 | 17 | 27 |
| Grilled Chicken, 3.7 oz | 220 | 12 | 16 |
| Regular, 2.8 oz | 130 | 7 | 9 |
| Turkey, 3.4 oz | 150 | 7 | 10 |
| **Salads:** Deluxe Beef Taco | 820 | 47 | 66 |
| Deluxe Chicken | 770 | 43 | 64 |
| **Desserts:** Cinn. Churro, 1.8 oz | 220 | 15 | 23 |
| Caramel Cheesecake Bites, 2 Bites, 4.3 oz | 460 | 28 | 43 |
| *Premium Shakes: Per 16 oz* | | | |
| Chocolate | 560 | 11 | 105 |
| Strawberry; Vanilla, average | 520 | 11 | 95 |

## Denny's® (Aug '15)

### Breakfast:

| | C | F | Cb |
|---|---|---|---|
| **Favorites:** *Without Side Choices* | | | |
| Banana Pecan Pancakes | 750 | 13 | 154 |
| Blueberry P'cakes w/ Scr. Eggs | 840 | 44 | 88 |
| Cinnamon P'cakes, Hash Browns, & Fried Eggs | 990 | 48 | 117 |
| Moons Over My Hammy | 980 | 65 | 55 |
| Peanut Butter Cup Pancakes, Hash Browns & Fried Egg | 1510 | 90 | 147 |
| **Omelettes:** *With Hash Browns, without Bread* | | | |
| Fantastic Four | 810 | 58 | 27 |
| Ham & Cheese | 790 | 59 | 21 |
| Meat Lovers | 1040 | 80 | 28 |
| Loaded Veggie | 600 | 43 | 25 |
| Ultimate | 830 | 66 | 25 |
| **Skillets:** *As Served* | | | |
| Hearty Breakfast | 1090 | 85 | 40 |
| Human Torch | 1130 | 87 | 54 |
| Santa Fe | 720 | 53 | 31 |
| Ultimate | 720 | 54 | 33 |
| Veggie, Fit Fare | 340 | 11 | 43 |
| **Slams:** | | | |
| All American, w/ Hash Browns | 990 | 83 | 20 |
| Fit Slam | 390 | 10 | 54 |
| French Toast | 810 | 48 | 66 |
| Invisible Woman w/ Bacon & Hash Browns | 760 | 33 | 89 |
| Lumberjack, w/o bread, 17oz | 1230 | 76 | 90 |
| The Grand Slamwich, with Hash Browns, 20 oz | 1390 | 96 | 82 |
| **Sides:** Buttermilk Biscuit (2) | 400 | 18 | 50 |
| English Muffin, w/o Margarine (1) | 140 | 1 | 29 |
| Hash Browns, 1 serve | 210 | 16 | 15 |
| **Pancakes:** | | | |
| Buttermilk, w/ Margarine, (2) | 370 | 8 | 68 |
| Hearty Wheat, 2 cakes | 310 | 2 | 64 |

### Burgers & Sandwiches:

| | | | |
|---|---|---|---|
| **Burgers:** *Without Sides, Unless Indicated* | | | |
| Bacon, Avocado Cheeseburger | 970 | 64 | 50 |
| Bacon Slamburger | 880 | 49 | 55 |
| Bourbon Bacon Burger | 1040 | 58 | 77 |
| Double Cheeseburger | 1120 | 67 | 49 |
| Spicy Sriracha Burger | 790 | 43 | 49 |
| The Thing Burger | 1920 | 131 | 121 |
| **Melts:** Chicken Philly | 800 | 49 | 56 |
| Prime Rib Philly | 970 | 57 | 60 |
| **Sandwiches:** *Without Sides* | | | |
| Cali Club | 1100 | 75 | 70 |
| Chicken Salad | 610 | 34 | 50 |
| Club | 810 | 39 | 75 |
| The Super Bird | 610 | 32 | 42 |

## Denny's® cont... (Aug '15)

*Dinners: W/out Sides Unless Indicated*

| | C | F | Cb |
|---|---|---|---|
| Bourbon Chicken Skillet, 22 oz | 840 | 26 | 78 |
| Brooklyn Spag. & Meatballs, 23 oz | 1230 | 61 | 111 |
| Chicken Strips, with Bread, 10 oz | 780 | 40 | 64 |
| Fish & Chips, w/ French Fries, 23 oz | 1050 | 75 | 131 |
| Slow-Cooked Pot Roast, 16 oz | 1390 | 37 | 166 |
| T-Bone Steak: With Bread, 12 oz | 840 | 38 | 23 |
| With Breaded Shrimp, 15 oz | 1030 | 46 | 43 |

*Dinner Sides:*

| | | | |
|---|---|---|---|
| Broccoli, 3 oz | 25 | 0 | 4 |
| French Fries, salted, 6 oz | 510 | 28 | 59 |
| Golden-Fried Shrimp, 6 pieces | 190 | 8 | 20 |
| Hash Browns, 1 serving | 210 | 16 | 15 |
| Mac 'n Cheese, 3 oz | 180 | 12 | 12 |
| Mashed Potatoes, 1 serving | 100 | 3 | 20 |
| Red-Skinned Potatoes, 4 oz | 200 | 9 | 27 |

*Soups: Per Bowl, Without Bread*

| | | | |
|---|---|---|---|
| Broccoli & Cheddar | 370 | 16 | 48 |
| Chicken Noodle | 140 | 4 | 17 |
| Clam Chowder | 300 | 14 | 16 |
| Vegetable Beef | 170 | 4 | 23 |

*Salads: Without Bread*

| | | | |
|---|---|---|---|
| Avocado Chicken Caesar, with Caesar Drssng | 660 | 49 | 15 |
| Cranb. Apple Chicken with Balsamic Vinaigrette | 360 | 9 | 36 |
| Prime Rib Cobb, with Fat-Free Italian Dressing | 665 | 47 | 25 |

*Dressings: Per 1 oz*

| | | | |
|---|---|---|---|
| Bleu Cheese | 110 | 11 | 1 |
| Caesar | 100 | 10 | 0 |
| French | 75 | 5 | 8 |
| Honey Mustard | 120 | 10 | 8 |
| Ranch | 130 | 14 | 1 |

*Desserts: As Served*

**Apple Pie:**

| | | | |
|---|---|---|---|
| with Caramel Topping | 780 | 40 | 102 |
| A La Mode (with Ice Cream) | 1090 | 57 | 137 |
| Banana Split | 810 | 31 | 125 |
| Caramel Apple Crisp | 740 | 21 | 134 |
| Chocolate Lava Cake | 730 | 36 | 84 |
| Doom Lava Cake | 820 | 40 | 102 |
| NY Style Cheesecake w/ Toppings | 560 | 34 | 57 |

*Beverages:*

| | | | |
|---|---|---|---|
| Hot Chocolate | 100 | 2 | 28 |
| Iced Cappuccino | 190 | 5 | 30 |
| Lemonade Iced Tea, 15 oz | 70 | 0 | 19 |
| Strawberry Lemonade, 15 oz | 200 | 0 | 50 |
| **Floats,** Coke/Root Beer, 16 oz | 430 | 17 | 69 |
| **Fruit Smoothies,** av. | 270 | 0 | 68 |
| **Milk Shakes:** Chocolate | 1090 | 57 | 132 |
| Vanilla | 750 | 37 | 95 |

*For Complete Nutritional Data ~ see CalorieKing.com*

## Dippin' Dots® (Aug '15)

*Flavored Ices: Per ½ Cup, 3 oz*

| | C | F | Cb |
|---|---|---|---|
| Rockin' Cherry with Popping Candy | 130 | 0.5 | 30 |
| Sour Blue Razz | 60 | 0 | 14 |
| Other varieties | 100 | 0 | 26 |

*Frozen Yogurt: Per ½ Cup*

| | | | |
|---|---|---|---|
| Strawberry Cheesecake, ½ cup | 100 | 0 | 21 |
| YoDots: Cookies 'N Cream | 100 | 1.5 | 16 |
| Chocolate & Vanilla | 70 | 0 | 12 |
| Cookie Dough | 110 | 2 | 19 |

*Ice Cream: Per ½ Cup*

| | | | |
|---|---|---|---|
| Banana Split | 160 | 8 | 20 |
| Choc. Chip Cookie Dough | 230 | 11 | 32 |
| Mint Chocolate | 170 | 8 | 21 |
| Strawberry | 160 | 8 | 18 |

## Donatos Pizza® (Aug '15)

*Pizzas:*

| | C | F | Cb |
|---|---|---|---|
| **Signature:** Thin Crust, ¼ Large Pizza | | | |
| Classic Trio | 630 | 32 | 51 |
| Founder's Favorite | 660 | 34 | 51 |
| Hawaiian | 540 | 24 | 52 |
| **Signatures:** Thicker Crust, ¼ Large Pizza | | | |
| Founder's Favorite | 730 | 33 | 70 |
| Mariachi Beef | 600 | 23 | 70 |
| Mariachi Chicken | 610 | 21 | 70 |
| Pepperoni | 670 | 30 | 69 |
| Serious Cheese | 650 | 23 | 69 |
| The Works | 690 | 32 | 70 |
| Vegy | 560 | 21 | 69 |

*Signature Subs: On White*

| | | | |
|---|---|---|---|
| Big Don: Italian | 670 | 33 | 63 |
| Marinara | 610 | 25 | 65 |
| Sausage Italian | 950 | 56 | 64 |
| Sausage Marinara | 890 | 48 | 66 |
| Buffalo Chicken | 680 | 27 | 66 |
| Chicken Bacon Cheddar | 810 | 39 | 65 |
| Meatball | 930 | 52 | 74 |

*Signature Subs: On Wheat*

| | | | |
|---|---|---|---|
| Buffalo Chicken | 680 | 27 | 67 |
| Steak Hoagie: Marinara Sauce | 670 | 30 | 66 |
| Mushroom Gravy | 650 | 30 | 64 |
| Turkey Club | 700 | 30 | 64 |
| **Stromboli:** Deluxe | 790 | 35 | 82 |
| Pepperoni | 930 | 46 | 83 |
| Three Meat | 920 | 44 | 83 |
| **Desserts:** Apple Timpano, 1 slice | 200 | 3.5 | 37 |
| Cinnamon Timpano, 1 slice | 260 | 10 | 37 |
| Cinnamon Twists (2 sticks) | 230 | 4 | 45 |

*For Complete Nutritional Data ~ see CalorieKing.com*

## Domino's® (Aug '15)

**12" Hand Tossed:**
*Per Slice, ⅛ Pizza, Includes Base Sauce and Cheese*

| | C | F | Cb |
|---|---|---|---|
| Bacon, Beef & Sausage | 275 | 14 | 27 |
| Beef, Green Pepp., On. & Mshrm | 200 | 8 | 25 |
| Black Olives, Green Peppers, Onions, Mushrooms, Tomatoes | 190 | 7 | 25 |
| Ham & Pineapple | 200 | 6.5 | 26 |
| Pepperoni | 215 | 9 | 25 |
| Pepperoni & Sausage | 240 | 11 | 26 |
| Sausage | 230 | 10 | 26 |
| Sliced Ital. Ssg, Beef & Pepperoni | 265 | 14 | 25 |

**14" Thin Crust:** *Per Slice, ⅛ Pizza, Includes Base Sauce and Cheese*

| | C | F | Cb |
|---|---|---|---|
| Bacon, Beef & Sausage | 325 | 19 | 21 |
| Beef, Green Pepp., On. & Mshrm | 220 | 12 | 19 |
| Black Olives, Green Peppers, Onions, Mushrooms & Tomatoes | 210 | 11 | 19 |
| Ham & Pineapple | 220 | 10 | 21 |
| Pepperoni | 240 | 13 | 19 |
| Pepperoni & Sausage | 275 | 16 | 20 |
| Sausage | 260 | 15 | 21 |

**14" Brooklyn:** *Per Slice, ⅙ Pizza, Includes Base Sauce and Cheese*

| | C | F | Cb |
|---|---|---|---|
| Beef, Green Pepp., On. & Mushroom | 270 | 13 | 26 |
| Black Olives, Green Peppers, Onions, Mushrooms, Tomatoes | 250 | 12 | 26 |
| Ham & Pineapple | 265 | 12 | 29 |
| Pepperoni | 290 | 15 | 26 |
| Pepperoni & Sausage | 340 | 19 | 27 |
| Sausage | 320 | 18 | 28 |

**12" Feast Hand-Tossed:** *Per Slice, ⅛ Pizza*

| | C | F | Cb |
|---|---|---|---|
| America's Favorite | 250 | 12 | 27 |
| Bacon Cheeseburger | 270 | 13 | 26 |
| Deluxe | 230 | 10 | 27 |
| ExtravaganZZa | 290 | 14 | 28 |
| MeatZZa | 280 | 14 | 27 |
| Ultimate Pepperoni | 260 | 13 | 25 |

**14" Feast Hand Tossed:** *Per Slice, ⅛ Pizza*

| | C | F | Cb |
|---|---|---|---|
| America's Favorite | 350 | 17 | 36 |
| Bacon Cheeseburger | 380 | 19 | 36 |
| Deluxe | 320 | 14 | 36 |
| ExtravaganZZa | 390 | 19 | 37 |
| MeatZZa Feast | 380 | 19 | 36 |
| Ultimate Pepperoni | 360 | 18 | 34 |

**12" Legends Thin Crust:** *Per ¼ Party Pizza*

| | C | F | Cb |
|---|---|---|---|
| Buffalo Chicken | 380 | 22 | 26 |
| Cali Chicken Bacon Ranch | 490 | 33 | 28 |
| Fiery Hawaiian | 390 | 22 | 32 |
| Memphis BBQ Chicken | 370 | 19 | 33 |
| Philly Cheese Steak | 360 | 21 | 26 |

## Domino's® cont... (Aug '15)

**Chicken Wings:** *W/out Dipping Sauce*

| | C | F | Cb |
|---|---|---|---|
| Barbeque, 4 wings | 250 | 13 | 14 |
| Hot, 4 wings | 200 | 13 | 5 |

**Chicken Dipping Cups:** *Per 1.5 oz Container*

| | C | F | Cb |
|---|---|---|---|
| Blue Cheese | 240 | 25 | 2 |
| Kicker Hot | 50 | 4.5 | 3 |
| Mango Habanero | 80 | 0 | 20 |
| Ranch | 200 | 21 | 2 |

**BreadBowl Pasta:** *Per ½ Bowl*

| | C | F | Cb |
|---|---|---|---|
| Chicken Alfredo, 10.85 oz | 700 | 26 | 93 |
| Chicken Carbonara, 11.6 oz | 740 | 28 | 94 |
| Italian Sausage Marinara, 11.85 oz | 730 | 27 | 97 |
| Pasta Primavera, 11 oz | 670 | 24 | 94 |

**Oven Baked Sandwiches:** *Per Sandwich*

| | C | F | Cb |
|---|---|---|---|
| Buffalo Chicken with Blue Cheese | 830 | 41 | 74 |
| Chicken Bacon Ranch | 870 | 45 | 72 |
| Chicken Parmesan | 750 | 30 | 73 |
| Italian | 820 | 41 | 70 |
| Italian Sausage & Peppers | 860 | 45 | 74 |
| Mediterranean Veggie | 680 | 29 | 72 |
| Philly Cheese Steak | 690 | 28 | 70 |
| Sweet & Spicy Chicken Habanero | 800 | 32 | 83 |

**Salads:** *Per Serving Without Dressing*

| | C | F | Cb |
|---|---|---|---|
| Garden Fresh | 70 | 3.5 | 5 |
| Grilled Chicken Caesar | 90 | 3.5 | 5 |

**Salad Dressings & Condiments:** *Per 1.5 oz Package*

| | C | F | Cb |
|---|---|---|---|
| Blue Cheese | 240 | 25 | 2 |
| Buttermilk Ranch | 230 | 24 | 2 |
| Creamy Caesar | 210 | 21 | 2 |
| Golden Italian | 210 | 22 | 2 |
| Light Italian | 20 | 1 | 3 |

**Bread Side Items:**

| | C | F | Cb |
|---|---|---|---|
| **Breadsticks:** 1 stick, without sauce | 110 | 6 | 11 |
| 8 sticks, without sauce | 880 | 48 | 88 |
| **Cheesy Bread:** | | | |
| 1 stick, without sauce | 120 | 6 | 11 |
| 8 sticks, without sauce | 960 | 48 | 88 |

**Bread Dipping Sauces:** *Per Container*

| | C | F | Cb |
|---|---|---|---|
| Garlic, 1 oz | 250 | 28 | 0 |
| Marinara, 2 oz | 25 | 0 | 5 |

**Cinna Stix:**

| | C | F | Cb |
|---|---|---|---|
| 1 stick, without icing | 120 | 6 | 14 |
| 8 sticks, without icing | 960 | 48 | 112 |
| **Sweet Icing,** Dipping Cup | 250 | 2.5 | 57 |
| **Dessert,** Chocolate Lava Crunch Cake | 350 | 17 | 47 |

Updated Nutrition Data ~ www.CalorieKing.com
Persons with Diabetes ~ See Disclaimer (Page 22)

## Don Pablos® (Aug '15)

*Start The Fiesta: Per Entire Plate*

| | C | F | Cb |
|---|---|---|---|
| **Don's Boneless Wings:** *Without Bleu Cheese Dressing* | | | |
| Buffalo | 750 | 48 | 49 |
| Chipotle Honey BBQ | 1010 | 59 | 94 |
| **Flautas,** without Guacamole | 505 | 29 | 40 |
| **Taquitos,** without Guacamole | 560 | 39 | 28 |
| **Optional Guacamole,** #30 scoop | 70 | 6 | 1 |
| **Nachos:** | | | |
| Cantina: With Chicken | 1060 | 46 | 108 |
| With Beef | 1185 | 55 | 109 |
| **Quesadillas:** *Without Guacamole* | | | |
| Cheese, small | 950 | 66 | 50 |
| Mesquite Grilled, Steak, small | 860 | 53 | 54 |
| **Dips:** *Without Chips or Tortillas* | | | |
| Bowls: Queso Blanco | 1080 | 88 | 14 |
| Prairie Fire Bean | 715 | 43 | 53 |
| *Entrees: Per Meal, Without Sides* | | | |
| **Burritos:** Chicken | 1025 | 53 | 79 |
| Fajita Steak | 1025 | 50 | 79 |
| **Carnitas:** Pork | 815 | 31 | 88 |
| Cold Set, Side | 185 | 11 | 24 |
| **Chimichangas:** Chicken | 785 | 37 | 64 |
| Spicy Beef De Oro | 1360 | 79 | 89 |
| **Don's Combos:** *Without Sides* | | | |
| Cinco Combo | 1175 | 66 | 64 |
| El Matador | 960 | 54 | 59 |
| Mexicano | 715 | 43 | 31 |
| Numero uno Favorito | 870 | 45 | 65 |
| Presidente | 1010 | 54 | 70 |
| **Enchiladas:** Cadillac Chicken | 875 | 43 | 60 |
| Cadillac Steak | 1015 | 53 | 65 |
| **Sizzlin' Fajitas:** *With Proteins, Onions & Peppers* | | | |
| Combo - Steak & Chicken | 580 | 28 | 34 |
| Mesquite-Grilled: Chicken | 485 | 20 | 32 |
| Steak | 680 | 36 | 36 |
| **Fajita Fixin's:** 7" Flour Tortilla (3) | 375 | 11 | 60 |
| Corn Tortillas (4) | 60 | 1 | 12 |
| Guacamole, #30 scoop | 70 | 6 | 4 |
| Pico de Gallo, #30 scoop | 5 | 0 | 2 |
| Sour Cream, #30 scoop | 80 | 8 | 2 |
| *Fresh Salads: Without Dressing* | | | |
| **Caesar:** With Chicken | 815 | 27 | 96 |
| With Steak | 945 | 38 | 99 |
| **Southwest:** *Without Extra Dressing* | | | |
| With Buffalo Sauce | 950 | 57 | 73 |
| With Chipotle-Honey BBQ Sauce | 1215 | 67 | 118 |
| *Sides:* | | | |
| Mexican Rice, 3 oz | 120 | 2 | 23 |
| Refritos, 5 oz | 215 | 7 | 27 |
| Seasoned French Fries, 7 oz | 345 | 16 | 46 |
| Seasoned Vegetables, 6 oz | 110 | 5 | 16 |

## Dunkin' Donuts® (Aug '15)

*Bagels:*

| | C | F | Cb |
|---|---|---|---|
| Plain; Onion, average | 310 | 1 | 64 |
| Cinnamon Raisin | 320 | 1 | 67 |
| Everything | 340 | 3 | 67 |
| Sesame Seed | 350 | 4.5 | 65 |
| Tomato Mozzarella Supreme | 390 | 6 | 66 |
| Whole Wheat | 320 | 2 | 61 |
| *Danish:* Apple Cheese | 330 | 16 | 41 |
| Cheese | 330 | 17 | 39 |
| Strawberry Cheese | 320 | 16 | 40 |
| *Donuts:* Apple 'n Spice | 270 | 14 | 32 |
| Bavarian Kreme | 270 | 15 | 31 |
| Boston Kreme | 310 | 16 | 39 |
| Bow Tie Donut | 310 | 15 | 39 |
| Chocolate Frosted Cake | 370 | 23 | 45 |
| Chocolate Kreme Filled | 370 | 21 | 42 |
| French Cruller | 220 | 15 | 18 |
| Jelly | 270 | 14 | 32 |
| Old Fashioned Cake | 320 | 22 | 33 |
| Powdered Cake | 340 | 22 | 38 |
| Strawberry Frosted | 280 | 15 | 32 |
| Sugar Raised | 230 | 14 | 22 |
| Vanilla Kreme Filled | 380 | 23 | 42 |
| *Muffins:* | | | |
| Blueberry: Regular | 460 | 15 | 76 |
| Reduced Fat | 410 | 10 | 75 |
| Chocolate Chip | 550 | 21 | 83 |
| Coffee Cake | 590 | 24 | 86 |
| Corn; Honey Bran Raisin, av. | 450 | 15 | 73 |
| *Munchkins:* Jelly Filled (4) | 320 | 16 | 36 |
| Plain Cake; Cinnamon Cake (4) | 240 | 14 | 24 |
| *Sandwiches: On French Roll Unless Indicated* | | | |
| Bacon Ranch Chicken | 660 | 27 | 69 |
| BBQ Chicken | 590 | 19 | 74 |
| Chicken on Pretzel Roll | 640 | 25 | 68 |
| Chicken Salad Croissant | 580 | 38 | 42 |
| Ham & Cheese | 440 | 14 | 54 |
| Roast Beef | 460 | 16 | 54 |
| Texas Toasted Grilled Cheese | 510 | 30 | 41 |
| Tuna Salad: Melt on Croissant | 680 | 47 | 42 |
| On a Plain Bagel | 570 | 24 | 69 |
| On English Muffin | 400 | 24 | 34 |
| Turkey Cheddar Bacon | 460 | 14 | 55 |

*Continued Next Page... . ...*

## Dunkin' Donuts® cont... (Aug '15)

*Breakfast:*

| | C | F | Cb |
|---|---|---|---|
| **Hash Browns,** 6 pieces | 130 | 7 | 15 |
| **Oatmeal:** | | | |
| Original, w/ Dried Fruit Topping | 270 | 4 | 54 |
| Brown Sugar Flavored Oatmeal, | | | |
| with Dried Fruit Topping | 300 | 4 | 61 |
| **Bagels:** | | | |
| Bacon, Egg & Cheese | 460 | 11 | 67 |
| Egg & Cheese | 410 | 7 | 67 |
| Ham, Egg & Cheese | 440 | 8 | 67 |
| Sausage, Egg & Cheese | 620 | 26 | 67 |
| **Big N' Toasted** | 530 | 28 | 43 |
| **Biscuits:** Bacon, Egg & Cheese | 470 | 27 | 38 |
| Sausage, Egg & Cheese | 630 | 43 | 38 |
| **Croissants:** Bacon, Egg & Cheese | 480 | 27 | 40 |
| Egg & Cheese | 440 | 24 | 40 |
| Ham, Egg & Cheese | 460 | 25 | 40 |
| Sausage, Egg & Cheese | 640 | 44 | 41 |
| **English Muffins:** | | | |
| Bacon, Egg & Cheese | 290 | 10 | 32 |
| Ham, Egg & Cheese | 280 | 8 | 34 |
| Sausage, Egg & Cheese | 450 | 26 | 32 |
| **Multigrain Flatbreads:** | | | |
| Bacon Guacamole | 360 | 17 | 34 |
| Egg White | 280 | 9 | 33 |
| Turkey Sausage | 410 | 20 | 35 |
| **Wake-Up Wraps:** | | | |
| Bacon, Egg & Cheese | 180 | 9 | 14 |
| Egg & Cheese | 150 | 8 | 13 |
| Ham, Egg & Cheese | 170 | 8 | 14 |
| Sausage, Egg & Cheese | 260 | 17 | 14 |
| Egg & Turkey Sausage | 210 | 11 | 14 |

*Hot Beverages: Per Medium Size*

| | C | F | Cb |
|---|---|---|---|
| **Chocolate:** Original | 320 | 11 | 58 |
| Mint | 310 | 10 | 52 |
| **Dunkaccino** | 350 | 16 | 51 |

*Cold Beverages: Per Medium Size*

| | C | F | Cb |
|---|---|---|---|
| **Coolatta:** Orange, 24 fl.oz | 310 | 0 | 80 |
| Strawberry Fruit, 24 fl.oz | 350 | 0 | 86 |
| Vanilla Bean, 24 fl.oz | 630 | 9 | 138 |
| **Iced Coffee:** *Per Medium Size, Without Cream* | | | |
| Regular, without sugar | 15 | 0 | 2 |
| Caramel Mocha | 180 | 0 | 41 |
| Peppermint Mocha | 190 | 0.5 | 46 |
| **Lattes:** *Per Medium, With Whole Milk* | | | |
| Caramel Mocha | 260 | 0.5 | 53 |
| Caramel Swirl | 350 | 9 | 55 |

## Eat 'N Park® (Aug '15)

*Breakfast:*

| | C | F | Cb |
|---|---|---|---|
| Bananas Foster French Toast, | | | |
| 2 slices | 495 | 15 | 82 |
| **Omelettes:** Ham & Cheese | 535 | 35 | 5 |
| Meat Lover's | 725 | 55 | 3 |
| **Pancakes:** | | | |
| Buttermilk: Plain (1) | 75 | 1 | 15 |
| Blueberry (1) | 85 | 1 | 16 |
| **Scramblers:** | | | |
| All-American w/ sausage | 705 | 39 | 55 |
| Skinny | 355 | 14 | 32 |
| **Waffles:** Belgian (1) | 280 | 12 | 35 |
| Strawberry (1) | 375 | 17 | 48 |

*Appetizers:*

| | C | F | Cb |
|---|---|---|---|
| Fried Cheese Sticks | 535 | 36 | 26 |
| Fried Ravioli | 455 | 31 | 30 |
| Grilled Chicken Quesadilla | 905 | 56 | 52 |
| Onion Rings Basket | 365 | 24 | 34 |

*Burgers:*

| | C | F | Cb |
|---|---|---|---|
| **Black Angus:** | | | |
| American Grill | 615 | 37 | 30 |
| Mushroom & Onion | 575 | 31 | 31 |
| Superburger | 1085 | 73 | 28 |
| **Classic:** Black Angus | 455 | 22 | 28 |
| Black Angus Bacon Cheeseburger | 570 | 31 | 28 |
| Black Angus Cheeseburger | 505 | 26 | 28 |
| Garden Burger | 290 | 5 | 43 |
| **Original,** Superburger | 565 | 38 | 27 |

*Sandwiches: With Menu Board Standard Add-Ins*

| | C | F | Cb |
|---|---|---|---|
| BLT | 490 | 15 | 65 |
| Buffalo Chicken Wrap | 835 | 48 | 61 |
| Chargrilled Chicken | 345 | 7 | 31 |
| Gourmet Grilled Cheese | 795 | 58 | 27 |
| Hot Turkey | 500 | 8 | 71 |
| Santa Fe Turkey | 740 | 50 | 31 |
| Shredded Pot Roast | 530 | 31 | 28 |
| Turkey Club | 835 | 49 | 51 |
| Whale of a Cod Fish | 880 | 42 | 76 |

*Dinners: Without Sides*

| | C | F | Cb |
|---|---|---|---|
| **Baked Chicken Parmigiana:** | | | |
| W/ Marinara Sauce | 960 | 38 | 99 |
| W/ Meat Sauce | 985 | 41 | 95 |
| Baked Lemon Sole, 2 fillets | 390 | 19 | 11 |
| Chicken Fillets, 5 pieces | 530 | 26 | 28 |
| Cod Floridian, 2 fillets | 240 | 3 | 8 |
| Mile-High Meatloaf | 900 | 57 | 59 |
| Smothered Ground Sirloin Steak | 445 | 27 | 8 |
| Spaghetti Marinara | 695 | 8 | 129 |
| Spaghetti with Meat Sauce | 835 | 16 | 146 |
| Whitefish w/ Mac & Cheese 2 fillets | 750 | 34 | 58 |

*Continued Next Page....*

## Eat 'N Park® cont... (Aug '15)

### Salads: Without Dressing

| | C | F | Cb |
|---|---|---|---|
| Buffalo Chicken | 610 | 33 | 42 |
| Garden | 95 | 3 | 16 |
| Grilled Chicken | 445 | 20 | 30 |
| Steak | 740 | 46 | 33 |

### Dressings: Per 2 oz

| | C | F | Cb |
|---|---|---|---|
| Bleu Cheese | 245 | 25 | 3 |
| Citrus Lime Vinaigrette | 70 | 6 | 13 |
| French, Fat Free | 75 | 0 | 18 |
| House Ranch | 215 | 21 | 4 |
| Poppy & Sesame Seed | 390 | 32 | 26 |

### Desserts:

| | C | F | Cb |
|---|---|---|---|
| Ice Cream, 2 scoops | 230 | 12 | 27 |
| Pies: Apple Pie, 1 slice | 525 | 27 | 67 |
| Blackberry Pie, 1 slice | 565 | 28 | 75 |
| Coconut Cream Pie, 1 slice | 490 | 27 | 55 |
| Dutch Apple Pie, 1 slice | 375 | 14 | 61 |
| Sundaes: Caramel Fudge | 400 | 19 | 56 |
| Oreo | 505 | 21 | 74 |

## Edo Japan® (Aug '15)

### Bento Box: Without Teriyaki Sauce

| | C | F | Cb |
|---|---|---|---|
| Beef Yakisoba, 20.3 oz | 840 | 29 | 102 |
| Chicken Yakisoba, 20.5 oz | 790 | 24 | 102 |
| Sizzling Shrimp, 22 oz | 790 | 15 | 122 |
| Sukiyaki Beef, 20.3 oz | 880 | 27 | 120 |

### Teriyaki Dishes: Without Teriyaki Sauce

| | C | F | Cb |
|---|---|---|---|
| Chicken, 15 oz | 570 | 11 | 80 |
| Chicken & Shrimp | 640 | 14 | 82 |
| Sukiyaki Beef, 14.8 oz | 580 | 15 | 80 |

### Soup: Per 33 oz Bowl

| | C | F | Cb |
|---|---|---|---|
| Beef Udon | 580 | 17 | 72 |
| Chicken Udon | 550 | 13 | 72 |

### Maki Sushi: Per 6 Pieces

| | C | F | Cb |
|---|---|---|---|
| California Roll, 7.6 oz | 430 | 17 | 61 |
| Spicy Tuna Roll, 6.5 oz | 300 | 2.5 | 54 |

### Nigiri Sushi: Per 1 Piece

| | C | F | Cb |
|---|---|---|---|
| Ebi (Steamed Prawn), 1.7 oz | 70 | 0.5 | 12 |
| Salmon Sashimi, 0.7 oz | 30 | 1.5 | 1 |

## Einstein Bros® (Aug '15)

### Bagels:

| | C | F | Cb |
|---|---|---|---|
| Bagels: Asiago Cheese | 300 | 4 | 54 |
| Blueberry | 290 | 1 | 60 |
| Chocolate Chip | 290 | 3 | 58 |
| Cinnamon Sugar | 320 | 6 | 59 |
| Cranberry | 290 | 1 | 61 |
| Garlic | 270 | 2.5 | 56 |
| Honey Whole Wheat | 260 | 3 | 50 |
| Onion | 270 | 1 | 59 |
| Plain; Everything, average | 270 | 2 | 55 |
| Potato | 280 | 4 | 52 |
| Sesame | 290 | 3 | 54 |
| Gourmet Bagels: Apple Cinnamon | 440 | 8 | 82 |
| Green Chile | 370 | 9 | 58 |
| Power Protein | 350 | 6 | 64 |
| Six-Cheese | 370 | 9 | 57 |
| Spinach Florentine | 380 | 11 | 58 |
| Bagel Dogs: Original | 610 | 32 | 57 |
| Asiago | 620 | 33 | 58 |

### Egg Sandwiches:

| | C | F | Cb |
|---|---|---|---|
| Applwd Bacon & Spinach Panini | 790 | 49 | 60 |
| Cinnamon Toast | 270 | 30 | 73 |
| Southwest Turkey Sausage | 400 | 13 | 45 |
| Spinach, Mshrm & Swiss, on Plain Bagel | 490 | 18 | 58 |
| Flatbreads: BBQ Chicken | 590 | 20 | 67 |
| Pepperoni | 590 | 31 | 51 |
| Roasted Veggie | 570 | 28 | 55 |

### Signature Sandwiches:

| | C | F | Cb |
|---|---|---|---|
| Albacore Tuna Salad | 570 | 24 | 62 |
| Harvest Chicken Salad | 570 | 21 | 69 |
| Honey Smoked Salmon | 560 | 16 | 65 |
| Hummus Veg Out | 440 | 12 | 72 |
| The: Einstein's Club | 990 | 50 | 84 |
| Farmhouse | 920 | 43 | 85 |
| Soup: Broccoli Cheddar, 14 oz | 470 | 33 | 24 |
| Chicken Noodle, 14 oz | 170 | 5 | 22 |
| Turkey Chilli, 14 oz | 260 | 7 | 35 |
| Tostinis: BBQ Chicken | 560 | 13 | 74 |
| Buffalo Chicken & Bacon | 570 | 20 | 57 |
| Iltalian Chicken | 660 | 32 | 57 |
| Roasted Veggie | 560 | 24 | 63 |
| Turkey Club | 760 | 41 | 62 |
| Wraps:Buffalo Chicken | 600 | 28 | 60 |
| Santa Fe | 650 | 32 | 60 |

### Cream Cheese: Per 1.3 oz Schmear

| | C | F | Cb |
|---|---|---|---|
| Reduced Fat: Garlic Herb/Garden Veggie | 130 | 10 | 6 |
| Honey Almond; Strawberry, av. | 150 | 10 | 13 |
| Plain | 150 | 14 | 2 |
| Onion and Chive | 140 | 12 | 5 |
| Sweets: Blueberry Muffin, 5.5 oz | 510 | 24 | 69 |
| Cinnamon Twist, 3.4 oz | 360 | 18 | 23 |
| Snickerdoodle Cookie, 2.9 oz | 350 | 14 | 31 |

# Fast - Foods & *Restaurants*

## El Pollo Loco® (Aug '15)

| | C | F | Cb |
|---|---|---|---|
| **Soup Starters:** *Per Small Serving* | | | |
| Chicken Tortilla w/ Tortilla Strips | 210 | 9 | 19 |
| Without Tortilla Strips | 140 | 5 | 10 |
| **Bowl:** Original Pollo | 610 | 10 | 87 |
| Mexican Caesar | 480 | 24 | 38 |
| **Burritos, Chicken/Shrimp::** | | | |
| Avocado, average | 950 | 53 | 74 |
| Poblano Avocado, average | 910 | 40 | 93 |
| Ranchero, average | 875 | 40 | 85 |
| Spicy Chipotle, average | 860 | 36 | 86 |
| **Flame-Grilled Chicken:** *Skin On* | | | |
| Breast; Thigh, av. | 220 | 12 | 0 |
| Leg; Wing, av. | 90 | 4.5 | 0 |
| **Quesadillas:** | | | |
| Avocado Chicken | 980 | 62 | 61 |
| Avocado Shrimp | 1020 | 63 | 67 |
| Bacon & Guacamole, Chkn; Shrimp | 880 | 51 | 56 |
| **Salads:** *Without Dressing* | | | |
| **Classic:** Chicken | 240 | 8 | 19 |
| With Shrimp | 290 | 14 | 22 |
| **Mexican Cobb:** With Chicken | 520 | 25 | 38 |
| With Shrimp | 560 | 32 | 40 |
| *Tacos,* Avocado Chkn/Shrimp, av. | 315 | 18 | 20 |
| **Tostada:** *Without Dressing* | | | |
| Chicken | 860 | 42 | 77 |
| Shrimp | 910 | 49 | 80 |
| Ultimate Double: Chicken | 1030 | 50 | 82 |
| Shrimp | 1070 | 61 | 85 |
| **Under 500 Calories:** *Without Dressing* | | | |
| Double Chicken Avocado | 380 | 15 | 14 |
| Grilled Chicken Mango | 470 | 35 | 56 |
| Skinny Chicken Quesadilla | 460 | 17 | 43 |
| **Dressings:** Creamy Cilantro: 1.3 oz | 190 | 20 | 1 |
| Light, 1.5 oz | 70 | 5 | 6 |
| Ranch, 1.5 oz | 230 | 24 | 2 |
| **Sides:** Black Beans, 6 oz | 200 | 0 | 35 |
| Cole Slaw, 4 oz | 130 | 10 | 9 |
| Cut Corn with Red Peppers, 5 oz | 160 | 5 | 24 |
| Gravy, 1 oz | 10 | 0 | 2 |
| Macaroni & Cheese, 5.5 oz | 250 | 15 | 22 |
| Mashed Potatoes, 5 oz | 110 | 1.5 | 23 |
| Pinto Beans, 6 oz | 200 | 4 | 29 |
| **Condiments:** Pico de Gallo, 1.5 oz | 15 | 1 | 2 |
| **Salsa:** Avocado, 1.5 oz | 30 | 2.5 | 2 |
| House; Roja, av.,1.5 oz | 15 | 0 | 3 |
| Sour Cream, 1.3 oz | 80 | 7 | 1 |
| **Dessert:** Mini Cheesecake Burrito | 380 | 21 | 39 |
| Chocolate Chip Brownie | 390 | 19 | 53 |
| Two Cinnamon Churros | 300 | 18 | 32 |

## Fatburger® (Aug '15)

| | C | F | Cb |
|---|---|---|---|
| **Burgers:** *Without Extras* | | | |
| Burgers: Small | 400 | 21 | 37 |
| Medium | 590 | 31 | 46 |
| Large | 850 | 41 | 69 |
| Turkeyburger | 480 | 21 | 50 |
| Veggieburger | 510 | 20 | 60 |
| **Hot Dogs:** *Without Extas* | | | |
| Chili Cheese | 480 | 27 | 35 |
| Regular Hot Dog | 320 | 15 | 32 |
| **Sandwiches:** *Without Extras* | | | |
| Chicken: Crispy | 560 | 27 | 53 |
| Grilled | 430 | 14 | 42 |
| Fish | 560 | 31 | 55 |
| **Fries:** Fat Fries | 380 | 18 | 47 |
| With Chili | 480 | 2 | 52 |
| With Chili & Cheese | 590 | 33 | 53 |
| **Add-Ons:** American Cheese, 1 slice | 70 | 5 | 1 |
| Cheddar Cheese, 1 slice | 110 | 9 | 1 |
| Mayonnaise, 1 serving | 90 | 10 | 1 |
| Relish, 1 serving | 20 | 0 | 5 |
| **Sides:** Chili Cup | 200 | 11 | 10 |
| With Cheese & Onions | 320 | 20 | 12 |
| Onion Rings | 540 | 29 | 64 |
| **Shakes:** Chocolate | 910 | 45 | 115 |
| Cookies & Ice Cream | 1180 | 59 | 163 |
| Maui-Banana | 940 | 44 | 126 |
| Peanut Butter | 950 | 53 | 114 |
| Strawberry; Vanilla, average | 885 | 44 | 112 |

*For Complete Nutritional Data ~ see CalorieKing.com*

## Fazoli's® (Aug '15)

| | C | F | Cb |
|---|---|---|---|
| **Oven-Baked Pasta:** *Per Serving* | | | |
| Baked Ziti | 660 | 27 | 70 |
| Chicken Broccoli Penne | 870 | 41 | 74 |
| Chicken Parmigano | 870 | 35 | 91 |
| Penne Romano | 850 | 42 | 74 |
| Penne with Creamy Basil Chicken | 870 | 42 | 72 |
| Twice-Baked Lasagna | 700 | 31 | 69 |
| **Top It Options:** | | | |
| Asiago Mushrooms, 2.5 oz | 120 | 11 | 3 |
| Broccoli, 2.5 oz | 60 | 4.5 | 3 |
| Italian Meatballs, 3 oz | 250 | 18 | 6 |
| Italian Sausage, 2 oz | 200 | 16 | 3 |
| Roasted Chicken, 3.6 oz | 110 | 2.5 | 1 |

*Continued Next Page....*

Updated Nutrition Data ~ www.CalorieKing.com
Persons with Diabetes ~ See Disclaimer (Page 22)

## Fazoli's® cont... (Aug '15)

*Lighter Options Baked Pasta:*

| | C | F | Cb |
|---|---|---|---|
| Baked Spaghetti | 330 | 10 | 43 |
| Chicken Mushroom Alfredo | 400 | 23 | 45 |
| Three Cheese Baked Ravioli | 430 | 28 | 25 |

*Samplers: Per Serving*

| | C | F | Cb |
|---|---|---|---|
| Classic Sampler | 870 | 25 | 121 |
| Spicy Sampler | 1010 | 34 | 125 |
| Ultimate Sampler Platter | 1120 | 29 | 165 |

*Submarinos:*

| | C | F | Cb |
|---|---|---|---|
| Fazoli's Original | 790 | 37 | 42 |
| Smoked Turkey Basil | 740 | 33 | 40 |
| Turkey Club Italiano | 730 | 28 | 41 |

*For Complete Nutritional Data ~ see CalorieKing.com*

## Firehouse Subs® (Aug '15)

*Hot Subs: Per Medium White Sub, With Standard Toppings and Dressings*

| | C | F | Cb |
|---|---|---|---|
| Ham | 740 | 37 | 71 |
| Roast Beef | 710 | 36 | 54 |
| Turkey | 670 | 35 | 58 |
| Veggie | 720 | 45 | 60 |
| **Specialty:** Club on a Sub | 780 | 43 | 64 |
| Engineer | 685 | 35 | 61 |
| Hero | 770 | 37 | 64 |
| Hook & Ladder | 700 | 37 | 64 |
| Italian | 915 | 57 | 64 |
| Meatball | 815 | 50 | 60 |
| *Sides,* Chili, Bowl | 335 | 18 | 25 |

*Under 500 Calorie Salads: With Dressing*

| | C | F | Cb |
|---|---|---|---|
| **Chopped:** With Chicken Salad | 425 | 26 | 23 |
| With Grilled Chicken | 335 | 16 | 19 |
| With Honey Ham | 405 | 19 | 33 |
| With Turkey | 345 | 17 | 21 |
| Hook & Ladder | 375 | 18 | 27 |
| House, without meat | 240 | 16 | 17 |
| Italian, with Grilled Chicken | 485 | 32 | 18 |

## Five Guys® (Aug '15)

*Burgers:*

| | C | F | Cb |
|---|---|---|---|
| Bacon Burger | 780 | 50 | 39 |
| Bacon Cheeseburger | 920 | 62 | 40 |
| Cheeseburger | 840 | 55 | 40 |
| Hamburger | 700 | 43 | 39 |

*Little Burgers:*

| | C | F | Cb |
|---|---|---|---|
| Little: Bacon Burger | 560 | 33 | 39 |
| Bacon Cheeseburger | 630 | 39 | 40 |
| Cheeseburger | 550 | 32 | 40 |
| Hamburger | 480 | 26 | 39 |

## Five Guys® cont... (Aug '15)

*Dogs:*

| | C | F | Cb |
|---|---|---|---|
| Bacon Dog; Cheese Dog | 620 | 42 | 40 |
| Bacon Cheese Dog | 695 | 48 | 41 |
| Hot Dog | 545 | 35 | 40 |

*Fries:*

| | C | F | Cb |
|---|---|---|---|
| Little Fry, 8 oz | 525 | 23 | 72 |
| Regular, 15 oz | 955 | 41 | 131 |

## Flame Broiler® (Aug '15)

*Bowls: With White Rice*

| | C | F | Cb |
|---|---|---|---|
| Beef | 620 | 11 | 74 |
| Chicken | 600 | 14 | 68 |
| Chicken & Veggie | 510 | 14 | 49 |
| Half & Half | 610 | 13 | 71 |
| The Works | 520 | 13 | 52 |

*Plates: With White Rice*

| | C | F | Cb |
|---|---|---|---|
| Beef | 840 | 18 | 94 |
| Rib | 1100 | 44 | 95 |
| The Works | 700 | 19 | 63 |

## Freshens® (Aug '15)

*Smoothies: 100% Juice (20 fl.oz)*

**Blended Fruit Classics:**

| | C | F | Cb |
|---|---|---|---|
| Bangin' Berry | 370 | 0 | 90 |
| Caribbean Craze; Maui Mango | 330 | 0 | 81 |
| Feelin' Peachy | 310 | 0 | 78 |
| Jmcn Jammer; Ornge Sunrise, av. | 320 | 2 | 70 |
| Peach On The Beach | 280 | 3 | 61 |
| Pom-Tastic; Purple Rein, av. | 320 | 0 | 80 |
| Tropical Therapy | 480 | 6 | 109 |
| Wild Strawberry | 340 | 0 | 87 |
| **Protein:** Peanut Butter | 500 | 12 | 76 |
| Power-Up | 560 | 14 | 73 |

*Crepes:*

| | C | F | Cb |
|---|---|---|---|
| Breakfast, Denver, with Bacon | 510 | 27 | 28 |

*Savory Golden Crepes:*

| | C | F | Cb |
|---|---|---|---|
| Chipotle Ranch Turkey | 430 | 24 | 27 |
| Pesto Chicken | 350 | 12 | 30 |

*Flatbreads:*

| | C | F | Cb |
|---|---|---|---|
| BBQ Chicken, 10.4 oz | 570 | 15 | 75 |
| California Club, 11 oz | 640 | 38 | 38 |
| Roasted Vegie, 10 oz | 440 | 22 | 41 |

*Rice Bowls:*

| | C | F | Cb |
|---|---|---|---|
| Bangkok Thai, 15.7 oz | 570 | 12 | 87 |
| KC BBQ, 16.8 oz | 620 | 22 | 79 |
| Mediterranean, 16 oz | 650 | 37 | 71 |

*Dessert Crepes:*

| | C | F | Cb |
|---|---|---|---|
| Cheesecake Supreme | 450 | 23 | 51 |
| Nutella Supreme | 520 | 21 | 75 |

# Fast - Foods & *Restaurants*

## Godfather's Pizza® (Aug '15)

*Golden Crust Pizza:* Per Slice

| | C | F | Cb |
|---|---|---|---|
| Cheese: Medium, 1/8 pizza | 220 | 8 | 25 |
| Large, 1/10 pizza | 250 | 9 | 28 |
| Combo: Medium, 1/8 | 290 | 13 | 27 |
| Large, 1/10 pizza | 330 | 15 | 30 |
| Super Combo: Medium, 1/8 pizza | 320 | 15 | 28 |
| Large, 1/10 pizza | 370 | 18 | 31 |

*Original Crust Pizza:*

| | C | F | Cb |
|---|---|---|---|
| Cheese: Mini, 1/4 pizza | 150 | 4 | 20 |
| Medium, 1/8 pizza | 260 | 7 | 34 |
| Jumbo, 1/12 pizza | 350 | 10 | 44 |
| Combo: Mini, 1/4 pizza | 200 | 8 | 21 |
| Medium, 1/8 pizza | 350 | 14 | 36 |
| Jumbo, 1/12 pizza | 480 | 20 | 47 |
| Super Combo: Mini, 1/4 pizza | 220 | 9 | 22 |
| Medium, 1/8 pizza | 350 | 14 | 36 |
| Jumbo, 1/12 pizza | 520 | 23 | 48 |

*Thin Crust Pizza:*

| | C | F | Cb |
|---|---|---|---|
| Cheese: Medium, 1/8 pizza | 170 | 8 | 15 |
| Large, 1/10 pizza | 210 | 10 | 17 |
| Combo: Medium, 1/8 pizza | 240 | 13 | 17 |
| Large, 1/10 pizza | 280 | 16 | 20 |
| Super Combo: Medium, 1/8 pizza | 290 | 16 | 19 |
| Large, 1/10 pizza | 330 | 19 | 20 |

*Calzones:* Per Medium Calzone

| | C | F | Cb |
|---|---|---|---|
| Cheese | 1660 | 52 | 200 |
| Combo | 1450 | 40 | 200 |
| Pepperoni | 1410 | 39 | 195 |

*Sides:*

| | C | F | Cb |
|---|---|---|---|
| Breadstick (1) | 110 | 2 | 20 |
| Cheesestick, medium, 1/8 | 200 | 7 | 24 |
| Garlic Toast: 1 piece | 150 | 9 | 15 |
| With Cheese, 1 piece | 210 | 12 | 16 |
| Chicken Wings, Buffalo (4) | 180 | 13 | 6 |
| Potato Wedges, 4 oz | 175 | 8 | 24 |

## Gold Star Chili® (Aug '15)

*Burritos & Burrito Bowls:*

| | C | L | CP |
|---|---|---|---|
| Gold Star Chili Burrito | 970 | 33 | 126 |
| Grilled Chicken Bowl | 905 | 29 | 111 |

*Coneys:*

| | C | L | CP |
|---|---|---|---|
| Cheese | 310 | 19 | 21 |
| Coney | 225 | 12 | 21 |
| Sriracha Coney | 315 | 19 | 22 |

*Ways,* Regular:

| | | | |
|---|---|---|---|
| 2-Way | 395 | 10 | 54 |
| 3-Way | 680 | 34 | 55 |
| 4-Way, Bean | 825 | 34 | 81 |
| 5-Way | 840 | 33 | 87 |
| **Ways,** Super 5-Way | 1180 | 48 | 122 |

*Chili By The Bowl:*

| | | | |
|---|---|---|---|
| Gold Star | 205 | 10 | 10 |
| Veggie | 200 | 3 | 34 |

## Gold Star Chili® cont... (Aug '15)

*Double Deckers:*

| | C | F | Cb |
|---|---|---|---|
| Ham & Bacon | 515 | 29 | 40 |
| Ham & Turkey | 620 | 26 | 48 |
| Turkey & Bacon | 590 | 30 | 44 |
| *Sandwich,* Crispy Chicken | 355 | 20 | 24 |

*Salads:* Without Dressing

| | | | |
|---|---|---|---|
| Cafe | 305 | 13 | 34 |
| Chili | 685 | 36 | 62 |
| Spring Harvest | 185 | 5 | 29 |
| *Fries:* Regular | 400 | 16 | 58 |
| Cheese | 575 | 30 | 59 |
| Chili Cheese | 680 | 36 | 63 |
| Sriracha | 425 | 16 | 64 |

## Golden Corral® (Aug '15)

*Breakfast:*

| | C | F | Cb |
|---|---|---|---|
| Bacon & Cheese Quiche, 1 slice | 290 | 21 | 15 |
| Corned Beef Hash, Grilled, 1 cup | 440 | 28 | 26 |
| Creamed Chipped Beef, 1 cup | 320 | 18 | 20 |
| French Toast, Plain, 1 slice | 200 | 6 | 29 |
| Hash Brown Casserole, 1 cup | 260 | 10 | 28 |
| Sausage Links (1) | 120 | 11 | 1 |

*Meals:* Without Sides

**Hot Buffet:**

| | | | |
|---|---|---|---|
| Awesome Pot Roast, 1 cup | 320 | 14 | 16 |
| Baked Fish w/ Shrimp & Sce, 3 oz | 160 | 10 | 2 |
| Baked Florentine Fish, 1 piece | 180 | 12 | 2 |
| BBQ: Chicken Leg Quarter, 1 pce | 490 | 22 | 21 |
| Pork, 3 oz | 170 | 8 | 5 |
| Bone-In Catfish, 3 oz | 210 | 14 | 7 |
| Bourbon Street Chicken, 3 oz | 170 | 9 | 4 |
| Lasagne, 1 piece | 430 | 26 | 21 |
| Pork Meatloaf, 1 sl. | 200 | 11 | 10 |
| Roast Beef, 3 oz | 110 | 3 | 0 |
| Salisbury Steak (1) | 130 | 4.5 | 9 |
| Sirloin Steak, 3 oz | 150 | 6 | 0 |

*Sides:* Baby Carrots; Baby Corn, av

| | | | |
|---|---|---|---|
| | 45 | 1 | 8 |
| BBQ Baked Beans, 1/2 cup | 160 | 1 | 35 |
| Breaded Okra (10) | 110 | 7 | 10 |
| Creamed Corn, 1/2 cup | 110 | 0.5 | 25 |
| Flamed Broiled Mixed Veg., 1/2 cup | 15 | 0 | 3 |
| Frield Cubed Potatoes, 1/2 cup | 160 | 9 | 19 |

*Salad Buffet:* Per 1/2 Cup Unless Indicated

| | | | |
|---|---|---|---|
| Caesar, without dressing, 1 cup | 110 | 8 | 8 |
| Cajun Potato | 230 | 17 | 15 |
| Chicken | 240 | 20 | 3 |
| Coleslaw | 110 | 9 | 6 |
| Seafood | 140 | 10 | 9 |
| Spinach Bacon, 1 cup | 120 | 9 | 4 |
| Tuna | 190 | 13 | 5 |

*Dressings:* Balsamic Vinaig., 2 T.

| | | | |
|---|---|---|---|
| | 20 | 0 | 5 |
| Caesar, 2 Tbsp | 150 | 15 | 2 |
| Ranch, 2 Tbsp | 110 | 12 | 2 |

202

## (The) Great American Bagel Co® (Aug '15)

| Bagels: | C | F | Cb |
|---|---|---|---|
| Asiago Cheese | 520 | 16 | 72 |
| Cheddar Herb | 390 | 8 | 66 |
| Cinnamon Raisin | 380 | 3.5 | 76 |
| Jalapeno Cheddar | 370 | 7 | 63 |
| Plain | 360 | 4 | 71 |
| Spinach Tomazzo | 640 | 20 | 86 |
| Tomazzo | 520 | 13 | 77 |

| *Paninis:* On Regular Baguette | | | |
|---|---|---|---|
| Chicken Pesto | 770 | 35 | 70 |
| Ham & Swiss | 600 | 26 | 58 |
| Philly Beef | 920 | 40 | 92 |
| Turkey Club | 680 | 29 | 67 |

| *Sandwiches:* Asiago Omelet | 720 | 29 | 80 |
|---|---|---|---|
| BLT | 550 | 17 | 72 |
| Chicken Parmigiana | 740 | 22 | 81 |
| Ham | 460 | 9 | 71 |
| Roast Beef | 465 | 9 | 71 |
| Turkey | 435 | 5 | 72 |

| *Cream Cheese Filling:* Per 1 oz | | | |
|---|---|---|---|
| Plain | 100 | 10 | 1 |
| Strawberry; Vegetable, average | 90 | 8 | 4 |

| Pastries: | | | |
|---|---|---|---|
| **Cookies:** Chocolate Chunk, 4 oz | 110 | 3.5 | 19 |
| Oatmeal Raisin, 4 oz | 120 | 5 | 18 |
| **Muffins:** Blueberry, 4.25 oz | 430 | 16 | 64 |
| Banana Nut, 4.25 oz | 430 | 18 | 61 |

## Green Burrito® (Aug '15)

| Burritos: | C | F | Cb |
|---|---|---|---|
| Bean & Cheese | 440 | 15 | 56 |
| Beef, Bean & Cheese | 470 | 18 | 52 |
| California: Chicken | 450 | 18 | 41 |
| Steak | 480 | 21 | 44 |
| Chicken Especial | 530 | 19 | 55 |
| Mexicano: Chicken | 500 | 16 | 54 |
| Steak | 540 | 19 | 56 |

| *Specialties:* | | | |
|---|---|---|---|
| **Super Nachos:** | | | |
| Chicken | 900 | 43 | 92 |
| Ground Beef | 970 | 51 | 95 |
| **Taco Salad:** Chicken | 770 | 39 | 67 |
| Ground Beef | 850 | 47 | 70 |
| Steak | 810 | 43 | 69 |

| *Tacos:* | | | |
|---|---|---|---|
| Ground Beef, hard taco | 210 | 12 | 16 |
| Southwest Chicken, soft | 300 | 19 | 17 |
| Street Tacos: Chicken | 140 | 6 | 13 |
| Steak | 160 | 7 | 14 |
| *Sides:* Beans, 6.25 oz | 250 | 6 | 34 |
| Chips, 2 oz | 300 | 17 | 35 |
| Guacamole, 1.4 oz | 60 | 5 | 3 |

## (The) Great Steak & Potato Company® (Aug '15)

| Breakfast Sandwiches: | C | F | Cb |
|---|---|---|---|
| Bacon, Egg & Cheese | 600 | 36 | 39 |
| Sausage, Egg & Cheese | 700 | 47 | 39 |
| Steak, Egg & Chse | 590 | 31 | 41 |

| Burgers: | | | |
|---|---|---|---|
| Bacon Cheeseburger | 680 | 45 | 33 |
| BBQ Cheeseburger | 570 | 28 | 50 |
| Cheeseburger | 600 | 39 | 33 |
| Chili Burger | 550 | 27 | 47 |
| Hamburger | 550 | 34 | 32 |
| Philly Cheeseburger | 570 | 32 | 37 |

| *Sandwiches:* 7" | | | |
|---|---|---|---|
| Bacon Cheddar Cheesesteak | 620 | 23 | 60 |
| Buffalo Chicken Philly | 800 | 42 | 66 |
| Chicagoland Cheesesteak | 640 | 25 | 61 |
| Chicken Bacon Ranch | 860 | 47 | 65 |
| Great Steak Cheesesteak | 720 | 34 | 60 |
| Gyro | 600 | 32 | 53 |
| Orig. Philly Cheesesteak | 540 | 17 | 60 |
| Pastrami Philly | 830 | 46 | 62 |
| Reuben Philly | 770 | 39 | 61 |
| Turkey Philly | 570 | 19 | 63 |
| Super Steak Cheesesteak | 720 | 34 | 62 |
| Ultimate Chicken Philly | 620 | 23 | 65 |
| Veggie Delight | 530 | 21 | 67 |
| Wisconsin Inside-Out | 550 | 26 | 55 |

| Baked Potatoes: | | | |
|---|---|---|---|
| Bacon & Cheese | 430 | 23 | 29 |
| Broccoli & cheese | 220 | 6 | 38 |
| **The Great Potato:** Chicken | 430 | 19 | 42 |
| Ham | 420 | 19 | 45 |
| Steak | 440 | 20 | 39 |
| Turkey | 390 | 16 | 41 |
| The King | 480 | 29 | 30 |

| Fries: | | | |
|---|---|---|---|
| **Great Fry:** Kids | 270 | 13 | 36 |
| Regular | 440 | 20 | 60 |
| Large | 540 | 25 | 72 |
| Coney Island Fry, Regular | 590 | 29 | 72 |
| King Fry, regular | 570 | 31 | 64 |
| Nacho Fry, regular | 490 | 23 | 64 |

| *Salads:* Without Dressing | | | |
|---|---|---|---|
| **Great Salad:** Grilled Chicken | 380 | 22 | 16 |
| Grilled Ham | 370 | 22 | 20 |
| Grilled Steak | 370 | 23 | 13 |
| Grilled Turkey | 340 | 19 | 15 |
| *Salad Dressings:* Ranch, 1 oz | 170 | 18 | 1 |
| Thousand Island, 1 oz | 130 | 12 | 4 |

## Haagen-Dazs® (Aug '15)

### *Classic Flavors: Per ½ Cup*

| | C | F | Cb |
|---|---|---|---|
| Butter Pecan | 300 | 22 | 20 |
| Caramel Cone | 320 | 20 | 30 |
| Chocolate Chocolate Chip | 300 | 19 | 26 |
| Chocolate Chip Cookie Dough | 300 | 18 | 30 |
| Chocolate Peanut Butter | 340 | 23 | 26 |
| Coffee; Green Tea | 250 | 17 | 20 |
| Dulce de Leche | 270 | 16 | 27 |
| Mint Chip | 280 | 18 | 25 |
| Pineapple Coconut | 230 | 13 | 25 |
| Rocky Road | 290 | 17 | 29 |
| Rum Raisin | 240 | 16 | 21 |
| Strawberry | 240 | 15 | 22 |
| Vanilla Swiss Almond | 290 | 19 | 24 |
| Vanilla Bean | 270 | 17 | 24 |
| White Chocolate Raspb. Truffle | 280 | 16 | 31 |

### *Frozen Yogurt: Per ½ Cup*

| | | | |
|---|---|---|---|
| Coffee | 180 | 2.5 | 31 |
| Vanilla | 170 | 2.5 | 29 |
| Vanilla Raspberry Swirl | 150 | 1 | 31 |

### *Gelato: Per ½ Cup*

| | | | |
|---|---|---|---|
| Black Cherry Amaretto; Limoncello | 240 | 9 | 35 |
| Cappuccino | 230 | 10 | 32 |
| Sea Salt Caramel | 270 | 11 | 38 |
| Stracciatella | 270 | 13 | 34 |

### *Sorbet: Per ½ Cup*

| | | | |
|---|---|---|---|
| Mango | 150 | 0 | 38 |
| Orchard Peach | 130 | 0 | 33 |
| Raspberry; Zesty Lemon, av. | 115 | 0 | 29 |

*Ice Cream Bars/Cones ~ See Page 109*

## Hardee's® (Aug '15)

### Burgers:

| | C | F | Cb |
|---|---|---|---|
| Cheeseburgers: Small | 330 | 15 | 32 |
| Double, 7 oz | 420 | 22 | 33 |
| Hamburger, Small | 280 | 12 | 32 |
| Original Turkey Burger | 390 | 17 | 31 |

### Thickburgers:

| | | | |
|---|---|---|---|
| Original, ⅓ lb | 850 | 54 | 56 |
| ½ lb Most American | 1190 | 78 | 71 |
| ⅓ lb Most American | 980 | 61 | 70 |
| ¼ lb Most American | 750 | 50 | 43 |
| Bacon Cheese, ⅓ lb | 890 | 59 | 54 |
| Double, ⅔ lb | 1200 | 81 | 58 |
| ⅓ lb El Diablo | 1170 | 75 | 83 |
| ½ lb El Diablo | 1380 | 92 | 84 |
| ¼ lb El Diablo | 940 | 61 | 63 |
| Frisco: ⅓ lb | 880 | 59 | 46 |
| ½ lb | 960 | 62 | 50 |

## Hardee's® cont... (Aug '15)

### *Burgers (Cont):*

### Thickburgers (Cont):

| | C | F | Cb |
|---|---|---|---|
| Little Thick Cheeseburger, 6 oz | 430 | 23 | 33 |
| Little Thickburger, ¼ lb | 580 | 39 | 33 |
| Low-Carb, ⅓ lb | 470 | 36 | 9 |
| Monster, ⅔ lb | 1330 | 95 | 51 |
| Mushroom 'N' Swiss: | | | |
| ⅓ lb | 710 | 41 | 52 |
| ½ lb | 820 | 46 | 56 |

### *Sandwiches:*

| | | | |
|---|---|---|---|
| Big Hot Ham 'N' Cheese | 410 | 18 | 31 |
| Big Roast Beef | 500 | 23 | 48 |
| **Chicken:** Charbroiled BBQ Chicken | 330 | 6 | 50 |
| Charbroiled Chicken Club | 540 | 31 | 38 |
| El Diablo Big Chicken | 1170 | 18 | 95 |
| Hand Breaded Chkn Tender Fillet | 530 | 32 | 38 |
| Spicy Chicken | 450 | 24 | 54 |
| The Bacon Swiss Big Chicken | 900 | 54 | 65 |
| The Big Chicken Fillet | 800 | 45 | 65 |
| **Fish,** Beer Battered Cod | 530 | 28 | 50 |

### *Breaded Chicken Tenders: Without Sauce*

| | | | |
|---|---|---|---|
| 3 pieces, 4.5 oz | 260 | 13 | 13 |
| 5 pieces, 7.5 oz | 440 | 21 | 21 |

### *Fried Chicken Pieces:*

| | | | |
|---|---|---|---|
| Breast, 5.2 oz | 370 | 15 | 29 |
| Leg, 2.4 oz | 170 | 7 | 15 |
| Thigh, 4.3 oz | 330 | 15 | 30 |
| Wing, 2.3 oz | 200 | 8 | 23 |

### *Sides:*

| | | | |
|---|---|---|---|
| Coleslaw, Small | 270 | 22 | 17 |
| **Crispy Curls:** Small | 360 | 18 | 46 |
| Medium | 470 | 23 | 60 |
| Large | 570 | 28 | 72 |
| Jalapeno Poppers | 470 | 25 | 48 |
| Mashed Potato & Gravy | 80 | 1 | 15 |
| Side Salad, without Dressing | 120 | 7 | 7 |

### *Fries & Onion Rings:*

| | | | |
|---|---|---|---|
| Beer Battered Onion Rings, 4.5 oz | 410 | 24 | 45 |
| **Natural Cut Fries:** Small, 4 oz | 360 | 18 | 47 |
| Medium, 5.85 oz | 490 | 24 | 63 |
| Large, 6.8 oz | 530 | 26 | 69 |

### *Kids Meals: Includes Kid's Fries*

| | | | |
|---|---|---|---|
| Cheeseburger | 550 | 26 | 61 |
| Chicken Tenders | 400 | 19 | 37 |
| Hamburger | 500 | 22 | 61 |

*Continued Next Page...*

## Hardee's® cont... (Aug '15)

### Breakfast:

| | C | F | Cb |
|---|---|---|---|
| **Biscuits:** Bacon, Egg & Cheese | 460 | 26 | 38 |
| Biscuit 'N' Gravy | 460 | 26 | 49 |
| Chicken Fillet | 550 | 32 | 47 |
| Cinnamon 'N Raisin | 340 | 15 | 49 |
| Country Steak | 510 | 31 | 44 |
| Grilled Pork Chop | 400 | 19 | 36 |
| With Egg & Cheese | 510 | 27 | 38 |
| Loaded Omelet | 490 | 28 | 40 |
| Made From Scratch | 300 | 15 | 36 |
| Mile High Bacon, Egg & Cheese | 670 | 42 | 41 |
| Monster | 730 | 49 | 40 |
| Sausage and Egg | 560 | 37 | 39 |
| **Bowl,** Low Carb | 660 | 52 | 10 |
| **Burrito,** Loaded | 580 | 30 | 46 |
| **Platter,** with Bacon | 750 | 43 | 67 |
| **Sandwiches:** Bacon Grilled Cheese | 480 | 23 | 45 |
| Frisco | 450 | 19 | 45 |
| Ham Grilled Cheese | 510 | 25 | 45 |
| Sausage Grilled Cheese | 670 | 41 | 46 |
| **Sunrise Croissant,** with Ham | 400 | 23 | 29 |

### Breakfast Sides:

| | C | F | Cb |
|---|---|---|---|
| Grits | 100 | 3 | 16 |
| **Hash Rounds:** Small, 2.9 oz | 260 | 15 | 23 |
| Medium, 4.2 oz | 370 | 22 | 33 |
| Large, 5.8 oz | 510 | 30 | 45 |

### Desserts:

| | C | F | Cb |
|---|---|---|---|
| Apple Turnover w/o Cinn. Sugar | 270 | 13 | 35 |
| Chocolate Chip Cookie (2), 2 oz | 240 | 10 | 36 |
| Single Scoop Ice Cream: | | | |
| Bowl, 4 oz | 240 | 13 | 27 |
| Cone, 4.4 oz | 290 | 13 | 37 |

### Drinks:

| | C | F | Cb |
|---|---|---|---|
| **Hot Chocolate** | 150 | 3 | 18 |
| **Ice Cream Malts:** | | | |
| Chocolate, 14 oz | 780 | 35 | 99 |
| Strawberry, 14 oz | 770 | 35 | 97 |
| Vanilla, 14 oz | 780 | 35 | 98 |
| **Ice Cream Shakes:** | | | |
| Choc.; Strawb., av., 14 oz | 705 | 34 | 86 |
| Vanilla, 14 oz | 700 | 33 | 86 |

## Hissho Sushi® (Aug '15)

### Starters: With White Rice

| | C | F | Cb |
|---|---|---|---|
| Baby Octopus Salad, 4 oz | 170 | 3 | 20 |
| Chicken Gyoza, 4 oz | 180 | 6 | 20 |
| Pork Gyoza, 4 oz | 230 | 11 | 23 |
| Spring Rolls: Regular, 7 oz | 185 | 4 | 30 |
| Ocean, 7 oz | 180 | 2 | 29 |
| Squid Salad, 4 oz | 95 | 2 | 7 |

### Maki Sushi: With White Rice

| | C | F | Cb |
|---|---|---|---|
| **Rolls:** Blazing California, 7 oz | 405 | 12 | 65 |
| California, 7 oz | 295 | 3 | 59 |
| Dynamaite Roll, 7 oz | 470 | 13 | 66 |
| Eel, 7 oz | 375 | 1 | 69 |
| Hissho Healthy, 6 oz | 210 | 1 | 46 |
| Nippon Favorite, 6 oz | 300 | 4 | 45 |
| Philadelphia, 7 oz | 385 | 12 | 60 |
| Snow Crab, 7 oz | 280 | 3 | 56 |
| Spicy, 7 oz | 430 | 11 | 62 |
| Sushicado,7 oz | 290 | 3 | 54 |
| Veggie Roll, 7 oz | 275 | 2 | 57 |

### Specialty Items:

**Rolls:** Per 7 oz Roll Unless Indicated

| | C | F | Cb |
|---|---|---|---|
| Caterpillar | 480 | 5 | 84 |
| Living Color | 370 | 5 | 51 |
| Mango Tango | 420 | 10 | 58 |
| Salmon Lover | 720 | 32 | 63 |
| Sriracha Party | 540 | 14 | 77 |
| Tempura Shrimp, 9 oz | 664 | 19 | 108 |
| TNT | 545 | 14 | 71 |
| Wasabi Crunch | 550 | 19 | 76 |

## Hot Dog on a Stick® (Aug '15)

### Menu Items:

| | C | F | Cb |
|---|---|---|---|
| American Cheese on a Stick | 260 | 16 | 21 |
| Beef Hot Dog on a Bun | 340 | 23 | 22 |
| Turkey Hot Dog on a Stick | 240 | 13 | 23 |
| Veggie Dog on a Stick | 220 | 8 | 24 |
| Pepperjack Cheese on a Stick | 240 | 14 | 19 |
| **Sides,** French Fries, 4.5 oz | 400 | 21 | 49 |
| **Dessert,** Funnel Cake Sticks, (10) | 210 | 8 | 31 |
| **Beverages:** Per Regular Size, 16 fl.oz | | | |
| Lemonade: Original | 150 | 0 | 38 |
| Sugar Free | 15 | 0 | 3 |
| Lime | 230 | 0 | 57 |

## Hungry Howie's Pizza® (Aug '15)

*Counts may vary in Florida.*

*Pizzas: Per Slice of Buttercrust Pizza*

| | C | F | Cb |
|---|---|---|---|
| BBQ Chicken: Small, ⅙ pizza | 210 | 6 | 27 |
| Medium, ⅛ pizza | 240 | 8 | 30 |
| Large, ⅒ pizza | 260 | 8 | 32 |
| X-Large, ⅟₁₂ pizza | 300 | 9 | 39 |

*Calzones: Per Regular 8" Calzone*

| | | | |
|---|---|---|---|
| Deluxe Italian | 660 | 23 | 81 |
| Ham & Cheese | 590 | 15 | 68 |
| Steak, Cheese & Mushroom | 610 | 18 | 81 |
| Turkey Club | 660 | 18 | 80 |
| Veggie | 610 | 19 | 83 |

*Wings:*

| | | | |
|---|---|---|---|
| Asian, 5 wings | 440 | 28 | 11 |
| Original Howie, 5 wings | 400 | 29 | 0 |

*Salads: Per Regular*

| | | | |
|---|---|---|---|
| Antipasto | 170 | 10 | 10 |
| Chef | 140 | 8 | 9 |
| Garden | 70 | 2 | 12 |
| Greek | 140 | 7 | 15 |

*Dressings: Per 1 oz*

| | | | |
|---|---|---|---|
| Creamy Italian | 120 | 12 | 2 |
| Greek | 110 | 11 | 2 |
| Ranch | 180 | 19 | 1 |
| Thousand Island | 140 | 14 | 4 |

## In-N-Out Burger® (Aug '15)

*Burgers:*

| | C | F | Cb |
|---|---|---|---|
| **Hamburger:** With Onion | 390 | 19 | 39 |
| With Mustard/Ketchup, w/o Spread | 310 | 10 | 41 |
| Protein Style w/ Lettuce Wrap, w/o Bun | 240 | 17 | 11 |
| **Cheeseburger:** With Onion | 480 | 27 | 39 |
| With Mustard/Ketchup, w/o Spread | 400 | 18 | 41 |
| Protein Style w/ Lettuce Wrap, w/o Bun | 330 | 25 | 11 |
| **Double Double:** With Onion | 670 | 41 | 39 |
| With Mustard/Ketchup, w/o Spread | 590 | 32 | 41 |
| Protein Style w/ Lettuce Wrap, w/o Bun | 520 | 39 | 11 |
| *French Fries*, 4.5 oz | 395 | 18 | 54 |
| *Drinks:* Milk, 10 fl.oz | 180 | 6 | 18 |
| Coca-Cola, 16 fl.oz | 195 | 0 | 54 |
| Dr Pepper; 7-Up, av., 16 fl.oz | 200 | 0 | 53 |
| Lemonade, 16 fl.oz | 180 | 0 | 40 |
| Root Beer, 16 fl.oz | 220 | 0 | 60 |
| **Shakes:** | | | |
| Chocolate, 15 fl.oz | 590 | 29 | 72 |
| Strawberry, 15 fl.oz | 590 | 27 | 81 |
| Vanilla, 15 fl.oz | 580 | 31 | 67 |

## IHOP® (Aug '15)

*Pancakes:*

| | C | F | Cb |
|---|---|---|---|
| **Buttermilk:** With Menu Toppings | | | |
| Full Stack (5) | 660 | 20 | 100 |
| Short Stack (3) | 410 | 14 | 60 |
| Chocolate Chocolate Chip (4) | 630 | 21 | 97 |
| Double Blueberry (4) | 620 | 15 | 106 |
| Strawberry Banana (4) | 690 | 15 | 126 |

*Condiments:*

| | | | |
|---|---|---|---|
| Syrup: Blueberry; Maple, 1 fl.oz | 110 | 0 | 27 |
| Boysenberry; Strawberry, 1 fl.oz | 100 | 0 | 26 |
| Sugar-Free Syrup, 1 fl.oz | 15 | 0 | 6 |

*French Toast & Waffles: W/ Toppings Unless Indicated*

| | | | |
|---|---|---|---|
| **French Toast:** Original | 720 | 30 | 92 |
| Berry Berry Brioche | 770 | 29 | 114 |
| Double Dipped: Cinnamon Sugar | 820 | 91 | 110 |
| Lemon Strawberry | 1580 | 91 | 137 |
| Strawberry Banana | 880 | 28 | 138 |
| **Waffle,** Belgian | 500 | 24 | 60 |

*Crepes:*

| | | | |
|---|---|---|---|
| **Cheese Blintzes:** | | | |
| With Blueberry Topping | 1000 | 58 | 95 |
| With Strawberry Topping | 990 | 58 | 94 |
| Chicken Florentine | 760 | 42 | 44 |
| German Crepes | 630 | 35 | 65 |
| Swedish Crepes | 650 | 34 | 71 |

*Made To Order Omelettes: Without Pancakes or Sides*

| | | | |
|---|---|---|---|
| Big Steak | 1260 | 90 | 48 |
| Garden | 930 | 76 | 18 |
| Hearty Ham & Cheese | 1040 | 79 | 17 |
| Spinach & Mushroom | 980 | 82 | 21 |

*Breakfast Combinations: As Served, w/o Syrup*

| | | | |
|---|---|---|---|
| Biscuits & Gravy Combo with Country Gravy | 1380 | 87 | 108 |
| Breakfast Sampler | 1150 | 73 | 73 |
| Chicken Fried Chicken & Eggs, with Country Gravy | 1130 | 64 | 90 |
| Chorizo & Eggs | 1420 | 91 | 98 |
| T-Bone Steak & Eggs, 12 oz | 1180 | 63 | 64 |

*Sandwiches: Without Sides*

| | | | |
|---|---|---|---|
| Chicken Clubhouse Super Stacker | 1130 | 74 | 62 |
| Double BLT | 670 | 46 | 40 |
| Ham & Egg Melt | 1270 | 74 | 79 |
| Turkey Berry Melt | 1200 | 68 | 81 |

*Dinner Classics: With Set Sides, excluding Baked Potato, Salad or Soup*

| | | | |
|---|---|---|---|
| Chkn Fried Chkn, w/ Country Gravy | 770 | 37 | 84 |
| Pot Roast | 980 | 52 | 80 |
| T-Bone Steak, 12 oz | 830 | 42 | 54 |

## Jack in the Box® (Aug '15)

### Sandwiches & Burgers:

| | C | F | Cb |
|---|---|---|---|
| Bacon Ultimate Cheeseburger | 905 | 56 | 44 |
| Black Pepper Cheeseburger | 795 | 48 | 55 |
| Classic Buttery Jack | 815 | 52 | 50 |
| Cheeseburger | 320 | 14 | 32 |
| Hamburger | 280 | 11 | 32 |
| Jumbo Jack: | | | |
| With Cheese | 570 | 30 | 45 |
| Without Cheese | 490 | 23 | 44 |
| Junior Bacon Cheeseburger | 385 | 21 | 32 |
| Sirloin Cheeseburger | 930 | 65 | 48 |
| Sourdough Jack | 660 | 41 | 40 |
| Ultimate Cheeseburger | 820 | 49 | 44 |

### Chicken & Fish:

| | C | F | Cb |
|---|---|---|---|
| Chicken Sandwich | 415 | 21 | 42 |
| With Bacon | 470 | 25 | 42 |
| Chicken Strips: Crispy, 4 pieces | 565 | 24 | 53 |
| Grilled, 4 pieces | 250 | 7 | 5 |
| Fish Sandwich | 380 | 14 | 45 |
| Jack's Spicy Chkn S'wich | 530 | 20 | 61 |
| With Cheese | 600 | 25 | 62 |
| Sourdough Gr. Chicken Club | 535 | 26 | 38 |

### Breakfast:

| | C | F | Cb |
|---|---|---|---|
| **Biscuit:** Bacon, Egg & Cheese | 410 | 25 | 26 |
| Sausage, Egg & Cheese | 535 | 38 | 27 |
| **Breakfast Jack:** Regular | 285 | 11 | 30 |
| With Bacon | 310 | 14 | 30 |
| **Burrito:** Meat Lovers | 790 | 50 | 50 |
| Steak & Egg | 850 | 50 | 67 |
| **Croissants:** Sausage | 560 | 39 | 32 |
| Supreme | 450 | 27 | 32 |
| **Hash Brown Plank** | 185 | 13 | 17 |
| **Meaty Burrito,** with salsa | 600 | 36 | 40 |
| **Sandwiches:** Extreme Sausage | 645 | 45 | 32 |
| Sourdough | 410 | 21 | 35 |
| Ultimate | 520 | 25 | 42 |

### Snacks & Sides:

| | C | F | Cb |
|---|---|---|---|
| Bacon Cheddar Potato Wedges | 600 | 41 | 58 |
| Chiquita Apple Bites, w/ Caramel Dip | 70 | 0 | 17 |
| Egg Rolls (3), w/o sauce | 440 | 22 | 46 |
| Mozzarella Cheese Sticks: | | | |
| 3 Pieces | 280 | 16 | 22 |
| 6 Pieces | 560 | 33 | 43 |
| Stuffed Jalapenos: | | | |
| 3 Pieces | 220 | 12 | 21 |
| 7 Pieces | 510 | 29 | 49 |
| Onion Rings (8), 4.3 oz | 450 | 28 | 45 |
| Seasoned Curly Fries, med., 4.5 oz | 430 | 25 | 46 |

## Jack in the Box® cont... (Aug '15)

### Better For You:

| | C | F | Cb |
|---|---|---|---|
| Chicken Fajita Pita, without Salsa | 365 | 13 | 42 |
| Chicken Teriyaki Bowl | 690 | 6 | 134 |
| Grilled Chicken Strips, | | | |
| w/ Teriyaki Dipping Sce | 310 | 8 | 15 |

### Salads: No Dressing or Condiments

| | C | F | Cb |
|---|---|---|---|
| Chicken Club with Grilled Chicken | 370 | 20 | 11 |
| Grilled Chicken | 250 | 10 | 13 |
| Southwest Chicken, | | | |
| with Grilled Chicken Strips | 355 | 15 | 27 |
| **Croutons** | 70 | 3 | 9 |
| **Dressings:** Creamy Southwest | 190 | 19 | 3 |
| Ranch | 250 | 25 | 5 |
| Low Fat Balsamic Vinaigrette | 30 | 1.5 | 4 |

### Sauces:

| | C | F | Cb |
|---|---|---|---|
| **Dipping Sauce:** Barbecue, 1 oz | 40 | 0 | 10 |
| Buttermilk, 1 oz | 130 | 13 | 3 |
| Frank's Red Hot Buffalo, 1 oz | 10 | 0 | 1 |
| Sweet & Sour, 1 oz | 45 | 0 | 11 |
| Tartar, 1 oz | 150 | 16 | 2 |
| **Sandwich Sauce:** | | | |
| Mayo-Onion, 0.5 oz | 90 | 10 | 0 |
| Peppercorn Mayo, 1.5 oz | 280 | 31 | 1 |
| Sundried Tomato Sauce, 0.6 oz | 80 | 8 | 1 |

### Desserts:

| | C | F | Cb |
|---|---|---|---|
| Chocolate Overload Cake | 300 | 7 | 57 |
| Churros, Mini (5) | 345 | 18 | 42 |
| New York Style Cheesecake | 310 | 17 | 32 |

### Shakes: 16 oz, with Whipped Topping

| | C | F | Cb |
|---|---|---|---|
| Chocolate | 780 | 38 | 103 |
| Oreo Cookie | 795 | 43 | 92 |
| Strawberry | 760 | 38 | 97 |
| Vanilla | 685 | 38 | 78 |

*For Complete Nutritional Data ~ see CalorieKing.com*

## Jack's® (Aug '15)

### Burgers & Sandwiches:

| | C | F | Cb |
|---|---|---|---|
| Big Bacon Burger | 610 | 41 | 31 |
| Big Jack Burger | 530 | 33 | 35 |
| Cheeseburger | 380 | 21 | 31 |
| Chicken Fillet Sandwich | 490 | 24 | 40 |
| Double Big Jack Cheese Burger | 850 | 59 | 35 |
| Double Cheeseburger | 540 | 33 | 31 |
| Grilled Chicken Sandwich | 380 | 16 | 32 |
| Hamburger | 340 | 18 | 31 |
| *Chicken,* Chicken Fingers, 3 pieces | 300 | 14 | 14 |
| *Fries,* regular | 310 | 13 | 42 |
| *Breakfast:* Egg & Cheese Biscuit | 360 | 21 | 31 |
| Sausage, Egg & Cheese Biscuit | 520 | 35 | 32 |
| Steak Biscuit | 480 | 28 | 43 |

*For Complete Menu & Data ~ see CalorieKing.com*

## Jamba Juice® (Aug '15)

*Freshly Squeezed Juice:* 16 fl.oz

| | C | F | Cb |
|---|---|---|---|
| Cucumber Orange Cooler | 190 | 1 | 46 |
| Purely Carrot | 130 | 0.5 | 30 |
| Purely Orange | 220 | 1 | 52 |
| Tropical Kick-Start | 210 | 1 | 50 |

*Smoothies:* Per 16 fl.oz

| | | | |
|---|---|---|---|
| Classic: Banana Berry | 280 | 1 | 67 |
| Mango-A-Go-Go | 300 | 1.5 | 69 |
| Peach Pleasure | 280 | 1 | 65 |
| Razzamatazz | 290 | 1 | 67 |
| Strawberry Surf Rider | 320 | 1 | 78 |
| Strawberry Wild | 260 | 0 | 62 |

**Make It Light:**

| | | | |
|---|---|---|---|
| Aloha Pineapple | 190 | 0 | 40 |
| Caribbean Passion | 150 | 0 | 34 |
| Razzmatazz | 180 | 0 | 41 |

*Tasty Bites:*

**Artisan Flat Bread:** *Per Flatbread*

| | | | |
|---|---|---|---|
| Four Cheese | 420 | 16 | 46 |
| Sweet 'n Spicy | 390 | 10 | 53 |

**Baked Goods:** *Per Item*

| | | | |
|---|---|---|---|
| Apple Cinnamon Pretzel | 380 | 4 | 76 |
| Cheddar Tomato Twist | 240 | 4.5 | 41 |
| Sourdough Parmesan Pretzel | 410 | 10 | 67 |
| Sweet Belgian Waffle | 310 | 15 | 41 |

**Breakfast Wraps:**

| | | | |
|---|---|---|---|
| Spinach 'n Cheese | 240 | 8 | 30 |
| Turkey Sausage 'n Cheese | 320 | 16 | 29 |

**Steel-Cut Oatmeal:** *With Soymilk*

| | | | |
|---|---|---|---|
| Plain | 180 | 2.5 | 35 |
| Add: Apple Cinnamon | 70 | 0 | 16 |
| Banana | 50 | 0 | 13 |
| Blueberries | 10 | 0 | 2 |
| Brown Sugar Crumble | 40 | 1 | 8 |
| Strawberries | 5 | 0 | 1 |

**Toasted Bistro Sandwiches:**

| | | | |
|---|---|---|---|
| Ham, Jarlsberg & Dijon | 290 | 8 | 33 |
| Roast Chkn, Cheddar & Hon. Dijon | 290 | 7 | 34 |
| Three Cheeses | 330 | 14 | 32 |

*Energy Bowls:* Per 16 fl.oz

| | | | |
|---|---|---|---|
| Acai Primo | 530 | 13 | 101 |
| Chunky Strawberry | 570 | 17 | 90 |
| Fruit & Greek Yogurt | 360 | 4 | 61 |

## Jersey Mike's Subs® (Aug '15)

*Cold Subs:* Per Regular, on White, without Vinegar, Oil or Mayo Unless Indicated

| | C | F | Cb |
|---|---|---|---|
| #1 BLT | 550 | 23 | 63 |
| #2 Jersey Shore Favorite | 565 | 15 | 70 |
| #3 American Classic | 560 | 15 | 69 |
| #5 Super Sub | 580 | 16 | 71 |
| #6 Roast Beef & Provolone | 720 | 22 | 67 |
| #7 Turkey Breast & Provolone | 535 | 12 | 67 |
| #8 Club Sub with Mayonnaise | 895 | 49 | 70 |
| #9 Club Supreme w/ Mayonnaise | 940 | 49 | 69 |
| #10 Albacore Tuna | 915 | 56 | 70 |
| #13 Original Italian | 680 | 24 | 72 |
| #14 Veggie | 670 | 29 | 69 |

*Hot Subs:* Per Regular on White Roll

| | | | |
|---|---|---|---|
| #15 Meatball & Cheese | 830 | 42 | 75 |
| #17: Chicken Philly | 720 | 23 | 71 |
| Steak Philly | 650 | 22 | 71 |
| #18 Grilled Chicken Parmesan | 545 | 14 | 64 |
| #19 BBQ Beef | 750 | 18 | 87 |
| #20 Pastrami & Swiss | 665 | 21 | 70 |
| #43: Chipotle Chicken, with Mayo | 1000 | 53 | 74 |
| Chipotle Steak, with Mayo | 930 | 52 | 74 |
| #56: Big Kahuna Steak | 710 | 26 | 73 |
| Big Kahuna Chicken | 770 | 27 | 72 |

*Cold Wraps:* With Flour Tortilla, w/o Vin./Oil or Mayo

| | | | |
|---|---|---|---|
| #1 BLT | 580 | 29 | 59 |
| #2 Jersey Shore Favorite | 580 | 22 | 64 |
| #3 American Classic | 580 | 22 | 63 |
| #5 Super Sub | 600 | 22 | 65 |

*Salads:* Without Dressing

| | | | |
|---|---|---|---|
| Chef, 16 oz | 255 | 10 | 16 |
| Grilled Chicken Caesar, 12.5 oz | 510 | 35 | 11 |
| Tossed, 12 oz | 50 | 0.5 | 11 |
| Tuna, 18 oz | 690 | 60 | 15 |

*Dressings:* Per 2 Tbsp, 1 oz

| | | | |
|---|---|---|---|
| Caesar | 150 | 15 | 2 |
| Chipotle Mayo | 180 | 20 | 0 |
| Golden Italian | 110 | 11 | 3 |
| Ranch | 120 | 12 | 2 |
| Russian | 160 | 16 | 4 |

*Desserts:* Cookie, Choc Chip, 1.5 oz

| | | | |
|---|---|---|---|
| Cookie, Choc Chip, 1.5 oz | 190 | 9 | 26 |
| Chocolate Brownie, 4 oz | 470 | 21 | 79 |

*Drinks:* Mountain Dew, 22 oz

| | | | |
|---|---|---|---|
| Mountain Dew, 22 oz | 310 | 0 | 84 |
| Mug Root Beer, 22 oz | 290 | 0. | 79 |
| Tropicana Twister Orange, 22 oz | 360 | 0 | 96 |

Updated Nutrition Data ~ www.CalorieKing.com
Persons with Diabetes ~ See Disclaimer (Page 22)

## Jimmy John's® (Aug '15)

*Subs: (8")* **C** **F** **Cb**

*Figures Based on French Bread w/ Standard Toppings & Mayo, Unless Indicated*

| | C | F | Cb |
|---|---|---|---|
| #1 Pepe | 600 | 31 | 58 |
| #2 Big John | 510 | 23 | 55 |
| #3 Totally Tuna, without mayo | 690 | 35 | 61 |
| #4 Turkey Tom | 480 | 21 | 56 |
| #5 Vito with Italian Vinaigrette | 610 | 32 | 60 |
| #6 Vegetarian | 660 | 39 | 60 |
| JJBLT | 570 | 32 | 55 |

*Giant Club Sandwiches: Figures Based on French Bread w/ Standard Toppings & Mayo, Unless Indicated*

| | C | F | Cb |
|---|---|---|---|
| #7 Gourmet Smoked Ham | 760 | 35 | 70 |
| #8 Billy Club | 790 | 37 | 68 |
| #9 Italian Night w/ Mayo & Vinaig. | 935 | 54 | 72 |
| #10 Hunter's Club | 800 | 38 | 66 |
| #11 Country Club | 750 | 34 | 69 |
| #12 Beach Club | 810 | 43 | 71 |
| #13 Gourmet Veggie Club | 970 | 60 | 72 |
| #14 Bootlegger | 660 | 27 | 66 |
| #15 Club Tuna w/o dressing | 1000 | 56 | 73 |
| #16 Club Lulu | 720 | 35 | 66 |
| #17 Ultimate Porker, with 9-grain wheat bread | 730 | 36 | 67 |

*Plain Slims: Figures Based on French Bread without Toppings, Dressing or Mayo*

| | C | F | Cb |
|---|---|---|---|
| Slim 1 Ham & Cheese | 540 | 13 | 76 |
| Slim 2 Roast Beef | 450 | 5.5 | 73 |
| Slim 3 Tuna Salad | 785 | 36 | 78 |
| Slim 4 Turkey Breast | 420 | 3 | 74 |
| Slim 5 Salami Capicola & Cheese | 625 | 23 | 75 |
| Slim 6 Double Provolone | 580 | 21 | 75 |

*Sides:*

| | C | F | Cb |
|---|---|---|---|
| **Jimmy Chips:** BBQ, 1 oz | 150 | 8 | 17 |
| Jalapeno, 1 oz | 150 | 8 | 17 |
| Regular, 1 oz | 150 | 9 | 16 |
| Sea Salt & Vinegar, 1 oz | 150 | 8 | 17 |
| Thinny, 1 oz | 130 | 5 | 19 |
| Jumbo Kosher Dill Pickle | 20 | 0 | 4 |

## Johnny Rockets® (Aug '15)

*Original Hamburgers:* **C** **F** **Cb**

| | C | F | Cb |
|---|---|---|---|
| Hamburger #12 | 950 | 60 | 57 |
| Original Burger | 900 | 59 | 54 |
| **Rocket:** Single | 950 | 60 | 56 |
| Double | 1420 | 97 | 56 |
| Route 66 | 1000 | 68 | 52 |
| **Smoke House:** Single | 1100 | 66 | 70 |
| Double | 1660 | 110 | 70 |
| Streamliner | 420 | 11 | 59 |

## Johnny Rockets® ...cont (Aug '15)

*Chicken Tenders:* **C** **F** **Cb**

| | C | F | Cb |
|---|---|---|---|
| 3 pieces, without sauce | 440 | 28 | 21 |
| 6 pieces, without sauce | 880 | 56 | 42 |
| *Hot Dogs:* Regular, w/out sauce | 410 | 22 | 34 |
| Chili Cheese Dog | 770 | 51 | 42 |

*Philly Cheese Steaks:*

| | C | F | Cb |
|---|---|---|---|
| With Cheddar, 11.7 oz | 780 | 40 | 55 |
| With Swiss, 12 oz | 830 | 42 | 57 |
| *Chicken Philly,* w/ Chedd, 11.7 oz | 660 | 24 | 58 |

*Sandwiches:*

| | C | F | Cb |
|---|---|---|---|
| BLT, on White Bread | 480 | 26 | 49 |
| Chicken Club, on White Bread | 920 | 36 | 77 |
| Grilled Chicken, on Hamburger Bun | 590 | 26 | 52 |
| Tuna Salad, on White Bread | 750 | 48 | 47 |

*Salads: Without Dressing*

| | C | F | Cb |
|---|---|---|---|
| Breaded Chicken Club | 660 | 45 | 23 |
| Egg Salad | 390 | 35 | 2 |
| Grilled Chkn Club | 510 | 28 | 12 |
| Garden Salad | 280 | 19 | 9 |
| Tuna Salad | 370 | 29 | 0 |

*Breakfast: With Menu Set Components*

| | C | F | Cb |
|---|---|---|---|
| 2 French Toast with Bacon | 600 | 29 | 56 |
| 2 Pancakes with Bacon | 380 | 19 | 36 |
| Patty & 2 Eggs, Beef & Potatoes | 1150 | 86 | 46 |
| Sandwiches: Egg, Bacon, White | 810 | 60 | 46 |
| Egg, Bacon Rye | 850 | 61 | 50 |
| Egg, Ham, English Muffin | 820 | 5 | 55 |
| The Works | 1000 | 70 | 55 |

*Starters:*

**Fries:**

| | C | F | Cb |
|---|---|---|---|
| American Fries, 7 oz | 480 | 19 | 69 |
| Bacon Cheese Fries, 13 oz | 830 | 44 | 82 |
| Cheese Fries, 12 oz | 740 | 37 | 82 |
| Chili Cheese Fries, 14 oz | 1000 | 56 | 93 |
| ½ Rings & ½ American Fries, 8 oz | 660 | 29 | 79 |
| Onion Rings, 9 oz | 880 | 40 | 90 |
| Rocket Wings, Traditional, without Dressing, 7 wings | 660 | 49 | 19 |
| *Desserts:* Apple Pie | 620 | 34 | 74 |
| Super Sundae w/ Hot Fudge, Almonds & Wh. Cream, 11 oz | 660 | 41 | 65 |

*Beverages:*

| | C | F | Cb |
|---|---|---|---|
| Coke, 20 oz | 240 | 0 | 67 |
| Fanta Orange, 20 oz | 270 | 0 | 74 |
| Minute Made Lemonade, 20 oz | 240 | 0 | 65 |

*Deluxe Shakes:*

| | C | F | Cb |
|---|---|---|---|
| Chocolate Vanilla Twist, 12 oz | 910 | 50 | 102 |
| Oreo Cookies & Cream, 12 oz | 1030 | 61 | 110 |
| Strawberry Banana, 11.5 oz | 900 | 50 | 99 |

## KFC® (Aug '15)

*Chicken Pieces: Per Piece*

| | C | F | Cb |
|---|---|---|---|
| **Original Recipe:** Breast, 5.8 oz | 320 | 14 | 13 |
| Drumstick, 1.8 oz | 120 | 7 | 3 |
| Thigh, 3.4 oz | 290 | 21 | 8 |
| Whole Wing, 2 oz | 140 | 8 | 5 |
| Original Recipe Bites: 6 Bites | 200 | 9 | 7 |
| 10 Bites | 330 | 15 | 12 |
| **Extra Crispy:** Breast, 6.4 oz | 490 | 29 | 20 |
| Drumstick, 2 oz | 160 | 10 | 5 |
| Tenders: 1 Tender, 1.8 oz | 130 | 7 | 6 |
| ½ Family Tray | 500 | 26 | 22 |
| Full Family Tray | 1010 | 53 | 45 |
| Thigh, 3.8 oz | 370 | 26 | 15 |
| Whole Wing, 2 oz | 210 | 15 | 8 |
| **Kentucky Grilled:** | | | |
| Breast, 4.3 oz | 220 | 7 | 0 |
| Drumstick, 1.5 oz | 90 | 4 | 0 |
| Thigh, 2.5 oz | 170 | 10 | 0 |
| Whole Wing, 1.3 oz | 80 | 4.5 | 1 |
| **Spicy Crispy:** | | | |
| Breast, 6.2 oz | 520 | 34 | 23 |
| Drumstick, 2 oz | 150 | 10 | 5 |
| Thigh, 3.5 oz | 350 | 27 | 11 |
| Whole Wing, 1.7 oz | 160 | 12 | 6 |
| **Go Cups:** Chicken Littles | 600 | 33 | 58 |
| Exta Crispy Tenders | 540 | 28 | 46 |
| Fiery Buff. Hot Wings | 510 | 28 | 50 |
| HBBQ Hot Wings | 540 | 28 | 58 |
| Hot Wings | 490 | 27 | 45 |
| Popcorn Nuggets | 570 | 31 | 53 |
| **Popcorn Nuggets:** Kids | 270 | 16 | 18 |
| Large | 570 | 33 | 37 |
| ½ Family Tray | 700 | 41 | 46 |
| Family Tray | 1410 | 83 | 92 |
| **Wings:** *Without Dipping Sauce* | | | |
| Fiery Buffalo, Hot | 70 | 4 | 5 |
| Honey BBQ, Hot | 80 | 4 | 8 |
| Hot | 70 | 4 | 3 |
| **Dipping Sauces:** *Per 0.9 oz Container* | | | |
| Buttermilk Ranch | 100 | 10 | 2 |
| Colonel's Buttery Spread | 30 | 3.5 | 0 |
| Creamy Buffalo | 70 | 7 | 2 |
| Honey Mustard | 120 | 10 | 6 |
| Summertime BBQ | 40 | 0 | 9 |
| Sweet & Tangy | 45 | 0 | 12 |

## KFC® cont... (Aug '15)

*KFC Famous Bowls & Pot Pie:*

| | C | F | Cb |
|---|---|---|---|
| **Famous Bowl:** Snack Size, 7 oz | 270 | 12 | 28 |
| 19 oz | 710 | 31 | 82 |
| **Chicken Pot Pie,** 14 oz | 790 | 45 | 66 |
| **Sandwiches:** *With Sauce* | | | |
| Chicken Littles | 310 | 18 | 23 |
| Colonal's Original | 500 | 23 | 47 |
| Crispy Twister | 630 | 34 | 49 |
| Doublicious | 580 | 29 | 47 |
| Honey BBQ | 320 | 3.5 | 47 |
| **Salads:** *Without Dressing or Croutons* | | | |
| Caesar, Side | 40 | 2 | 2 |
| Crispy Chicken BLT | 350 | 18 | 18 |
| Crispy Chicken Caesar | 330 | 17 | 16 |
| House Side Salad | 15 | 0 | 3 |
| **Dressings & Add-Ins:** | | | |
| Creamy Parmesan Caesar, 2 oz | 260 | 26 | 4 |
| Light Italian, 1 oz | 15 | 0.5 | 2 |
| Original Ranch Fat Free, 1.5 oz | 35 | 0 | 8 |
| Croutons, Parm. Garlic, 1 pouch | 70 | 3 | 8 |
| **Homestyle Sides:** *Per Single Portion* | | | |
| BBQ Baked Beans, 4.5 oz | 230 | 1.5 | 39 |
| Biscuit, 2 oz | 180 | 8 | 23 |
| Cole Slaw, 4.2 oz | 170 | 10 | 19 |
| Corn on the Cob (3"), 2.5 oz | 70 | 0.5 | 16 |
| Cornbread Muffin, 2 oz | 210 | 9 | 28 |
| Macaroni & Cheese, 4.8 oz | 170 | 6 | 22 |
| Mashed Potatoes, with Gravy, 5 oz | 120 | 4 | 19 |
| Potato Wedges, 3.8 oz | 290 | 15 | 35 |
| Sweet Kernel Corn | 100 | 0.5 | 21 |
| **Homestyle Sides:** *Per Family Portion* | | | |
| Baked Beans | 750 | 5 | 22 |
| Coleslaw | 620 | 36 | 69 |
| Green Beans | 90 | 0.5 | 17 |
| Macaroni & Cheese | 560 | 22 | 74 |
| Mashed Potatoes & Gray | 570 | 20 | 90 |
| Potato Wedges | 1210 | 63 | 145 |
| **Desserts:** | | | |
| Apple Turnover, 2.9 oz | 230 | 10 | 32 |
| Cafe Valley Choc. Chip cake, 1 slice | 300 | 15 | 39 |
| Oreo Cookies & Creme Pie | 290 | 16 | 34 |
| Reese's Peanut Butter Pie, 2.6 oz | 310 | 19 | 31 |

## Kilwins® ~ *see CalorieKing.com*

## Kolache® ~ *see CalorieKing.com*

Updated Nutrition Data ~ www.CalorieKing.com
Persons with Diabetes ~ See Disclaimer (Page 22)

## Krispy Kreme® (Aug '15)

| Doughnuts: | C | F | Cb |
|---|---|---|---|
| Apple Fritter, 3.5 oz | 390 | 20 | 50 |
| Chocolate Iced Cake, 2.5 oz | 280 | 16 | 32 |
| Chocolate Iced Custard Filled, 3 oz | 350 | 22 | 35 |
| Choc. Iced, Kreme Filled, 3.2 oz | 340 | 17 | 42 |
| Cinnamon Apple Filled | 330 | 21 | 31 |
| Cinnamon Bun | 220 | 12 | 27 |
| Cinnamon Twist | 230 | 12 | 30 |
| Dulce de Leche | 310 | 17 | 37 |
| **Glazed:** Chocolate Cake | 330 | 22 | 32 |
| Chocolate Iced, 2.2 oz | 240 | 12 | 32 |
| With Sprinkles | 250 | 12 | 34 |
| Choc. Iced Glazed Cruller, 2.5 oz | 300 | 18 | 34 |
| Cinnamon | 190 | 10 | 23 |
| Cruller | 250 | 17 | 23 |
| Kreme Filled | 370 | 23 | 38 |
| Lemon Filled | 340 | 21 | 35 |
| Maple Iced | 230 | 11 | 31 |
| Original | 190 | 11 | 21 |
| Sour Cream | 360 | 22 | 42 |
| **Powdered:** Cake | 260 | 16 | 26 |
| Strawberry Filled | 330 | 22 | 30 |
| Sugar | 180 | 11 | 19 |
| Traditional Cake | 230 | 15 | 20 |
| **Doughnut Holes:** Orig. Glazed (5) | 200 | 9 | 27 |
| Glazed Cake, Chocolate (4) | 190 | 10 | 24 |

*Kool Kreme:*

| **Doughnut Shakes:** Per 17 oz | | | |
|---|---|---|---|
| Chocolate | 750 | 24 | 117 |
| Vanilla | 730 | 23 | 113 |
| **Doughnut Sundae,** | | | |
| Original Glazed, 7 oz | 450 | 17 | 69 |

*Chiller Beverages: Without Whipped Cream Topping*

| Orange You Glad; Very Berry, average: | | | |
|---|---|---|---|
| 12 fl.oz | 175 | 0 | 43 |
| 20 fl.oz | 295 | 0 | 71 |

*Chiller Beverages: With Whipped Topping*

| Lotta Latte: 12 oz | 640 | 25 | 102 |
|---|---|---|---|
| 20 oz | 980 | 36 | 163 |
| Mocha Dream: 12 oz | 670 | 28 | 105 |
| 20 oz | 1050 | 41 | 171 |

*Kremey Chillers: Includes Whipped Cream Topping*

| Berries & Kreme: 12 fl.oz | 620 | 28 | 92 |
|---|---|---|---|
| 20 fl.oz | 960 | 40 | 150 |
| Oranges & Kreme: 12 fl.oz | 630 | 28 | 92 |
| 20 fl.oz | 970 | 40 | 150 |

*For Complete Menu & Data ~ See CalorieKing.com*

## Krystal® (Aug '15)

| Burgers: | C | F | Cb |
|---|---|---|---|
| **Big Angus:** Original | 550 | 35 | 46 |
| Dble, w/ Bacon & Cheese | 850 | 59 | 48 |
| **Krystal:** | | | |
| Original | 130 | 6 | 20 |
| Double | 290 | 13 | 33 |
| Bacon Cheese | 200 | 11 | 20 |
| Chik Club | 320 | 16 | 29 |
| Double Cheese | 350 | 17 | 34 |
| **Pups:** Chili Cheese | 230 | 14 | 16 |
| Corn | 240 | 14 | 22 |
| Plain | 150 | 8 | 15 |

*Fries:*

| Chili Cheese, 8.25 oz | 570 | 29 | 62 |
|---|---|---|---|
| Regular, Medium, 4.25 oz | 310 | 13 | 46 |
| *Chik'n Bites,* Small, 3 oz | 200 | 7 | 20 |
| *Salad,* Crispy Chicken, 11 oz | 370 | 21 | 20 |

*Breakfast Items:*

| Biscuits: | | | |
|---|---|---|---|
| Bacon, Egg & Cheese | 440 | 24 | 34 |
| Chik | 400 | 18 | 43 |
| Gravy | 350 | 18 | 41 |
| Plain | 260 | 13 | 32 |
| Sausage | 420 | 28 | 32 |
| **Sandwich,** Krystal Sunriser | 200 | 11 | 16 |
| **Scramblers:** | | | |
| Original: With Bacon | 330 | 16 | 27 |
| With Sausage | 420 | 26 | 27 |
| 4-Carb Scrambler, | | | |
| With Sausage | 620 | 52 | 3 |

*Desserts:*

| Apple Turnover, fried | 220 | 8 | 34 |
|---|---|---|---|
| Lemon Icebox Pie | 320 | 9 | 56 |

*Drinks: Per 16 fl.oz, with ¼ ice*

| Coca-Cola, Classic | 120 | 0 | 32 |
|---|---|---|---|
| Diet Coke | 0 | 0 | 0 |

*For Complete Menu & Data ~ see CalorieKing.com*

**For Menu Updates,
Check Author's Website
www.CalorieKing.com**

## LaRosa's Pizzeria® (Aug '15)

### Pizzas:

| | C | F | Cb |
|---|---|---|---|
| **Focaccia Style:** *Per Slice, 1/10 of Medium Pizza* | | | |
| Florentine | 240 | 13 | 24 |
| Roma | 300 | 18 | 23 |
| **Hand Tossed:** *Per Slice, 1/8 of Medium Pizza* | | | |
| Cheese | 230 | 8 | 29 |
| Double Pepperoni | 300 | 14 | 29 |
| Big 4: Meat | 325 | 15 | 29 |
| Pick 4 | 280 | 11 | 30 |
| Veggie | 240 | 7 | 30 |
| **Multigain Wheat:** *Per 1/2 of 12" Pizza* | | | |
| Pepperoni-Sausage | 190 | 11 | 14 |
| Average other varieties | 125 | 5 | 15 |
| **Pan Crust:** *Per Slice, 1/8 of Medium Pizza* | | | |
| Cheese | 300 | 16 | 30 |
| Double Pepperoni | 370 | 22 | 30 |
| Big 4: Meat | 325 | 15 | 29 |
| Pick 4 | 280 | 11 | 30 |
| Veggie | 240 | 7 | 30 |
| **Traditional Crust:** *Per Slice, 1/8 of Medium Pizza* | | | |
| Cheese | 200 | 10 | 19 |
| Double Pepperoni | 280 | 16 | 20 |
| Big 4: Meat | 285 | 16 | 20 |
| Pick 4 | 240 | 12 | 20 |
| Veggie | 200 | 8 | 21 |

### Calzones: *Per Calzone, No Dipping Sauce*

| | C | F | Cb |
|---|---|---|---|
| Cheese & Pepperoni | 960 | 45 | 101 |
| Cheese | 840 | 34 | 101 |
| Philly Cheesesteak | 870 | 39 | 90 |
| Sausage Pelucci | 1040 | 52 | 92 |

### Classic Hoagys:

| | C | F | Cb |
|---|---|---|---|
| Baked Meatball | 700 | 29 | 75 |
| Original Steak | 740 | 33 | 69 |

### Pasta Dinner: *Without Bread, Soup or Salad*

| | C | F | Cb |
|---|---|---|---|
| Cheese Ravioli | 660 | 26 | 80 |
| Lasagna, with Meat Sauce | 735 | 38 | 61 |
| Spaghetti: With Alfredo Sauce | 975 | 50 | 104 |
| With Meatballs | 870 | 28 | 119 |
| With Meat Sauce | 700 | 18 | 104 |
| With Traditional Sauce | 640 | 12 | 113 |
| Ziti Chicken Alfredo | 980 | 42 | 102 |
| Ziti Sausage Pelucci | 765 | 20 | 115 |

### Fresh Salad: *Without Dressing*

| | C | F | Cb |
|---|---|---|---|
| Antipasto For One | 470 | 345 | 13 |
| Crispy Chicken | 400 | 22 | 29 |
| Grilled Salad | 290 | 12 | 15 |
| JoJo's BLT | 150 | 9 | 10 |
| Tossed Salad | 160 | 10 | 11 |

### Soup: Baked Onion

| | C | F | Cb |
|---|---|---|---|
| Baked Onion | 180 | 9 | 19 |
| Minestrone | 110 | 1 | 22 |

### Salad Dressings: Bleu Cheese

| | C | F | Cb |
|---|---|---|---|
| Bleu Cheese | 220 | 24 | 2 |
| Caesar | 160 | 17 | 1 |
| Honey French | 210 | 18 | 14 |
| La Rosa Italian | 230 | 26 | 2 |

## LaRosa's Pizzeria® cont... (Aug '15)

### Appetizers:

| | C | F | Cb |
|---|---|---|---|
| Garlic Fries, 11 oz | 630 | 34 | 74 |
| Four Taste Sampler, 6.6 oz | 475 | 26 | 48 |
| Fried Cheesesticks, 6.2 oz | 450 | 22 | 45 |
| Garlic Bread, 2 pcs, 2.6 oz | 300 | 14 | 38 |
| Kitchen Chips, 10 oz | 570 | 27 | 71 |
| Onion Twists, 10 oz | 910 | 57 | 91 |
| Rondo: Pepperoni, 4.6 oz | 545 | 36 | 35 |
| Spinach/Cheese, average, 4.5 oz | 405 | 22 | 35 |

## La Salsa Fresh Mexican® (Aug '15)

### Appetizers:

| | C | F | Cb |
|---|---|---|---|
| **Salsa & Chips:** Regular, 14.5 oz | 700 | 32 | 87 |
| W/ Guacamole, 14.5 oz | 970 | 55 | 103 |
| Chips (15), 1.4 oz | 200 | 10 | 25 |
| **Nachos:** | | | |
| Black Beans: With Carnitas | 1570 | 83 | 141 |
| With Chicken | 1600 | 83 | 148 |
| With Steak | 1580 | 84 | 142 |
| Pinto Beans: With Carnitas | 1560 | 83 | 139 |
| With Chicken | 1590 | 83 | 146 |
| With Steak | 1565 | 84 | 139 |
| **Burritos:** *Without Chips* | | | |
| **Black Beans & Cheese** | 1100 | 48 | 132 |
| With Carnitas | 1205 | 51 | 132 |
| With Chicken | 1240 | 52 | 139 |
| **Pinto Beans & Cheese** | 1070 | 48 | 115 |
| With Chicken | 1200 | 52 | 122 |
| With Steak | 1175 | 54 | 115 |
| Baja Fish Burrito | 875 | 53 | 58 |
| California Steak w/ Black Beans | 815 | 35 | 89 |
| **Overstuffed Grilled Burrito:** | | | |
| With Carnitas | 1200 | 59 | 108 |
| With Chicken | 1260 | 59 | 110 |
| With Steak | 1290 | 66 | 109 |
| **Grande, Black Beans:** | | | |
| With Carnitas or Chicken, average | 810 | 34 | 92 |
| With Steak | 820 | 35 | 91 |
| **Tacos:** *Without Chips* | | | |
| Baja Fish | 395 | 22 | 29 |
| Baja Shrimp | 320 | 19 | 30 |
| Guadalajara Carnitas | 320 | 15 | 30 |
| Mexico City, Chicken or Steak, av. | 190 | 4 | 27 |
| **Quesadillas:** *Without Chips* | | | |
| **Classic:** Carnitas | 960 | 58 | 57 |
| Chicken | 955 | 57 | 58 |
| Steak | 965 | 59 | 57 |
| **Grande,** Pinto Beans, with choice of meat, average | 1130 | 61 | 90 |
| **Grande,** Black Beans, with choice of meat, average | 1140 | 61 | 91 |

*Continued Next Page...*

Updated Nutrition Data ~ www.CalorieKing.com
Persons with Diabetes ~ See Disclaimer (Page 22)

## La Salsa® cont... (Aug '15)

*Favorites: Without Chips*

| | C | F | Cb |
|---|---|---|---|
| **Stuffed Fajita Quesadilla:** | | | |
| With Carnitas or Chicken, av. | 860 | 51 | 54 |
| With Shrimp | 800 | 49 | 54 |
| With Steak | 885 | 55 | 53 |
| **Fire Roasted Bowls:** | | | |
| Black Beans: W/ Chicken | 730 | 32 | 74 |
| With Steak | 735 | 34 | 73 |
| Without Meat | 630 | 29 | 71 |
| Pinto Beans: W/ Chicken | 730 | 32 | 73 |
| With Steak | 720 | 34 | 70 |
| Without Meat | 620 | 29 | 69 |

## Little Caesars® (Aug '15)

*14" Pizza: Per Slice, ⅛ Pizza*

| | C | F | Cb |
|---|---|---|---|
| **Optional:** 3 Meat Treat | 340 | 17 | 32 |
| Hula Hawaiian: W/ Ham | 280 | 9 | 35 |
| W/ Canadian Bacon | 280 | 9 | 35 |
| Ultimate Supreme | 320 | 13 | 33 |
| Veggie | 270 | 10 | 33 |
| **Hot-N-Ready:** | | | |
| Deep Deep Dish: Cheese | 360 | 15 | 41 |
| Pepperoni | 390 | 18 | 41 |
| Round Pizza: | | | |
| Cheese | 250 | 9 | 32 |
| Pepperoni | 280 | 11 | 32 |

*Caesar Wings: Per Wing*

| | | | |
|---|---|---|---|
| BBQ: Regular | 80 | 5 | 3 |
| Spicy | 70 | 5 | 1 |
| Buffalo, Mild or Hot | 70 | 5 | 0 |
| Garlic Parmesan | 90 | 7 | 1 |
| Lemon Pepper | 90 | 8 | 0 |
| Oven Roasted | 70 | 5 | 0 |

*Caesar Dips: Per 1 oz Container Unless Indicated*

| | | | |
|---|---|---|---|
| BBQ; Buffalo Ranch | 160 | 17 | 2 |
| Buffalo | 100 | 10 | 2 |
| Buttery Garlic, 0.5 oz | 130 | 14 | 0 |
| Cheezy Jalapeno | 140 | 15 | 2 |
| Ranch | 170 | 18 | 2 |

*Bread: Per Piece*

| | | | |
|---|---|---|---|
| Crazy Bread, 1 stick | 100 | 3 | 15 |
| Crazy Sauce, 4 oz | 45 | 0 | 10 |
| Italian Cheese Bread | 130 | 6 | 13 |
| Pepperoni Cheese Bread | 150 | 8 | 13 |

## Lone Star Steakhouse® (Oct '12)

*Appetizers: Per Serving*

| | C | F | Cb |
|---|---|---|---|
| Lone Star Wings, mild, 3.5 oz | 305 | 20 | 5 |
| Spin. & Artichoke Dip, 3.5 oz | 160 | 13 | 4.5 |
| Texas Rose, 3.5 oz | 285 | 19 | 25 |
| **Meals:** *Without Sides, Toppings & Sauce* | | | |
| Chopped Steak, 9.6 oz | 710 | 52 | 0 |
| NY Strip, 9.6 oz | 525 | 28 | 0 |
| Texas Ribeye, 12.5 oz | 710 | 40 | 5.5 |
| **Ribs Combo:** | | | |
| Baby Back Ribs, with Chicken | 740 | 30 | 46 |
| **Seafood:** | | | |
| Fried Shrimp Entree, 11.7 oz | 865 | 40 | 97 |
| Grilled Shrimp: 3.5 oz | 60 | 2 | 5.5 |
| 11 oz | 190 | 7 | 17 |
| Sweet Bourbon Salmon: 6oz | 240 | 11 | 0 |
| 9 oz | 360 | 16 | 0 |
| **Burgers:** | | | |
| Bubba, 15.7 oz | 1085 | 57 | 67 |
| Swiss & Mushroom, 15.2 oz | 845 | 38 | 53 |
| **Salads:** *Per Serving, Includes Dressing* | | | |
| Dinner, Caesar, 6.3 oz | 145 | 11 | 8 |
| Grilled Chicken Caesar | 480 | 24 | 19 |
| Lettuce Wedge | 395 | 34 | 10 |
| **Sides:** *Per Serving* | | | |
| Garlic Mashed Potatoes, ½ cup | 130 | 5 | 19 |
| Steak Fries, 8 oz | 610 | 26 | 86 |
| Texas Seasoned Rice, 8 oz | 100 | 3.5 | 14 |

## Long John Silver's® (Aug '15)

| | C | F | Cb |
|---|---|---|---|
| Chicken Tenders, 1 piece 2 oz | 170 | 8 | 11 |
| **Sandwiches & Tacos:** | | | |
| Ciabatta Jack: Chicken Sandwich | 660 | 33 | 57 |
| Fish Sandwich | 550 | 30 | 48 |
| Baja: Fish Taco (1), 7oz | 580 | 39 | 41 |
| Chicken Taco (1), 6.2 oz | 530 | 33 | 40 |
| **Seafood:** | | | |
| Baked Cod, 1 piece, 6 oz | 160 | 1 | 1 |
| Battered: Alaskan Pollock, 1 piece, 3.2 oz | 230 | 14 | 14 |
| Cod, 1 piece, 3 oz | 280 | 19 | 6 |
| Shrimp, 3 pieces, 1.5 oz | 130 | 7 | 5 |
| Crab Cake, 1 cake, 2.2 oz | 280 | 15 | 26 |
| Snack Box: Breaded Clam Strips | 280 | 16 | 20 |
| Popcorn Shrimp, 3 oz | 330 | 12 | 20 |

*Continued Next Page....*

## Long John's® cont... (Aug '15)

*Sauces & Condiments:*

| | C | F | Cb |
|---|---|---|---|
| **Dipping Sauces:** BBQ, 1 oz | 40 | 0 | 10 |
| Cocktail, 1 oz | 25 | 0 | 6 |
| Honey Mustard, 1 oz | 100 | 6 | 12 |
| Ketchup, 1 pouch, 1 oz | 30 | 0 | 8 |
| Louisiana Hot Sauce, 1 tsp | 0 | 0 | 0 |
| Malt Vinegar, 0.5 oz | 0 | 0 | 0 |
| Tartar, 0.5 oz packet | 40 | 4 | 2 |

*Sides:*

| | | | |
|---|---|---|---|
| Breaded Mozzarella Sticks (3) | 170 | 10 | 12 |
| Broccoli Cheese Soup, 1 bowl, 7.5 oz | 220 | 18 | 8 |
| Clam Chowder, 1 bowl | 230 | 16 | 16 |
| Cole Slaw, 4 oz | 200 | 15 | 15 |
| Corn Cobbette w/ Butter Oil, 3.5 oz | 150 | 10 | 14 |
| Crumblies, 1 oz | 150 | 13 | 8 |
| Fries, 3.7oz | 350 | 17 | 44 |
| Hushpuppy, 2 pups, 1.5 oz | 160 | 13 | 18 |
| Jalapeno Cheddar Bites (5), 1 oz | 240 | 16 | 18 |
| Rice, 5 oz | 180 | 1 | 37 |

*For Complete Menu & Data ~ see CalorieKing.com*

## Macaroni Grill® (Aug '15)

*Tappas & Antipasti:*
*Per Whole Appetizer as Served*

| | C | F | Cb |
|---|---|---|---|
| Calamari Fritti | 760 | 55 | 33 |
| Goat Cheese Peppadew Peppers | 350 | 11 | 56 |
| Mac & Chse Bites w/ Dip | 920 | 70 | 44 |
| Spicy Ricotta Meatballs | 440 | 30 | 14 |
| Stuffed Mushrooms | 500 | 37 | 19 |

*Meals: Per Whole Entree, as Served*

| | | | |
|---|---|---|---|
| **Carne:** Calabrese Steak | 1650 | 153 | 41 |
| Chianti Pork Chop | 960 | 71 | 38 |
| **Chicken:** Marsala | 790 | 32 | 61 |
| Milanese | 1410 | 98 | 80 |
| Scallopine | 1110 | 74 | 51 |
| Under a Brick | 1590 | 145 | 20 |
| **Classics:** Eggplant Parmesan | 1340 | 90 | 103 |
| Fettuccine Alfredo | 1040 | 59 | 86 |
| Lasagne Bolognese | 1110 | 67 | 69 |
| Mom's Meatballs: W/ Bologn. | 1130 | 62 | 83 |
| With Pomodoro | 970 | 51 | 79 |

## Macaroni Grill® cont... (Aug '15)

*Meals (Cont): Per Whole Entree*

| | C | F | Cb |
|---|---|---|---|
| **Pasta:** Cannelloni Bolognese | 930 | 67 | 38 |
| Carmela's Chicken | 1030 | 60 | 82 |
| Lobster Ravioli | 600 | 35 | 36 |
| Mama's Trio | 2040 | 127 | 123 |
| Mushroom Ravioli | 930 | 66 | 53 |
| Penne Rustica | 930 | 43 | 78 |
| **Pesce:** Grilled Salmon | 1030 | 66 | 53 |
| Parmesan-Crusted Sole | 1330 | 94 | 94 |

*Artisan Pizzas: Per Whole Meal, as Served*

| | | | |
|---|---|---|---|
| Farmhouse | 1370 | 60 | 147 |
| Margherita | 1280 | 52 | 148 |
| Pesto Primavera | 1210 | 47 | 149 |
| Smashed Meatball | 1420 | 59 | 149 |
| *Kids:* Chkn Tenders w/ Broccolini | 860 | 45 | 46 |
| Macaroni & Cheese | 540 | 31 | 44 |
| Pepperoni Pizza | 630 | 25 | 72 |
| Spaghetti & Meatballs, w/ Sauce | 460 | 21 | 45 |

*Salads: Includes Dressing*

| | | | |
|---|---|---|---|
| Bibb & Blue | 520 | 42 | 17 |
| Parmesan Crusted Chicken | 1080 | 48 | 100 |
| Side Caesar | 240 | 21 | 8 |
| Warm Spinach & Shrimp | 370 | 24 | 14 |
| *Soups:* Minestrone, 8 oz bowl | 160 | 3 | 28 |
| Pomodorina, 8 oz bowl | 170 | 12 | 12 |
| *Dessert:* Gelato, Vanilla | 310 | 13 | 42 |
| Homemade Choc. Cake | 940 | 58 | 101 |
| Lemon Passion | 740 | 45 | 77 |
| New York Style Cheesecake | 690 | 41 | 70 |
| Tiramisu | 600 | 39 | 54 |

## Manhattan Bagel® (Aug '15)

*Bagels: Per Bagel*

| | C | F | Cb |
|---|---|---|---|
| Blueberry, 3.8 oz | 300 | 1 | 65 |
| Chocolate Chip, 3.8 oz | 290 | 3 | 58 |
| Cinnamon Raisin, 4 oz | 330 | 1 | 70 |
| Egg; Jalapeno Cheddar, av., 4 oz | 320 | 2 | 67 |
| Everything; Poppy, av 4.3 oz | 335 | 3 | 68 |
| Pumpernickel, 3.5 oz | 240 | 2 | 53 |
| Salt, 4.3 oz | 320 | 1 | 68 |
| *Cream Cheese:* Plain, 1.3 oz | 120 | 12 | 2 |
| Scallion, 1.3 oz | 120 | 11 | 5 |

*Continued Next Page...*

**214**

## Manhattan Bagel® cont... (Aug '15)
*Breakfast:* On Plain Bagel

| | C | F | Cb |
|---|---|---|---|
| Egg & Cheese | 480 | 13 | 69 |
| Egg Bacon & Cheese | 620 | 25 | 70 |
| Egg, Pork Roll & Cheese | 710 | 31 | 71 |
| Omelet Wrap, Egg, Cheese & Ham | 640 | 29 | 54 |

*Deli Sandwich:*

| | | | |
|---|---|---|---|
| Big City BLT on Multigrain bread | 500 | 25 | 48 |
| Roast Beef on Cheddar Roll | 490 | 8 | 76 |
| *Signature Lunch:* Bronx Bomber | 430 | 14 | 49 |
| Chelsea Chicken | 760 | 31 | 75 |
| Village Veggie Wrap | 470 | 21 | 62 |

*Salad:* Without Dressing

| | | | |
|---|---|---|---|
| Garden Market, 10 oz | 350 | 26 | 25 |
| NY Deli Chef, 14 oz | 690 | 49 | 25 |

## Marie Callender's® (Aug '15)
*Appetizers:* Per Serving

| | C | F | Cb |
|---|---|---|---|
| Crispy Chicken Tenders, 12.9 oz | 870 | 47 | 72 |
| Crispy Green Beans, 10.5 oz | 810 | 52 | 75 |
| Mozzarella Sticks, 8.6 oz | 690 | 42 | 46 |

*Burgers and Sandwiches:* With Fries

| | | | |
|---|---|---|---|
| Original Burger | 1290 | 87 | 84 |
| Albacore Tuna Melt | 1430 | 92 | 99 |
| French Dip Supreme | 1110 | 53 | 105 |
| Roasted Turkey Croissant Club | 1450 | 97 | 95 |

*Main Meals:* Per Complete Meal as Served

**Comfort Classics:**

| | | | |
|---|---|---|---|
| Artichoke & Mushroom Chicken | 1010 | 71 | 29 |
| Home-Style Meatloaf | 650 | 38 | 33 |

**From The Grill:**

| | | | |
|---|---|---|---|
| Grilled Atl. Salmon, Cajun Style | 570 | 34 | 16 |
| St. Louis BBQ Ribs | 1090 | 72 | 58 |

*Pasta Perfecto:* Includes Garlic Bread

| | | | |
|---|---|---|---|
| Chicken & Broccoli Fettuccini | 1540 | 87 | 119 |
| Double Shrimp Pasta | 1500 | 96 | 97 |
| **Pies,** Chicken Pot Pie, w/out sides | 1140 | 79 | 70 |

*Fresh Crisp Salads:* Includes Dressing

| | | | |
|---|---|---|---|
| Chinese Chicken | 910 | 33 | 107 |
| Gorgonzola, Pecan & Field Greens | 990 | 53 | 79 |
| Traditional Caesar, with Chicken | 700 | 43 | 28 |

*Sides:* Cornbread,

| | | | |
|---|---|---|---|
| with Honey Butter, 3 oz | 340 | 21 | 33 |
| French Fries, 4 oz | 380 | 20 | 45 |
| Loaded Mashed Potatoes, 6.2 oz | 340 | 23 | 23 |
| Macaroni & Cheese, 6.4 oz | 230 | 9 | 26 |

*Soups:* Per Bowl

| | | | |
|---|---|---|---|
| Chicken Noodle | 130 | 0.5 | 22 |
| Clam Chowder | 270 | 13 | 22 |
| Hearty Vegetable | 90 | 3 | 13 |
| Split Pea & Ham | 220 | 13 | 17 |

## Marie Callender's® cont... (Aug '15)
*Breakfast:* As Served

| | C | F | Cb |
|---|---|---|---|
| **Griddle Greats:** | | | |
| Belgian Waffles | 600 | 19 | 99 |
| Buttermilk Pancake Stack | 720 | 30 | 99 |
| Old Fashioned French Toast | 830 | 31 | 123 |
| **Hashers:** Country | 1320 | 82 | 90 |
| Tex-Mex | 1180 | 71 | 99 |
| **Homestyle Choices:** | | | |
| Country Fried Steak & Eggs | 1580 | 70 | 179 |
| Grilled Ham & Eggs | 1170 | 47 | 146 |
| Marie's Magnificent Six: | | | |
| With Bacon | 750 | 36 | 80 |
| With Sausage | 910 | 52 | 81 |
| **Omelettes:** BTA | 1610 | 84 | 160 |
| Denver | 1380 | 65 | 149 |
| Spanish | 1550 | 78 | 165 |
| **Quiche:** Bacon, 1 slice | 990 | 79 | 45 |
| Ham, 1 slice | 1030 | 83 | 39 |

*Desserts:* Per Slice Unless Indicated

| | | | |
|---|---|---|---|
| **Pies:** Apple | 630 | 39 | 66 |
| Banana Cream, with Meringue | 510 | 24 | 66 |
| Chocolate Cream, with Meringue | 570 | 26 | 77 |
| Coconut Cream with Meringue | 590 | 29 | 75 |
| Razzleberry | 650 | 39 | 71 |

*For Complete Nutritiona Data ~ see CalorieKing.com*

## Max & Erma's® (Aug '15)
*Shareables:* As Served

| | C | F | Cb |
|---|---|---|---|
| **Black Bean Roll-Ups:** Original | 680 | 31 | 90 |
| Crispy | 890 | 54 | 90 |
| Boneless Buffalo Wings | 1320 | 99 | 49 |
| Potato Skin Appetizers, Erma | 650 | 51 | 28 |

*Burgers:* Without Sides

| | | | |
|---|---|---|---|
| Cheeseburger, Erma | 790 | 51 | 47 |
| Daily Double | 990 | 68 | 47 |
| Garbage, Erma | 1260 | 92 | 53 |

*Salads:* Entrée Size, w/ Dressing, w/out Breadstick

| | | | |
|---|---|---|---|
| Buffalo Chicken | 1280 | 95 | 62 |
| Grilled Chicken Santa Fe | 1090 | 73 | 54 |
| Sthrn Fried Chicken | 1260 | 81 | 78 |
| *Sides:* Baked Potato | 190 | 2.5 | 38 |
| French Fries, 5 oz | 460 | 28 | 47 |
| Fresh Fruit Salad | 120 | 0 | 31 |
| Herb Rice | 240 | 2.5 | 49 |

*Sweet And Treats:*

| | | | |
|---|---|---|---|
| Banana Cream Pie | 890 | 69 | 68 |
| Chocolate Cake Ala Mode | 1270 | 66 | 154 |

*For Complete Menu & Data ~ See CalorieKing.com*

## McAlister's Deli® (Aug '15)

*Sandwiches: Per Whole Sandwich*

| | C | F | Cb |
|---|---|---|---|
| **Classic:** Grilled Chicken | 650 | 36 | 45 |
| Harvest Chicken Salad | 760 | 53 | 51 |
| The Italian | 760 | 36 | 51 |
| Tuna Salad | 540 | 27 | 45 |
| Veggie Pita | 590 | 40 | 45 |
| **Club:** Black Angus | 810 | 40 | 68 |
| Grilled Chicken | 740 | 33 | 72 |
| McAlister | 770 | 36 | 73 |
| **Grilled Sandwiches:** | | | |
| Four Cheese Griller | 800 | 43 | 64 |
| Smoky Pepper Jack Turkey | 800 | 39 | 72 |
| Spicy Southwest Chicken | 920 | 52 | 74 |
| Sweet Chipotle Chicken | 640 | 19 | 75 |
| **Hot Sandwiches:** | | | |
| California Turkey Reuben | 850 | 50 | 66 |
| French Dip | 540 | 20 | 43 |
| Ham Melt | 590 | 25 | 44 |
| Reuben | 780 | 41 | 62 |
| Roast Beef Melt | 580 | 25 | 41 |
| The Big Nasty | 780 | 24 | 67 |
| The New Yorker | 740 | 30 | 51 |

## McDonald's® (Aug '15)

*Beef Burgers/Sandwiches:*

| | C | F | Cb |
|---|---|---|---|
| **Bacon Clubhouse Burger** | 720 | 40 | 52 |
| **BBQ Ranch Burger** | 340 | 15 | 37 |
| **Big Mac Burger** | 530 | 27 | 47 |
| **Cheeseburger** | 290 | 11 | 33 |
| **Double:** Cheeseburger | 430 | 21 | 35 |
| Daily Double | 430 | 22 | 34 |
| Jalapeno Double | 430 | 23 | 35 |
| **Hamburger** | 240 | 8 | 32 |
| **McDouble:** Regular | 380 | 17 | 34 |
| Bacon | 440 | 22 | 35 |
| **McRib** | 500 | 26 | 44 |
| **Quarter Pounder:** | | | |
| With Cheese | 520 | 26 | 42 |
| Deluxe | 540 | 27 | 45 |
| Double, with Cheese | 740 | 42 | 43 |
| **Steakhouse Sirloin:** 1/3 lb | 730 | 36 | 62 |
| With Lettuce & Tomato | 750 | 39 | 63 |

*Chicken & Fish Sandwiches:*

| | C | F | Cb |
|---|---|---|---|
| **Artisan Grilled Chicken** | 360 | 6 | 43 |
| **Filet-O-Fish** | 390 | 19 | 39 |
| **McChicken** | 370 | 17 | 40 |
| **Premium:** | | | |
| Crispy Chicken Bacon Clubhouse | 750 | 38 | 65 |
| Grilled Chicken Bacon Clubhouse | 610 | 26 | 50 |

## McDonald's® cont... (Aug '15)

*Premium McWraps:*

| | C | F | Cb |
|---|---|---|---|
| **Crispy:** Chicken & Bacon | 630 | 32 | 56 |
| Chicken & Ranch | 610 | 31 | 56 |
| Chicken Sweet Chili | 540 | 23 | 61 |
| **Grilled:** Chicken & Bacon | 490 | 19 | 41 |
| Chicken & Ranch | 460 | 18 | 42 |
| Chicken Sweet Chili | 400 | 10 | 47 |

*Snack Wraps:*

| | C | F | Cb |
|---|---|---|---|
| Crispy Chicken, Ranch | 360 | 20 | 32 |
| Grilled Chicken, Ranch | 290 | 13 | 25 |

*Chicken McNuggets:*

| | C | F | Cb |
|---|---|---|---|
| 6 pieces | 280 | 18 | 18 |
| 10 pieces | 470 | 30 | 30 |

*French Fries:* Kids, 1.3 oz

| | C | F | Cb |
|---|---|---|---|
| French Fries: Kids, 1.3 oz | 110 | 5 | 15 |
| Small, 2.6 oz | 230 | 11 | 30 |
| Medium, 3.9 oz | 340 | 16 | 44 |
| Large, 5.9 oz | 510 | 24 | 67 |
| Ketchup, packet | 10 | 0 | 2 |

*Sauces:* Chipotle BBQ, 1 oz

| | C | F | Cb |
|---|---|---|---|
| Sauces: Chipotle BBQ, 1 oz | 50 | 0 | 11 |
| Creamy Ranch, 0.8 oz | 110 | 12 | 1 |
| Spicy Buffalo, 0.8 oz | 35 | 3 | 1 |
| Sweet 'N Sour; Tangy BBQ, 1 oz | 50 | 0 | 12 |

*Breakfast:*

| | C | F | Cb |
|---|---|---|---|
| **Bagel,** Steak, Egg & Cheese | 670 | 35 | 56 |
| **Big Breakfast:** With Regular Biscuit | 740 | 48 | 51 |
| With Hotcakes | 1090 | 56 | 111 |
| **Biscuits:** | | | |
| Bacon Egg & Cheese: Reg. Bisc. | 460 | 26 | 38 |
| Large Biscuit | 520 | 30 | 43 |
| Sausage with Egg: Regular Bisc. | 510 | 33 | 36 |
| With Large Biscuit | 570 | 37 | 42 |
| Southern Style Chicken: | | | |
| Regular Biscuit | 410 | 20 | 41 |
| Large Biscuit | 470 | 24 | 46 |
| Steak & Egg, regular biscuit | 540 | 32 | 38 |
| **Burrito,** Sausage | 300 | 16 | 26 |
| **Cinnamon Melts,** 4 oz | 460 | 19 | 66 |
| **Fruit & Yogurt Parfait** | 150 | 2 | 30 |
| **Fruit & Maple Oatmeal:** | | | |
| With Brown Sugar | 290 | 4 | 58 |
| Without Brown Sugar | 260 | 4 | 49 |

*continued Next Page...*

## McDonald's® cont... (Aug '15)

*Breakfast (Cont):*

| | C | F | Cb |
|---|---|---|---|
| **Hash Browns,** (1), 2 oz | 150 | 9 | 15 |
| **Hotcakes:** Plain (3) | 350 | 9 | 60 |
| With 1 Pat Margarine & Syrup | 570 | 13 | 105 |
| With 2 Pats Margarine & Syrup | 610 | 17 | 105 |
| **McGriddles:** Bacon, Egg & Cheese | 460 | 21 | 48 |
| Sausage | 420 | 22 | 44 |
| Sausage, Egg & Cheese | 550 | 31 | 48 |
| **McMuffins:** Egg | 300 | 13 | 31 |
| Egg White Delight | 250 | 8 | 30 |
| Sausage | 370 | 23 | 29 |
| Sausage with Egg | 450 | 28 | 30 |
| Steak & Egg | 430 | 23 | 31 |

*Happy Meals:*

| | C | F | Cb |
|---|---|---|---|
| **4 Chicken McNuggets:** | | | |
| + Fries + Apple Slices | 320 | 17 | 31 |
| + Fries + 1% Low Fat Milk | 410 | 20 | 39 |
| +Apple Slices +1% Low Fat Milk | 310 | 14 | 28 |
| **Hamburger:** | | | |
| +Fries + Apple Juice | 440 | 13 | 67 |
| +Fries + Fat Free Choc Milk | 480 | 13 | 50 |
| + Apple Slices + GoGurt Strawb Yog. | 380 | 8 | 61 |
| **Cheeseburger:** | | | |
| +Fries + Apple Juice | 480 | 16 | 69 |
| +Fries + Fat Free Choc Milk | 530 | 16 | 71 |
| + Apple Slices & Fat-Free Choc Milk | 435 | 11 | 60 |

*Mighty Kids Meals:*

| | C | F | Cb |
|---|---|---|---|
| **With 6 Chicken McNuggets:** | | | |
| +Fries+ Apple Juice | 470 | 23 | 54 |
| + Apple Slices+ Fat-Free Choc Milk | 425 | 18 | 45 |
| **With McDouble:** | | | |
| +Fries + Apple Juice | 570 | 23 | 70 |
| + Apple Slices + 1% Low-Fat Milk | 495 | 20 | 50 |

*Premium Salads: Without Dressing*

| | C | F | Cb |
|---|---|---|---|
| **Bacon Ranch:** Without Chicken | 150 | 8 | 10 |
| With Crispy Chicken | 400 | 22 | 24 |
| With Grilled Chicken | 260 | 10 | 10 |
| **Southwest:** | | | |
| With Crispy Chicken | 480 | 24 | 43 |
| With Grilled Chicken | 340 | 11 | 28 |

*Salad Dressings: Per Package*

| | C | F | Cb |
|---|---|---|---|
| **Newman's Own:** Ranch, 2 fl.oz | 200 | 17 | 11 |
| **Low-Fat:** Balsamic Vinaig., 1.5 fl.oz | 35 | 1.5 | 3 |
| Family Recipe Italian, 1.5 fl.oz | 50 | 1.5 | 7 |
| *Snacks:* Apple Slices | 15 | 0 | 4 |
| Yoplait Go-Gurt, Strawberry | 50 | 0 | 9 |

## McDonald's® cont... (Aug '15)

*Desserts & Shakes:*

| | C | F | Cb |
|---|---|---|---|
| **Baked Apple Pie,** 2.7 oz | 250 | 13 | 32 |
| **Cookies:** Choc. Chip Cookie (1) | 160 | 8 | 21 |
| Oatmeal Raisin (1), 1 oz | 150 | 6 | 22 |
| **Pie,** Strawberry & Creme | 310 | 17 | 36 |
| **McFlurry:** M&M Candies, 12 fl.oz | 650 | 23 | 96 |
| Oreo Cookies, 12 fl.oz cup | 510 | 17 | 80 |
| **Soft Serve:** Kiddie Cone | 45 | 1.5 | 7 |
| Vanilla Reduced Fat, Cone | 170 | 4.5 | 27 |
| **Sundaes:** | | | |
| Hot Caramel, 6.4 oz | 340 | 8 | 60 |
| Hot Fudge, 6.3 oz | 330 | 9 | 53 |
| Strawberry, 6.3 oz | 280 | 6 | 49 |
| **Shakes:** Chocolate; Strawberry, average: | | | |
| 12 fl.oz cup | 555 | 16 | 91 |
| 16 fl.oz cup | 695 | 20 | 114 |
| 22 fl.oz cup | 850 | 24 | 140 |
| Vanilla: 12 fl.oz cup | 530 | 15 | 86 |
| 16 fl.oz cup | 660 | 19 | 109 |
| 22 fl.oz cup | 820 | 23 | 135 |
| **Smoothies, all flavors:** | | | |
| Small, 12 fl oz cup | 210 | 0.5 | 50 |
| Medium, 16 fl oz cup | 260 | 1 | 60 |
| Large, 22 fl oz cup | 340 | 1 | 77 |
| *Milk:* 1% Low-Fat, 8 fl.oz cup | 100 | 2.5 | 12 |
| Fat-Free Chocolate Milk, 8 fl.oz | 130 | 0 | 23 |
| *Juice:* Apple, 6.8 fl.oz box | 100 | 0 | 23 |
| Orange: Small, 12 fl.oz | 150 | 0 | 34 |
| Medium, 16 fl.oz cup | 190 | 0 | 44 |
| Large, 22 fl.oz cup | 280 | 0 | 65 |
| *Frappe,* Oreo, medium, 18.3 oz | 650 | 24 | 102 |
| *Soda: With Ice, approx. 30%* | | | |
| **Coca-Cola or Sprite:** | | | |
| Extra Small, 12 fl.oz cup | 100 | 0 | 29 |
| Small, 16 fl.oz cup | 140 | 0 | 38 |
| Medium, 21 fl.oz cup | 205 | 0 | 55 |
| Large, 30 fl.oz cup | 280 | 0 | 76 |
| **Diet Coke** | 0 | 0 | 0 |
| **Hi-C Orange Lavaburst:** | | | |
| Extra Small, 12 fl.oz cup | 110 | 0 | 31 |
| Small, 16 fl.oz cup | 160 | 0 | 43 |
| Medium, 21 fl.oz cup | 230 | 0 | 61 |
| Large, 30 fl.oz cup | 310 | 0 | 84 |
| **Powerade,** Mountain Berry Blast: | | | |
| Extra Small, 12 fl.oz cup | 60 | 0 | 15 |
| Small, 16 fl.oz cup | 80 | 0 | 21 |
| Medium, 21 fl.oz cup | 120 | 0 | 30 |
| Large, 30 fl.oz cup | 160 | 0 | 42 |
| *Iced Tea,* medium, 21 fl.oz cup | 0 | 0 | 0 |
| *Sweet Tea,* small, 16 fl oz cup | 150 | 0 | 36 |

*McCafe Coffees ~ Next Page*

## McDonald's® cont... (Aug '15)
*McCafe:*

| | C | F | Cb |
|---|---|---|---|
| **Hot Chocolate:** | | | |
| Whole Milk: Small, 12 fl oz | 360 | 13 | 50 |
| Medium, 16 fl oz cup | 440 | 16 | 61 |
| Large, 20 fl oz cup | 540 | 20 | 73 |
| Nonfat Milk: Small, 12 fl oz | 280 | 3.5 | 50 |
| Medium, 16 fl oz cup | 340 | 3.5 | 61 |
| **Hot Mocha:** | | | |
| Whole Milk: | | | |
| Small, 12 fl oz | 340 | 11 | 49 |
| Medium, 16 fl oz cup | 410 | 14 | 60 |
| Large, 20 fl.oz cup | 500 | 17 | 72 |
| Nonfat Milk: Small, 12 fl oz | 270 | 3.5 | 49 |
| Medium, 16 fl oz cup | 330 | 3.5 | 60 |
| Large, 20 fl.oz cup | 390 | 4 | 73 |
| *Iced Coffee:* | | | |
| **Regular:** Small, 16 fl.oz cup | 140 | 4.5 | 23 |
| Large, 22 fl.oz cup | 190 | 7 | 31 |
| **Mocha:** Small, 12 fl.oz cup | 290 | 11 | 41 |
| Large, 22 fl.oz cup | 480 | 16 | 70 |

## Mimi's Cafe® (Aug '15)
*Breakfast:*

| | C | F | Cb |
|---|---|---|---|
| **Benedicts:** *With Potatoes* | | | |
| Original | 1030 | 68 | 55 |
| Smoked Salmon | 810 | 52 | 52 |
| **Omelets:** *With Potatoes Unless Indicated* | | | |
| Andouille Sausage & Red Pepper | 800 | 52 | 36 |
| Bacon Avocado | 900 | 66 | 35 |
| Egg White & Veggie, with Fruit | 300 | 12 | 21 |
| Hickory-Smoked Ham & Cheese | 730 | 49 | 31 |
| **Griddle:** *Includes Fresh Fruit* | | | |
| Brioche French Toast | 800 | 22 | 132 |
| Cinnamon Roll French Toast | 1120 | 37 | 179 |
| Orange Crème French Toast | 620 | 22 | 97 |
| *Appetizers:* | | | |
| Artichoke Frites, 6.5 oz | 600 | 49 | 28 |
| Baked Brie To Share, 10.5 oz | 650 | 29 | 68 |
| Warm Spinach Artich. Dip, 15 oz | 990 | 57 | 89 |
| *Lunch & Dinner: Without Side Choices* | | | |
| **Burgers:** | | | |
| Bacon Avocado Sourdough | 1160 | 73 | 76 |
| Brioche Cheeseburger | 650 | 36 | 54 |
| Brioche, Bacon & Egg Chseburger | 980 | 63 | 56 |
| **Craft Sandwiches:** | | | |
| Chicken Cordon Bleu | 990 | 49 | 74 |
| West Coast Reuben | 1270 | 72 | 80 |
| **Entrees:** | | | |
| Bouillabasse | 610 | 25 | 57 |
| French Pot Roast | 830 | 47 | 56 |
| Grilled Atlantic Salmon | 750 | 52 | 32 |
| Slow-Roasted Turkey | 680 | 25 | 58 |
| *Sides:* Broccoli/Green Beans, av. | 80 | 6 | 6 |
| Mashed Potatoes | 300 | 14 | 37 |

## Mr. Goodcents® (Aug '15)
*Cold Subs:*

| | C | F | Cb |
|---|---|---|---|
| *Per 8" Wheat Bread Sub With Standard Toppings* | | | |
| Centsable | 440 | 17 | 55 |
| Italian Sub | 630 | 37 | 52 |
| Mr. Goodcents Original | 510 | 24 | 54 |
| Oven Roasted Chicken Breast | 340 | 6 | 52 |
| Penny Club | 350 | 5 | 53 |
| Pepperoni | 685 | 42 | 52 |
| Tuna Salad | 475 | 20 | 59 |
| Veggie Sub | 295 | 4 | 57 |
| **Toasted Sub:** *Per 8" Wheat Bread Sub With Standard Toppings* | | | |
| Chicken Bacon Ranch, w/ Cheddar | 665 | 30 | 57 |
| Meatball with Mozzarella | 760 | 37 | 70 |
| *Pasta:* | | | |
| Alfredo Sauce | 1235 | 42 | 183 |
| Chicken Alfredo | 1380 | 45 | 187 |
| Chicken Parmesan | 1090 | 12 | 190 |
| Marinara Sauce, with Meatballs | 1205 | 27 | 197 |
| *Bread Stick,* 1 piece, 2 oz | 170 | 8 | 23 |

## Mr. Hero® (Aug '15)
*7" Hot Subs & Burgers:*

| | C | F | Cb |
|---|---|---|---|
| **Burgers:** Cheeseburger | 775 | 55 | 47 |
| Mushroom & Swiss | 785 | 55 | 48 |
| Romanburger | 860 | 62 | 48 |
| *Subs:* | | | |
| **Chicken,** | | | |
| Grilled Chicken Philly | 540 | 22 | 48 |
| **Deli Subs:** *Per 7" Sub with Menu Board Toppings* | | | |
| Original Italian | 640 | 39 | 47 |
| Tuna & Cheese | 725 | 54 | 44 |
| Turkey | 470 | 20 | 46 |
| Ultimate Italian | 675 | 40 | 46 |
| **Steak Subs:** | | | |
| Hot Buttered Cheesesteak | 670 | 42 | 45 |
| Zesty Bacon & Swiss | 615 | 32 | 42 |
| **Taste Buddies:** *Per 4 ½" Sandwich with Menu Board Toppings* | | | |
| Bacon Cheeseburger | 430 | 30 | 33 |
| Grilled Italiano | 440 | 32 | 32 |
| Tuna 'n Cheese | 485 | 38 | 31 |
| Zesty Chicken | 495 | 25 | 48 |
| *Sides:* | | | |
| Mozzarella Sticks, w/ Marinara Sce | 565 | 43 | 12 |
| Onion Petals, w/ Tangy Sce, 5.8 oz | 595 | 37 | 58 |
| **Fries:** Potato Waffer, w/o Sce, 5.8 oz | 430 | 30 | 38 |
| With Cheese Sauce, 1.5 oz | 485 | 34 | 42 |
| Zesty Fries, 5.6 oz | 595 | 37 | 58 |
| *Desserts:* Oreo Cookie Cheesecake | 260 | 17 | 24 |
| Snickers Cheesecake | 270 | 18 | 23 |
| Strawb. Swirl Cheesecake | 280 | 19 | 22 |

Updated Nutrition Data ~ www.CalorieKing.com
Persons with Diabetes ~ See Disclaimer (Page 22)

## Mrs Fields Cookies® (Aug '15)

| | C | F | Cb |
|---|---|---|---|
| *Brownies: Per 2.15 oz Brownie* | | | |
| Butterscotch Blondie | 260 | 10 | 38 |
| Double Fudge; Pecan Fudge, av. | 265 | 14 | 33 |
| Special Walnut Fudge & Blondie | 260 | 13 | 35 |
| Toffee Fudge; Walnut Fudge, av. | 265 | 14 | 33 |
| *Brownie Bites:* | | | |
| Double Fudge (3) | 200 | 10 | 27 |
| Toffee Fudge (3) | 200 | 11 | 26 |
| *Coffee Cake,* | | | |
| Choc. Chip, small, 2.35 oz | 240 | 11 | 30 |
| *Cookies:* | | | |
| **Bite Size Nibblers:** Cinn. Sugar (3) | 180 | 8 | 25 |
| Peanut Butter (3) | 170 | 9 | 19 |
| Semi-Sweet Chocolate (3) | 170 | 8 | 23 |
| Triple Chocolate (3) | 160 | 8 | 22 |
| White Chunk Macadamia (3) | 180 | 9 | 22 |
| Butter (1) | 200 | 8 | 29 |
| Cut Out (1) | 280 | 11 | 44 |
| Debra's Special (1) | 200 | 9 | 27 |
| Oatmeal, Raisins and Walnuts (1) | 200 | 9 | 27 |
| Peanut Butter (1) | 200 | 12 | 24 |
| Semi-Sweet: Chocolate (1) | 210 | 10 | 29 |
| With Walnuts (1) | 220 | 11 | 28 |
| Triple Chocolate (1) | 210 | 10 | 28 |
| White Chunk Macadamia (1) | 230 | 12 | 28 |
| *Muffins: Per 2 oz* | | | |
| Blueberry | 190 | 9 | 24 |
| Chocolate Chip | 200 | 10 | 26 |

*For Complete Nutritional Data ~ see CalorieKing.com*

## My Favorite Muffin® (Aug '15)

| | C | F | Cb |
|---|---|---|---|
| *Jumbo Muffins: Per 5.8 oz* | | | |
| **Regular:** Blueberry | 505 | 24 | 66 |
| Choc. Chip; Cinn Swirl Cheesecake | 635 | 33 | 82 |
| Deep Dish Apple Pie | 530 | 24 | 75 |
| Pumpkin Spice | 545 | 24 | 78 |
| **Fat Free:** Blueberry | 325 | 0 | 78 |
| Chocolate Marble | 375 | 0 | 87 |
| Cinnamon Bun | 505 | 0 | 126 |

## Nathan's Famous® (Aug '15)

| | C | F | Cb |
|---|---|---|---|
| *Burgers:* | | | |
| Bacon Cheeseburger, 5 oz | 900 | 61 | 43 |
| Double Beefburger, 10 oz | 1030 | 73 | 41 |
| Hamburger, 5 oz | 620 | 38 | 41 |
| Super Cheeseburger, 5 oz | 960 | 67 | 48 |
| *Nathan's Famous Hot Dogs: With Natural Casings* | | | |
| Original, 3.5 oz | 290 | 17 | 24 |
| Cheese Dog, 5.5 oz | 390 | 25 | 30 |
| Chili Dog, 5.5 oz | 420 | 28 | 30 |
| Chili Cheese, 6.5 oz | 460 | 31 | 33 |
| *Corn Dog,* on a stick, 3.2 oz | 380 | 21 | 39 |

## Nathan's Famous® cont... (Aug '15)

| | C | F | Cb |
|---|---|---|---|
| *Chicken:* | | | |
| Chicken Tenders, Krispy, | | | |
| 3 pieces, 6.3 oz | 520 | 31 | 32 |
| Grilled: Chicken Sandwich, 8.2 oz | 470 | 21 | 43 |
| Chicken Caesar Wrap, 9.2 oz | 570 | 22 | 57 |
| Krispy: Chicken Sandwich, 8.8 oz | 620 | 32 | 59 |
| Homestyle Sandwich, 8.5 oz | 660 | 37 | 58 |
| *Fries:* | | | |
| **French:** Regular, 7.5 oz | 510 | 34 | 42 |
| Large, 11.5 oz | 780 | 52 | 64 |
| Family, 15.5 oz | 1050 | 70 | 86 |
| **Cheese:** Regular, 9 oz | 570 | 38 | 46 |
| Large, 13.5 oz | 860 | 58 | 70 |
| Philly Cheesesteak, 14.4 oz | 680 | 33 | 52 |

## New York Fries® ~ See CalorieKing.com

## Ninety Nine (Aug '15)

| | C | F | Cb |
|---|---|---|---|
| *Standout Starters: As Served* | | | |
| Boneless Wings & Skins Sampler | 1890 | 125 | 107 |
| Fried Mozzarella | 770 | 45 | 57 |
| Outrageous Potato Skins | 1470 | 101 | 84 |
| *Burgers: Without Sides* | | | |
| Bacon & Cheese Steakburger | 900 | 58 | 48 |
| BBQ BLT Crunch Burger | 1260 | 76 | 89 |
| Vermont Cheddar Burger | 1040 | 69 | 54 |
| West Coast Turkey Burger | 810 | 47 | 47 |
| *Sandwiches: Without Sides* | | | |
| Honey BBQ Chicken Wrap | 850 | 33 | 100 |
| Triple-Decker Turkey Club | 700 | 31 | 58 |
| *Meals: Served With Menu Set Sides Unless Indicated* | | | |
| Fish & Chips | 1570 | 105 | 107 |
| Macadamia Crusted Chicken | 1120 | 71 | 88 |
| New England Shoreline Combo | 1890 | 126 | 132 |
| Original Crispy Chicken Tenders | 1750 | 112 | 128 |
| Prime Rib: 12 oz, without sides | 550 | 27 | 2 |
| 18 oz, without sides | 830 | 41 | 3 |
| Smothered Sirloin Tips, w/o sides | 1050 | 62 | 18 |
| *Salads: As Served* | | | |
| Chicken Caesar | 830 | 54 | 50 |
| Fire Grilled SW Cobb | 890 | 58 | 30 |
| Tropical Chicken | 740 | 40 | 58 |
| *Sides:* | | | |
| Double Bleu Iceberg Wedge | 460 | 42 | 11 |
| Honey Butter Bisc., w/ Honey Butter | 230 | 11 | 29 |
| Baked Potato with Sour Cream | 310 | 8 | 52 |
| *Dessert,* | | | |
| Towering Midnight Fudge Cake | 790 | 40 | 96 |

# Fast - Foods & *Restaurants*

## Noodles & Company® (Aug '15)

*Noodles & Pasta: Regular Size*

| | C | F | Cb |
|---|---|---|---|
| Buttered Noodles | 930 | 39 | 115 |
| Bangkok Curry | 480 | 14 | 78 |
| Indonesian Peanut Saute | 810 | 17 | 150 |
| Japanese Pan Noodles | 620 | 15 | 111 |
| Mushroom Stroganoff | 930 | 44 | 105 |
| Pad Thai | 800 | 19 | 145 |
| Penne Rosa, with Parmesan | 700 | 25 | 97 |
| Spaghetti & Meatballs | 1020 | 54 | 98 |
| Steak Stroganoff | 1170 | 59 | 107 |
| Wisconsin Mac & Cheese | 1040 | 42 | 125 |
| *Sandwiches:* BBQ Pork | 540 | 16 | 69 |
| Mmmeatball | 790 | 49 | 57 |
| Spicy Chkn Caesar, without Dressing | 370 | 14 | 40 |
| The Veggie Med | 320 | 12 | 43 |
| *Salads: Per Regular Size* | | | |
| Chinese Chicken Chop Salad | 510 | 26 | 42 |
| Grilled Chicken Caesar | 550 | 34 | 25 |
| Pork Med Salad | 340 | 13 | 44 |
| Spinach & Fresh Fruit Salad | 600 | 38 | 46 |
| *Soups: Per Regular Size* | | | |
| Chicken Noodle | 350 | 10 | 43 |
| Thai Curry | 450 | 15 | 65 |
| Tomato Basil Bisque | 450 | 31 | 36 |
| *Extras:* Cheesy Garlic Bread (3) | 300 | 16 | 28 |
| Cucumber Tomato Salad | 90 | 0 | 21 |
| Margherita Flatbread | 330 | 14 | 37 |
| Potsticker (6), without sauce | 340 | 10 | 45 |

## Nothing But Noodles® (Aug '15)

*Noodle Bowls:*

| | C | F | Cb |
|---|---|---|---|
| **American:** Beef Stroganoff | 510 | 31 | 33 |
| Buttery Noodles | 650 | 44 | 46 |
| Santa Fe Pasta | 705 | 54 | 40 |
| Southwest Chipotle | 715 | 58 | 41 |
| Spicy Cajun Pasta | 660 | 50 | 44 |
| **Asian:** Pad Thai Noodles | 600 | 10 | 118 |
| Sesame Lo Mein | 410 | 11 | 64 |
| Spicy Japanese Noodles | 420 | 8 | 74 |
| Thai Peanut | 570 | 20 | 89 |
| **Italian:** Basil Pesto | 575 | 42 | 36 |
| Cappelini Primavera | 500 | 28 | 56 |
| Fettuccini Alfredo | 725 | 56 | 36 |
| Margherita Pasta | 475 | 31 | 36 |
| Marinara Pasta | 485 | 11 | 77 |
| Three-Cheese Macaroni | 445 | 21 | 45 |

*For Complete Menu & Data ~ see CalorieKing.com*

## O'Charley's® (Aug '15)

*Appetizers: As Served*

| | C | F | Cb |
|---|---|---|---|
| Chicken Tenders, Chipotle | 1160 | 40 | 107 |
| Over-Loaded Potato Skins | 1400 | 109 | 44 |
| Spicy Jack Cheese Wedges (7) | 720 | 48 | 44 |
| Top Shelf Combo Platter | 1880 | 132 | 74 |
| *Chicken & Pasta: Without Sides Unless Indicated* | | | |
| Bruschetta Chicken | 340 | 10 | 14 |
| Cajun Chicken Pasta | 1150 | 59 | 97 |
| Chkn Tenders, Buffalo w/o sides | 1070 | 64 | 31 |
| Prime Rib Pasta | 1400 | 94 | 80 |
| *Classic Combos: Without Sides* | | | |
| Panko-Crusted Shrimp, with Battered Cod | 1060 | 58 | 69 |
| Steak & Chicken Tenders, 6 oz | 1030 | 67 | 26 |
| Steak & Grilled Atl. Salmon, 6 oz | 750 | 47 | 3 |
| Steak & Panko-Crstd Shrimp, 9 oz | 780 | 42 | 41 |
| Steak & Shrimp Scampi, 9 oz | 700 | 51 | 9 |
| *Hand-Crushed Burgers: Without Sides* | | | |
| Better Cheddar Bacon | 1000 | 68 | 49 |
| Wild West Burger | 1290 | 94 | 64 |
| *Steaks & Ribs: Without Sides* | | | |
| **O'Charley's:** | | | |
| Baby Back Ribs: Full Rack | 1460 | 85 | 96 |
| Half Rack | 730 | 43 | 48 |
| **Slow Roasted Prime Rib:** | | | |
| 8oz | 830 | 70 | 3 |
| 16 oz | 1460 | 120 | 3 |
| *Coastal Favorites: Without Sides* | | | |
| Grilled Atlantic Salmon, 9 oz | 500 | 31 | 2 |
| Hand Battered Fish & Chips: Reg. | 1460 | 91 | 85 |
| Large | 1810 | 127 | 106 |
| Panko Crusted Shrimp Dinner | 560 | 24 | 56 |
| *Sides:* Baked Potato | 200 | 1 | 50 |
| Broccoli | 110 | 8 | 6 |
| French Fries, side | 400 | 24 | 40 |
| Loaded Baked Potato | 490 | 27 | 53 |
| Sweet Potato Fries | 280 | 19 | 27 |
| *Salads: Per Full Salad, With Dressing Unless Indicated* | | | |
| California Chicken, w/out Dressing | 980 | 63 | 68 |
| Southern Fried Chicken Salad | 1620 | 114 | 50 |
| Southern Pecan Chicken Tender | 1600 | 114 | 89 |
| *Signature Soup: Per Cup* | | | |
| Chicken Harvest | 120 | 7 | 11 |
| Chicken Tortilla | 100 | 4 | 11 |
| *Desserts:* | | | |
| Double Crust Peach Pie, 1 slice | 570 | 35 | 64 |
| Ooey Gooey Caramel Pie, 1 slice | 640 | 39 | 76 |

*For Complete Menu & Data ~ see CalorieKing.com*

Updated Nutrition Data ~ www.CalorieKing.com
Persons with Diabetes ~ See Disclaimer (Page 22)

## Olive Garden® (Aug '15)

| Appetizers: | C | F | Cb |
|---|---|---|---|
| Bruschetta Caprese | 660 | 19 | 97 |
| Classic Calamari | 680 | 44 | 47 |
| Spicy Shrimp Scampi Fritta | 560 | 37 | 34 |
| Stuffed Mushrooms | 380 | 30 | 13 |
| *Entrees:* | | | |
| **Lunch:** | | | |
| Chicken Alfredo | 1030 | 70 | 59 |
| Eggplant Parmigiana | 520 | 26 | 68 |
| Fettuccine Alfredo | 700 | 45 | 56 |
| Five Cheese Ziti al Forno | 740 | 42 | 62 |
| Lasagna Classico | 610 | 37 | 34 |
| Spaghetti with Meatballs | 740 | 35 | 67 |
| Seafood Alfredo | 760 | 46 | 58 |
| **Dinner:** | | | |
| Eggplant Parmigiana | 1050 | 52 | 85 |
| Fettuccini Alfredo | 1090 | 68 | 92 |
| Five Cheese Ziti al Forno | 1250 | 73 | 105 |
| Lasagna Classico | 960 | 58 | 54 |
| Ravioli di Portobello | 810 | 47 | 73 |
| Spaghetti with Chicken M'balls | 1010 | 32 | 110 |
| Tour of Italy | 1500 | 93 | 91 |
| *Desserts:* Black Tie Mousse Cake | 770 | 52 | 77 |
| Tiramisu | 470 | 27 | 52 |
| Zeppoli | 810 | 28 | 119 |

## Old Spaghetti Factory® (Aug '15)

| Appetizers: As Served | C | F | Cb |
|---|---|---|---|
| Shrimp, Spinach & Artichoke Dip | 590 | 40 | 39 |
| Sicilian Garlic Cheese Bread | 1220 | 78 | 97 |
| *Entrees, Lunch/Dinner:* | | | |
| **Classics:** | | | |
| Spaghetti: With Clam Sauce, 15 oz | 810 | 31 | 107 |
| With Marina Sauce, 15 oz | 560 | 5 | 108 |
| With Meat Sauce, 15 oz | 650 | 11 | 108 |
| With Sicilian Meatballs, 21 oz | 1040 | 36 | 115 |
| **Factory Favorites:** | | | |
| Chicken Parmigiana, 18 oz | 750 | 29 | 70 |
| Spinach & Cheese Ravioli, 11 oz | 470 | 16 | 63 |
| Spinach Tortellini w/ Alfredo Sce | 940 | 56 | 86 |
| **Managers Favorites:** | | | |
| Marinara: Clam, 15 oz | 690 | 18 | 107 |
| Meat, 15 oz | 600 | 8 | 108 |
| Mushroom, 16.5 oz | 610 | 10 | 109 |
| **Signature Selection:** | | | |
| Chicken Penne, 18.8 oz | 870 | 38 | 102 |
| Baked Chicken, 16.5 oz | 950 | 55 | 61 |
| Crab Ravioli, 11 oz | 810 | 45 | 73 |

## On the Border® (Aug '15)

| Appetizers: As Served | C | F | Cb |
|---|---|---|---|
| Border Sampler | 2090 | 143 | 101 |
| Fajita Quesadillas: Chicken | 1190 | 83 | 55 |
| Steak | 1220 | 89 | 54 |
| *Burritos: Includes Rice, Without Beans & Sauce* | | | |
| Classic Chicken | 910 | 36 | 96 |
| Classic Shredded Beef | 1070 | 41 | 95 |
| *Chimichangas: Includes Rice, Without Beans & Sauce* | | | |
| Chicken Tinga | 1430 | 90 | 104 |
| Ground Beef | 1580 | 105 | 106 |
| *Enchiladas: With rice, Without Beans* | | | |
| Barbacoa | 1090 | 48 | 99 |
| La Bandera | 920 | 39 | 95 |
| Suiza | 960 | 44 | 99 |
| *Fajita Grill: Without Rice, Beans, Tortillas or Condiments* | | | |
| Monterey Ranch Chicken | 660 | 44 | 11 |
| The Ultimate | 1040 | 85 | 20 |
| *Fresh Grill: Served As Listed* | | | |
| Carne Asada | 980 | 59 | 64 |
| Queso Chicken | 700 | 29 | 59 |
| Jalapeno- BBQ Salmon | 570 | 15 | 54 |
| *Salads: Without Dressing* | | | |
| House, side size | 160 | 6 | 22 |
| **Grande Taco Salad:** Chkn Tinga | 780 | 45 | 63 |
| With Ground Beef | 870 | 55 | 64 |
| *Sides: Per Serving* | | | |
| Black Beans | 170 | 1.5 | 29 |
| Mexican Rice | 280 | 4.5 | 54 |
| Pico de Gallo | 10 | 0 | 1 |
| Sour Cream | 60 | 5 | 2 |
| *Dressings: Per Serving* | | | |
| Ranch Dressing | 230 | 24 | 2 |
| Smoked Jalapeno Vinaigrette | 250 | 24 | 8 |

*For Complete Nutritional Data ~ see CalorieKing.com*

## Orange Julius® (Aug '15)

| Julius Originals: Per Small Size | C | F | Cb |
|---|---|---|---|
| Berry Pomegranate | 330 | 0 | 83 |
| Mango Pineapple | 350 | 0 | 87 |
| OrangeBerry | 250 | 0 | 63 |
| Strawberry Banana | 400 | 6 | 87 |
| *Premium Fruit Smoothies: Per Medium Size* | | | |
| Berry Pomegranate | 380 | 0 | 91 |
| Pina Colada | 340 | 0 | 80 |
| Strawberry | 300 | 0.5 | 71 |
| *Light Smoothies: Per Medium Size* | | | |
| Orange | 170 | 0 | 41 |
| Strawberry | 200 | 0 | 50 |
| Tripleberry | 210 | 0 | 55 |
| *Boost,* Banana, Small drink | 30 | 0 | 7 |

## Outback Steakhouse® (Aug '15)

*Aussie-Tizers: Per Whole Dish, With Selected Dressing/Sauce*

| | C | F | Cb |
|---|---|---|---|
| Alice Springs Chicken Quesadillas | 1590 | 96 | 92 |
| Aussie Cheese Fries: Small | 770 | 87 | 63 |
| Regular | 1740 | 120 | 114 |
| Bloomin' Onion | 1945 | 156 | 120 |
| Coconut Shrimp | 615 | 34 | 54 |
| Wings | 1750 | 132 | 40 |

*Burgers & Sandwiches: Without Sides*

| | C | F | Cb |
|---|---|---|---|
| Cripsy Chicken Sandwich | 775 | 42 | 68 |
| Double Burger | 930 | 62 | 44 |
| Outback Burger: | | | |
| Without Cheese | 625 | 38 | 33 |
| With American Cheese | 725 | 46 | 34 |
| With Cheddar or Swiss Chse, av. | 790 | 52 | 34 |
| Ribeye Melt | 1215 | 78 | 71 |
| The Bloomin' Burger | 1075 | 78 | 48 |
| Wood Grilled, California Chicken Sandwich | 580 | 26 | 44 |

*Chicken, Ribs, Chops: Without sides*

| | C | F | Cb |
|---|---|---|---|
| Alice Springs Chicken, lunch, 5 oz | 490 | 31 | 11 |
| Chicken Tender Platter | 1015 | 68 | 58 |
| Grilled Chicken On The Barbie | | | |
| Lunch, 5 oz | 200 | 2 | 11 |
| Maple Mustard Glazed Pork Chops | 365 | 14 | 13 |
| New Zealand Lamb Chops | 595 | 39 | 1 |
| No Rules Parmesan Pasta, | | | |
| No Protein: Lunch | 575 | 31 | 54 |
| Dinner | 900 | 51 | 78 |
| Ribs & Chicken On The Barbie | 660 | 32 | 23 |
| Signature Chop Steak | 645 | 46 | 9 |

*Combinations: Without Sides*

| | C | F | Cb |
|---|---|---|---|
| Filet, 6 oz & Lobster Tail, 4 oz | 620 | 41 | 3 |
| Sirloin: 6 oz, with Coconut Shrimp | 595 | 30 | 36 |
| 9 oz, with Coconut Shrimp | 725 | 36 | 36 |
| 9 oz, with Grilled Shrimp | 650 | 40 | 5 |
| 12 oz, with Grilled Shrimp | 780 | 47 | 5 |

*Straight From The Sea: Without Sides*

| | C | F | Cb |
|---|---|---|---|
| Firecracker Salmon | 480 | 25 | 25 |
| Lobster Tails, 4 oz | 435 | 26 | 2 |
| Simply Grilled Mahi | 380 | 5 | 33 |
| Tilapia, with Pure Lump Crab Meat | 545 | 31 | 10 |
| Add Ons: Blue Cheese Crumblees | 105 | 9 | 0 |
| Baby Back Ribs, ⅓ | 540 | 31 | 29 |
| Grilled Shrimp | 270 | 21 | 5 |
| Sauteed Mushrooms | 130 | 6 | 10 |

## Outback Steakhouse® cont... (Aug '15)

*Signature Outback Classic Cuts: Without Sides*

| | C | F | Cb |
|---|---|---|---|
| New York Strip, 14 oz | 765 | 49 | 0 |
| Outback Special: 6 oz Sirloin | 255 | 13 | 0 |
| 9 oz Sirloin | 380 | 19 | 0 |
| 12 oz Sirloin | 510 | 25 | 0 |
| Ribeye: 10 oz | 545 | 35 | 0 |
| 13 oz | 710 | 45 | 0 |
| Victoria's Filet: 6 oz | 220 | 9 | 0 |
| 8 oz | 300 | 12 | 0 |

*Soup & Salads:*

**Salads:** *Full Size, without dressing unless indicated*

| | C | F | Cb |
|---|---|---|---|
| Aussie Chicken Cobb: | | | |
| Crispy Chicken | 850 | 52 | 46 |
| Grilled Chicken | 525 | 25 | 19 |
| Caesar: Chicken, with dressing | 420 | 25 | 12 |
| Shrimp, with dressing | 575 | 37 | 26 |
| Steakhouse, with dressing | 950 | 66 | 46 |
| **Soup,** Clam Chowder, 1 Bowl | 700 | 45 | 46 |

*Sides: As Per Menu Description*

| | C | F | Cb |
|---|---|---|---|
| Blue Cheese Pecan Chopped Salad | 665 | 47 | 48 |
| Classic Blue Cheese Wedge Salad | 490 | 39 | 27 |
| Dressed Baked Potato | 355 | 12 | 53 |
| Fresh Seasonal Mixed Veggies | 95 | 3 | 11 |
| Garlic Mashed Potatoes | 275 | 15 | 30 |
| Sweet Potato, w/ Butter & Sugar | 290 | 2 | 63 |

*Desserts: Per Whole Dish*

| | C | F | Cb |
|---|---|---|---|
| Carrot Cake | 640 | 30 | 90 |
| Chocolate Thunder | 1635 | 108 | 148 |
| Sweet Adventure Trio | 1710 | 104 | 180 |

*Mini Milkshakes:*

| | C | F | Cb |
|---|---|---|---|
| Chocolate | 575 | 36 | 57 |
| Oreo | 645 | 36 | 73 |
| Strawberry | 440 | 22 | 54 |
| Vanilla | 475 | 27 | 50 |

*For Complete Menu & Data ~ see CalorieKing.com*

## Panda Express® (Aug '15)

*Appetizers:*

| | C | F | Cb |
|---|---|---|---|
| Chicken Egg Roll (3), 3.3 oz | 160 | 6 | 20 |
| Chicken Potsticker (3), 3.3 oz | 160 | 6 | 20 |
| Cream Cheese Rangoon (3), 2.4 oz | 190 | 8 | 24 |
| Veggie Spring Rolls (2), 3.4 oz | 190 | 8 | 27 |

*Continued Next Page...*

Updated Nutrition Data ~ www.CalorieKing.com
Persons with Diabetes ~ See Disclaimer (Page 22)

## Panda Express® cont... (Aug '15)

*Entrees:*

| | C | F | Cb |
|---|---|---|---|
| **Beef:** Beijing Beef, 5.6 oz | 470 | 26 | 46 |
| Broccoli Beef, 5.4 oz | 150 | 7 | 13 |
| Shanghai Angus Beef, 5.4 oz | 310 | 19 | 16 |
| **Chicken Breast:** | | | |
| String Bean, 5.6 oz | 190 | 9 | 13 |
| Sweet & Sour, 5.8 oz | 300 | 12 | 40 |
| SweetFire, 5.8 oz | 380 | 15 | 47 |
| **Shrimp:** Crispy Shrimp (6), 3.5 oz | 260 | 13 | 26 |
| Honey Walnut Shrimp, 3.7 oz | 360 | 23 | 35 |

*Rice & Noodles: Per Serving*

| | C | F | Cb |
|---|---|---|---|
| Chow Mein, 5.2 oz | 280 | 12 | 36 |
| Fried Rice, 6.2 oz | 350 | 11 | 55 |
| Steamed White Rice, 5.1 oz | 240 | 0 | 54 |

## Panera Bread® (Aug '15)

*Bagels:*

| | C | F | Cb |
|---|---|---|---|
| Asiago Cheese | 330 | 6 | 55 |
| Cinnamon Crunch | 420 | 6 | 81 |

*Breakfast Sandwiches, Grilled:*

| | C | F | Cb |
|---|---|---|---|
| Bacon, Egg & Cheese on Ciabatta | 520 | 25 | 43 |
| Sausage, Egg & Cheese on Ciabatta | 550 | 29 | 44 |
| Steak & Egg on Everthing Bagel | 550 | 18 | 60 |

*Sandwiches: Per Full Sandwich*

| | C | F | Cb |
|---|---|---|---|
| Asiago Steak on Asiago Chse Demi | 810 | 38 | 67 |
| Bacon Turkey Bravo | | | |
| on Tomato Basil | 790 | 27 | 85 |
| Mediterranean Chkn Flatbread (1) | 310 | 11 | 36 |
| Southwest Chicken (1) | 380 | 17 | 41 |
| Napa Almond Chicken Salad, | | | |
| on Sesame Semolina | 690 | 26 | 93 |
| Sierra Turkey, | | | |
| on Asiago Cheese Foccacia | 740 | 27 | 82 |
| Smoked Turkey Breast on Country | 430 | 3.5 | 67 |
| Tuna Salad on Honey Wheat | 510 | 16 | 65 |

*Hot Paninis: Per Full Panini*

| | C | F | Cb |
|---|---|---|---|
| Chipotle Chicken on French | 840 | 38 | 72 |
| Frontega Chicken on Focaccia | 740 | 24 | 87 |

*Salads: Full Size, With Dressing, without Bread*

| | C | F | Cb |
|---|---|---|---|
| Asian Sesame Chicken | 420 | 21 | 27 |
| BBQ Chicken | 450 | 20 | 38 |
| Chicken Caesar | 440 | 26 | 19 |
| Greek | 350 | 31 | 12 |
| Steak & Blue Cheese | 680 | 48 | 29 |

## Panera Bread® cont... (Aug '15)

*Soups: Per Bowl, w/o Bread*

| | C | F | Cb |
|---|---|---|---|
| All Natural Turkey Chili | 280 | 12 | 34 |
| Baked Potato | 340 | 24 | 27 |
| Broccoli Cheddar | 330 | 21 | 23 |
| Cream of Chicken & Wild Rice | 310 | 20 | 24 |
| New England Clam Chowder | 720 | 62 | 31 |
| Vegetarian Creamy Tomato | 450 | 32 | 33 |

*Pastries & Sweets:*

| | C | F | Cb |
|---|---|---|---|
| Bear Claw, 4.5 oz | 570 | 28 | 69 |
| Cheese Pastry, 3.8 oz | 400 | 22 | 44 |
| Chocolate Pastry, 3.5 oz | 410 | 23 | 47 |
| Cobblestone, 7 oz | 570 | 15 | 100 |
| Oatmeal Raisin Cookie, 3.3 oz | 400 | 14 | 62 |
| *Muffins:* Apple Crunch, 5 oz | 450 | 12 | 80 |
| Pumpkin, 6 oz | 590 | 22 | 91 |
| Wild Blueberry, 4.5 oz | 440 | 17 | 66 |

## Papa Gino's® (Aug '15)

*Appetizers: Per Small Serving*

| | C | F | Cb |
|---|---|---|---|
| BBQ Chicken Tender (2), 5.2 oz | 360 | 18 | 33 |
| Buffalo Chicken Tender (2), 5.4 oz | 390 | 25 | 22 |
| Chicken Tender (2), 4.4 oz | 350 | 20 | 24 |
| Toasted Ravioli (2), 7.9 oz | 570 | 32 | 62 |
| *Burgers:* Cheeseburger, 6.7 oz | 570 | 32 | 37 |
| Classic Double, 12.8 oz | 1040 | 67 | 43 |
| Hamburger, 6.3 oz | 520 | 28 | 36 |
| *French Fries,* small, 5 oz | 230 | 10 | 33 |

*Pastas: Per ⅙ of Order*

| | C | F | Cb |
|---|---|---|---|
| Mac & Cheese, 8.8 oz | 520 | 30 | 44 |
| Ravioli, 10 oz | 450 | 17 | 56 |
| Spaghetti & Meatballs, 10.5 oz | 540 | 29 | 52 |

*Pizzas:*

**Thin Crust:** *Per lice, ⅛ of Large Pizza*

| | C | F | Cb |
|---|---|---|---|
| Boss BBQ Chicken | 320 | 12 | 38 |
| Cheese | 230 | 7 | 32 |
| Meat Combo | 330 | 16 | 32 |
| PapaRoni | 340 | 16 | 32 |
| Pepperoni | 280 | 11 | 32 |
| Super Veggie | 250 | 8 | 35 |
| Works | 330 | 14 | 34 |

*Subs: Per Small Sub*

| | C | F | Cb |
|---|---|---|---|
| BLT | 690 | 35 | 67 |
| Italian | 590 | 24 | 64 |
| Meatball Parmesan | 790 | 38 | 79 |
| Steak & Cheese | 710 | 33 | 63 |
| Super Steak | 750 | 33 | 72 |
| Tuna | 730 | 39 | 64 |
| Turkey Club | 600 | 22 | 67 |

## Papa John's® (Aug '15)

**Pizzas:**

| | C | F | Cb |
|---|---|---|---|
| **Original Crust (14"):** *Per 1/8 of Large 14" Pizza* | | | |
| Double Bacon 6 Cheese | 350 | 14 | 38 |
| Spicy Italian, 5.25 oz | 370 | 18 | 38 |
| Spinach Alfredo, 4 oz | 280 | 10 | 36 |
| The Meats, 3.8 oz | 370 | 17 | 38 |
| The Works, 5.5 oz | 330 | 14 | 39 |
| **Thin Crust (14"):** *Per 1/8 of Large 14" Pizza* | | | |
| Double Bacon 6 Cheese | 290 | 16 | 22 |
| Spicy Italian, 4 oz | 310 | 20 | 23 |
| Spinach Alfredo, 2.8 oz | 220 | 12 | 21 |
| The Meats, 3.8 oz | 310 | 19 | 22 |
| The Works, 4.3 oz | 270 | 15 | 23 |
| ***Wings:*** *Without Dipping Sauce* | | | |
| BBQ, 2 wings, 2.75 oz | 190 | 12 | 6 |
| Spicy Buffalo, 2 wings, 2.75 oz | 140 | 9 | 1 |
| ***Dipping Sauces:*** *Per 1 oz Container* | | | |
| Barbeque | 45 | 0 | 11 |
| Blue Cheese | 160 | 16 | 1 |
| Buffalo | 15 | 0.5 | 2 |
| Ranch | 100 | 10 | 1 |
| ***Sides:*** *Without Dipping Sauce* | | | |
| Breadsticks (2) | 290 | 4.5 | 53 |
| Cheesesticks (4) | 330 | 16 | 41 |
| Parmesan Breadsticks (2) | 340 | 10 | 54 |

## Papa Murphy's® (Aug '15)

**Pizzas:**

| | C | F | Cb |
|---|---|---|---|
| **Original Crust:** *Per 1/12 of Family Size Pizza* | | | |
| BBQ Chicken | 330 | 12 | 36 |
| Cheese | 270 | 10 | 29 |
| Chicken Garlic | 320 | 13 | 30 |
| Classic Italian | 350 | 18 | 31 |
| Cowboy | 335 | 16 | 30 |
| Gourmet Vegetarian | 300 | 13 | 31 |
| Hawaiian | 295 | 11 | 33 |
| Murphy's Combo | 350 | 17 | 31 |
| Papa's Favorite | 350 | 17 | 31 |
| Pepperoni | 320 | 15 | 31 |
| Rancher | 325 | 15 | 30 |
| Specialty of the House | 310 | 14 | 30 |
| Vegetarian | 280 | 12 | 32 |
| **Stuffed Pizzas:** *Per 1/16 of Family Size Pizza* | | | |
| 5 Meat | 370 | 15 | 38 |
| Big Murphy | 370 | 15 | 39 |
| Chicago Style | 365 | 15 | 39 |
| Chicken and Bacon | 370 | 12 | 38 |

## Papa Murphy's® cont... (Aug '15)

**Pizzas (Cont):**

| | C | F | Cb |
|---|---|---|---|
| **Thin Crust:** *Per 1/8 of Large Pizza* | | | |
| Cheese | 180 | 9 | 16 |
| Hawaiian | 195 | 9 | 19 |
| Pepperoni | 215 | 12 | 16 |
| ***Salads:*** *Per Whole Salad, w/out Dressing or Croutons* | | | |
| Club, 13 oz | 280 | 16 | 12 |
| Garden, 14.5 oz | 190 | 11 | 15 |
| Italian, 13 oz | 265 | 19 | 13 |

## Pei Wei Asian Diner (Aug '15)

| | C | F | Cb |
|---|---|---|---|
| ***Perfect Additions:*** *W/out Sauce* | | | |
| Crab Wontons (4) | 340 | 20 | 26 |
| Crispy Potstickers (4) | 300 | 16 | 25 |
| Traditional Edamame, small | 160 | 7 | 10 |
| Vegetable Spring Rolls (4) | 460 | 20 | 52 |
| **Sauces:** Potsticker, 2 oz | 35 | 1.5 | 3 |
| Sweet Chile, 2 oz | 140 | 0 | 34 |
| Thai Peanut Dipping Sauce, 2 oz | 230 | 15 | 20 |
| ***Lettuce Wraps:*** *With Sauce* | | | |
| Thai Chicken | 540 | 30 | 31 |
| Traditional Chicken | 720 | 36 | 66 |
| Sauce, 2 oz | 70 | 3.5 | 4 |
| ***Wok Fresh Classic Entrees:*** *Per Small Serving with Rice* | | | |
| **Honey Seared:** With Chicken | 1010 | 30 | 149 |
| With Shrimp | 1010 | 30 | 161 |
| With Steak | 1080 | 33 | 164 |
| Original: | | | |
| With Chicken | 1500 | 48 | 206 |
| With shrimp | 1380 | 46 | 199 |
| With Steak | 1520 | 51 | 206 |
| **Fried Rice:** | | | |
| With Chicken | 750 | 23 | 95 |
| With Shrimp | 670 | 21 | 93 |
| With Steak | 780 | 27 | 98 |
| Pei Wei Spicy: | | | |
| With Chicken | 900 | 21 | 145 |
| With Steak | 1080 | 30 | 176 |
| *Soup:* Hot & Sour, 1 Cup | 70 | 2.5 | 6 |
| Thai Wanton, 1 Cup | 80 | 2 | 11 |
| ***Salads:*** *Per Per Small, Without Dressing* | | | |
| Asian Chopped Chicken | 250 | 8 | 22 |
| Pei Wei Spicy Chicken | 700 | 27 | 91 |
| *Cookies,* Choc. Chip; Snickerdoodle | 370 | 16 | 53 |
| **Pepe's Mexican•** ~ *see CalorieKing.com* | | | |

## Perkins® (Aug '15)

*Breakfast:* With Menu Set Items **C** **F** **Cb**

| | C | F | Cb |
|---|---|---|---|
| **Classic:** Eggs Benedict | 1220 | 54 | 148 |
| Eggs & Canadian Bacon | 670 | 40 | 48 |
| **Griddle Greats:** | | | |
| Belgian Waffles: Plain, | | | |
| with whipped topping | 470 | 23 | 57 |
| Blueberry, w/ Wh. Topping | 640 | 18 | 112 |
| Strawberry, w/ Wh. Topping | 580 | 18 | 97 |
| Berry Blueb. P'cakes w/ Topping | 860 | 24 | 150 |
| Brioche French Toast Platter | 890 | 47 | 74 |
| Cinnamon Roll French Platter | 870 | 51 | 71 |
| Potato Pancakes (3) | 990 | 43 | 130 |
| Short Stack, without syrup | 420 | 22 | 48 |
| The Buttermilk Five, w/o syrup | 640 | 30 | 80 |
| **Pancake Syrup,** 2 oz | 140 | 0 | 35 |
| **Omelettes:** *With Fruit Cup & White Bread Toast* | | | |
| Everything | 840 | 46 | 67 |
| Farmers | 730 | 54 | 27 |
| Granny's Country | 1260 | 53 | 151 |
| **Hearty Extras:** | | | |
| Breakfast Potatoes, 5 oz | 250 | 12 | 32 |
| English Muffin, w/ butter, 2.7 oz | 230 | 11 | 28 |
| Fruit Cup, 4 oz | 50 | 0 | 12 |
| Hash Browns, 4 oz | 490 | 13 | 87 |
| Oatmeal, | | | |
| w/ 2% Milk & Br. Sugar | 330 | 6 | 60 |
| Sausage Links (4) | 460 | 44 | 2 |
| **Burgers:** *With Standard Toppings w/out Fruit Cup* | | | |
| BBQ Bacon Supreme | 980 | 62 | 56 |
| Cheeseburger | 870 | 56 | 46 |
| Hamburger | 710 | 42 | 44 |
| Tangler | 1040 | 69 | 56 |
| **Melts:** *With Standard Toppings, Without Fruit Cup* | | | |
| Chicken Strips | 1290 | 80 | 88 |
| Country Club | 1050 | 64 | 66 |
| Reuben Melt on Rye | 1100 | 63 | 75 |
| **Sandwiches:** *With Standard Toppings, w/o Fruit Cup* | | | |
| Kickin' Chicken | 990 | 57 | 80 |
| Triple Decker Club | 910 | 56 | 57 |
| **Sides,** French Fries, 7 oz | 570 | 36 | 56 |
| **Wrap,** Ham & Turkey BLT | | | |
| with French Fries | 1080 | 69 | 89 |

## Perkins® cont... (Aug '15)

*Lunch & Dinners:* **C** **F** **Cb**

**Fork Worthy Entrees:** *W/- Dinner Roll & Two Menu Set Sides Unless Indicated.*

| | C | F | Cb |
|---|---|---|---|
| Chicken Pot Pie, w/o sides | 1570 | 104 | 101 |
| Chicken Strips | 1120 | 63 | 85 |
| Country Fried Steak | 1120 | 63 | 85 |
| Grilled Pork Chops | 880 | 52 | 35 |
| Homestyle Pot Roast | 590 | 33 | 32 |
| Mushroom 'n Swiss Chkn on Rice | 930 | 43 | 76 |
| Tilapia Grille, with Tartar Sauce | 690 | 38 | 36 |
| Turkey & Dressing | 810 | 37 | 69 |
| Tuscan Gr. Chicken on Herb Rice | 590 | 21 | 61 |
| *Sides:* | | | |
| Baked Potato, with Sour Cream, | | | |
| & Whipped Butter, 8.6 oz | 390 | 22 | 42 |
| Broccoli Florets, 4 oz | 35 | 0 | 5 |
| French Fries, 7 oz | 570 | 36 | 56 |
| Green Beans & Bacon, 4 oz | 45 | 2.5 | 4 |
| Macaroni & Five Cheese, 5.2 oz | 300 | 16 | 26 |
| Mashed Potatoes, 4 oz | 290 | 16 | 32 |
| With Brown Gravy, 8.6oz | 290 | 16 | 32 |
| Sauteed Spinach, 4.1 oz | 70 | 3.5 | 4 |
| Side Salad with Croutons, | | | |
| and Ranch Dressing, 6.5 oz | 300 | 25 | 15 |
| Vegetable Medley, side, 4 oz | 110 | 8 | 6 |
| **Soups:** *Per Bowl, Includes Crackers* | | | |
| Homestyle Chicken Noodle | 260 | 6 | 37 |
| Tomato Basil | 460 | 26 | 46 |
| **Salads:** *Includes Dinner Roll* | | | |
| Chef Deluxe, without dressing | 660 | 39 | 34 |
| Chicken & Spinach, w/out dressng | 970 | 66 | 40 |
| Honey Mustard Chicken Crunch | | | |
| with Honey Mustard Dressing | 1220 | 79 | 83 |
| *Dessert:* | | | |
| **Muffins:** *Includes Whipped Butter Blend* | | | |
| Apple Cinnamon | 570 | 31 | 66 |
| Banana Nut | 700 | 40 | 78 |
| Blueberry, | 600 | 31 | 72 |
| **Pies:** *Per Slice* | | | |
| Caramel Apple, 7.2 oz | 500 | 22 | 68 |
| Chocolate French Silk, | | | |
| with Whipped Cream, 6 oz | 760 | 54 | 66 |
| Southern Pecan, 5.5 oz | 670 | 33 | 86 |
| Wildberry, no sugar added, 7 oz | 470 | 27 | 50 |

## Peter Piper Pizza® (Aug '15)

*Appetizers:*

| | C | F | Cb |
|---|---|---|---|
| **Boneless Wings:** *Per 10 oz Serving* | | | |
| Mild Buffalo | 1010 | 67 | 56 |
| Sweet BBQ | 1130 | 58 | 110 |
| Cheddar Bacon Roll (1) | 350 | 18 | 34 |
| Garlic Cheese Bread, 3.25 oz | 390 | 17 | 45 |
| Handmade Breadsticks, with Marinara Sauce (6) | 1000 | 9 | 198 |

*Dipping Sauces:*

| | C | F | Cb |
|---|---|---|---|
| BBQ | 240 | 0 | 60 |
| Buffalo | 120 | 9 | 6 |
| Ranch | 320 | 36 | 2 |
| Sweet Chili | 200 | 0 | 46 |
| Xtra Hot Buffalo | 90 | 6 | 5 |

*Signature Pizzas: Per Slice*

| **Original Crust:** *Per ⅛ of Large 14" Pizza* | C | F | Cb |
|---|---|---|---|
| 5 Meat Supreme | 390 | 18 | 39 |
| Buffalo Ranch | 400 | 20 | 37 |
| California Veggie | 290 | 9 | 41 |
| Cheddar & Bacon | 540 | 28 | 45 |
| Cheese | 310 | 11 | 39 |
| Chicago Classic | 330 | 12 | 40 |
| Double Pepperoni Parmesan | 310 | 15 | 27 |
| Extreme Pepperoni | 260 | 13 | 26 |
| New York 3 Cheese w/ Pepperoni | 480 | 25 | 40 |
| Pizza Mexicana | 390 | 18 | 39 |
| The Werx | 340 | 14 | 40 |

| **Original Crust:** *Per ½ of Extra Large 16" Pizza* | C | F | Cb |
|---|---|---|---|
| 5 Meat Supreme | 340 | 16 | 34 |
| Buffalo Ranch | 340 | 17 | 32 |
| California Veggie | 250 | 7 | 36 |
| Cheddar & Bacon | 480 | 25 | 39 |
| Cheese | 270 | 9 | 33 |
| Chicago Classic | 290 | 11 | 35 |
| Double Pepperoni Parmesan | 400 | 19 | 35 |
| Extreme Pepperoni | 340 | 16 | 34 |
| New York 3 Cheese w/ Pepperoni | 410 | 21 | 34 |
| Pizza Mexicana | 340 | 15 | 34 |
| The Werx | 290 | 11 | 35 |

| **Salads:** *Without Dressing* | C | F | Cb |
|---|---|---|---|
| Apple Harvest with Walnuts | 270 | 16 | 27 |
| Caesar, small | 320 | 14 | 35 |
| Chopped House, small | 210 | 6 | 35 |
| Mandarin Cranberry, small | 150 | 6 | 26 |

## Peter Piper® ...cont (Aug '15)

*Dessert:*

| | C | F | Cb |
|---|---|---|---|
| Cinnamon Crunch, 3 pieces | 380 | 9 | 69 |
| Vanilla Soft Serve: Cone | 200 | 6 | 35 |
| Cup | 180 | 6 | 31 |

## P.F. Chang's® (Aug '15)

| **Starters:** *Per Whole Dish* | C | F | Cb |
|---|---|---|---|
| Crispy Green Beans, without sauce | 760 | 55 | 63 |
| Crispy Bean Sauce, 2 oz | 310 | 33 | 3 |
| Egg Rolls (4), without sauce | 560 | 20 | 75 |
| Egg Roll Sauce, 2 oz | 70 | 1.5 | 13 |
| Lettuce Wraps: Chicken (4) | 530 | 24 | 47 |
| Vegetarian (4) | 610 | 36 | 39 |
| Pork Dumplings: | | | |
| Pan-Fried, with sauce, (6) | 420 | 20 | 39 |
| Steamed, with sauce, (6) | 390 | 17 | 39 |
| Salt & Pepper Calamari | 710 | 37 | 68 |
| Shrimp Dumplings: | | | |
| Pan-Fried, with sauce, (6) | 300 | 11 | 34 |
| Steamed, with sauce, (6) | 290 | 6 | 37 |
| Veg. Spring Rolls, w/out Sauce, (4) | 330 | 11 | 50 |

*Specialties:*

| **Beef:** *Per Whole Meal, Without Rice* | C | F | Cb |
|---|---|---|---|
| A La Sichuan | 680 | 32 | 54 |
| Mongolian | 720 | 39 | 31 |
| Shaking | 800 | 49 | 42 |

| **Chicken:** *Per Whole Dish, Without Rice* | C | F | Cb |
|---|---|---|---|
| Almond & Cashew | 640 | 25 | 46 |
| Cantonese-Style Lemon | 750 | 37 | 47 |
| Chang's Spicy | 820 | 34 | 73 |
| Korean BBQ Chicken Stir-Fry | 870 | 44 | 70 |

| **Seafood:** *Per Whole Meal, Without Rice* | C | F | Cb |
|---|---|---|---|
| Asian Grilled Salmon | 610 | 35 | 17 |
| Hunan-Style Hot Fish | 650 | 32 | 42 |
| Oolong Chilean Sea Bass | 560 | 38 | 10 |
| Salt & Pepp. Prwns | 590 | 30 | 34 |
| Sauce, 2 oz | 70 | 1.5 | 13 |
| Walnut Shrimp with Melon | 1380 | 104 | 74 |

| **Vegetarian Plates:** *Without Rice* | C | F | Cb |
|---|---|---|---|
| Coconut Curry Vegetables | 1050 | 77 | 47 |
| Ma Po Tofu | 1030 | 70 | 44 |

*Continued Next Page...*

## P.F. Chang's® cont... (Aug '15)

| *Wok Classics:* Without Rice | C | F | Cb |
|---|---|---|---|
| Crispy Honey Chicken | 1140 | 49 | 114 |
| Crispy Honey Shrimp | 760 | 28 | 108 |
| Kung Pao Combo | 830 | 49 | 46 |
| Kung Pao Scallops | 830 | 48 | 44 |
| Sweet & Sour Pork | 710 | 25 | 94 |
| *Noodles Meins & Rice:* | | | |
| Fried Rice, with Beef | 1240 | 28 | 203 |
| Lo Mein Pork | 760 | 25 | 100 |
| Singapore Street Noodles | 920 | 21 | 127 |
| *Sides:* Per Small Dish | | | |
| Brown Rice, 6 oz | 310 | 2 | 66 |
| Shanghai Cucumbers | 70 | 3 | 7 |
| Sichuan-Style Asparagus | 90 | 4 | 11 |
| Spinach with Garlic | 120 | 8 | 8 |
| White Rice, 6 oz | 300 | 1 | 68 |
| **Soups:** | | | |
| **Hot & Sour:** 1 cup | 80 | 2.5 | 11 |
| 1 bowl | 380 | 11 | 48 |
| **Egg Drop:** 1 cup | 50 | 2 | 8 |
| 1 bowl | 260 | 9 | 39 |

## Pita Pit® ~ See CalorieKing.com

## Pizza Hut® (Aug '15)

| *Hand-Tossed Style:* Per ⅛ of 12" Pizza | C | F | Cb |
|---|---|---|---|
| Cheese | 210 | 8 | 25 |
| Hot & Twisted | 200 | 7 | 26 |
| Meat Lover's | 280 | 15 | 25 |
| Pepperoni | 220 | 9 | 25 |
| Pepperoni Lover's | 270 | 13 | 26 |
| Supreme | 240 | 10 | 26 |
| Sweet Sriracha Dynamite | 210 | 6 | 30 |
| Ultimate Cheese Lover's | 230 | 10 | 25 |
| Veggie Lover's | 190 | 6 | 26 |
| *Pan:* Per ⅛ of 12" Pizza | | | |
| Cheese | 240 | 10 | 28 |
| Meat Lover's | 310 | 17 | 27 |
| Pepperoni | 260 | 12 | 27 |
| Pepperoni Lover's | 310 | 16 | 28 |
| Pretzel Piggy | 260 | 12 | 28 |
| Supreme | 270 | 13 | 28 |
| Ultimate Cheese Lover's | 270 | 13 | 27 |
| Veggie Lover's | 220 | 9 | 28 |

## Pizza Hut® cont... (Aug '15)

| *Personal Pan:* Per 6" Pizza | C | F | Cb |
|---|---|---|---|
| BBQ Lover's | 740 | 36 | 74 |
| Meat Lover's | 850 | 48 | 69 |
| Pepperoni | 620 | 28 | 67 |
| Pepperoni Lover's | 730 | 37 | 68 |
| Supreme | 730 | 37 | 69 |
| Sweet Sriracha Dynamite | 600 | 21 | 77 |
| Ultimate Cheese Lover's | 680 | 32 | 68 |
| Veggie Lover's | 550 | 20 | 70 |
| *Thin 'n Crispy:* Per ⅛ of 12" Pizza | | | |
| Cheese | 190 | 8 | 22 |
| Cherry Pepper Bombshell | 200 | 8 | 24 |
| Meat Lover's | 270 | 15 | 22 |
| Old Fashioned Meatbrawl | 210 | 9 | 23 |
| Pepperoni | 210 | 10 | 21 |
| Pepperoni Lover's | 260 | 14 | 22 |
| Supreme | 220 | 10 | 23 |
| Ultimate Cheese Lover's | 220 | 11 | 21 |
| Veggie Lover's | 180 | 6 | 23 |
| *Stuffed Crust:* Per ⅛ 14" Pizza | | | |
| Cheese | 310 | 13 | 35 |
| Meat Lover's | 430 | 24 | 35 |
| Supreme | 360 | 18 | 36 |
| Ultimate Cheese Lover's | 340 | 16 | 34 |
| Veggie Lover's | 300 | 12 | 36 |
| *Pastas, Tuscani:* Per ½ Pan | | | |
| Creamy Chicken Alfredo | 510 | 26 | 47 |
| Meaty Marinara | 450 | 19 | 48 |
| *Appetizers/Sides:* | | | |
| Baked Hot Wings, average all flavors, | | | |
| 2 pieces | 105 | 7 | 1 |
| Breadstick (1) | 130 | 4.5 | 19 |
| Cheese Sticks (1) | 160 | 6 | 20 |
| Flavor Sticks (1), av. all flavors | 130 | 4 | 20 |
| Flavor Sticks, toasted (1), all flav. | 140 | 4 | 19 |
| Waffle Fries, side order, 7 oz | 660 | 41 | 66 |
| *Desserts:* Cinnamon Sticks, 2 pcs | 160 | 4.5 | 26 |
| Hershey's: Choc. Dunkers, 2 pcs | 190 | 8 | 26 |
| Chocolate Sauce, 1.5 oz | 120 | 2.5 | 25 |
| White Icing Dipping Cup, 2 oz | 170 | 0 | 44 |

## Pizza Ranch® (Aug '15)

*Pizza:*

| | C | F | Cb |
|---|---|---|---|
| **Breakfast,** average all varieties | | | |
| ⅛ of medium pizza | 250 | 11 | 28 |
| **Original Crust:** *Per ¹⁄₁₀ Slice of Medium Buffet Pizza* | | | |
| Bacon Cheeseburger | 240 | 9 | 29 |
| BLT | 280 | 14 | 29 |
| Bronco | 250 | 10 | 29 |
| Buffalo Chicken | 240 | 9 | 28 |
| California Chicken | 260 | 11 | 28 |
| Chicken Bacon Ranch | 270 | 12 | 28 |
| Chicken Broccoli Alfredo | 230 | 8 | 28 |
| Garlic Cheese | 240 | 11 | 27 |
| Italian Sausage | 230 | 8 | 29 |
| Pepperoni | 240 | 9 | 29 |
| Prairie (Veggie) | 220 | 7 | 30 |
| Roundup | 240 | 9 | 30 |
| Stampede | 250 | 9 | 30 |
| Sweet Swine | 220 | 6 | 30 |
| Texan Taco | 270 | 9 | 37 |
| **Thin Crust:** *Per ⅛ Slice of Medium Carry Out Pizza* | | | |
| BBQ Chicken | 180 | 7 | 16 |
| Beef & Blue | 220 | 13 | 13 |
| BLT | 250 | 16 | 14 |
| Cheese | 190 | 10 | 12 |

*For Complete Menu & Data ~ see CalorieKing.com*

## Pollo Tropical® ~ *See CalorieKing.com*

## Popeye's® (Aug '15)

*Chicken Pieces: Mild & Spicy With Skin*

| | C | F | Cb |
|---|---|---|---|
| Breast, average | 430 | 27 | 14 |
| Leg, average | 165 | 10 | 5 |
| Thigh, average | 270 | 20 | 8 |
| Wing | 210 | 14 | 8 |
| **Nuggets:** 4 pieces, 1.8 oz | 150 | 9 | 10 |
| 6 Pieces 2.7 oz | 230 | 14 | 14 |
| **Tenders:** Mild, 3 pieces, 4.5 oz | 340 | 14 | 26 |
| Spicy, 3 pieces, 4.5 oz | 310 | 15 | 16 |
| **Sandwiches & Wraps:** *Each* | | | |
| Blackened BBQ Chicken Po'Boy | 340 | 7 | 49 |
| Chicken & Sausage Jambalaya | 220 | 11 | 20 |
| Chicken Po'Boy | 660 | 34 | 61 |
| Loaded Chicken Wrap | 310 | 13 | 33 |
| Shrimp Po' Boy | 690 | 42 | 66 |
| **Seafood:** Catfish Fillets, 5 oz | 460 | 29 | 27 |
| Butterfly Shrimp (8) | 290 | 17 | 21 |
| Popcorn Shrimp, 3 oz | 330 | 9 | 28 |

## Popeye's® ... cont (Aug '15)

*Sides:*

| | C | F | Cb |
|---|---|---|---|
| Biscuit, 2 oz | 260 | 15 | 26 |
| Cajun Fries, regular, 3 oz | 260 | 14 | 30 |
| Cajun Rice, regular, 4.3 oz | 170 | 5 | 25 |
| Cole Slaw, regular, 4.9 oz | 220 | 15 | 19 |
| Corn on the Cob (1), 7.8 oz | 190 | 2 | 37 |
| Mashed Potatoes, regular, 5 oz | 110 | 4 | 18 |
| Onion Rings (12) | 560 | 38 | 50 |
| Red Beans & Rice, regular, 5.2 oz | 230 | 14 | 23 |
| *Breakfast:* | | | |
| **Biscuits:** Bacon | 400 | 25 | 37 |
| Chicken | 490 | 26 | 47 |
| Egg | 510 | 29 | 41 |
| Egg & Sausage | 690 | 45 | 43 |
| Sausage | 540 | 36 | 41 |
| Sausage & Gravy | 510 | 33 | 42 |
| Grits | 370 | 5 | 80 |
| Hashbrowns | 360 | 20 | 41 |
| *Desserts:* | | | |
| Hot Sweet Potato Pie 3.4 oz | 350 | 19 | 41 |
| Mardi Gras Cheesecake, 3 oz | 310 | 19 | 32 |
| Mississippi Mud Pie, 3 oz | 280 | 7 | 51 |
| Sliced Pecan Pie, 3.4 oz | 410 | 21 | 52 |

## Port of Subs® (Aug '15)

*Figures Based on West Coast Outlets*

*Cold Submarine S'wiches: Per 5" Sub with Cheese, Lettuce, Tomato Vinegar, Oil, Salt & Oregano*

| | C | F | Cb |
|---|---|---|---|
| #1 Ham, Salami, Capicolla Pepperoni, Provolone | 435 | 18 | 42 |
| #2 Ham & Turkey, Provolone | 355 | 9 | 42 |
| #3 Salami & Turkey, Provolone | 390 | 13 | 43 |
| #4 Ham, Salami, Provolone | 385 | 14 | 42 |
| #5 Smoked Ham, Turkey, Cheddar | 370 | 10 | 43 |
| #6 Vegetarian, 3 Chse | 450 | 21 | 45 |
| #7 Roast Beef, Prov. | 365 | 10 | 42 |
| #8 Turkey, Provolone | 360 | 8 | 44 |
| #10 Rstd Chicken Breast, Provolone | 350 | 8 | 42 |
| #11 Ham, American Cheese | 405 | 14 | 44 |
| #12 Salami, Provolone | 395 | 16 | 42 |
| #13 Peppered Pastrami Turkey, Swiss | 375 | 12 | 43 |
| #15 Salami, Pepperoni, Provolone | 405 | 18 | 42 |
| #16 BLT | 470 | 26 | 39 |
| #17 Tuna, Provolone | 475 | 25 | 43 |
| #18 Roast Beef,Turkey, Provolone | 360 | 9 | 43 |

*Continued Next Page...*

# Fast - Foods & *Restaurants*

## Port of Subs® ...cont (Aug '15)

*Figures Based on West Coast Outlets* **C** **F** **Cb**

**Wraps:** *With 12" Flour Tortilla, Cheese, Lettuce, Tomato, Onion, Vinegar, Oil, Salt & Oregano*

| | C | F | Cb |
|---|---|---|---|
| #4 Ham, Salami, with Provolone | 600 | 28 | 56 |
| # 8 Turkey, with Provolone | 565 | 21 | 59 |
| #11 Ham, with American Cheese | 615 | 27 | 58 |

**Fresh Salads:** *With Lettuce, Tomato & Onion, w/o Dressing*

| | C | F | Cb |
|---|---|---|---|
| Caesar: With Parmesan, 6 oz | 35 | 0 | 11 |
| Add Grilled Chicken, 10 oz | 190 | 3 | 10 |
| Garden, 10 oz | 70 | 2 | 11 |
| Grilled Chicken, 10 oz | 190 | 3 | 10 |

**Salad Dressings:**

| | C | F | Cb |
|---|---|---|---|
| Blue Cheese, 1.5 oz | 220 | 23 | 2 |
| Ranch, 1.5 oz | 260 | 28 | 2 |
| Fat Free Ranch, 1.5 oz | 50 | 0 | 13 |

**Sides:** *Per Regular, 8 oz*

| | C | F | Cb |
|---|---|---|---|
| Caesar Bow Tie Pasta Salad, 8 oz | 355 | 18 | 37 |
| Potato Salad | 325 | 13 | 52 |

**Desserts:**

| | C | F | Cb |
|---|---|---|---|
| Brownie, 4.5 oz | 535 | 12 | 96 |
| Chocolate Chunk Cookie, 4.5 oz | 560 | 29 | 72 |
| Oatmeal Raisin Cookie | 500 | 23 | 68 |

**Fountain Beverages:** *Without Ice*

| | C | F | Cb |
|---|---|---|---|
| Coca Cola: 22 oz | 270 | 0 | 74 |
| 32 oz | 395 | 0 | 108 |
| Barq's Root Beer: 22 oz | 305 | 0 | 83 |
| 32 oz | 445 | 0 | 120 |
| Cherry Coke: 22 oz | 285 | 0 | 77 |
| 32 oz | 415 | 0 | 112 |

**Smoothies:** *Strawb. Bomb, 8 oz* 250, 0, 63

| | C | F | Cb |
|---|---|---|---|
| Mand. Orange Passion Fruit, 8 oz | 240 | 1 | 59 |
| Average other flavors, 8 oz | 220 | 1 | 53 |

## Pret A Manger® (Aug '15)

**Baguettes:** *Per Pack*

| | C | F | Cb |
|---|---|---|---|
| Albacore Tuna & Cucumber | 490 | 28 | 35 |
| Brie, Tomato & Basil | 540 | 17 | 72 |
| Chicken Mozzarella | 620 | 19 | 73 |
| Roast Beef & Parmesan | 350 | 15 | 70 |

**Hot Food:** *Per Pack*

| | C | F | Cb |
|---|---|---|---|
| Crispy Bacon Mac & Cheese | 470 | 26 | 38 |
| Melts: Chicago's Angus Beef | 610 | 23 | 55 |
| Toasties: Ham & Cheese | 540 | 24 | 49 |
| Mozzarella & Pesto | 450 | 16 | 52 |
| Wraps: BBQ Pulled Pork | 650 | 20 | 96 |
| Holiday Turkey | 540 | 12 | 79 |
| New York Meatball | 600 | 22 | 60 |
| Pret's Buffalo Chicken | 560 | 24 | 55 |

## Pret A Manger® ...cont (Aug '15)

**Sandwiches:** *Per Pack*

| | C | F | Cb |
|---|---|---|---|
| Albacore Tuna Salad | 510 | 29 | 39 |
| California Club | 490 | 25 | 44 |
| Crayfish & Arugula | 360 | 16 | 36 |
| Lebanese Chicken Flatbread | 380 | 16 | 40 |
| Pret's: Egg Salad & Arugula | 420 | 25 | 37 |
| Holiday Lunch | 490 | 9 | 74 |

**Soups:** *Per Medium*

| | C | F | Cb |
|---|---|---|---|
| Butternut Squash & Apple | 225 | 12 | 30 |
| Chicken Noodle | 150 | 4 | 14 |
| Creamy Chicken & Veggie | 225 | 11 | 26 |
| Moroccan Lentil | 450 | 18 | 53 |
| Thai Chicken Curry | 140 | 5 | 18 |
| Tomato Feta | 195 | 11 | 18 |

**Salads:** *Per Pack, Without Dressing*

| | C | F | Cb |
|---|---|---|---|
| Baja Crayfish Pot | 170 | 7 | 15 |
| California Tuna | 490 | 30 | 32 |
| Kale Chicken Caesar | 360 | 15 | 22 |
| Pret's Cobb | 430 | 22 | 35 |

**Dressings:**

| | C | F | Cb |
|---|---|---|---|
| Balsamic Vinaigrette | 140 | 15 | 2 |
| Caesar | 170 | 17 | 3 |
| Lemon Shallot Vinaigrette | 100 | 10 | 2 |
| Skinny | 50 | 0 | 10 |

**Bakery:** *Per Pack*

| | C | F | Cb |
|---|---|---|---|
| Croissants: Almond | 410 | 23 | 41 |
| Pain au Chocolate | 300 | 15 | 34 |
| Muffins: Blueberry | 420 | 20 | 54 |
| Cranberry Orange | 370 | 12 | 62 |
| Yogurt Pots: Banana & Honey | 310 | 9 | 41 |
| Blueberry & Granola | 320 | 12 | 33 |
| Pomegranate & Honey | 150 | 3 | 21 |

## Pretzelmaker® (Aug '15)

**Pretzels:** *Per Serving*

| | C | F | Cb |
|---|---|---|---|
| Bites: Plain, salted, large, 3.5 oz | 250 | 1 | 52 |
| Cinnamon Sugar, 3.8 oz | 330 | 4 | 65 |
| Whole: Caramel Crunch, 4.2 oz | 300 | 4 | 58 |
| Cinnamon Sugar, 3.9 oz | 330 | 4 | 65 |
| Garlic; Salted, average, 4.2 oz | 310 | 4 | 60 |
| Iced Cinnamon Swirl, 3.9 oz | 330 | 4 | 65 |
| Ranch, 4.2 oz | 320 | 4.5 | 60 |
| Pretzel Dogs: Mini (6) | 300 | 19 | 23 |
| Jalapeno, 6.4 oz | 410 | 19 | 32 |

*Continued Next Page...*

**229**

# Fast - Foods & *Restaurants*

## Pretzelmaker® cont... (Aug '15)

*Sauces: Per Single Portion*

| | C | F | Cb |
|---|---|---|---|
| Caramel | 140 | 0 | 35 |
| Cheddar Cheese | 80 | 5 | 4 |
| Cream Cheese | 200 | 20 | 2 |
| Honey Mustard | 80 | 0 | 20 |
| Icing | 180 | 0 | 45 |
| Ketchup | 20 | 0 | 4 |
| Mustard | 10 | 0 | 1 |
| Nacho Cheese | 80 | 5 | 4 |
| Pizza | 20 | 0.5 | 6 |

*Beverages: Per 20 fl.oz Unless Indicated*

**Blended Drinks:**

| | C | F | Cb |
|---|---|---|---|
| Cool Cappuccino | 640 | 21 | 107 |
| Lemon Twist | 540 | 16 | 99 |
| Mango Madness | 520 | 16 | 89 |
| Mocha Mania | 620 | 20 | 106 |
| Power Pomegranate | 490 | 16 | 86 |
| Strawberry Bananza | 650 | 20 | 115 |
| **Lemonade:** Original, 44 oz | 380 | 0 | 91 |
| Strawberry; Raspberry, 20 oz | 290 | 0 | 74 |

## Qdoba® (Aug '15)

*Burritos: Each with Flour Tortilla, Cilantro-Lime Rice, Black Beans, Salsa Verde, Sour Cream, Lettuce and Shredded Cheese*

| | C | F | Cb |
|---|---|---|---|
| Grilled Chicken | 1075 | 39 | 122 |
| Pulled Pork | 1045 | 33 | 131 |
| Seasoned Ground Beef | 1125 | 45 | 123 |

**Signature Flavors:** *With Flour Tortilla, 3-Cheese Queso, Pinto Beans, Lettuce, Guacamole & Sour Cream*

| | | | |
|---|---|---|---|
| Grilled Chicken | 925 | 40 | 91 |
| Grilled Steak | 935 | 41 | 91 |
| Pulled Pork | 895 | 34 | 100 |
| Seasoned Ground Beef | 975 | 46 | 92 |

*Grilled Quesadillas: With Flour Tortilla, Shredded Cheese, Pice de Gallo and Fajita Vegetables*

| | | | |
|---|---|---|---|
| Grilled Chicken | 980 | 54 | 61 |
| Shredded Beef | 980 | 51 | 66 |

*3-Cheese Nachos: Per Serving, with Tortilla Chips, 3-Cheese Queso, Salsa Roja, Guacamole & Sour Cream*

| | | | |
|---|---|---|---|
| Grilled Chicken | 1120 | 64 | 95 |
| Pulled Pork | 1090 | 58 | 104 |

## Qdoba® cont... (Aug '15)

*Tacos: Each, With Lettuce, Cheese, Guacamole, Pico de Gallo & Sour Cream*

| | C | F | Cb |
|---|---|---|---|
| **Crispy Shell:** Grilled Chicken | 250 | 16 | 12 |
| Pulled Pork | 235 | 14 | 15 |
| Seasoned Ground Beef | 265 | 19 | 13 |
| Shredded Beef | 245 | 16 | 14 |

*Taco Salads: With Crunchy Flour Tortilla Bowl, Lettuce, Black Bean & Corn Salsa, Shredded Cheese, Sour Cream, Guacamole & Cilantro Lime Dressing*

| | | | |
|---|---|---|---|
| Grilled Chicken | 1035 | 64 | 70 |
| Pulled Pork | 985 | 58 | 78 |
| Seasoned Ground Beef | 1085 | 70 | 71 |

*Chips & Dip: Includes Tortilla Chips*

| | | | |
|---|---|---|---|
| 3- Cheese Queso | 750 | 42 | 81 |
| 3-Cheese Queso, Guac. & Salsa Roja | 955 | 56 | 98 |

*Breakfast Burritos: With Flour Tortilla*

**Chorizo, Egg & Potato:**

| | | | |
|---|---|---|---|
| With 3-Cheese Queso Sauce | 925 | 42 | 87 |
| With Shred. Chse & Salsa Roja | 1070 | 52 | 89 |

## Quiznos Subs® (Aug '15)

*Subs: Per Regular Size On Japaleno Cheddar Sub, with Standard Menu Toppings Unless Indicated*

**All Natural Chicken:**

| | C | F | Cb |
|---|---|---|---|
| Baja Chicken | 860 | 38 | 74 |
| Carbonara | 950 | 48 | 71 |
| Honey Mustard | 910 | 41 | 77 |
| Mesquite Chicken | 910 | 43 | 72 |
| Pesto Caesar on Rosemary Parm | 780 | 33 | 62 |

**Steak:**

| | | | |
|---|---|---|---|
| Black Angus Steak | | | |
| On Rosemary Parmesan | 720 | 26 | 76 |
| Chipotle Steak & Cheddar | 830 | 44 | 66 |
| Peppercorn Steak | 830 | 43 | 69 |
| Steak, Bacon & Swiss | 790 | 34 | 69 |

**Deli Classics:**

| | | | |
|---|---|---|---|
| Classic Italian | 870 | 47 | 74 |
| Honey Bacon Club | 860 | 39 | 85 |
| Italian Meatball | 1110 | 59 | 86 |
| Spicy Monterey | 630 | 20 | 78 |
| The Traditional | 760 | 37 | 73 |
| Tuna | 790 | 37 | 74 |
| Veggie Guacamole | 760 | 43 | 71 |

*Grilled Flatbreads: Per Small*

| | | | |
|---|---|---|---|
| Basil Pesto Chicken | 360 | 15 | 37 |
| Chicken Bacon Ranch | 480 | 25 | 37 |
| Honey Bourbon Chkn | 290 | 6 | 45 |
| Sonoma Turkey | 450 | 26 | 36 |

*Continued Next Page...*

**230**

# Fast - Foods & *Restaurants*

## Quiznos Subs® cont... (Aug '15)

*Wraps: Includes Dressing*

| | C | F | Cb |
|---|---|---|---|
| BBQ Ranch Chicken | 510 | 15 | 64 |
| Honey Mustard Chicken | 580 | 21 | 63 |

*Salads: Per Large, without Dressing*

| | C | F | Cb |
|---|---|---|---|
| Honey Mustard Chicken | 290 | 14 | 13 |
| Peppercorn Caesar Chicken | 180 | 6 | 13 |

*Savory Soups: Per Regular Bowl, with 2 Crackers*

| | C | F | Cb |
|---|---|---|---|
| Broccoli Cheese | 180 | 9 | 17 |
| Chicken Noodle | 140 | 4.5 | 19 |

*Desserts:*

| | C | F | Cb |
|---|---|---|---|
| Choc. Chunk Cookie | 390 | 19 | 54 |
| Chocolate Brownie | 310 | 16 | 40 |
| Cinnamon Sugar Cookie | 400 | 17 | 58 |
| Oatmeal Raisin Cookie | 360 | 12 | 58 |

## Rally's/Checkers® (Aug '15)

*Burgers/Sandwiches:*

| | C | F | Cb |
|---|---|---|---|
| Big Buford | 570 | 36 | 31 |
| Bacon Double Cheese | 650 | 42 | 32 |
| Cheese Double Cheese | 510 | 31 | 31 |
| Chili Cheeseburger | 320 | 15 | 30 |
| Rallyburger | 390 | 22 | 32 |

*Classic Wings: Buffalo, 5 pieces*

| | C | F | Cb |
|---|---|---|---|
| | 335 | 18 | 2 |
| Honey BBQ, 5 pieces | 390 | 17 | 18 |
| Parmesan Garlic, 5 pieces | 480 | 35 | 1 |

*Fries:*

| | C | F | Cb |
|---|---|---|---|
| Fries, medium, 4.2 oz | 420 | 27 | 40 |
| Chili Cheese, 7.8 oz | 550 | 34 | 48 |
| Fully Loaded, 7.4 oz | 640 | 44 | 51 |

## Ranch One® (Aug '15)

*Sandwiches:*

| | C | F | Cb |
|---|---|---|---|
| Chicken & Cheese | 390 | 12 | 40 |
| Chkn Philly, 9.3 oz | 410 | 13 | 40 |
| Grilled Classic Chicken, 9.4 oz | 680 | 47 | 37 |
| Original Crispy Chicken, 11.5 oz | 640 | 31 | 60 |

*Other Favorites:*

| | C | F | Cb |
|---|---|---|---|
| Chicken Fajita, 10 oz | 540 | 24 | 53 |
| Chicken Platter, with Rice, 11.9 oz | 270 | 6 | 28 |
| Popcorn Chicken: Small, 5.5 oz | 310 | 10 | 30 |
| Large, 7.5 oz | 420 | 14 | 40 |
| Kids, 2 oz | 120 | 4 | 11 |

*Salads: Completed*

| | C | F | Cb |
|---|---|---|---|
| Grilled Chicken Caesar, 13.3 oz | 430 | 30 | 14 |
| Southwest Chicken, 17.5 oz | 680 | 43 | 44 |
| *Fries:* Medium, 5.8 oz | 380 | 19 | 43 |
| Kids, 4.3 oz | 280 | 14 | 31 |
| Cheese: Medium, 7.3 oz | 490 | 27 | 46 |
| Large, 11 oz | 760 | 44 | 66 |

## Red Hot & Blue® (Aug '15)

*Entrees: Per Serving*

| | C | F | Cb |
|---|---|---|---|
| Delta Double: | | | |
| With Memphis Chicken | 900 | 54 | 12 |
| With Pulled Pork | 795 | 60 | 9 |
| Five Meat Treat | 935 | 63 | 15 |
| Ribs, Half Slab: Dry | 935 | 72 | 14 |
| Sweet | 950 | 71 | 22 |

*Sandwiches: Regular, Without Sides*

| | C | F | Cb |
|---|---|---|---|
| Beef Brisket | 390 | 15 | 37 |
| Carolina Chopped Pork | 360 | 14 | 34 |
| Pulled Pork | 370 | 15 | 37 |

*Salads: Without Dressing*

| | C | F | Cb |
|---|---|---|---|
| Grilled Chicken Caesar Salad | 770 | 46 | 47 |
| Pulled Chicken Salad | 295 | 8 | 14 |
| Smokehouse Salad | 670 | 36 | 36 |
| Southern Fried Chicken Salad | 710 | 31 | 60 |

*Soup, Memphis Corn Chowder,*

| | C | F | Cb |
|---|---|---|---|
| 1 bowl | 270 | 12 | 23 |

*Sides:*

| | C | F | Cb |
|---|---|---|---|
| BBQ Beans | 255 | 2 | 48 |
| Mashed Potatoes with Gravy | 310 | 14 | 44 |
| Memphis Fries, 6 oz | 345 | 19 | 38 |
| Potato Salad | 405 | 28 | 33 |

## Red Lobster® (Aug '15)

*Seaside Starters:*

| | C | F | Cb |
|---|---|---|---|
| Chilled Jumbo Shrimp Cocktail | 100 | 0.5 | 0.5 |
| Crispy Calamari & Vegetables | 1660 | 109 | 132 |
| Lobster, Artich. & Seafood Dip | 1040 | 61 | 93 |
| Lobster, Crab & Seafood, | | | |
| Stuffed Mushrooms | 430 | 26 | 20 |
| Lobster Pizza | 680 | 31 | 66 |
| Mozzarella Cheesesticks | 780 | 43 | 64 |
| Shrimp Nachos | 1200 | 72 | 98 |
| Sweet Chili Shrimp | 1140 | 79 | 79 |

**Lunch Classics:** *Without Condiments, Dipping Sauces or Optional Side Dishes.*

| | C | F | Cb |
|---|---|---|---|
| Cajun Chicken Linguini Alfredo, | | | |
| lunch serve | 720 | 35 | 55 |
| Crab Linguine, lunch serve | 810 | 46 | 64 |
| Crunchy Popcorn Shrimp | 380 | 18 | 38 |
| Garlic Shrimp Scampi | 100 | 4.5 | 1 |
| Sailor's Platter | 320 | 10 | 6 |
| Walleye: | | | |
| Beer-Battered | 590 | 37 | 26 |
| Blackened | 220 | 4.5 | 2 |
| Fried | 290 | 15 | 6 |

*Continued Next Page...*

## Red Lobster® cont... (Aug '15)

*Dinner Menu: Without Condiments, Dipping Sauces Or Optional Side Dishes Unless Indicated*

| Soup: Per Cup | C | F | Cb |
|---|---|---|---|
| Creamy Potato & Bacon | 250 | 18 | 19 |
| Lobster Bisque | 290 | 23 | 15 |
| New England Clam Chowder | 200 | 15 | 11 |
| **Lobster & Signature Combinations:** | | | |
| Live Main Lobster, steamed, with Corn & Potatoes | 420 | 4.5 | 35 |
| Rock Lobster Tail | 170 | 1 | 1 |
| Ultimate Feast w/- Rice Pilaf | 650 | 25 | 62 |
| **Shrimp & Classic Combinations:** | | | |
| Parrot Isle Jumbo C'nut Shrimp | 860 | 57 | 64 |
| Shrimp Linguini Alfredo, full | 1250 | 66 | 107 |
| Walt's Favorite Shrimp | 580 | 28 | 57 |
| *Side Dishes:* | | | |
| Baked Potato: Plain | 200 | 0.5 | 43 |
| Cheddar Bay Biscuit | 160 | 10 | 16 |
| Coleslaw | 260 | 20 | 17 |
| Creamy Lobster Mashed Potatoes | 380 | 24 | 30 |
| Fresh Broccoli | 50 | 0.5 | 7 |
| French Fries | 360 | 17 | 47 |
| Garden Salad | 70 | 1.5 | 13 |
| Wild Rice Pilaf | 170 | 3 | 32 |
| *Salads: Includes Dressing* | | | |
| Caesar Salad: With Chicken | 660 | 53 | 15 |
| With Shrimp | 640 | 53 | 16 |
| *Sauces: Per Dinner Menu* | | | |
| 100% Pure Melted Butter | 300 | 33 | 0 |
| Cocktail Sauce | 45 | 0 | 11 |
| Honey Mustard Dipping Sauce | 190 | 17 | 8 |
| Marinara | 35 | 2 | 4 |
| *Lighthouse/Fresh Fish Menu: Without Sides* | | | |
| Maine Lobster, steamed | 230 | 1.5 | 0 |
| Parmesan Crusted Tilapia | 320 | 15 | 10 |
| Snow Crab Legs | 180 | 2 | 0 |
| Wood-Grilled Peppercorn Sirloin & Shrimp | 300 | 11 | 3 |
| *Desserts:* | | | |
| Carrot Cake | 600 | 36 | 63 |
| Chocolate Wave | 1490 | 81 | 172 |
| Key Lime Pie | 580 | 22 | 88 |
| New York-Style Cheesecake with Strawberries | 590 | 41 | 48 |
| Warm Apple Crostada | 620 | 30 | 79 |
| Warm Chocolate Chip Lava Cookie | 1070 | 51 | 142 |

*For Complete Nutritional Data ~ see CalorieKing.com*

## Red Robin® (Aug '15)

*Nutritional Information varies between restaurants. Please refer to Red Robin's website for further information*

| Appetizers: | C | F | Cb |
|---|---|---|---|
| Chili Chili Con Queso | 650 | 34 | 51 |
| Creamy Artichoke & Spinach Dip | 685 | 41 | 52 |
| Guacamole, Salsa & Chips | 430 | 22 | 43 |
| Red's Tavern Fries | 1355 | 87 | 107 |
| Towering Onion Rings, w/ Ranch Dressing & Mayo | 1935 | 125 | 173 |
| Warm Pretzel Bites, w/ Beer Chse | 635 | 19 | 96 |
| *Jump Starters:* | | | |
| Jalepeno Coins, fried, w/out Dress. | 490 | 33 | 45 |
| Swt Potato Fries, w/out Dressing | 285 | 15 | 35 |
| Zucchini, Breaded & Fried, without Dressing | 215 | 15 | 17 |
| *Entrees: With Standard Menu Components* | | | |
| Arctic Cod Fish & Chips | 1050 | 65 | 74 |
| Clucks & Fries | 1320 | 78 | 102 |
| Ensenada Chicken Platter, 1 piece | 215 | 9 | 11 |
| Prime Rib Dip | 765 | 29 | 76 |
| Red's Nantucket Seafood Scatter | 1205 | 72 | 92 |
| *Finest Burgers:* Black & Bleu | 1115 | 69 | 65 |
| DGB | 1165 | 81 | 50 |
| Smoke & Pepper | 1030 | 51 | 74 |
| Southern Charm | 1220 | 61 | 98 |
| *Gourmet Burgers:* | | | |
| A.1. Peppercorn | 1365 | 82 | 93 |
| All American Patty Melt | 1175 | 80 | 72 |
| Bleu Ribbon | 1360 | 84 | 97 |
| Burnin' Love | 895 | 53 | 60 |
| Chili Chili Chsebgr | 915 | 49 | 61 |
| Garden Burger | 550 | 23 | 72 |
| Guacamole Bacon | 990 | 61 | 50 |
| Keep It Simple | 1995 | 115 | 151 |
| Prime Chophouse | 1385 | 83 | 105 |
| Red Robin Cheeseburger | 835 | 51 | 48 |
| Royal Red Robin | 1205 | 83 | 47 |
| Sauteed Mushroom | 840 | 49 | 52 |
| Whiskey River BBQ | 1390 | 89 | 94 |
| *Sandwiches & Wraps:* | | | |
| BLTA Croissant | 695 | 39 | 45 |
| Caesars Chkn Wrap | 765 | 42 | 54 |
| Whiskey River BBQ Chicken Wrap | 995 | 54 | 68 |

*Continued Next Page... ...*

## Red Robin® cont... (Aug '15)

| Soups: | C | F | Cb |
|---|---|---|---|
| **Chicken Tortilla:** *Includes Tortilla Strips* | | | |
| 1 Cup | 205 | 11 | 17 |
| 1 Bowl | 410 | 20 | 35 |
| **Clam Chowder:** *Includes Croutons* | | | |
| 1 Cup | 250 | 16 | 19 |
| 1 Bowl | 470 | 31 | 34 |
| **French Onion:** *Includes Baguette, Au Jus & Croutons* | | | |
| 1 Cup | 200 | 13 | 13 |
| 1 Bowl | 465 | 25 | 40 |
| *Salads: Without Bread or Dressing* | | | |
| Avo-Cobb-O | 500 | 28 | 20 |
| Crispy Chicken Tender | 875 | 49 | 53 |
| Simply Grilled Chicken | 235 | 8 | 16 |
| Spicy Sombrero | 620 | 40 | 32 |
| Whiskey Rio BBQ Chicken | 295 | 10 | 28 |
| *Desserts:* | | | |
| Gooey Chocolate Brownie Cake | 795 | 28 | 132 |
| Mountain High Mudd Pie | 1390 | 59 | 194 |
| *Milkshakes:* | | | |
| **Classic:** Banana | 530 | 21 | 77 |
| Chocolate | 535 | 21 | 77 |
| **Smoothie:** Groovy | 340 | 2 | 81 |
| Hawaiian Heart Throb | 375 | 2 | 91 |

## Roly Poly® (Aug '15)

| Wraps: | C | F | Cb |
|---|---|---|---|
| *Per 6" White Tortilla Unless Indicated* | | | |
| **Chicken:** Basil Cashew Chicken | 300 | 10 | 30 |
| Catalina Chicken | 315 | 11 | 28 |
| Chicken Caesar | 310 | 11 | 30 |
| Chicken Fajita | 315 | 9 | 28 |
| Cobb Salad | 255 | 12 | 27 |
| Oriental Chicken | 230 | 4 | 29 |
| Santa Fe Chicken | 305 | 11 | 28 |
| **Ham & Smoked Pork:** | | | |
| Italian Classic | 335 | 12 | 32 |
| Key West Cuban Mix | 330 | 9 | 44 |
| Peachtree Melt | 310 | 11 | 27 |
| Pork Melt | 310 | 11 | 26 |
| Porky's Nightmare | 320 | 12 | 28 |
| **Tuna:** Classic Tuna Melt | 340 | 17 | 26 |
| Popeyes Tuna on Wheat | 305 | 10 | 31 |
| Texas Tuna | 310 | 12 | 30 |
| Thai Hot Tuna | 290 | 11 | 30 |
| **Turkey:** California | 330 | 12 | 30 |
| Tuscan | 220 | 2 | 31 |

## Round Table Pizza® (Aug '15)

| Appetizers: | C | F | Cb |
|---|---|---|---|
| Boneless Wings: | | | |
| With BBQ Sauce, | | | |
| 8 pieces | 565 | 14 | 73 |
| With Buffalo Sauce, av., 6 pcs | 440 | 14 | 42 |
| Garlic Bread: 1 piece | 60 | 3 | 12 |
| With Cheese, 1 piece | 90 | 6 | 12 |
| Garlic Parmesan Twists, 1 twist | 170 | 5 | 24 |
| *Pizzas: Per ½ of Large 14" Pizza* | | | |
| **Original Crust:** Cheese | 230 | 9 | 25 |
| Chicken & Garlic Gourmet | 250 | 11 | 25 |
| Gourmet Veggie | 240 | 10 | 27 |
| Guinevere's Garden Delight | 220 | 8 | 26 |
| Hawaiian | 220 | 8 | 27 |
| Italian Garlic Supreme | 270 | 14 | 25 |
| King Arthur Supreme | 270 | 13 | 26 |
| Maui Zaui, with Polynesian Sce | 260 | 10 | 29 |
| Montague's All Meat Marvel | 290 | 15 | 25 |
| Smokehouse Combo, Chicken | 290 | 14 | 26 |
| Triple Play Pepperoni | 250 | 12 | 24 |
| **Pan Crust:** Cheese | 300 | 11 | 38 |
| Chicken & Garlic Gourmet | 340 | 13 | 39 |
| Gourmet Veggie | 320 | 12 | 41 |
| Guinevere's Garden Delight | 300 | 10 | 39 |
| Hawaiian | 300 | 10 | 40 |
| Italian Garlic Supreme | 360 | 16 | 39 |
| King Arthur Supreme | 340 | 14 | 39 |
| Maui Zaui w/ Polynesian Sauce | 340 | 12 | 43 |
| Montague's All Meat Marvel | 350 | 15 | 37 |
| Smokehouse Combo, Chicken | 370 | 16 | 40 |
| Triple Play Pepperoni | 330 | 14 | 36 |
| **Skinny Crust:** Cheese | 190 | 9 | 17 |
| Chicken & Garlic Gourmet | 220 | 11 | 18 |
| Gourmet Veggie | 200 | 10 | 20 |
| Guinevere's Garden Delight | 180 | 8 | 19 |
| Hawaiian | 190 | 8 | 20 |
| Italian Garlic Supreme | 240 | 14 | 18 |
| King Arthur Supreme | 240 | 13 | 19 |
| Maui Zaui w/ Polynesian Sauce | 220 | 10 | 22 |
| Montague's All Meat Marvel | 260 | 15 | 18 |
| Smokehouse Combo, Chicken | 250 | 14 | 20 |
| Triple Play Pepperoni | 220 | 12 | 17 |
| *Sandwiches:* | | | |
| Chicken Club | 800 | 43 | 59 |
| Ham Club | 740 | 40 | 60 |
| RT Veggie | 630 | 32 | 65 |
| Turkey Club | 720 | 38 | 59 |
| Turkey Sante-Fe | 730 | 40 | 57 |

*For Complete Nutritional Data ~ see CalorieKing.com*

# Fast - Foods & *Restaurants*

## Rubio's Mexican Grill® (Aug '15)

*Burritos:* Each With Flour Tortilla, without Chips

| | C | F | Cb |
|---|---|---|---|
| **Beef:** | | | |
| Baja Grilled, with Steak | 640 | 28 | 52 |
| Especial, w/ Steak | 890 | 34 | 107 |
| **Chicken:** | | | |
| Baja Grilled, w/ Chkn | 600 | 25 | 52 |
| Especial, with Chicken | 860 | 31 | 106 |
| **Seafood:** Beer Battered Fish | 850 | 53 | 68 |
| Blackened Atlantic Salmon | 700 | 32 | 74 |
| Classic Grilled Shrimp | 690 | 33 | 70 |
| Grilled Pacific Mahi Mahi | 690 | 31 | 74 |
| **Veggies & More:** Bean & Cheese | 710 | 31 | 74 |
| Veggie | 820 | 33 | 113 |

*Enchiladas:* With Black Beans & Citrus Rice

| | | | |
|---|---|---|---|
| Two Cheese, with Fire-Rstd Sauce | 800 | 38 | 83 |
| Two Chicken, with Fire-Rstd Sauce | 770 | 30 | 84 |
| Two Shrimp, with Verde Sauce | 810 | 33 | 90 |

*Tacos:* Each, with Corn Tortilla

| | | | |
|---|---|---|---|
| **Grilled Gourmet:** Chicken | 320 | 19 | 19 |
| Steak | 330 | 20 | 19 |
| **Seafood, Blackened:** | | | |
| Atlantic Salmon | 220 | 10 | 22 |
| Pacific Mahi Mahi | 220 | 10 | 22 |
| **Seafood, Grilled:** | | | |
| Atlantic Salmon | 220 | 10 | 21 |
| Pacific Mahi Mahi | 220 | 10 | 22 |
| Regal Springs Tilapia | 220 | 11 | 17 |

*Sides:*

| | | | |
|---|---|---|---|
| **Black Beans:** Regular, 4 oz | 130 | 2 | 22 |
| Large, 12 oz | 380 | 4 | 64 |
| **Chips:** Regular, 1.8 oz | 210 | 2 | 43 |
| Large, 4 oz | 460 | 5 | 96 |
| **Citrus Rice:** Regular, 3 oz | 150 | 2 | 29 |
| Large, 8 oz | 400 | 6 | 78 |
| **Mexican Rice:** Regular, 3 oz | 140 | 2 | 27 |
| Large, 8 oz | 360 | 5 | 71 |
| **No Fried Pinto Beans:** Reg., 4 oz | 130 | 1 | 21 |
| Large, 12 oz | 370 | 3 | 62 |

*Salad & Bowls:* Entree Size, Includes Dressing

| | | | |
|---|---|---|---|
| **Chipotle Ranch:** With Grilled Chkn | 480 | 34 | 20 |
| With Grilled Mahi Mahi | 490 | 35 | 20 |
| With Grilled Tilapia | 510 | 38 | 19 |

*Salsas:* Per 1 oz

| | | | |
|---|---|---|---|
| Mango, Picante, Tomatillo, average | 20 | 0.5 | 3 |
| Other Varieties | 10 | 0 | 1 |

## Ruby Tuesday® (Aug '15)

*Shareables:* Per Serve, w/out Sauce

| | C | F | Cb |
|---|---|---|---|
| BBQ Chicken Flatbread | 130 | 6 | 12 |
| Cheese Fries | 270 | 19 | 22 |
| Fire Wings | 180 | 11 | 4 |
| Fried Mozzarella | 135 | 8 | 11 |
| Shrimp Fondu, with chips | 300 | 18 | 25 |
| Spinach Artichoke Dip, with chips | 285 | 18 | 25 |
| Thai Spring Rolls | 130 | 6 | 14 |

*Burgers:* With Fries

| | | | |
|---|---|---|---|
| Avocado Turkey | 1380 | 77 | 112 |
| Buffalo Chicken | 1235 | 63 | 123 |
| Chicken BLT | 1245 | 61 | 123 |
| Ruby's Classic | 1305 | 76 | 104 |
| Smokehouse | 1600 | 92 | 129 |
| Turkey | 1215 | 65 | 110 |
| Triple Prime: Original | 1355 | 80 | 109 |
| Bacon Cheddar | 1575 | 97 | 109 |
| Cheddar | 1515 | 92 | 109 |

*Fit & Trim Choices:* Without Sides

| | | | |
|---|---|---|---|
| Chicken Bella | 425 | 20 | 17 |
| Grilled Salmon | 425 | 23 | 9 |
| Hickory Bourbon: | | | |
| Chicken | 355 | 10 | 25 |
| Salmon | 485 | 23 | 25 |
| Top Sirloin | 445 | 27 | 15 |
| **Sides:** Green Beans | 70 | 4 | 5 |
| Grilled Zucchini | 40 | 2 | 4 |
| Roasted Spaghetti Squash | 55 | 3 | 6 |
| Steamed Broccoli | 50 | 2 | 7 |

*Fresh All Natural Chicken:* Without Sides

| | | | |
|---|---|---|---|
| Chicken Bella | 330 | 15 | 7 |
| Chicken Fresco | 350 | 20 | 8 |
| Hickory Bourbon Chicken | 250 | 5 | 16 |
| Smoky Mountain Chicken | 550 | 28 | 16 |

*Ribs & Chops:* Without Sides

| | | | |
|---|---|---|---|
| BBQ Baby-Back Ribs, Half-Rack | 470 | 24 | 21 |
| Hickory Bourbon-Glazd Pork Chops | 885 | 42 | 57 |

*Seafood:* Without Sides

| | | | |
|---|---|---|---|
| Grilled Salmon | 330 | 18 | 0 |
| Herb-Crusted Tilapia | 400 | 24 | 11 |
| Jumbo Skewered Shrimp | 275 | 15 | 0 |
| New Orleans Seafood | 315 | 14 | 6 |

*Smart Eating:* Without Sides

| | | | |
|---|---|---|---|
| Blackened Tilapia | 200 | 7 | 2 |
| Grilled Chicken Wrap | 495 | 17 | 47 |
| Plain Grilled Chicken | 190 | 5 | 0 |
| Turkey Burger Wrap | 585 | 28 | 45 |

*Continued Next Page...*

Updated Nutrition Data ~ www.CalorieKing.com
Persons with Diabetes ~ See Disclaimer (Page 22)

# Fast - Foods & *Restaurants*

## Ruby Tuesday® cont... (Aug '15)

| Pasta & More: *Without Sides* | C | F | Cb |
|---|---|---|---|
| Cajan Jambalaya | 960 | 44 | 88 |
| Chicken & Broccoli | 1435 | 87 | 100 |
| Chicken & Mushroom Alfredo | 1170 | 58 | 95 |
| Parmesan Chicken | 1285 | 67 | 113 |
| Parmesan Shrimp | 1015 | 47 | 97 |

| Steakhouse Steaks: *Without Sides* | | | |
|---|---|---|---|
| Black Fire New York Strip | 505 | 28 | 6 |
| Rib Eye | 840 | 67 | 6 |
| Top Sirloin | 350 | 22 | 6 |

| Salads: *Without Dressing* | | | |
|---|---|---|---|
| Carolina Chicken | 1115 | 68 | 56 |
| Grilled: Chicken | 765 | 49 | 49 |
| Salmon | 730 | 40 | 37 |

| Dressing: *Per 1 oz* | | | |
|---|---|---|---|
| Balsamic Vinaigrette | 40 | 2 | 5 |
| Blue Cheese | 180 | 19 | 1 |
| Honey Mustard; Thsnd Island, av. | 85 | 8 | 5 |
| Italian; Signature Parmesan, av. | 140 | 15 | 1 |
| Ranch | 90 | 9 | 1 |

| Fresh Sides: | | | |
|---|---|---|---|
| Baked Potato: Plain | 250 | 3 | 51 |
| Loaded | 560 | 35 | 53 |
| French Fries | 480 | 24 | 54 |
| Garlic Cheese Biscuit | 110 | 5 | 12 |
| Mashed Potatoes | 265 | 15 | 29 |
| Onion Rings | 340 | 19 | 37 |
| Rice Pilaf | 160 | 3 | 30 |
| Sweet Potato Fries | 330 | 12 | 54 |

| Kid's Menu: *Includes Fries* | | | |
|---|---|---|---|
| Chicken Breast | 335 | 14 | 27 |
| Chicken Tenders | 585 | 24 | 36 |
| Cheese Pizza | 470 | 14 | 61 |

| Desserts: | | | |
|---|---|---|---|
| Blondie | 980 | 42 | 141 |
| Cookies: Chocolate Chip | 180 | 9 | 24 |
| White Choc. Macadamia Nut | 200 | 12 | 23 |
| Cupcakes: Carrot Cake (1) | 325 | 16 | 45 |
| Red Velvet (1) | 285 | 11 | 45 |
| New York Cheesecake | 760 | 60 | 89 |
| Tiramisu | 555 | 30 | 69 |

*For Complete Menu ~ see CalorieKing.com*

## Runza® (Aug '15)

| Burgers: | C | F | Cb |
|---|---|---|---|
| ¼ lb BBQ Bacon & Swiss | 530 | 32 | 26 |
| ¼ lb Bacon Cheeseburger | 510 | 31 | 26 |
| Deluxe | 540 | 34 | 26 |
| ¼ lb French Onion | 490 | 29 | 26 |
| ¼ lb Jalap.; Legend Supreme, av. | 525 | 34 | 26 |
| ¼ lb Spicy Jack Hamburger | 570 | 38 | 23 |
| ¼ lb Swiss Mushroom | 480 | 29 | 24 |
| Runza Way: ¼ lb Cheeseburger | 420 | 22 | 28 |
| ¼ lb Hamburger | 370 | 18 | 26 |
| ½ lb Double Cheeseburger | 670 | 39 | 30 |
| ½ lb Double Hamburger | 570 | 31 | 26 |

| Sandwiches: | | | |
|---|---|---|---|
| Grilled: BBQ Chicken | 400 | 11 | 40 |
| Buffalo Chicken | 360 | 11 | 37 |
| Deluxe Chicken | 360 | 10 | 37 |

| Sides: | | | |
|---|---|---|---|
| French Fries: Small | 220 | 11 | 29 |
| Medium | 320 | 15 | 41 |
| Large | 460 | 23 | 60 |
| Frings: Medium | 330 | 18 | 39 |
| Large | 470 | 25 | 55 |
| Onion Rings: Medium | 320 | 19 | 35 |
| Large | 550 | 31 | 58 |

| Salads: | | | |
|---|---|---|---|
| Asian Grilled Chicken w/ dressing | 410 | 7 | 59 |
| Southwest Chicken Salad w/ Salsa | 330 | 16 | 31 |
| Sweet Berry Chicken w/o dressing | 370 | 19 | 21 |
| Dressings: Honey Mustard | 290 | 27 | 13 |
| Ranch | 270 | 27 | 4 |

| Soups: *Per Bowl* | | | |
|---|---|---|---|
| Boston Clam Chowder | 280 | 15 | 29 |
| Broccoli Cheese | 240 | 16 | 20 |
| Chicken Tortilla | 150 | 6 | 16 |
| Homemade Chili | 320 | 15 | 23 |
| Wisconsin Cheese | 340 | 23 | 29 |

| Kids: | | | |
|---|---|---|---|
| Junior: Cheeseburger, plain | 250 | 13 | 18 |
| Hamburger, plain | 200 | 9 | 16 |
| Swiss Cheese Mushroom Burger | 300 | 17 | 17 |
| Runza Way: Cheeseburger | 270 | 13 | 22 |
| Hamburger | 220 | 9 | 20 |

| Desserts: | | | |
|---|---|---|---|
| Ice Cream Cones, all flavors | 260 | 7 | 40 |
| Ice Cream Dish, all flavors | 230 | 7 | 34 |
| Sundaes: Caramel; Chocolate | 300 | 7 | 51 |
| Turtle | 360 | 13 | 53 |

| Shakes: *Per Regular, 16 oz* | | | |
|---|---|---|---|
| Cappuccino | 490 | 12 | 82 |
| Chocolate | 480 | 12 | 81 |
| Vanilla | 430 | 12 | 66 |

## Ryan's Grill Buffet & Bakery® (Aug '15)

*Entrees: Without Sides*

| | C | F | Cb |
|---|---|---|---|
| **Beef:** BBQ'd, 4 oz | 140 | 5 | 16 |
| Country Fried Steak, w/ gravy, 2.6 oz | 220 | 13 | 16 |
| Meatloaf, 3 oz | 180 | 11 | 7 |
| Perfect Pot Roast, 5 oz | 160 | 7 | 9 |
| Salisbury Steak, 3.5 oz | 150 | 9 | 8 |
| **Chicken:** | | | |
| Breasts: Country BBQ, 5.8 oz | 310 | 16 | 6 |
| Rotisserie, 5.3 oz | 310 | 17 | 1 |
| Chicken & Dumplings, 5 oz | 160 | 5 | 17 |
| New Orleans Bourbon Street, 3 oz | 180 | 8 | 9 |
| Orange Chicken, 3 oz | 340 | 22 | 26 |
| **Fish/Seafood:** Baked Fish, 2 oz | 90 | 4.5 | 0 |
| Butter Crumb Alaskan Pollock, 1.8 oz | 110 | 5 | 2 |
| Butterfly Shrimp (6), 2.3 oz | 210 | 9 | 24 |
| Carved Salmon Filet, 3 oz | 190 | 11 | 0 |
| Clam Strips, 3 oz | 320 | 20 | 28 |
| Fried: Fish, 3 pieces, 3 oz | 240 | 12 | 27 |
| Shrimp (22), 3 oz | 240 | 12 | 24 |
| Wood Seared Salmon, 1 pce, 3 oz | 220 | 16 | 0 |
| **Pasta/Spaghetti:** *Per 5 oz Serving* | | | |
| Country Pasta Gratine | 160 | 4 | 24 |
| Creamy Penne Carbonara | 260 | 17 | 17 |
| Fire Grilled Chicken Alfredo | 220 | 14 | 14 |
| Grilled Italian Sausage Penne | 180 | 11 | 14 |
| **Pork:** | | | |
| Carved: Grilled Loin, 3 oz | 140 | 10 | 0 |
| Ham, 3 oz | 100 | 5 | 0 |
| Honey Glazed Baked, 1 sl, 3 oz | 120 | 5 | 1 |
| Ribs, BBQ/County-Style (3), 3.5 oz | 420 | 27 | 15 |
| Steak: Grilled, 2 oz | 140 | 9 | 0 |
| BBQ, grilled, 2 oz | 150 | 9 | 3 |
| **Salads:** *Without Dressing* | | | |
| Asian Chopped, 3.5 oz | 90 | 4 | 13 |
| Caesar, 1 cup, 2.5 oz | 70 | 6 | 4 |
| Greek, 2.6 oz | 120 | 8 | 10 |
| Seafood, 4.2 oz | 310 | 26 | 15 |
| **Sides:** | | | |
| Baked Potato, plain, 4.3 oz | 150 | 0 | 36 |
| BBQ Baked Beans, 3 oz | 130 | 3 | 26 |
| Cauliflower Au Gratin, 3 oz | 50 | 2 | 8 |
| French Fries, 2 oz | 170 | 9 | 23 |
| Fried Okra, 3 oz | 220 | 12 | 28 |
| Mashed Potatoes, 4 oz | 70 | 0.5 | 13 |
| **Desserts:** Cheesecake, plain, 1 sl. | 230 | 12 | 28 |
| Key Lime Pie, scratch, 1 sl., 2.5 oz | 220 | 9 | 31 |
| Lemon Meringue Pie, 2.3 oz | 130 | 4.5 | 23 |

## 7-Eleven® (Aug '15)

*7-Select Burritos:*

| | C | F | Cb |
|---|---|---|---|
| Bean and Cheese, 5 oz | 320 | 10 | 47 |
| Beef & Bean, 5 oz | 360 | 16 | 44 |
| Beef, Bean & Green Chile, 5 oz | 360 | 15 | 44 |
| Red Hot Beef, 5 oz | 340 | 15 | 41 |
| **Big Bites:** *Without Bun or Toppings* | | | |
| Big Bite Hot Dog, 2 oz | 180 | 17 | 1 |
| Breakfast Bite Sausage, 3 oz | 250 | 21 | 2 |
| Cheeseburger Bite Link, 4.2 oz | 440 | 38 | 2 |
| Qtr Pound Big Bite Hot Dog, 4 oz | 360 | 34 | 2 |
| **Breakfast Sandwiches:** | | | |
| Biscuits: | | | |
| Egg, Cheese & Ssg, 5.5 oz | 460 | 32 | 31 |
| Sausage, 3.3 oz | 330 | 22 | 28 |
| Croissant, Egg, Cheese & Ssg, 4.8 oz | 410 | 30 | 20 |
| Eng. Muffin, Egg, Chse & Ssg, 5 oz | 390 | 25 | 24 |
| **Fresh:** | | | |
| Cilantro Lime Chicken Flatbread | 570 | 25 | 51 |
| Southwest Turkey Sandwich | 560 | 28 | 48 |
| Very Berry Salad | 210 | 15 | 12 |
| Yoplait Yogurt Parfait | 230 | 2.5 | 47 |
| **Other Selections:** | | | |
| Chicken Tenders (1), 3.3 oz | 160 | 5 | 11 |
| Maple Pancake Sausage (1), 2.6 oz | 270 | 19 | 19 |
| Pepperoni Pizza, 1 slice, 3.9 oz | 300 | 14 | 30 |
| **Rollers:** Buffalo Chicken (1), 3 oz | 190 | 7 | 16 |
| Corn Dog (1), 3.4 oz | 320 | 21 | 23 |
| **Taquitos:** *Per 1.3 oz Taquito* | | | |
| Bacon, Egg, Cheese & Potato | 190 | 8 | 23 |
| Jalapeno Cream Cheese | 240 | 13 | 27 |
| Monterey Jack & Chicken | 280 | 14 | 30 |
| Steak & Cheese | 210 | 11 | 22 |
| **Wings,** Bone In, Spicy Wing Zings, | | | |
| 1 wing | 80 | 4.5 | 3 |
| **Sides:** Hash Browns (1), 2 oz | 100 | 5 | 12 |
| Potato Wedges (6), 0.7 oz | 240 | 4.5 | 27 |
| **Slurpees,** average all flavors: | | | |
| 12 oz cup | 95 | 0 | 26 |
| 22 oz cup | 175 | 0 | 44 |
| 28 oz cup | 220 | 0 | 56 |
| Sugar Free, 12 oz cup | 30 | 0 | 9 |

Updated Nutrition Data ~ www.CalorieKing.com
Persons with Diabetes ~ See Disclaimer (Page 22)

# Fast - Foods & *Restaurants*

## Saladworks® (Aug '15)

*Salads: Without Dressing*

| | C | F | Cb |
|---|---|---|---|
| Autumn Harvest | 300 | 12 | 40 |
| Bently | 245 | 10 | 11 |
| Buffalo Bleu | 250 | 7.5 | 24 |
| Chicken Caesar | 285 | 4 | 19 |
| Cobb | 270 | 16 | 13 |
| Fire Roasted Cabo Jack | 390 | 19 | 31 |
| Greek | 185 | 10 | 18 |
| Nuevo Nicoise | 230 | 4 | 31 |
| Sophie's Salad | 310 | 14 | 35 |
| Tivoli | 430 | 19 | 31 |

*Focaccia Fusion: Without Spread*

| | | | |
|---|---|---|---|
| BLT | 345 | 13 | 32 |
| Chicken Monterey | 385 | 12 | 35 |
| Fajitalicious | 380 | 12 | 33 |
| Turkey Ranch | 365 | 10 | 33 |

*Dressings & Spreads: Per 1 oz Ladle*

| | | | |
|---|---|---|---|
| Balsamic Vinaigrette | 170 | 18 | 4 |
| Classic French; Green Goddess, av | 140 | 14 | 5 |
| Dijon Lemon Capri | 130 | 13 | 4 |
| Mayonnaise | 45 | 5 | 2 |
| Oriental Sesame | 90 | 4.5 | 12 |
| Parmesan Caesar: Thousand Isl., av. | 145 | 15 | 3 |
| Salsa Mayo Spread | 20 | 1 | 2 |

*Extra Menu Items ~ See CalorieKing.com*

## Sandella's® (Aug '15)  C  F  Cb

*Grilled Flatbread: With Standard Toppings*

| | | | |
|---|---|---|---|
| Brazilian Bacon | 560 | 17 | 79 |
| Brazilian Chicken | 510 | 10 | 73 |
| Pesto Chicken | 610 | 28 | 56 |
| Spinach & Bacon | 660 | 39 | 52 |

*Paninis: With Standard Toppings*

| | | | |
|---|---|---|---|
| Philly Cheese | 590 | 25 | 55 |
| Spin., Ham & Swiss | 550 | 20 | 61 |
| Tuscan Chicken | 540 | 21 | 55 |

*Quesadillas: With Standard Toppings*

| | | | |
|---|---|---|---|
| California | 500 | 23 | 53 |
| Mediterranean | 400 | 16 | 53 |

*Salads: Includes ½ Flatbread & Dressing*

| | | | |
|---|---|---|---|
| Fiesta | 360 | 8 | 54 |
| Greek | 310 | 15 | 37 |

*Rice Bowls: Includes Flatbread & Standard Toppings*

| | | | |
|---|---|---|---|
| Black Bean & Rice | 840 | 20 | 130 |
| Chicken Fajita | 750 | 20 | 104 |

*Wraps: With Standard Toppings*

| | | | |
|---|---|---|---|
| California Turkey | 410 | 10 | 55 |
| Chipotle Chicken | 350 | 7 | 55 |
| Pesto Turkey | 460 | 15 | 54 |
| Sweet & Spicy Chicken | 400 | 7 | 64 |

## Sarku Japan® (Aug '15)

*D'Lite Meals:*

| | C | F | Cb |
|---|---|---|---|
| Rice & Chicken Tempura, 15 oz | 970 | 58 | 81 |
| Rice & Shrimp Tempura, 11 oz | 540 | 21 | 70 |
| Vegetarian, 14 oz | 360 | 0.5 | 79 |
| Vegetarian Soba Noodle, 14 oz | 710 | 24 | 106 |

*Combos:*

| | | | |
|---|---|---|---|
| **Tempura:** Chicken, 23 oz | 1270 | 78 | 102 |
| Chicken & Shrimp, 20 oz | 980 | 53 | 95 |
| **Teriyaki:** Beef, 19 oz | 690 | 26 | 81 |
| Beef & Shrimp, 21 oz | 630 | 11 | 85 |
| Chicken, 22 oz | 640 | 13 | 90 |
| Chkn & Shrimp, 24 oz | 700 | 14 | 90 |
| Shrimp, 19 oz | 500 | 2.5 | 83 |
| *Sauce,* Teriyaki, 1.5 oz | 45 | 0 | 9 |
| *Sides:* Maki Roll, 2 oz | 140 | 11 | 9 |
| Rice: Steamed, 9 oz | 290 | 0 | 64 |
| Fried, 9 oz | 330 | 4.5 | 62 |
| Tempura Chicken, 1 piece, 2 oz | 230 | 19 | 8 |
| Tempura Shrimp, 1 piece, 0.8 oz | 90 | 7 | 4 |

## Schlotzsky's® (Aug '15)

*Oven-Toasted Sandwiches: Per Medium Size*

**Angus:**

| | C | F | Cb |
|---|---|---|---|
| Beef & Cheese | 760 | 29 | 78 |
| Corned Beef | 510 | 9 | 72 |
| Corned Beef Reuben | 890 | 38 | 81 |
| Pastrami Reuben | 900 | 40 | 84 |
| Pastrami & Swiss | 830 | 33 | 79 |
| BLT | 540 | 17 | 74 |
| Chicken & Pesto | 560 | 11 | 79 |
| Chicken Breast | 490 | 3 | 82 |
| Chipotle Chicken | 530 | 9 | 78 |
| Homestyle Tuna | 580 | 16 | 75 |
| Santa Fe Chicken | 660 | 19 | 78 |
| Smoked Turkey Reuben | 850 | 35 | 83 |
| Turkey & Guacamole | 520 | 11 | 78 |
| Turkey Bacon Club | 770 | 29 | 81 |

**Original Style:**

| | | | |
|---|---|---|---|
| The Original | 780 | 33 | 79 |
| Deluxe | 980 | 46 | 81 |
| Ham & Cheese | 730 | 25 | 81 |
| Turkey | 820 | 33 | 82 |

*Wraps: Per Medium Size*

| | | | |
|---|---|---|---|
| Chicken & Pesto | 510 | 18 | 54 |
| Homestyle Tuna | 540 | 22 | 55 |
| Santa Fe Chicken | 590 | 24 | 55 |

*Continued Next Page...*

# Fast - Foods & Restaurants

## Schlotzsky's® cont... (Aug '15)

### 10" Pizzas: Per Pizza

| | C | F | Cb |
|---|---|---|---|
| BBQ Chicken & Jalapeno | 920 | 19 | 148 |
| Combination Special | 960 | 37 | 119 |
| Double Cheese | 830 | 326 | 115 |
| Fresh Veggie | 920 | 34 | 118 |
| Grilled Chicken & Pesto | 910 | 28 | 114 |
| Pepperoni & Double Cheese | 980 | 40 | 116 |

### Salads: Without Dressing or Breadsticks

| | C | F | Cb |
|---|---|---|---|
| Cranberry, Apple, Pecan & Chicken | 640 | 27 | 68 |
| Hearts of Romaine, Chicken Caesar | 400 | 17 | 29 |
| Garden | 40 | 2 | 9 |
| Potato | 240 | 13 | 29 |
| Turkey Avocado Cobb | 610 | 33 | 42 |
| Turkey Chef | 415 | 25 | 17 |
| Garlic Breadsticks, entree portion (2) | 60 | 2 | 10 |

### Dressings: Per 3 oz

| | C | F | Cb |
|---|---|---|---|
| Butttermilk Ranch | 320 | 33 | 4 |
| Chunky Blue Cheese | 455 | 49 | 3 |
| Red Wine Vinaigrette | 430 | 43 | 9 |
| Robusto Italian | 285 | 28 | 3 |
| Tuscan Caesar | 425 | 45 | 2 |

### Soup: Per Bowl

| | C | F | Cb |
|---|---|---|---|
| Broccoli Cheese | 210 | 14 | 17 |
| Chicken & Wild Rice | 320 | 17 | 29 |
| Potato with Bacon | 440 | 36 | 35 |
| Timberline Chili | 450 | 24 | 32 |
| Tomato Basil | 370 | 30 | 25 |

### Chips:

| | C | F | Cb |
|---|---|---|---|
| Baked: Regular; BBQ, average | 130 | 3 | 25 |
| Other varieties, average | 230 | 14 | 24 |

### Kid's Meals: Without Cookie or Drink

| | C | F | Cb |
|---|---|---|---|
| Cheese Pizza | 540 | 16 | 78 |
| Cheese Sandwich | 390 | 14 | 49 |
| Ham Sandwich | 340 | 2 | 73 |
| Pepperoni Pizza | 590 | 21 | 78 |
| Turkey Sandwich | 350 | 2 | 74 |

### Desserts:

| | C | F | Cb |
|---|---|---|---|
| Brownie (1) | 370 | 19 | 49 |
| Creamy Cheesecake, 1 slice | 540 | 33 | 50 |
| Cookies: Per Cookie | | | |
| Chocolate/Fudge Choc. Chip, av. | 160 | 7 | 23 |
| Oatmeal Raisin; Sugar, average | 150 | 6 | 24 |
| Macadamia Nut | 170 | 9 | 22 |

## Second Cup® ~ see CalorieKing.com

## Shakey's® (Aug '15)

### Pizzas: Per Slice, 1/12 Large Pizza

| | C | F | Cb |
|---|---|---|---|
| **Cheese:** | | | |
| Pan Crust | 185 | 6 | 26 |
| Thin Crust | 150 | 5.5 | 18 |
| **Firehouse:** Pan Crust | 255 | 12 | 27 |
| Thin Crust | 220 | 12 | 19 |
| **Garden Veggie:** Pan Crust | 185 | 5.5 | 27 |
| Thin Crust | 150 | 5 | 19 |
| **Margherita:** | | | |
| Pan Crust | 175 | 5 | 26 |
| Thin Crust | 135 | 4.5 | 18 |
| **Rustic Garlic Chicken:** Pan Crust | 190 | 5.5 | 26 |
| Thin Crust | 155 | 5.5 | 18 |
| **Shakey's Special:** Pan Crust | 210 | 6.5 | 31 |
| Thin Crust | 195 | 10 | 18 |
| **Texas BBQ Chicken:** Pan Crust | 205 | 5 | 29 |
| Thin Crust | 170 | 5 | 21 |
| **Ultimate Meat:** Pan Crust | 280 | 14 | 26 |
| Thin Crust | 245 | 13 | 18 |
| **Additional Toppings:** Beef | 35 | 3 | 0 |
| Cheese | 15 | 1 | 1 |
| Chicken | 15 | 0.5 | 0 |
| Pepperoni | 25 | 2.5 | 0 |
| Sausage | 45 | 4 | 1 |

### Shareables: Per Serving, Unless Indicated

| | C | F | Cb |
|---|---|---|---|
| Chicken Strips (5) | 620 | 31 | 48 |
| Mojo Potatoes (5) | 215 | 11 | 25 |
| Mojo Supreme, serves 4-6 | 1950 | 120 | 160 |
| Shakey's Spicy Wings (6) | 495 | 29 | 27 |

### Shakey's Famous Chicken: Per Piece

| | C | F | Cb |
|---|---|---|---|
| **Fried Chicken:** Breast | 475 | 26 | 16 |
| Leg | 170 | 19 | 6 |
| Thigh | 350 | 24 | 10 |
| Wing | 130 | 9 | 4 |

## Shari's® (Aug '15)

### Breakfast:

| | C | F | Cb |
|---|---|---|---|
| **Favorites:** | | | |
| Farmhouse Platter | 1170 | 73 | 94 |
| The Breakfast Sampler Platter | 1060 | 74 | 55 |
| Traditional Eggs Benedict, with Hashbrowns | 810 | 46 | 61 |
| **Fruit Crepes:** Apples; Strawb., av. | 685 | 36 | 79 |
| Burst O Berry | 630 | 36 | 68 |
| **Omelettes:** | | | |
| BMP | 930 | 77 | 8 |
| Chicken Fajita | 720 | 52 | 13 |
| Denver; Spring Spinach, average | 655 | 52 | 11 |
| **Pancakes:** Buttermilk | 370 | 5 | 73 |
| Potato Pancakes | 570 | 17 | 96 |

Continued Next Page...

## Shari's® cont... (Aug '15)

*Breakfast (Cont):*

| Specialties: | C | F | Cb |
|---|---|---|---|
| Breakfast Panini | 930 | 60 | 64 |
| Classic Quiche: BMP | 550 | 28 | 57 |
| Lorraine | 590 | 30 | 56 |
| Meat Lover's Skillet, without side choices | 1140 | 91 | 34 |

*Lunch:*

| **Flame-Grilled Burgers:** *Without Sides* | C | F | Cb |
|---|---|---|---|
| Bavarian | 1030 | 47 | 59 |
| Cheddar Cheesebuger | 660 | 34 | 46 |
| Garlic-Mushroom Swiss | 1030 | 72 | 50 |
| Hamburger | 600 | 29 | 46 |
| Pepperjack Cheese | 700 | 38 | 46 |
| Sriracha Burger | 730 | 40 | 50 |
| Trail Boss | 1030 | 57 | 54 |

| **Flatbread Paninis:** *Without Sides* | | | |
|---|---|---|---|
| All American | 740 | 33 | 62 |
| Pastrami | 760 | 32 | 58 |

| **Salads:** *Entrée Size* | | | |
|---|---|---|---|
| American Chopped, w/o Dress. | 590 | 28 | 39 |
| Northwest Steak | 660 | 30 | 53 |
| Spinach Cobb | 780 | 44 | 46 |

| **Sandwiches:** *Per Whole Sandwich, w/o Side Choices* | | | |
|---|---|---|---|
| Baja Chipotle Chicken | 870 | 49 | 59 |
| Cuban, on Ciabatta | 600 | 27 | 46 |
| Prime Rib Dip | 670 | 37 | 48 |

*Dinner:*

| **Distrinctive:** Chicken Penne Alfr. | 1100 | 55 | 94 |
|---|---|---|---|
| Chimichurri Chicken | 1110 | 65 | 87 |
| Sthn Style Chicken & Waffles | 1430 | 86 | 113 |

| **Flame Grilled Classics:** *With Garlic Herb Bread & Onion Rings* | | | |
|---|---|---|---|
| Center Cut NY Strip Steak | 940 | 64 | 33 |
| T-Bone Steak, 16 oz | 1100 | 67 | 35 |
| Steak: W/ Golden Fried Shrimp | 1040 | 50 | 89 |
| With Shrimp Scampi | 930 | 62 | 36 |
| With Shrimp Skewers | 760 | 43 | 35 |

| **Homestyle Favorite,** | | | |
|---|---|---|---|
| Country Fried Steak & Gravy | 1250 | 71 | 119 |

| **Seafood Favorites:** *As Served* | | | |
|---|---|---|---|
| Alaskan Cod with Shrimp & Chips | 1280 | 79 | 119 |
| Hand Cut Alaskan Cod & Chips | 1220 | 77 | 111 |

## Shari's® cont... (Aug '15)

| *Sides:* | C | F | Cb |
|---|---|---|---|
| Baked Potato w/ Butter& Sour Crm | 280 | 13 | 38 |
| Country Vegetables | 120 | 9 | 8 |
| French Fries | 390 | 25 | 40 |
| Rice Pilaf | 90 | 4.5 | 10 |
| Tater Tots | 370 | 26 | 33 |

*Desserts:*

| **Classic Pies:** *Per Slice, as Served* | | | |
|---|---|---|---|
| Banana Cream Dream | 410 | 19 | 55 |
| Chocolate Cream Supreme | 590 | 33 | 67 |

| **Gourmet Pies:** *Per Slice, As Served* | | | |
|---|---|---|---|
| Creamy Caramel Pecan Crunch | 710 | 45 | 71 |
| Peanut Butter Chocolate Silk | 660 | 45 | 60 |
| S'mores Galore | 570 | 31 | 68 |
| Velvet Chocolate Silk | 640 | 46 | 55 |

## Sheetz® (Aug '15)

| *Breakfast Sandwiches:* | C | F | Cb |
|---|---|---|---|
| Walker Breakfast Ranger | 580 | 22 | 68 |

| *Burgerz:* | | | |
|---|---|---|---|
| Atomic Burger | 380 | 20 | 22 |
| Big Mozz Burger | 530 | 27 | 32 |
| Boss Bacon Burger | 530 | 33 | 23 |
| Carolina Slaw Burger | 400 | 19 | 26 |
| Twisted Brunch Burger | 620 | 31 | 5 |

| **Hot Dogz:** *With Hot Dog Sausage* | | | |
|---|---|---|---|
| BLT | 450 | 27 | 34 |
| Firehouse | 390 | 22 | 35 |
| Junkyard | 330 | 16 | 39 |
| Philly | 460 | 25 | 44 |
| Shmokehouse | 380 | 18 | 40 |

| *Sidez:* | | | |
|---|---|---|---|
| Coleslaw | 80 | 3.5 | 11 |
| Crispy Chicken Stripz: 3 pieces | 130 | 6 | 11 |
| 5 pieces | 220 | 10 | 18 |
| Fryz, 1 cup | 730 | 36 | 95 |
| Hard Cooked Eggs, 1 order | 70 | 4.5 | 0 |
| Jalapeno Poppers, 1 order | 350 | 19 | 37 |
| Loaded Fryz | 870 | 43 | 113 |
| Mac & Cheese, 1 order | 130 | 6 | 15 |
| Onion Rings, 1 cup | 560 | 32 | 62 |
| Popcorn Chicken: Regular | 330 | 15 | 30 |
| Large | 660 | 30 | 59 |

*Continued Next Page...*

**239**

# Fast - Foods & *Restaurants*

## Sheetz® cont... (Aug '15)

### Donuts:

| | C | F | Cb |
|---|---|---|---|
| Apple/Blueberry Fritter, average | 485 | 24 | 61 |
| Chocolate Cake Donut | 530 | 33 | 54 |
| Cotton Candy Pink/Blue Donut | 400 | 19 | 52 |
| Cream Filled: Chocolate Iced Donut | 400 | 18 | 56 |
| Glazed Donut | 360 | 16 | 48 |
| Custard Filled Chocolate Iced D'nut | 350 | 15 | 50 |
| Glazed Ring Donut | 300 | 14 | 37 |
| P'nut Butter Filled Choc Iced D'nut | 380 | 19 | 50 |
| Sour Cream Cake Donut | 480 | 26 | 57 |
| *Muffin,* Blueberry (1) | 460 | 26 | 56 |

### Beverages:

| | C | F | Cb |
|---|---|---|---|
| **Cupo'ccino:** Cake Batter, 16 oz | 260 | 6 | 54 |
| Creme Brulee, 16 oz | 280 | 8 | 50 |
| French Vanilla, 16 oz | 285 | 10 | 50 |
| **Hot Chocolate,** 16 oz | 250 | 4 | 52 |

## Sizzler® (Aug '15)

### Burgers:

| | C | F | Cb |
|---|---|---|---|
| Mega Bacon Cheeseburger, ½ lb | 1010 | 61 | 48 |
| Sizzler Burger: ⅓ lb | 620 | 30 | 47 |
| ½ lb | 760 | 40 | 47 |

### Sandwiches:

| | C | F | Cb |
|---|---|---|---|
| Grilled Chicken Club | 645 | 28 | 48 |
| Malibu Chicken | 705 | 37 | 59 |

### Hot Entrees: *Without Condiments, Sides or Sauces Unless Indicated*

| | C | F | Cb |
|---|---|---|---|
| **Chicken:** Hibachi Chicken, Single | 180 | 4 | 7 |
| Lemon-Herb Chicken, Single | 170 | 6 | 0 |
| Malibu Chicken, Single | 360 | 25 | 11 |
| **Pasta:** Fettuccine Alfredo | 995 | 64 | 73 |
| Cajun Fettuccine Alfredo | 1035 | 64 | 82 |
| **Pork Chop**, Single, w/ Apple Sauce | 420 | 27 | 15 |
| **Ribs:** | | | |
| Half Rack | 625 | 39 | 37 |
| Full Rack | 1155 | 79 | 51 |
| **Seafood:** | | | |
| Grilled Salmon with Rice Pilaf | 530 | 20 | 40 |
| Ultimate Shrimp Platter | 1010 | 39 | 103 |
| **Steaks:** Bacon Wrapped Sirloin Filet | 555 | 35 | 5 |
| Burgundy M'shroom Sirloin Tips, with Rice Pilaf | 870 | 36 | 85 |
| Chopped Steak, 8 oz | 520 | 30 | 17 |
| Classic, 8 oz | 395 | 21 | 1 |
| NY Strip, 12 oz | 810 | 57 | 1 |
| **Combos:** Classic Trio | 860 | 47 | 36 |
| Steak & Hibachi Chicken | 475 | 20 | 7 |
| Steak & Lobster Tail | 410 | 17 | 2 |
| Steak & Malibu Chicken | 660 | 41 | 12 |

## Sizzler® cont... (Aug '15)

### Prepared Salads: *W/out Dressing*

| | C | F | Cb |
|---|---|---|---|
| Seafood, 4 oz | 160 | 11 | 11 |
| Sicilian Pasta, 2 oz | 65 | 4 | 6 |
| Three Bean, 1 oz | 25 | 1 | 5 |
| Tuna Pasta, 4 oz | 205 | 19 | 1 |
| Waldorf, 4 oz | 130 | 8 | 16 |

### Salad Dressings: *Per 1 oz*

| | C | F | Cb |
|---|---|---|---|
| Blue Cheese | 105 | 11 | 1 |
| Honey Mustard | 110 | 8 | 9 |
| Italian | 80 | 8 | 2 |
| Ranch | 115 | 12 | 2 |
| Thousand Island | 95 | 9 | 5 |

### Sides:

| | C | F | Cb |
|---|---|---|---|
| Baked Potato, plain | 265 | 4 | 51 |
| Broccoli, 5 oz | 50 | 0.5 | 7 |
| French Fries, 5 oz | 285 | 13 | 42 |
| Rice Pilaf, 5 oz | 225 | 4 | 39 |

*For Complete Menu & Data ~ see CalorieKing.com*

## Skyline Chili® (Aug '15)

### Burritos:

| | C | F | Cb |
|---|---|---|---|
| Chili Deluxe | 640 | 33 | 44 |
| Vegetarian Black Bean Deluxe | 700 | 32 | 73 |

### Ways: *Per Regular Serving*

**Chili & Cheddar Cheese Spaghetti:**

| | C | F | Cb |
|---|---|---|---|
| 3 Way | 730 | 47 | 49 |
| 4 Way Onion | 750 | 47 | 53 |
| 4 Way Bean | 820 | 48 | 65 |
| 5 Way | 830 | 48 | 69 |
| **Bowls:** Coney | 780 | 61 | 8 |
| Loaded Chili | 480 | 29 | 21 |
| Vegetarian Black Beans & Rice | 400 | 15 | 49 |
| **Chili** , Deluxe | 640 | 33 | 44 |
| **Potatoes:** | | | |
| 3-Way Potato | 610 | 25 | 65 |
| Cheddar Potato | 700 | 42 | 61 |
| Sour Cream Potato | 460 | 19 | 66 |

### Salads: *Without Dressing Unless Indicated*

| | C | F | Cb |
|---|---|---|---|
| Buffalo Chicken | 200 | 10 | 11 |
| Garden, with Croutons | 80 | 5 | 5 |
| Greek, regular size, with dressing | 390 | 37 | 9 |
| Dressings: Blue Cheese, 1.5 oz | 210 | 21 | 2 |
| Buttermilk Ranch, 1.5 oz | 210 | 22 | 2 |
| Greek, 1.5 oz | 260 | 28 | 1 |
| Thousand Island, 1.5 oz | 220 | 21 | 6 |

### Wraps:

| | C | F | Cb |
|---|---|---|---|
| Buffalo Chicken, w/ Ranch Dress. | 720 | 40 | 59 |
| Classic Chkn w/ Chili Ranch Dress. | 650 | 36 | 56 |
| Greek Chicken, w/ Greek Dressing | 680 | 36 | 56 |

### Sides:

| | C | F | Cb |
|---|---|---|---|
| Fries: Chili Cheese | 750 | 40 | 66 |
| French | 390 | 13 | 63 |

## Smoothie King® (Aug '15)

*Fruit Smoothies: Per 20 oz Cup*  **C**  **F**  **Cb**
*Figures Include Turbinado. Without Turbinado, deduct 100 calories and 23 carbs.*

**Fitness Blends:**

| | C | F | Cb |
|---|---|---|---|
| High Protein: Almond Mocha | 345 | 9 | 42 |
| Chocolate | 365 | 9 | 42 |
| Peanut Power Plus: | | | |
| Chocolate | 700 | 26 | 98 |
| Strawberry | 680 | 21 | 112 |
| The Activator: Chocolate | 340 | 1 | 67 |
| Strawberry | 495 | 1 | 105 |
| Vanilla | 345 | 1 | 67 |
| The Hulk: Chocolate | 800 | 31 | 108 |
| Strawberry | 965 | 32 | 145 |
| Vanilla | 800 | 32 | 105 |

**Take A Break Blends:**

| | | | |
|---|---|---|---|
| Banana Boat | 475 | 4 | 101 |
| Caribbean Way | 395 | 0 | 97 |
| Muscle Punch | 360 | 1 | 84 |
| Pineapple Surf | 460 | 1 | 104 |
| Yogurt D-Lite | 275 | 4 | 46 |

**Wellness Blends:** Acai Adventure 435 5 92

| | | | |
|---|---|---|---|
| Mangosteen Madness | 380 | 0 | 94 |
| Orange Ka-BAM | 470 | 0 | 117 |

*32 fl.oz Cup: Multiply 20 fl.oz figures by 1.5*
*40 fl.oz Cup: Multiply 20 fl.oz figures by 2*

**Kids Cup Smoothies:** *Per 12 fl.oz Cup*

| | | | |
|---|---|---|---|
| Apple Kiwi Bunga | 155 | 0 | 37 |
| Choc-A-Laka | 210 | 4 | 32 |
| Lil' Angel | 210 | 0 | 52 |
| Strawberry Bluegurt Blitz | 175 | 0 | 70 |

## Snappy Tomato (Aug '15)

*Pizza: Per Slice, ⅛ of Large Pizza*  **C**  **F**  **Cb**

| | C | F | Cb |
|---|---|---|---|
| Buffalo Grilled Chicken | 250 | 5 | 32 |
| Cheese | 220 | 7 | 30 |
| Hawaiian | 370 | 18 | 33 |
| Pepperoni | 340 | 17 | 31 |
| Ranch | 370 | 21 | 31 |
| Snapperoni | 390 | 22 | 31 |
| Snappy Ultimate | 460 | 26 | 33 |
| Supreme | 340 | 17 | 32 |
| Veggie | 240 | 8 | 33 |
| Snappetizers, Snappy Wings, | | | |
| Plain, without sauce (3), 2.6 oz | 160 | 11 | 0 |

## Sonic Drive-In® (Aug '15)

*Burgers:*  **C**  **F**  **Cb**

| | C | F | Cb |
|---|---|---|---|
| Cheeseburger: w/ Mayo | 750 | 48 | 44 |
| with Ketchup | 720 | 43 | 47 |
| Double Cheeseburger w/ Mayo | 1170 | 81 | 44 |
| Bacon Cheeseburger | 820 | 54 | 43 |
| Bacon Double Cheeseburger | 1240 | 87 | 44 |
| Jr. Burger | 340 | 17 | 32 |
| Jr. Double Cheeseburger | 520 | 33 | 31 |
| Jr. Deluxe Burger | 360 | 20 | 32 |
| Jr. Deluxe Cheeseburger | 420 | 25 | 32 |
| Toaster, Bacon Cheeseburger | 850 | 50 | 59 |

*Chicken Sandwiches:*

| | | | |
|---|---|---|---|
| Classic Crispy Chicken | 580 | 29 | 57 |
| Classic Grilled Chicken | 450 | 17 | 44 |
| Grilled Asiago Caesar Chicken | 530 | 24 | 44 |

**Breakfast:** Breakfast Toaster 500 29 39

**Burrito:** Breakfast w/ Bacon 480 26 39

| | | | |
|---|---|---|---|
| SuperSonic Breakfast | 580 | 32 | 49 |
| Jr. Breakfast Burrito | 280 | 15 | 23 |

**CroiSonic Sandwich:** with Bacon 550 37 31

| | | | |
|---|---|---|---|
| with Sausage | 630 | 45 | 31 |

**Cinnasnacks,** (3) with Frosting 630 33 75

**French Toast Sticks,** (4) with Syrup 590 31 71

*Coneys & Hot Dogs:*

| | | | |
|---|---|---|---|
| All American Dog | 380 | 18 | 40 |
| Chili Cheese | 420 | 26 | 30 |
| Footlong, ¼ pound | 830 | 55 | 54 |
| New York Dog | 340 | 19 | 30 |

*Chicken:*

| | | | |
|---|---|---|---|
| Chicken Strips with BBQ Sauce (5) | 590 | 26 | 52 |
| Jumbo Popcorn Chicken: | | | |
| Small, without Sauce, 4 oz | 380 | 22 | 27 |
| Large, without Sauce, 6 oz | 640 | 37 | 47 |

*Wraps:* Crispy Chicken 510 22 57

| | | | |
|---|---|---|---|
| Grilled Chicken | 430 | 14 | 42 |

*Sides:*

| | | | |
|---|---|---|---|
| **Apple Slices** | 35 | 0 | 9 |
| **Fries:** Small | 280 | 13 | 39 |
| Medium | 370 | 13 | 39 |
| Large | 510 | 24 | 68 |
| **Cheese Fries,** medium | 500 | 26 | 53 |
| **Mozzarella Sticks,** without sauce | 440 | 22 | 40 |
| **Onion Rings,** Medium | 440 | 21 | 55 |
| **Tater Tots:** Plain, med. | 360 | 19 | 43 |
| Cheese Tots, med. | 450 | 28 | 43 |
| Chili & Cheese Tots, medium | 540 | 34 | 48 |

*Continued Next Page…*

# Fast - Foods & *Restaurants*

## Sonic Drive-In® cont... (Aug '15)

| *Sundaes:* | C | F | Cb |
|---|---|---|---|
| **Banana Split** | 490 | 18 | 76 |
| **Ice Cream,** Caramel; Fudge, av. | 520 | 24 | 67 |
| **Molten Cake Sundae,** Fudge | 800 | 34 | 117 |
| *Cones:* | | | |
| **Vanilla Cone** | 250 | 13 | 31 |
| **Waffle Cone:** Vanilla | 320 | 15 | 43 |
| with Candy Pieces | 470 | 20 | 66 |
| *Floats:* | | | |
| Barq's/Coca-Cola, av: Small | 340 | 14 | 50 |
| Medium | 520 | 23 | 73 |
| *Java Chillers:* | | | |
| Caramel/Choc.: Small | 770 | 37 | 99 |
| Medium | 880 | 40 | 120 |
| *Shakes: Small* | | | |
| Banana; Caramel, av. | 620 | 31 | 80 |
| Pineapple; Strawberry, av. | 580 | 32 | 68 |
| *Slushes: Average all Flav.* | | | |
| Small | 180 | 0 | 48 |
| Medium | 260 | 0 | 68 |
| *CreamSlush Treats: Average all Flavors* | | | |
| Small | 420 | 20 | 60 |
| Medium | 600 | 28 | 85 |
| *Sonic Blast: Av. all Types* | | | |
| Small | 900 | 48 | 106 |
| Medium | 1230 | 65 | 146 |
| *Sonic Energy:* | | | |
| A.M./Berry: Small | 170 | 0 | 45 |
| Medium | 230 | 0 | 62 |
| *Sonic Master Blast:* | | | |
| Triple Choc: Small | 900 | 47 | 112 |
| Medium | 1370 | 68 | 178 |
| Large | 2000 | 99 | 259 |
| *Limeade:* | | | |
| Small | 140 | 0 | 38 |
| Medium | 170 | 0 | 45 |
| *Tea:* | | | |
| Black, Sweetened, Medium | 180 | 0 | 45 |
| Iced Green, Sweet, Medium | 120 | 0 | 30 |

*For Complete Nutritional Data ~ see CalorieKing.com*

## Souplantation® (Aug '15)

| *Soups: Per Cup* | C | F | Cb |
|---|---|---|---|
| Chesapeake Corn Chowder | 290 | 17 | 30 |
| Chunky Chicken Noodle | 100 | 3 | 10 |
| Classical Minestrone | 120 | 2 | 20 |
| Cream of Mushroom | 250 | 20 | 14 |
| New Orleans Jambalaya | 210 | 11 | 18 |
| Texas Red Chili | 190 | 7 | 24 |
| Vegetarian Harvest | 130 | 8 | 14 |

## Souplantation® cont... (Aug '15)

| *Hot Pastas: Per 1 Cup* | C | F | Cb |
|---|---|---|---|
| Carbonara Pasta, with Bacon | 290 | 10 | 43 |
| Creamy Cilantro Lime Pesto | 360 | 20 | 37 |
| Fettuccine Alfredo | 390 | 18 | 41 |
| Garden Vegetable with Meatballs | 310 | 10 | 44 |
| Macaroni & Cheese | 330 | 13 | 40 |
| Vegetarian Marinara with Basil | 260 | 4 | 44 |
| *Prepared Salads: Per ½ Cup* | | | |
| BBQ Potato | 170 | 9 | 21 |
| Carrot Raisin | 90 | 3 | 17 |
| Dijon Potato with Garlic Dill Vinegar | 150 | 12 | 9 |
| Lemon Rice with Cashews | 160 | 7 | 23 |
| Thai Noodle w/ Chkn & Peanut Sce | 190 | 10 | 19 |
| *Muffins:* Blueberry | 160 | 7 | 22 |
| Choc. Chip/Brownie | 190 | 8 | 26 |
| Fruit Medley Bran | 130 | 0.5 | 29 |
| Tangy Lemon | 170 | 6 | 27 |
| *Breads & Focaccia: Per Piece* | | | |
| Bruschetta Focaccia | 80 | 3 | 12 |
| Buttermilk Cornbread Muffin | 190 | 7 | 28 |
| Cheesy Garlic Focaccia | 75 | 3 | 9 |
| Indian Grain | 200 | 1.5 | 35 |
| Sourdough | 150 | 0.5 | 27 |
| *Desserts: Per ½ Cup* | | | |
| Apple Medley | 70 | 0 | 18 |
| Banana Royale | 80 | 0 | 20 |
| Caramel Apple Cobbler | 390 | 12 | 68 |
| Tapioca Pudding | 140 | 3 | 24 |
| *Soft Serve: Per ½ Cup* | | | |
| Chocolate | 90 | 2 | 19 |
| Vanilla | 100 | 3 | 19 |

*For Complete Nutritional Data ~ see CalorieKing.com*

## Southern Tsunami® (Aug '15)

| *Rolls:* | C | F | Cb |
|---|---|---|---|
| **Hybrid:** *With White Rice* | | | |
| Berry, 6 oz | 250 | 6 | 46 |
| Blueberry: Salmon, 8 oz | 360 | 15 | 47 |
| Shrimp, 8 oz | 340 | 12 | 47 |
| Done Deal, 7 oz | 350 | 14 | 41 |
| Happy Mango, 8 oz | 440 | 19 | 56 |
| Jalapeno, 8 oz | 310 | 7 | 50 |
| Mango Shrimp, 6 oz | 380 | 21 | 42 |
| Red Rock Fujisan, 7 oz | 380 | 13 | 44 |
| Spicy Mango Roll, 8 oz | 390 | 17 | 47 |
| Ultimate Chili Combo, 6 oz | 290 | 9 | 43 |
| **Chef Samplers:** A, 9.5 oz | 360 | 8 | 52 |
| B, 7.5 oz | 310 | 6 | 44 |

*Continued Next Page... ...*

## Southern Tsunami® cont... (Aug '15)

*Rolls (Cont):*

**Plus Rolls:** *White Rice, 6 oz Servings*

| | C | F | Cb |
|---|---|---|---|
| California | 250 | 5 | 46 |
| Cream Cheese Plus: Salmon | 300 | 11 | 40 |
| Shrimp | 280 | 8 | 40 |
| Tuna | 280 | 8 | 40 |
| Eel | 300 | 8 | 50 |
| Seaside Plus: Eel | 360 | 12 | 53 |
| Salmon | 310 | 7 | 47 |
| Shrimp | 260 | 15 | 48 |
| Steelhead | 260 | 6 | 40 |
| Tuna | 270 | 15 | 47 |
| Spicy Plus: Salmon | 290 | 10 | 40 |
| Shrimp | 250 | 6 | 40 |
| Steelhead | 260 | 6 | 40 |
| Tuna | 260 | 6 | 40 |
| Vegetable | 240 | 5 | 46 |

**Wraps:** Avocado Salad Roll, 4.6 oz

| | C | F | Cb |
|---|---|---|---|
| Avocado Salad Roll, 4.6 oz | 130 | 4.5 | 23 |
| Berry, 4.6 oz | 180 | 7 | 28 |
| California, 6.6 oz | 310 | 16 | 34 |
| Smoked Salmon Salad Roll, 4.6 oz | 300 | 18 | 21 |

*Salads: Without Dressing*

| | C | F | Cb |
|---|---|---|---|
| Edamame, 3.1 oz | 90 | 5 | 3 |
| Sea Breeze, 4 oz | 90 | 2 | 16 |

*Dressings/Sauces:* Eel Sauce, 1 T.

| | C | F | Cb |
|---|---|---|---|
| Eel Sauce, 1 T. | 30 | 0 | 7 |
| Ginger Dressing, 2 Tbsp | 50 | 1.5 | 8 |
| Peanut Sauce, 1.4 oz | 60 | 0 | 12 |
| Sweet Chili, 1.4 oz | 100 | 0 | 24 |
| Wasabe Dressing, 2 Tbsp | 35 | 2 | 2 |

## Starbucks® (Aug '15)

**Brewed Coffee:** *Figures based on 16 fl.oz Grande without Whipped Cream*

| | C | F | Cb |
|---|---|---|---|
| Caffe Misto (Au Lait): W/ Whole Milk | 130 | 7 | 10 |
| With Nonfat Milk | 70 | 0 | 10 |
| With Soy Milk | 100 | 3 | 13 |

*Chocolate: Per Grande, 16 fl.oz Without Whipped Cream*

**Hot Chocolate:**

| | C | F | Cb |
|---|---|---|---|
| With Whole Milk | 360 | 13 | 47 |
| With 2% Milk | 320 | 9 | 47 |
| With Soy | 320 | 8 | 51 |

**Peppermint Hot Chocolate:**

| | C | F | Cb |
|---|---|---|---|
| With Whole Milk | 420 | 13 | 65 |
| With 2% Milk | 390 | 9 | 66 |
| With Soy Milk | 390 | 7 | 69 |

## Starbucks® cont... (Aug '15)

**Hot Espresso Beverages:**
*Per Grande, 126 fl.oz without Whipped Cream*

| | C | F | Cb |
|---|---|---|---|
| **Caffe Latte:** With Whole Milk | 220 | 11 | 18 |
| With Nonfat Milk | 130 | 0 | 19 |
| With Soy Milk | 170 | 4.5 | 23 |
| **Cappuccino:** With Whole Milk | 140 | 7 | 12 |
| With Nonfat Milk | 80 | 0 | 12 |
| With Soy Milk | 120 | 3.5 | 16 |
| **Caramel Macchiato:** W/ Whole Milk | 270 | 11 | 34 |
| With Nonfat Milk | 190 | 1 | 35 |
| **Cinn. Dolce Latte:** With Whole Milk | 300 | 10 | 40 |
| With Nonfat Milk | 210 | 0 | 40 |
| **Espresso:** 1 Doppio, 2 fl.oz | 10 | 0 | 2 |
| 1 Solo, 1 fl.oz | 5 | 0 | 1 |
| Espresso Con Panna, 1 Solo, 1 fl.oz | 30 | 2.5 | 2 |

*Iced Espresso: Per 16 fl.oz Grande without Whipped Cream*

**Caffe Latte:**

| | C | F | Cb |
|---|---|---|---|
| With Whole Milk | 150 | 7 | 13 |
| With Nonfat Milk | 90 | 0 | 13 |
| With Soy Milk | 130 | 3.5 | 17 |

**Vanilla Latte:**

| | C | F | Cb |
|---|---|---|---|
| With Whole Milk | 210 | 6 | 30 |
| With Nonfat Milk | 160 | 0 | 31 |
| With 2% Milk | 190 | 4 | 30 |

*Fizzios: Per Grande, 16 fl.oz*

Ginger Ale; Lemon Ale,

| | C | F | Cb |
|---|---|---|---|
| Spiced Root Beer | 100 | 0 | 27 |

*Frappuccino: Cold, Per 16 fl.oz Grande With Whole Milk, With Whipped Cream*

| | C | F | Cb |
|---|---|---|---|
| Caffe Vanilla | 430 | 14 | 72 |
| Caramel | 410 | 15 | 66 |
| Cinnamon Dolce | 380 | 14 | 60 |
| Hazelnut | 390 | 14 | 62 |
| Java Chip | 470 | 18 | 72 |
| Mocha | 410 | 15 | 65 |
| White Chocolate Mocha | 440 | 16 | 69 |

*Frappuccino Creme: Cold, Per 16 fl.oz Grande with Whole Milk and Whipped Cream*

| | C | F | Cb |
|---|---|---|---|
| Double Chocolaty Chip | 420 | 20 | 57 |
| Lemon Bar Creme | 350 | 13 | 56 |
| Vanilla Bean Creme | 400 | 16 | 59 |

*Refreshers:* Cool Lime, 16 oz

| | C | F | Cb |
|---|---|---|---|
| Cool Lime, 16 oz | 50 | 0 | 13 |
| Strawberry Acai, 16 oz | 90 | 0 | 22 |
| Very Berry Hibiscus, 16 oz | 70 | 0 | 17 |

*Smoothies: Per16 fl.oz Grande with 2% Milk, without Whipped Cream*

| | C | F | Cb |
|---|---|---|---|
| Chocolate | 320 | 5 | 53 |
| Orange Mango | 270 | 1.5 | 53 |
| Strawberry | 300 | 2 | 60 |

*Continued Next Page... ...*

## Starbucks® cont... (Aug '15)

*Teas:* *Grande, With Whole Milk*

| | C | F | Cb |
|---|---|---|---|
| **Hot Tea Latte:** | | | |
| Classic Chai | 270 | 7 | 45 |
| Teavana: Earl Grey | 210 | 7 | 30 |
| Green Tea, unsweetened | 390 | 13 | 56 |
| Oprah Cinnamon Chai | 220 | 7 | 23 |
| **Iced Tea Latte:** Classic Chai | 260 | 7 | 44 |
| Teavana: Green Tea | 310 | 9 | 50 |
| Oprah Cinnamon Chai | 220 | 7 | 33 |
| **Drink Extras:** | | | |
| **Caramel Drizzle,** 1 teaspoon | 15 | 0.5 | 2 |
| **Flavored Syrup:** 1 Pump | 20 | 0 | 5 |
| Sugar-Free, 1 Pump | 0 | 0 | 0 |
| **Mocha Syrup,** 1 Pump | 25 | 0.5 | 6 |
| **Sweetened Whipped Cream:** | | | |
| Grande/Venti, cold drinks, average | 110 | 11 | 3 |
| Grande/Venti, hot drinks | 75 | 7 | 3 |
| **Breakfast, Hot:** | | | |
| Bacon, Gouda & Parmesan Frittata, on Artisan Roll | 350 | 18 | 30 |
| Egg & Cheddar Sandwich | 280 | 13 | 27 |
| Sausage & Cheddar Sandwich | 500 | 28 | 41 |
| **Bistro Boxes:** | | | |
| Cheese & Fruit | 480 | 28 | 39 |
| Edamame Hummus | 460 | 25 | 47 |
| Protein | 380 | 19 | 37 |
| Thai Style Peanut Chicken Wrap | 430 | 20 | 51 |
| **Paninis:** | | | |
| Chicken Artichoke/Ancient Grain | 510 | 27 | 37 |
| Chicken Santa Fe/Ancient Grain | 370 | 15 | 32 |
| Ham & Swiss | 340 | 10 | 42 |
| Roasted Tomato & Mozzarella | 390 | 18 | 44 |
| Turkey Rustico Panini | 480 | 18 | 53 |
| **Sandwich,** Turkey & Havarti | 450 | 22 | 31 |
| **Brownie,** Double Chocolate Chunk | 380 | 23 | 41 |
| **Cakes:** Per Slice | | | |
| Banana Nut Bread, 4.4 oz | 420 | 21 | 52 |
| Classic Coffee Cake | 390 | 16 | 57 |
| Iced Lemon Pound Cake | 470 | 20 | 68 |
| **Reduced Fat Cake,** | | | |
| Cinnamon Swirl Coffee Cake | 370 | 9 | 67 |
| **Cookies:** | | | |
| Chocolate Chip | 310 | 15 | 42 |
| Flourless Chewy Chocolate Chip | 170 | 4.5 | 32 |

## Starbucks® cont... (Aug '15)

*Croissants:*

| | C | F | Cb |
|---|---|---|---|
| Butter | 260 | 14 | 28 |
| Chocolate | 330 | 17 | 39 |
| **Doughnuts:** Devil's Food | 430 | 23 | 53 |
| Old-Fashioned Glazed | 480 | 27 | 56 |
| **Muffin,** Blueberry, with Yogurt & Honey | 380 | 16 | 53 |
| **Sweet Rolls & Danish:** | | | |
| Cheese Danish | 320 | 16 | 36 |
| Morning Bun | 350 | 15 | 54 |
| **Yogurt Parfaits:** | | | |
| Greek Yogurt with Berries & Honey | 250 | 7 | 34 |
| Greek Raspberry and Sweet Cherry | 280 | 7 | 39 |

*Bottled Drinks ~ See Page 37*
*Coffee Mix (VIA) ~ See Page 35*
*Ice Cream ~ See Page 107*

## Steak Escape® (Aug '15)

*Sandwiches:* *With Menu Board Toppings*

| | C | F | Cb |
|---|---|---|---|
| **Regular:** Cajun Chicken | 660 | 23 | 68 |
| Grand: Chicken | 620 | 19 | 68 |
| Escape | 660 | 19 | 68 |
| Gobbler | 530 | 13 | 68 |
| Turkey Club | 550 | 14 | 65 |
| Vegetarian | 550 | 20 | 71 |
| Wild West BBQ | 700 | 20 | 75 |

*Wraps:* *With Menu Board Toppings*

| | | | |
|---|---|---|---|
| Cajun Chicken | 470 | 17 | 50 |
| Grand: Chicken | 490 | 18 | 51 |
| Escape | 520 | 18 | 50 |
| Gobbler | 440 | 14 | 51 |
| Turkey Club | 440 | 15 | 49 |
| Vegetarian | 430 | 17 | 52 |
| Wild West BBQ | 550 | 19 | 56 |

*Salads:*

| | | | |
|---|---|---|---|
| **Grilled:** Chicken | 410 | 25 | 14 |
| Ham | 360 | 22 | 17 |
| Steak | 440 | 24 | 15 |
| Turkey | 360 | 21 | 15 |
| Without Meat | 280 | 20 | 13 |
| **Loaded Potatoes:** Bacon & Ranch | 670 | 46 | 51 |
| Cheddar & Bacon | 430 | 17 | 56 |

*For Complete Nutritional Data ~ see CalorieKing.com*

## Steak 'n Shake® (Aug '15)

### The Original Steakburgers:

| | C | F | Cb |
|---|---|---|---|
| Single, without Cheese | 280 | 11 | 30 |
| **Double:** With Cheese | 440 | 25 | 31 |
| Bacon 'n Cheese | 480 | 28 | 31 |
| Cheesy Cheddar | 480 | 27 | 32 |
| Guacamole | 670 | 44 | 47 |
| Wisconsin Buttery | 700 | 47 | 45 |
| Triple, without cheese | 510 | 30 | 30 |

### Chili:

| | C | F | Cb |
|---|---|---|---|
| 3-Way (1) | 830 | 36 | 94 |
| 5-Way (1) | 1170 | 63 | 99 |
| Deluxe, bowl | 1220 | 74 | 81 |

### Sandwiches:

| | C | F | Cb |
|---|---|---|---|
| Guacamole Gr. Chicken | 550 | 28 | 59 |
| Jalap. Crunch Chicken | 580 | 28 | 66 |
| Spicy Chicken | 460 | 18 | 51 |

### Signature Steak Franks:

| | C | F | Cb |
|---|---|---|---|
| Regular | 380 | 27 | 22 |
| Cheesy Cheddar | 490 | 36 | 24 |
| Chicago Style | 420 | 27 | 30 |
| Chili Cheese | 620 | 44 | 31 |

### Salads: Without Dressing

| | C | F | Cb |
|---|---|---|---|
| Apple Harvest Grilled Chicken | 480 | 19 | 56 |
| Fried Chicken | 470 | 26 | 34 |
| Grilled Chicken | 270 | 10 | 30 |

### Sides:

### French Fries:

| | C | F | Cb |
|---|---|---|---|
| Regular | 440 | 21 | 60 |
| Large | 640 | 30 | 87 |
| **Onion Rings:** Regular | 440 | 25 | 48 |
| Large | 880 | 50 | 95 |

### Breakfast:

| | C | F | Cb |
|---|---|---|---|
| **Bagels Sandwich:** With Bacon | 450 | 16 | 51 |
| With Sausage | 570 | 29 | 50 |
| **Biscuits:** Bacon, Egg & Cheese | 520 | 35 | 32 |
| Egg & Cheese | 450 | 30 | 31 |
| Sausage & Egg | 600 | 44 | 31 |
| Sausage, Egg & Cheese | 650 | 48 | 31 |
| With Sausage Gravy: Half order | 540 | 37 | 43 |
| Full Order | 1070 | 74 | 86 |
| **Hash Browns:** Shredded | 320 | 26 | 19 |
| Side order, 5 pieces | 260 | 17 | 23 |
| **Perfect Start Oatmeal** | 340 | 11 | 57 |
| **Skillets:** Country | 1240 | 94 | 63 |
| Portobello & Swiss | 1020 | 83 | 28 |

### Hand Dipped Milk Shakes: Per Regular

| | C | F | Cb |
|---|---|---|---|
| Banana; Mocha | 630 | 21 | 103 |
| Butterfinger | 850 | 30 | 138 |
| Chocolate | 650 | 21 | 106 |
| Oreo Cookies 'n Cream | 780 | 26 | 107 |

## Subway® (Aug '15)

**6" Sandwich:** 6g Fat Or Less

Figures Based on 9 grain wheat bread, lettuce, tomatoes, onions, green peppers and cucumbers. Oil or mayo not included.

| | C | F | Cb |
|---|---|---|---|
| Black Forest Ham | 290 | 4.5 | 46 |
| Oven Roasted Chicken | 320 | 5 | 47 |
| Roast Beef | 320 | 5 | 45 |
| Subway Club | 310 | 4.5 | 46 |
| Sweet Onion Chicken Teriyaki | 370 | 4.5 | 57 |
| Turkey Breast | 280 | 3.5 | 46 |
| Turkey Breast & Black Forest Ham | 280 | 4 | 46 |
| Veggie Delite | 230 | 2.5 | 44 |

**6" Sandwiches:** Figures based on 9-grain wheat bread, lettuce, tomatoes, onion, green peppers, cucumbers. Oil or mayo not included.

| | C | F | Cb |
|---|---|---|---|
| Chkn & Bacon Ranch Melt w/ Chse | 570 | 28 | 47 |
| Cold Cut Combo | 360 | 12 | 46 |
| Italian B.M.T. | 410 | 16 | 46 |
| Meatball Marinara | 480 | 18 | 59 |
| Spicy Italian | 480 | 24 | 46 |
| Steak & Cheese | 380 | 10 | 48 |
| Tuna | 480 | 25 | 44 |
| Turkey Breast | 280 | 3.5 | 46 |

**Kids Meal Sandwiches:** Figures based on 9-grain wheat bread, lettuce, tomatoes, onions, green peppers and cucumbers. Oil or mayo not included.

| | C | F | Cb |
|---|---|---|---|
| Black Forest Ham | 180 | 2.5 | 30 |
| Roast Beef | 200 | 3 | 30 |
| Turkey Breast | 180 | 2 | 30 |
| Veggie Delite | 150 | 1.5 | 29 |

**Condiments & Sauces:** For 6" Sandwiches

| | C | F | Cb |
|---|---|---|---|
| Chipotle Southwest, 0.8 oz | 100 | 10 | 1 |
| Honey Mustard, Fat-Free, 0.8 oz | 30 | 0 | 7 |
| Mayonnaise: 1 Tbsp, 0.5 oz | 110 | 12 | 0 |
| Light, 1 Tbsp, 0.5 oz | 50 | 5 | 1 |
| Mustard, Yellow or Deli Brown. 2 tsp | 5 | 0 | 1 |
| Olive Oil Blend, 1 tsp | 45 | 5 | 0 |
| Ranch Dressing | 110 | 11 | 1 |
| Sweet Onion, Fat-Free, 0.8 oz | 40 | 0 | 9 |

**Extras:** For 6" Sandwiches

| | C | F | Cb |
|---|---|---|---|
| Bacon Strips (2) | 45 | 3.5 | 0 |
| Cheese: American, 2 triangles, 0.3 oz | 40 | 3.5 | 1 |
| Cheddar, 2 triangles, 0.3 oz | 60 | 5 | 0 |
| Swiss, 2 triangles, 0.3 oz | 50 | 4.5 | 0 |

**Continued Next Page....**

## Subway® cont... (Aug '15)

*Flatizza:* Figures Based on 9-Grain Wheat Bread, Lettuce, Tomatoes, Onions, Green Peppers and Cucumbers. Oil or Mayo not included

| | C | F | Cb |
|---|---|---|---|
| Cheese | 390 | 16 | 42 |
| Pepperoni; Spicy Italian, average | 495 | 26 | 43 |
| Veggie | 410 | 17 | 44 |

**Breakfast:**

**6" Egg White Omelet Sandwiches:** *Includes 9-grain Wheat Bread*

| | | | |
|---|---|---|---|
| Bacon, Egg White & Cheese | 370 | 11 | 45 |
| Egg White & Cheese | 320 | 8 | 44 |
| Egg White & Cheese with Ham | 350 | 9 | 45 |
| Steak, Egg White & Cheese | 390 | 10 | 47 |

**6" Regular Egg Omelet Sandwiches:** *Includes 9-grain Wheat Bread*

| | | | |
|---|---|---|---|
| Bacon, Egg & Cheese | 410 | 16 | 45 |
| Egg & Cheese | 360 | 12 | 44 |
| Egg & Chse with Ham | 390 | 13 | 45 |
| Steak, Egg & Cheese | 430 | 15 | 47 |

**Egg White Omelet on 6" Flatbread:**

| | | | |
|---|---|---|---|
| Bacon, Egg White & Cheese | 380 | 13 | 43 |
| Egg White & Cheese | 330 | 10 | 42 |
| With Ham | 360 | 11 | 43 |
| Mega Melt | 520 | 24 | 44 |
| Steak, Egg White & Cheese | 400 | 12 | 45 |

**Regular Egg Omelet On 6" Flatbreads:**

| | | | |
|---|---|---|---|
| Bacon, Egg & Cheese | 420 | 18 | 42 |
| Black Forest Ham, Egg & Cheese | 400 | 15 | 43 |
| Egg & Cheese | 370 | 14 | 42 |
| Mega Melt | 560 | 29 | 43 |
| Steak, Egg & Cheese | 440 | 17 | 44 |

*Salads (6g Fat or Less):* Figures based on lettuce, tomatoes, onions, green peppers, olives & cucumbers. Dressing or croutons not included.

| | | | |
|---|---|---|---|
| Black Forest Ham | 110 | 3 | 12 |
| Oven Roasted Chicken | 140 | 2.5 | 10 |
| Roast Beef; Subway Club, av. | 140 | 3.5 | 11 |
| Sweet Onion Chicken Teriyaki, with Sweet Onion dressing | 230 | 3 | 32 |
| Turkey Breast & Ham | 110 | 2.5 | 12 |
| Veggie Delite | 60 | 1 | 10 |

**Salad Dressings:**

| | | | |
|---|---|---|---|
| Chipotle Southwest, 1.5 oz | 190 | 20 | 2 |
| Ranch, 1.5 oz | 220 | 23 | 2 |

## Subway® cont... (Aug '15)

*Soups:* Per 8 oz Bowl

| | C | F | Cb |
|---|---|---|---|
| Beef Chili | 350 | 24 | 17 |
| Chicken Noodle | 110 | 3 | 14 |
| Clam Chowder | 200 | 11 | 20 |
| Loaded Baked Potato | 210 | 13 | 15 |
| Minestrone | 90 | 1 | 17 |
| Poblano Corn Chowder | 150 | 7 | 18 |
| Vegetable Beef | 90 | 2 | 15 |

**Cookies & Desserts:**

| | | | |
|---|---|---|---|
| Apple Slices, 1 package, 2.5 oz | 35 | 0 | 9 |
| Chocolate Chip Cookie, 1.5 oz | 200 | 10 | 30 |
| Oatmeal Raisin Cookie, 1.5 oz | 200 | 8 | 30 |
| Raspberry Cheesecake, 1.6 oz | 200 | 9 | 29 |

## Sweet Tomatoes®

**Same Menu & Data as Souplantation ~ See Page 242**

## Swiss Chalet® (Aug '15)

*Starters:*

| | C | F | Cb |
|---|---|---|---|
| Caesar Salad without Dressing | 90 | 3 | 13 |
| Chalet Chicken Wings (8), with sauce | 550 | 34 | 23 |
| Cheese Perogies (7) | 420 | 10 | 69 |
| Garlic Cheese Loaf, 10.5 oz | 910 | 58 | 73 |

*BBQ Back Ribs:* With Sauce

| | | | |
|---|---|---|---|
| Half Rack | 460 | 29 | 17 |
| Full Rack | 920 | 59 | 34 |

*Burgers:* Without Sides, with Mayo

| | | | |
|---|---|---|---|
| Ultimate Bacon Cheeseburgr | 730 | 42 | 46 |
| Veggie | 440 | 15 | 50 |

*Chicken Pot Pie,* 1 pie | 610 | 35 | 43 |

*Rotisserie Chicken:* Meat Only

| | | | |
|---|---|---|---|
| Double Leg, with Skin | 490 | 31 | 0 |
| Half Chicken, with Skin | 530 | 27 | 0 |

Quarter Chicken:

| | | | |
|---|---|---|---|
| Dark meat, without Skin | 160 | 8 | 0 |
| Dark meat, with Skin | 240 | 16 | 0 |
| White meat, without Skin | 220 | 6 | 0 |
| White meat, with Skin | 290 | 11 | 0 |

*Sandwiches: Without Sides*

| | | | |
|---|---|---|---|
| Classic Hot Chicken, white meat | 520 | 11 | 51 |
| Crispy Fish | 1130 | 65 | 95 |
| Flatbread, Hickory Chicken | 700 | 31 | 71 |

*Continued Next Page...*

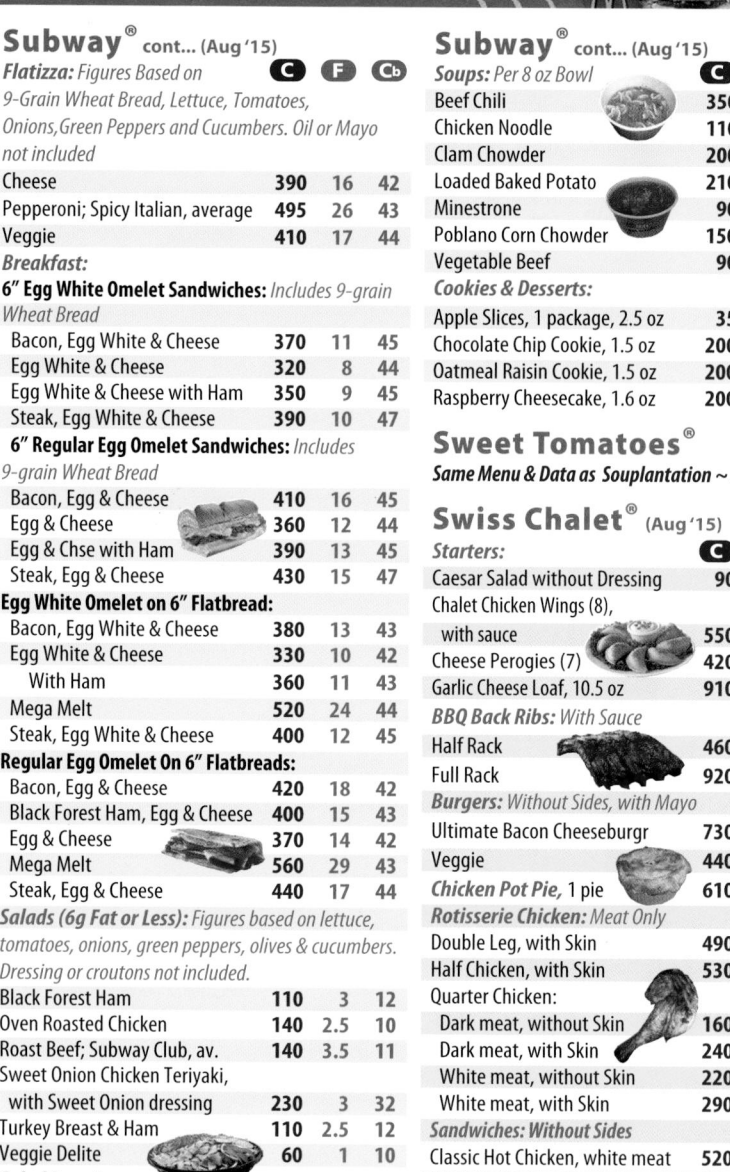

Updated Nutrition Data ~ www.CalorieKing.com
Persons with Diabetes ~ See Disclaimer (Page 22)

## Swiss Chalet® cont...(Aug '15)

| Wrap, | C | F | Cb |
|---|---|---|---|
| Rotisserie Chicken Club | 710 | 32 | 57 |

**Entree Salads:** *Without Dressing*

| | C | F | Cb |
|---|---|---|---|
| Spinach & Mandarin Chicken Salad | 400 | 16 | 28 |
| Sweet Heat Salad with Chicken | 340 | 9 | 30 |
| West Coast Salad with Chicken | 460 | 21 | 21 |

**Dressings/Sauces:**

| | C | F | Cb |
|---|---|---|---|
| Caesar Dressing, 1 oz | 180 | 18 | 2 |
| Chalet Dressing, 1 Tbsp, 1 oz | 160 | 14 | 6 |
| Chalet Dipping Sauce, 3.5 oz | 25 | 0.5 | 5 |

**Sides:**

| | C | F | Cb |
|---|---|---|---|
| Gravy, 4 oz | 45 | 1.5 | 7 |
| Mashed Potatoes, 5 oz | 170 | 5 | 27 |
| Sauteed Mushrooms, 6 oz | 140 | 1 | 30 |
| Seasoned Rice, 6 oz | 250 | 3.5 | 50 |

**Desserts/Pies:**

| | C | F | Cb |
|---|---|---|---|
| Apple Pie | 440 | 19 | 65 |
| Coconut Cream Pie | 540 | 33 | 57 |
| Lemon Meringue Pie | 400 | 11 | 73 |
| Pecan Pie | 590 | 29 | 79 |
| Sticky Toffee Pudding with Ice Crm | 540 | 20 | 88 |

## Taco Bell® (Aug '15)

| Burritos: | C | F | Cb |
|---|---|---|---|
| ½ lb Cheesy Potato | 510 | 24 | 56 |
| ½ lb Combo | 450 | 18 | 51 |
| 7-Layer | 430 | 16 | 57 |
| Beefy 5-Layer | 510 | 20 | 64 |
| Chicken | 400 | 18 | 45 |
| Chili Cheese | 370 | 16 | 39 |
| Smothered Shredded Chicken | 640 | 27 | 65 |
| Smothered Steak | 660 | 29 | 65 |
| Supreme: Beef | 410 | 15 | 51 |
| Chicken; Steak, av. | 390 | 13 | 50 |
| **XXL Grilled Stuft:** Beef | 860 | 41 | 91 |
| Chicken; Steak, av. | 820 | 35 | 88 |

**Fresco Menu:**

| | C | F | Cb |
|---|---|---|---|
| **Tacos:** Crunchy Beef | 150 | 8 | 13 |
| Soft Tacos: Beef | 160 | 7 | 18 |
| Shrd Chicken; Grilled Steak, av. | 145 | 4 | 16 |

**Fresco Style:**

| | C | F | Cb |
|---|---|---|---|
| **Chalupas:** Supreme Beef | 360 | 21 | 31 |
| Supreme Chicken | 340 | 17 | 30 |
| **Gorditas:** Cheesy Crunch | 500 | 29 | 40 |
| Supreme: Beef | 290 | 12 | 31 |
| Chicken | 260 | 9 | 30 |
| Steak | 270 | 10 | 29 |
| **Soft Tacos:** Chicken | 160 | 5 | 16 |
| Spicy Potato | 240 | 12 | 27 |
| Supreme Beef | 210 | 10 | 19 |

## Taco Bell® cont... (Aug '15)

| Fresco Style (Cont.): | C | F | Cb |
|---|---|---|---|
| **Cantina Power Bowls:** Chicken | 490 | 20 | 49 |
| Steak | 500 | 21 | 47 |
| Veggie | 460 | 19 | 58 |
| Loaded Potato Griller | 410 | 18 | 50 |

**Specialities:**

| | C | F | Cb |
|---|---|---|---|
| Cheese Roll-Up | 180 | 9 | 15 |
| Crunchwrap Supreme | 540 | 21 | 71 |
| MexiMelt | 250 | 14 | 19 |
| Mexican Pizza, 7.5 oz | 550 | 30 | 49 |
| **Nachos:** BellGrande | 760 | 38 | 84 |
| Supreme | 440 | 23 | 46 |
| **Quesadillas:** Cheese | 460 | 26 | 37 |
| Steak | 520 | 28 | 38 |

**Tacos:**

| | C | F | Cb |
|---|---|---|---|
| **Crunchy:** Regular | 170 | 10 | 13 |
| Supreme | 190 | 11 | 15 |
| **Double Decker:** Regular | 320 | 14 | 36 |
| Supreme | 340 | 15 | 38 |
| **Soft:** Beef | 190 | 9 | 17 |
| Beef Supreme | 210 | 10 | 19 |
| Chicken | 160 | 5 | 16 |

**Taco Salads:**

| | C | F | Cb |
|---|---|---|---|
| Express Fiesta | 570 | 26 | 62 |
| **Fiesta:** Beef | 770 | 41 | 76 |
| Chicken | 730 | 33 | 74 |
| Steak | 740 | 35 | 72 |

**Sides:** *Per Serve*

| | C | F | Cb |
|---|---|---|---|
| Cheesy Fiesta Potato | 230 | 12 | 28 |
| Chips & Guacamole | 320 | 20 | 32 |
| Pintos 'n Cheese, 4.3 oz | 190 | 7 | 21 |

**Condiments & Sauces:**

| | C | F | Cb |
|---|---|---|---|
| Avocado Ranch Dressing, 0.5 oz | 80 | 8 | 1 |
| Creamy Jalapeno Sauce, 0.5 oz | 70 | 7 | 1 |
| Green Tomatillo Sauce, 1 oz | 10 | 0 | 2 |
| Guacamole, 0.8 oz | 35 | 3 | 2 |
| Sour Cream, Reduced Fat, 0.8 oz | 30 | 2 | 2 |

**Breakfast:**

| | C | F | Cb |
|---|---|---|---|
| AM Crunchwrap: Bacon | 670 | 42 | 51 |
| Sausage | 710 | 47 | 51 |
| AM Grilled Taco: Bacon | 230 | 14 | 15 |
| Sausage | 280 | 19 | 16 |
| Biscuit Tacos: Bacon, Egg & Cheese | 380 | 23 | 30 |
| Egg & Cheese | 310 | 17 | 29 |
| Sausage & Cheese | 370 | 23 | 29 |
| Sausage, Egg & Cheese | 430 | 28 | 30 |

*Continued Next Page...*

## Taco Bell® cont... (Aug '15)

*Breakfast (Cont):*

| | C | F | Cb |
|---|---|---|---|
| Cheesy Burritos: Bacon | 490 | 28 | 37 |
| Sausage | 530 | 33 | 37 |
| Cinnabon Delights, 2 pack | 160 | 9 | 17 |
| Hash Brown, 1.9 oz | 160 | 12 | 13 |

*Sweets:*

| | | | |
|---|---|---|---|
| Cap'n Crunch Delights (4) | 330 | 22 | 29 |
| Caramel Apple Empanada | 310 | 15 | 39 |
| Cinnabon Delights: | | | |
| 2 Pack | 160 | 9 | 17 |
| 4 Pack | 310 | 18 | 35 |
| 12 Pack | 930 | 53 | 104 |
| Cinnamon Twists | 170 | 6 | 27 |

*Note: Nutritional data in New York outlets may vary slightly. Please check Taco Bell website*

## Taco Cabana® (Aug '15)

*Cabana Burritos:*
Includes Flour Burrito & Menu Set Toppings

| | C | F | Cb |
|---|---|---|---|
| Beef | 980 | 47 | 97 |
| Chicken, Stewed | 900 | 37 | 98 |
| Steak Fajita | 910 | 39 | 96 |

*Quesadillas:* Personal, with Guacamole & Sour Cream

| | | | |
|---|---|---|---|
| Cheese | 710 | 39 | 61 |
| Chicken Breast Fajita; Steak, av. | 765 | 41 | 62 |
| Shrimp Tampico | 820 | 45 | 63 |

*Sizzling Skillets:* Includes Flour Tortilla, Grilled Onion, Bell Pepper, Rice, Shredded Cheese, Sour Cream, Guacamole, Lettuce & Pico de Gallo

| | | | |
|---|---|---|---|
| ½ lb, 1 serving: Brisket | 960 | 46 | 95 |
| Chicken Fajita | 775 | 26 | 95 |
| Mixed Fajita Steak & Chicken | 785 | 28 | 95 |
| Shrimp Tampico; Steak Fajita, av. | 795 | 30 | 97 |

*Tacos:*

| | | | |
|---|---|---|---|
| Black Bean | 190 | 4 | 34 |
| Carne Guisada | 190 | 6 | 20 |
| **Crispy:** Ground Beef | 200 | 12 | 12 |
| Stewed Chicken | 160 | 7 | 12 |

*Soft:*

| | | | |
|---|---|---|---|
| Chicken, Stewed | 200 | 7 | 22 |
| Ground Beef | 240 | 12 | 22 |

*Sides & Add-Ons:* Per Serving

| | | | |
|---|---|---|---|
| Black Beans, 4 oz | 80 | 1 | 15 |
| Borracho Beans, 4 oz | 140 | 3 | 20 |
| Guacamole, 3 oz | 110 | 9 | 7 |
| Queso, 3 oz | 110 | 8 | 5 |
| Refried Beans with Cheese, 4 oz | 260 | 14 | 25 |
| Rice, 4 oz | 120 | 0.5 | 25 |
| Salsa: Fuego; Roja, 1 oz | 5 | 0 | 1 |
| Verde, 1 oz | 10 | 0 | 1 |
| Sour Cream, 3 oz | 160 | 15 | 3 |

## Taco Del Mar® (Aug '15)

*Baja Bowls:* Per Regular Bowl, with Standard Menu Toppings, without Guacamole, Sour Cream, Jalapenos or Sauce

| | C | F | Cb |
|---|---|---|---|
| Mondo: Beef Steak Asada | 500 | 14 | 63 |
| Chicken; Shredded Beef | 520 | 17 | 62 |
| Fish | 590 | 36 | 47 |
| Ground Beef | 570 | 23 | 62 |
| Pork | 500 | 15 | 61 |

*Burritos:* With Standard Menu Toppings, without Guacamole, Sour Cream, Jalapenos or Sauce

**Mondito:**

| | | | |
|---|---|---|---|
| Beef Steak Asada | 460 | 12 | 67 |
| Chicken; Shredded Beef, av. | 475 | 14 | 67 |
| Fish | 530 | 24 | 63 |
| Ground Beef | 500 | 17 | 67 |
| Pork | 470 | 13 | 66 |

**Mondo:** *Per Regular Size*

| | | | |
|---|---|---|---|
| Beef Steak Asada | 810 | 21 | 115 |
| Chicken; Shredded Beef | 840 | 24 | 113 |
| Fish | 910 | 44 | 98 |
| Ground Beef | 880 | 30 | 114 |
| Pork | 830 | 24 | 113 |

*Platters:*

**Enchilada:** *Per 2 Corn Tortillas and Standard Menu Toppings, without Jalapenos or Sauce*

| | | | |
|---|---|---|---|
| Beef Steak Asada | 810 | 27 | 107 |
| Cheese | 810 | 32 | 105 |
| Chicken; Shredded Beef, average | 845 | 31 | 106 |
| Ground Beef | 890 | 37 | 106 |
| Pork | 830 | 30 | 104 |

**Enchilada/Taco:** *Includes Corn & Flour Tortillas, Standard Menu Toppings, without Jalapenos or Sauce*

| | | | |
|---|---|---|---|
| Beef Steak Asada | 830 | 28 | 109 |
| Chicken; Shredded Beef, average | 865 | 31 | 107 |
| Ground Beef | 900 | 38 | 109 |
| Pork | 830 | 30 | 108 |

*Quesadillas:* Includes Flour Tortilla, Standard Menu Toppings, without Jalapenos and Sauce

| | | | |
|---|---|---|---|
| **Mondito, Small:** Beef Steak Asada | 390 | 17 | 40 |
| Chicken; Shredded Beef, average | 415 | 19 | 39 |
| Ground Beef | 430 | 22 | 40 |
| Pork | 410 | 19 | 39 |

*Continued Next Page...*

Updated Nutrition Data ~ www.CalorieKing.com
Persons with Diabetes ~ See Disclaimer (Page 22)

# Fast - Foods & *Restaurants*

## Taco Del Mar® cont... (Aug '15)

*Nachos: Includes Chips, Standard Menu Toppings, without Jalapenos and Sauce*

| | C | F | Cb |
|---|---|---|---|
| **Mondo, Regular:** Cheese | 1050 | 62 | 95 |
| Beef Steak Asada | 1150 | 64 | 98 |
| Chicken; Shredded Beef, av. | 1180 | 68 | 97 |
| Ground Beef | 1220 | 74 | 97 |
| Pork | 1170 | 67 | 96 |

*Salads: Includes Shell, Standard Menu Toppings, without Guacamole, Sour Cream or Jalapenos*

| | C | F | Cb |
|---|---|---|---|
| **Mondo, Regular:** Chicken | 640 | 32 | 56 |
| Fish | 670 | 34 | 67 |
| Pork | 620 | 31 | 56 |
| Veggie | 720 | 29 | 96 |

*Note: Nutritional Information varies from state to state. Please refer to Taco Del Mar Website*

## Taco John's® (Aug '15)

**Burritos:**

| | C | F | Cb |
|---|---|---|---|
| Bean Burrito | 370 | 11 | 53 |
| Beef Grilled Burrito | 590 | 32 | 53 |
| Beefy Burrito | 440 | 21 | 42 |
| Chicken Grilled Burrito | 590 | 30 | 50 |
| Combination Burrito | 410 | 16 | 47 |
| Crunchy Chicken & Potato Burrito | 580 | 27 | 67 |
| Meat & Potato Burrito | 520 | 25 | 57 |
| Super Burrito | 450 | 20 | 50 |

**Tacos:**

| | C | F | Cb |
|---|---|---|---|
| Cripsy Taco | 170 | 10 | 11 |
| Fish Taco | 280 | 14 | 29 |
| Soft Shell, Chicken | 190 | 6 | 21 |
| Taco Bravo | 330 | 13 | 38 |
| Taco Burger | 280 | 12 | 29 |

**Specialties:**

| | C | F | Cb |
|---|---|---|---|
| **Crunchy Chicken,** without sauce | 370 | 18 | 29 |
| **Quesadilla Melt:** Cheesy | 450 | 24 | 40 |
| Fajita Beef | 550 | 29 | 46 |
| Fajita Chicken | 520 | 25 | 45 |
| **Super Nachos:** Small | 420 | 25 | 37 |
| Regular | 790 | 47 | 72 |
| **Super Potato Oles:** | | | |
| Small | 650 | 40 | 59 |
| Regular | 1090 | 67 | 98 |
| **Taco Salads:** Chicken, w/o dressing | 500 | 27 | 39 |
| Crunchy Chicken, without dressing | 630 | 36 | 53 |
| Plain, without dressing | 540 | 33 | 40 |

## Taco John's® cont... (Aug '15)

**Sides:**

| | C | F | Cb |
|---|---|---|---|
| Chips & Queso | 430 | 25 | 43 |
| Cilantro Lime Rice, 6 oz | 220 | 6 | 39 |
| Potato Oles: Small | 480 | 27 | 52 |
| Medium | 670 | 38 | 73 |
| Large | 860 | 49 | 94 |
| **Refried Beans:** With Cheese | 320 | 7 | 46 |
| Without Cheese | 260 | 2.5 | 45 |

**Condiments:**

| | C | F | Cb |
|---|---|---|---|
| Bacon Ranch, 1.5 oz | 120 | 9 | 10 |
| House Dressing, 1.5 oz | 70 | 7 | 2 |
| Nacho Cheese, 3 oz | 110 | 9 | 5 |
| Salsa, 2 oz | 10 | 0 | 2 |
| Sour Cream, 2 oz | 120 | 10 | 3 |

**Dessert:**

| | C | F | Cb |
|---|---|---|---|
| Churro, 2 oz | 200 | 9 | 29 |
| Mexican Donut Bites, 3.2 oz | 290 | 12 | 47 |

## Taco Mayo® (Aug '15)

**Burritos:**

| | C | F | Cb |
|---|---|---|---|
| Bean | 495 | 16 | 71 |
| Beef | 490 | 23 | 41 |
| Super: Beef | 540 | 23 | 57 |
| Chicken | 405 | 16 | 39 |

**Melts:**

| | C | F | Cb |
|---|---|---|---|
| Tamale | 615 | 34 | 50 |
| Tostada | 525 | 32 | 35 |

**Quesadillas:**

| | C | F | Cb |
|---|---|---|---|
| Chicken | 675 | 37 | 46 |
| Fajita Chicken | 700 | 39 | 47 |
| Fajita Steak | 725 | 40 | 47 |

**Tacos:**

| | C | F | Cb |
|---|---|---|---|
| Crispy Taco, Beef | 160 | 9 | 10 |
| Soft Taco: Beef | 230 | 11 | 17 |
| Chicken | 185 | 6 | 16 |

*Salads: As Per Menu Description*

**Acapulco:**

| | C | F | Cb |
|---|---|---|---|
| Chicken, 12.4 oz | 680 | 50 | 35 |
| Steak, 12.4 oz | 705 | 51 | 35 |
| SalsaLita Steak, 12 oz | 305 | 8 | 33 |
| Taco Steak, 11.3 oz | 445 | 25 | 30 |

**Sides:**

| | C | F | Cb |
|---|---|---|---|
| Mexicali Rice | 160 | 1 | 36 |
| Refried Beans | 295 | 9 | 43 |
| Potato Locos, Small | 380 | 24 | 36 |

## Taco Time® (Aug '15)

| Burritos: | C | F | Cb |
|---|---|---|---|
| Beef, Bean & Cheese | 490 | 17 | 55 |
| Chicken B.L.T. | 690 | 39 | 43 |
| **Big Juan:** Chicken | 580 | 16 | 70 |
| Ground Beef | 630 | 23 | 73 |
| **Casita:** Chicken | 490 | 17 | 42 |
| Ground Beef | 540 | 24 | 46 |
| **Crisp Burrito:** | | | |
| Chicken | 380 | 17 | 33 |
| Ground Beef | 430 | 21 | 36 |
| Pinto Bean | 360 | 14 | 47 |
| **Soft Burrito:** Ground Beef | 430 | 16 | 43 |
| Pinto Bean | 370 | 10 | 54 |
| Veggie | 520 | 17 | 73 |
| *Tacos:* | | | |
| **Soft Tacos:** *Per 7 oz* | | | |
| Chicken | 360 | 9 | 40 |
| Ground Beef | 420 | 16 | 43 |
| Country, 13.25 oz | 720 | 54 | 20 |
| Nacho, 15.5 oz | 740 | 48 | 26 |
| *Other Favorites:* Cheddar Melt | 250 | 12 | 25 |
| Nachos Grande | 930 | 43 | 96 |
| **Tostada:** Bean | 230 | 13 | 21 |
| Chicken | 320 | 13 | 22 |
| Ground Beef | 380 | 20 | 25 |
| *Breakfast:* | | | |
| Burritos: Egg & Bacon, 7.5 oz | 510 | 24 | 49 |
| Egg & Cheese, 5.75 oz | 370 | 16 | 40 |
| Ultimate, 11 oz | 860 | 58 | 52 |
| Omelet, Cheese, 8 oz | 490 | 36 | 6 |
| *Sides:* | | | |
| Chips, Taco, 2 oz | 150 | 3.5 | 27 |
| Fries: Cheddar, medium, 7 oz | 500 | 35 | 39 |
| Mexi, medium, 6 oz | 390 | 26 | 38 |
| Stuffed, medium, 7 oz | 460 | 28 | 42 |
| Mexi-Rice, 3.5 oz | 80 | 0.5 | 17 |
| Refritos, with Chips, 6 oz | 230 | 7 | 29 |
| *Salads:* | | | |
| Regular: Chicken Taco, 9.5 oz | 310 | 13 | 22 |
| Ground Beef Taco, 9 oz | 370 | 20 | 24 |
| Tostada Delight: Chicken, 9 oz | 450 | 19 | 35 |
| Ground Beef, 9 oz | 490 | 26 | 36 |
| *Desserts:* Crustos | 290 | 6 | 58 |
| Churro: Plain | 210 | 16 | 17 |
| With Cinnamon & Sugar | 250 | 16 | 27 |

## TCBY® (Aug '15)

| Soft Sve Frozen Yogurt: Per 4 fl.oz | C | F | Cb |
|---|---|---|---|
| Bananas Foster | 100 | 0 | 24 |
| Cake Batter | 120 | 2 | 23 |
| Caramel Supreme | 130 | 1.5 | 27 |
| Cheesecake | 110 | 2 | 23 |
| Chocolate | 110 | 1.5 | 23 |
| Coffee; Golden Vanilla | 120 | 2 | 23 |
| Dutch Chocolate | 100 | 0 | 24 |
| Peanut Butter | 130 | 2 | 26 |
| Silk Almond Nog | 110 | 5 | 31 |
| **No Sugar Added,** Fat Free, | | | |
| average all flavors | 80 | 0 | 22 |
| *Sorbet,* average all flavors, 4 fl.oz | 100 | 0 | 25 |
| *Hand-Scooped Frozen Yogurt:* | | | |
| **Butter Pecan:** Kid's, 4 fl.oz | 120 | 4 | 16 |
| Small, 6.4 fl.oz | 190 | 6.5 | 26 |
| Regular, 12.8 fl.oz | 385 | 13 | 51 |
| **Chunky Choc. Cookie Dough:** | | | |
| Kid's, 4 fl.oz | 160 | 5 | 24 |
| Small, 6.4 fl.oz | 255 | 8 | 38 |
| Regular,12.8 fl.oz | 510 | 16 | 77 |
| **Cookies & Cream:** | | | |
| Kid's,4 fl.oz | 100 | 3.5 | 19 |
| Small, 6.4 fl.oz | 160 | 5 | 30 |
| Regular, 12.8 fl.oz | 320 | 11 | 61 |
| **Peanut Butter Delight:** Kid's, 4 fl.oz | 170 | 8 | 20 |
| Small, 6.4 fl.oz | 270 | 13 | 32 |
| Regular, 12.8 fl.oz | 540 | 26 | 64 |
| **Pralines & Cream:** Kid's 4 fl.oz | 130 | 4 | 19 |
| Small, 6.4 fl.oz | 210 | 6.5 | 30 |
| Regular, 12.8 fl oz | 415 | 13 | 60 |
| **Vanilla Bean:** Kid's,4 fl.oz | 110 | 2.5 | 16 |
| Small, 6.4 fl.oz | 175 | 4 | 26 |
| Regular, 12.8 fl.oz | 350 | 8 | 52 |
| *Cakes:* Per ⅒ Cake | | | |
| Chocolate Lovers Cake | 220 | 6 | 36 |
| Red Velvet Mousse Cake | 190 | 6 | 30 |
| *Pies:* Per ⅒ Pie | | | |
| Cookies & Creme Pie | 320 | 15 | 42 |
| Peanut Buttery Fudge Pie | 340 | 17 | 42 |

Updated Nutrition Data ~ www.CalorieKing.com
Persons with Diabetes ~ See Disclaimer (Page 22)

## TGI Friday's® (Aug '15)

*Appetiers: As Served*

| | C | F | Cb |
|---|---|---|---|
| **Individual:** | | | |
| Crispy Green Bean Fries | 900 | 65 | 69 |
| Mozzarella Sticks | 1100 | 75 | 62 |
| Pan Seared P'stickers | 590 | 25 | 72 |
| Sesame Jack Chicken Strips | 1090 | 35 | 159 |
| **Taste & Share:** | | | |
| Ahi Tuna Crisps | 330 | 24 | 15 |
| Bacon Mac & Cheese Bites | 600 | 40 | 41 |
| Corned Beef & Swiss Sliders | 510 | 24 | 46 |
| Garlic & Basil Bruschetta | 350 | 21 | 33 |
| Hibachi Skewers: Chicken | 470 | 15 | 63 |
| Sirloin | 490 | 20 | 58 |
| Parmesan Meatballs | 790 | 61 | 39 |
| Thai Pork Tacos | 280 | 14 | 25 |
| **Hand-Crafted Burgers:** *As Served* | | | |
| Cheeseburger | 1240 | 84 | 78 |
| Jack Daniel's Burger | 1490 | 86 | 132 |
| NY Cheddar & Bacon Burger | 1480 | 100 | 88 |
| Sedona Black Bean Burger | 1240 | 76 | 105 |
| Turkey Burger | 930 | 50 | 77 |
| **Sandwiches:** *Without Sides* | | | |
| California Club | 750 | 46 | 41 |
| Jack Daniel's Chicken | 1230 | 66 | 109 |
| Triple Stack Reuben | 1040 | 55 | 76 |
| **Steaks:** *Without Sides* | | | |
| Flat Iron | 380 | 26 | 3 |
| Sirloin: 6 oz | 370 | 23 | 3 |
| With Half Rack Ribs | 850 | 43 | 41 |
| Sirloin: 10 oz | 590 | 44 | 3 |
| With Grilled Lobster Tail | 710 | 46 | 6 |
| **Chicken & Pasta:** *As Served* | | | |
| Crispy Chicken Fingers | 1000 | 66 | 68 |
| **Pasta:** | | | |
| Bruschetta Chicken | 930 | 45 | 90 |
| Cajun Shrimp & Chicken | 1110 | 59 | 86 |
| Hibachi Chicken Skewers | 1230 | 34 | 185 |
| **Jack Daniels Grill:** *Without Sides* | | | |
| Chicken | 540 | 15 | 56 |
| Chicken & Shrimp | 530 | 14 | 65 |
| Flat Iron Steak | 500 | 16 | 57 |
| Ribs & Shrimp | 1730 | 75 | 180 |
| Sirloin & Crispy Shrimp | 920 | 41 | 79 |
| **Salads:** *Includes Dressing* | | | |
| Balsamic-Glazed Chicken Caesar | 500 | 31 | 25 |
| Chipotle Yucatan Chicken | 840 | 60 | 46 |
| Pecan-Crusted Chicken | 1080 | 71 | 76 |
| **Dressing:** *Per 2 oz* | | | |
| Balsamic Vinaigrette | 300 | 31 | 7 |
| Bleu Cheese | 320 | 34 | 2 |
| Honey Mustard | 310 | 29 | 12 |
| Ranch | 210 | 22 | 2 |

## TGI Friday's® cont... (Aug '15)

| | C | F | Cb |
|---|---|---|---|
| **Sides:** | | | |
| Ginger-Lime Slaw | 80 | 4.5 | 9 |
| Jasmin Rice Pilaf | 420 | 11 | 72 |
| Mashed Potatoes | 210 | 10 | 21 |
| Parmesan Steak Fries | 660 | 49 | 47 |
| Sweet Potato Fries | 390 | 20 | 50 |
| **Soups:** *Per 10 oz Bowl* | | | |
| Broccoli Cheese | 290 | 20 | 18 |
| French Onion | 310 | 18 | 21 |
| **Soup Of The Day:** Chicken Noodle | 250 | 7 | 33 |
| New England Clam Chowder | 500 | 30 | 45 |
| Tomato Basil | 300 | 24 | 20 |
| Tortilla | 250 | 13 | 23 |
| **Desserts:** | | | |
| Brownie Obsession, ½ serve | 600 | 30 | 77 |
| Oreo Madness, 1 serving | 500 | 21 | 76 |
| Vanilla Bean Cheesecake, 1 serving | 920 | 57 | 88 |
| **Signature Slushes:** *Per 22 oz Tumbler* | | | |
| Blue Raspberry | 310 | 0 | 75 |
| Mango Peach Lemonade | 150 | 0 | 41 |
| Red Bull Passion | 220 | 0 | 54 |
| Red Bull Ruby | 200 | 0 | 51 |

## Thundercloud Subs® (Aug '15)

*Subs: Small, w/ Standard Toppings*

| | C | F | Cb |
|---|---|---|---|
| **Classic:** BLT | 405 | 17 | 40 |
| Smoked Chicken | 295 | 4 | 40 |
| Turkey | 280 | 4 | 41 |
| **Low Fat:** Hot Pastrami | 430 | 13 | 41 |
| Roast Beef | 315 | 4 | 40 |
| **Signature Subs:** Club | 480 | 19 | 43 |
| California Club | 510 | 23 | 45 |
| NY Italian | 570 | 30 | 42 |
| Office Favorite | 850 | 40 | 81 |
| Texas Tuna | 700 | 45 | 44 |
| Veggie Delite, with Hummus | 360 | 10 | 53 |

## T.J. Cinnamons® (Aug '15)

| **Bakery:** | C | F | Cb |
|---|---|---|---|
| Cinnamon Roll, Original, 5.3 oz | 505 | 10 | 73 |
| Cinnamon Twist (1), 2.5 oz | 260 | 14 | 33 |
| Sticky Bun Smear w/ Pecans, 1.3 oz | 180 | 12 | 18 |
| T.J. Cream Cheese Icing, 1 oz | 115 | 5 | 18 |
| **Beverages:** | | | |
| **Mocha Chill,** w/o Whipped Cream, | | | |
| 12 fl.oz | 265 | 4 | 46 |

## Tim Hortons® (Aug '15)

| Breakfast: | C | F | Cb |
|---|---|---|---|
| **Bagel BELT,** Plain Bagel, with Ssg. Egg Omelette & Cheese | 630 | 29 | 65 |
| **Homestyle Biscuit:** | | | |
| Bacon Egg Omelette & Cheese | 420 | 23 | 33 |
| Sausage, Egg Omelette & Cheese | 530 | 34 | 33 |
| **English Muffins:** | | | |
| Bacon, Egg Omelette & Cheese | 340 | 16 | 30 |
| Turkey Ssg, Egg Omelette & Chse | 350 | 16 | 31 |
| **Wraps:** | | | |
| Bacon, Egg Omelette & Cheese | 290 | 17 | 19 |
| Egg Omelette & Cheese | 230 | 12 | 19 |
| Sausage, Egg Omelette & Cheese | 400 | 28 | 19 |
| **Sandwich,** Aged Cheddar Biscuit | 540 | 37 | 30 |
| *Hash Brown,* Regular | 130 | 7 | 16 |
| *Grilled Paninis:* With White Bread | | | |
| Buffalo Chicken | 520 | 16 | 62 |
| Grilled Cheese | 450 | 15 | 57 |
| Tuscan Chicken | 580 | 22 | 63 |
| *Sandwiches:* Per Regular With White Bun | | | |
| BLT | 370 | 13 | 46 |
| Crispy Chicken | 490 | 20 | 57 |
| Ham & Swiss | 400 | 12 | 48 |
| Turkey Bacon Club | 420 | 11 | 53 |
| *Wrap Snackers:* Per 3.5 oz Wrap | | | |
| Chicken Ranch | 190 | 7 | 17 |
| Chipotle Chicken | 200 | 9 | 17 |
| *Donuts:* | | | |
| **Cake:** Chocolate, glazed | 280 | 14 | 37 |
| Old Fashioned Plain | 210 | 10 | 25 |
| Sour Cream Glazed | 340 | 16 | 46 |
| **Filled:** Boston Cream | 220 | 6 | 35 |
| Canadian Maple | 210 | 6 | 35 |
| Strawberry Vanilla | 290 | 8 | 51 |
| **Honey Cruller** | 310 | 18 | 37 |
| **Yeast:** Apple Fritter | 290 | 8 | 48 |
| Chocolate/Maple Dip | 190 | 7 | 29 |
| Vanilla Dip with sprinkles | 270 | 9 | 45 |
| *Timbits:* | | | |
| **Cake:** Chocolate, glazed | 70 | 3 | 10 |
| Old Fashion, plain | 50 | 2.5 | 7 |
| Sour Cream, glazed | 90 | 4.5 | 12 |
| **Filled,** all varieties | 50 | 1 | 8 |
| **Yeast,** Apple Fritter; Honey Dip, av. | 50 | 1.5 | 9 |

## Tim Hortons® cont... (Aug '15)

| Cookies: | C | F | Cb |
|---|---|---|---|
| Chocolate Chunk | 210 | 9 | 32 |
| Oatmeal Raisin Spice | 210 | 8 | 32 |
| Peanut Butter | 250 | 15 | 24 |
| *Greek Yogurt with Berries,* Strawberry or Vanilla | 250 | 5 | 29 |
| *Beverages:* Per Medium Size | | | |
| Cafe Mocha | 240 | 9 | 38 |
| Hot Chocolate | 300 | 7 | 57 |
| **Iced Cappuccinos:** Per Small, 12 fl.oz | | | |
| Original: With milk | 180 | 1.5 | 39 |
| With cream | 310 | 16 | 40 |

## Togo's Eatery® (Aug '15)

| Sandwiches: | C | F | Cb |
|---|---|---|---|
| **Cold:** Per Regular White Bread With Standard Toppings, Without Dressing | | | |
| Albacore Tuna | 550 | 17 | 73 |
| Roast Beef | 580 | 9 | 66 |
| The Italian | 870 | 47 | 67 |
| Turkey & Avocado | 530 | 15 | 74 |
| Turkey, Bacon Club | 530 | 16 | 67 |
| Turkey, Ham & Cheese | 540 | 13 | 67 |
| Vegetarian: Avocado & Cheese | 630 | 29 | 73 |
| Hummus | 650 | 27 | 85 |
| **Hot:** Chicken | 500 | 8 | 67 |
| Meatball | 690 | 27 | 78 |
| Pastrami | 770 | 37 | 67 |
| Roast Beef | 580 | 9 | 66 |
| **Toasted Sandwiches:** Per Regular With Menu Board | | | |
| *Featured Bread* | | | |
| Clubhouse | 660 | 23 | 80 |
| Pepper Jack Pastrami | 1000 | 60 | 67 |
| Triple Dip | 1110 | 52 | 67 |
| *Salad Wraps:* Includes Spinach Wrap, Standard Toppings , With Dressing | | | |
| Asian Chicken | 590 | 24 | 70 |
| Chicken Caesar | Apr | 20 | 65 |
| Santa Fe Chicken | 660 | 31 | 70 |
| *Salads:* Per Full Salad, Without Dressing | | | |
| Chicken Caesar | 210 | 8 | 17 |
| Farmer's Market | 160 | 6 | 20 |
| Santa Fe Chicken | 410 | 21 | 35 |

## Tropical Smoothie Cafe® (Aug '15)

*Breakfast:*

| | C | F | Cb |
|---|---|---|---|
| **Omelet Wraps:** All American | 555 | 33 | 37 |
| Peanut Banana Crunch Flatbread | 775 | 39 | 85 |
| Southwest | 620 | 39 | 40 |
| Spinach & Feta | 495 | 30 | 40 |

*Toasted Sandwiches: Sandwich Only With Set Menu Components*

| | | | |
|---|---|---|---|
| Cranberry Pecan Chicken Salad, on Seedilicious Bread | 495 | 18 | 64 |
| Turkey Bacon Ranch on Ciabatta | 575 | 20 | 53 |
| Ultimate Club on Ciabatta | 645 | 28 | 52 |

*Toasted Wraps: Wrap Only, With Set Menu Components*

| | | | |
|---|---|---|---|
| Hummus Veggie | 675 | 32 | 79 |
| King Caesar | 625 | 32 | 53 |
| Totally Turkey | 615 | 26 | 54 |

*Fresh Salads: Includes Standard Dressing*

| | | | |
|---|---|---|---|
| Chicken Caesar | 495 | 40 | 11 |
| Loaded Spinach | 575 | 34 | 70 |
| Thai Chicken | 330 | 9 | 39 |

*Classic Smoothies: Per 24 oz with Turbinado*

| | | | |
|---|---|---|---|
| Blimey Limey | 370 | 0 | 99 |
| Blueberry Bliss | 310 | 1 | 78 |
| Jetty Punch | 340 | 0 | 86 |
| Peaches 'N Silk | 315 | 0 | 79 |
| Rockin' Raspberry | 400 | 0 | 100 |
| Sunny Day | 435 | 0 | 108 |
| Sunrise Sunset | 320 | 0 | 81 |

*Indulgent Smoothies: 24 oz with Turbinado*

| | | | |
|---|---|---|---|
| Bahama Mama | 475 | 4 | 107 |
| Beach Bum | 520 | 4 | 122 |
| Mocha Madness | 590 | 5 | 126 |
| Peanut Butter Cup | 695 | 20 | 121 |

*Supercharged: Per 24 oz With Turbinado*

| | | | |
|---|---|---|---|
| Health Nut, with Soy | 495 | 5 | 88 |
| Lean Machine | 440 | 0 | 112 |
| Muscle Blaster, with Whey | 440 | 2 | 88 |
| Peanut Paradise, with Whey | 675 | 18 | 101 |

*With Splenda, deduct 200 calories & 50g carbs*

## Tubby's® (Aug '15)

*Subs: Per 8" Regular Wheat Bun, without Dressing or Sauce*

**Deli-Subs:**

| | C | F | Cb |
|---|---|---|---|
| Ham & Cheese | 500 | 10 | 76 |
| Turkey Breast & Cheese | 530 | 12 | 76 |

**Grilled Burger Subs:** Big Tub

| | | | |
|---|---|---|---|
| Big Tub | 630 | 25 | 75 |
| Burger Special | 760 | 33 | 78 |
| Cheeseburger Italiano | 740 | 33 | 76 |
| Pizza Burger | 630 | 25 | 75 |

**Grilled Chicken Subs:**

| | | | |
|---|---|---|---|
| Chicken, Grilled | 440 | 4.5 | 73 |
| Chicken & Broccoli | 520 | 10 | 75 |
| Chicken & Cheddar | 510 | 10 | 73 |
| Chicken Fajita | 520 | 10 | 75 |

**Grilled Steak Subs:**

| | | | |
|---|---|---|---|
| Portabella Mushroom Steak | 600 | 17 | 80 |
| Pepper Steak & Cheese | 570 | 15 | 76 |
| Steak & Cheese | 560 | 15 | 74 |
| Steak Special | 590 | 16 | 76 |

**Specialty Subs:** BLT

| | | | |
|---|---|---|---|
| BLT | 580 | 23 | 73 |
| Cold Veggie | 470 | 9 | 79 |
| Italian Sausage | 630 | 26 | 77 |
| Pulled Pork | 610 | 25 | 68 |
| Tuna | 530 | 9 | 74 |

## Uno Chicago Grill® (Aug '15)

*Appetizers: Per Whole Dish*

| | C | F | Cb |
|---|---|---|---|
| Mozzarella Sticks, 11.4 oz | 850 | 47 | 80 |
| Pizza Skins, 25 .4 oz | 2070 | 140 | 147 |
| Shrimp & Crab Dip, 16.4 oz | 1120 | 81 | 64 |

*Burgers: Without Sides*

| | | | |
|---|---|---|---|
| BBQ, with Bacon & Cheddar | 1100 | 60 | 33 |
| Cheeseburger, Buffalo Cheddar | 970 | 51 | 29 |
| Uno | 860 | 42 | 28 |

*Entrees:*

**Chicken:** *Without Sides Or Breadstick*

| | | | |
|---|---|---|---|
| Baked Stuffed Spinoccoli, 11.8 oz | 360 | 14 | 10 |
| Chicken Milanese, 22.5 oz | 850 | 56 | 46 |
| Chicken Thumb Platter, 10.5 oz | 480 | 17 | 34 |

**Steak & Seafood:** *Without Sides Or Breadstick*

| | | | |
|---|---|---|---|
| Baked Haddock, 11.8 oz | 580 | 35 | 12 |
| Brewmasters Grill NY Sirloin | 510 | 14 | 21 |
| Grilled Shrimp & Sirloin, 11.3 oz | 440 | 21 | 4 |

*Sides:*

| | | | |
|---|---|---|---|
| Farro Salad, 7.5 oz | 180 | 7 | 31 |
| French Fries, 5.5 oz | 350 | 27 | 25 |
| Red Bliss Mashed Potatoes | 270 | 14 | 34 |
| Roasted Seasonal Veggies, 7.2 oz | 80 | 4.5 | 10 |

## Villa Fresh Italian® (Aug '15)

*Pizzas: Per Slice*

| | C | F | Cb |
|---|---|---|---|
| **Neapolitan:** | | | |
| Plain, 7 oz | 430 | 15 | 54 |
| Deluxe, 9 oz | 510 | 21 | 56 |
| Sausage & Pepperoni, 8.5 oz | 565 | 26 | 56 |
| **Stuffed:** Baked Ziti | 920 | 37 | 109 |
| Meat | 910 | 39 | 96 |
| Spinach and Mushroom | 735 | 33 | 80 |
| *Entrees:* | | | |
| Baked Ziti | 865 | 40 | 89 |
| Chicken Marsala | 745 | 20 | 107 |
| Chiken Parmigiana | 825 | 25 | 116 |
| Chicken Scampi | 840 | 33 | 103 |
| Fettuccini Alfredo | 930 | 52 | 88 |
| Mac & Cheese | 1160 | 77 | 83 |
| *Vegetables:* Roasted Potatoes | 210 | 12 | 23 |
| Sauteed, Fresh, 6oz | 85 | 6 | 6 |

## Vocelli Pizza® (Aug '15)

*Pizzas:*

| | C | F | Cb |
|---|---|---|---|
| **Artisan:** *Per ⅛ of Medium Pizza* | | | |
| Basil Pesto Primavera | 240 | 10 | 28 |
| Buffalo Chicken | 220 | 9 | 26 |
| Chicken Carbonara | 250 | 10 | 27 |
| Chicken Spinaci | 220 | 8 | 27 |
| Deluxe | 260 | 10 | 29 |
| Hawaiian | 280 | 11 | 30 |
| Meat Magnifico | 280 | 12 | 26 |
| Mexican | 300 | 15 | 28 |
| Philly Steak | 270 | 13 | 25 |
| Quattro Cheese | 270 | 11 | 28 |
| Spring Veggie | 210 | 7 | 28 |
| **Pasta:** Chicken Alfredo, 18 oz | 1080 | 55 | 100 |
| Chicken Parmesan, 20 oz | 1030 | 35 | 132 |
| Chicken Pesto, 18 oz | 1110 | 59 | 99 |
| *House Baked Subs:* On Ciabatta | | | |
| Buffalo Chicken, 7oz | 310 | 15 | 28 |
| Chicken Parmesan, 7.2 oz | 440 | 18 | 45 |
| Meatball, 7.2 oz | 460 | 23 | 36 |
| *Salads:* Per Regular Size, Without Dressing | | | |
| Antipasta, 16 oz | 270 | 16 | 17 |
| Caesar, 8 oz | 130 | 3 | 5 |
| Mediterranean, 16 oz | 270 | 18 | 17 |
| Tuscan Grilled Chicken, 14 oz | 290 | 13 | 12 |
| *Wings:* Bone In | | | |
| BBQ, hot, 9 oz | 760 | 53 | 14 |
| Buffalo, 9 oz | 720 | 54 | 2 |
| Garlic, 9 oz | 960 | 81 | 3 |
| Hot Vesuvius, 9 oz | 720 | 54 | 2 |

## Wahoo's Fish Taco® (Aug '15)

*Bowls: With White Rice & Black Beans*

| | C | F | Cb |
|---|---|---|---|
| #7 Blackened/Charbroiled Chkn, av. | 860 | 15 | 127 |
| # 8 Charbroiled/Teriyaki Fish, av. | 930 | 22 | 126 |
| #9 Veggie | 760 | 11 | 141 |
| #10 Carnitas/Kahlua Pig, average | 1025 | 25 | 131 |
| *Burritos:* With Brown Rice & White Beans | | | |
| **Banzai:** | | | |
| Blackened or Charbroiled: | | | |
| Chicken | 575 | 16 | 77 |
| Fish, average | 620 | 21 | 77 |
| Mushroom | 490 | 14 | 81 |
| Carne Asada | 565 | 17 | 79 |
| Carnitas | 685 | 23 | 79 |
| Shrimp | 475 | 14 | 77 |
| Vegetarian | 485 | 14 | 82 |
| *Side Kicks,* Corn Tortillas, each | 145 | 2 | 29 |
| *Salads: Chips Not Included* | | | |
| Blackened Chicken | 415 | 22 | 14 |
| Charbroiled Chicken | 415 | 21 | 14 |
| Charbroiled Fish | 485 | 29 | 14 |
| *Sandwiches: Blackened or Charbroiled* | | | |
| Chicken | 510 | 18 | 51 |
| Fish, average | 555 | 22 | 51 |
| Carne Asada | 500 | 19 | 52 |

**For Complete Nutritional Data ~ see CalorieKing.com**

## WAWA® (Aug '15)

*Breakfast:*

| | C | F | Cb |
|---|---|---|---|
| **Bagels:** Plain | 260 | 1 | 55 |
| With Reg. Butter | 310 | 7 | 55 |
| Cinnamon Raisin | 290 | 1 | 63 |
| With Regular Cream Cheese | 380 | 10 | 64 |
| Everything | 310 | 6 | 56 |
| *Bowls: Without Syrup* | | | |
| Creamed Chipped Beef On White | 230 | 6 | 36 |
| French Toasts: Plain | 340 | 13 | 54 |
| With Bacon | 420 | 19 | 55 |
| With Sausage Crumble | 540 | 32 | 55 |
| With Turkey Sausage Patty | 430 | 20 | 55 |
| Scrambled Egg: With Bacon | 470 | 34 | 10 |
| With Sausage Crumble | 590 | 47 | 10 |
| **Burritos:** *With Scrambled Egg* | | | |
| Bacon | 420 | 23 | 35 |
| Beef Steak & Cheddar Cheese | 450 | 23 | 37 |
| Chicken Steak with Cheddar Chse | 450 | 22 | 37 |
| **Sizzlis:** *Per Sizzli* | | | |
| Bagels: Bacon, Egg & Cheese | 410 | 18 | 43 |
| Pork Roll, Egg & Cheese | 420 | 19 | 42 |

**Continued Next Page...**

## WAWA® cont... (Aug '15)

| Breaded Chicken Strips: | C | F | Cb |
|---|---|---|---|
| 3 piece | 240 | 13 | 16 |
| 5 piece | 400 | 22 | 27 |

**Cold Hoagies:** *On Shorti Roll without Toppings*

| | | | |
|---|---|---|---|
| Egg Salad | 650 | 37 | 61 |
| Tuna Salad | 690 | 39 | 63 |
| Turkey | 370 | 5 | 59 |

**Hot Dogs:** *Without Toppings, Mustard or Sauce*

| | | | |
|---|---|---|---|
| All Beef: ¼ Pound | 420 | 28 | 21 |
| Big Bacon Cheese Dog | 810 | 47 | 57 |

**Hot Hoagies:** *On Shorti Roll without Toppings*

| | | | |
|---|---|---|---|
| Beef Steak & Cheddar Cheese | 550 | 19 | 59 |
| Chicken Steak & Cheddar Cheese | 550 | 17 | 59 |
| Meatballs & Cheddar Cheese | 730 | 34 | 75 |

**Soups:** *Per Medium Serving*

| | | | |
|---|---|---|---|
| Baked Potato w/ Cheddar & Bacon | 450 | 32 | 28 |
| Chicken Noodle | 150 | 3 | 23 |
| Lobster Bisque | 470 | 38 | 20 |
| Italian Wedding | 210 | 7 | 21 |
| New England Clam Chowder | 330 | 21 | 24 |

**Quesadillas:** *Without Toppings*

| | | | |
|---|---|---|---|
| Beef & Cheddar Cheese | 450 | 22 | 36 |
| Cheddar Cheese | 370 | 20 | 35 |
| Chicken & Cheddar Cheese | 450 | 20 | 36 |

**Sides:** *Per Medium Serving*

| | | | |
|---|---|---|---|
| Chili | 350 | 16 | 35 |
| Macaroni & Beef | 350 | 11 | 43 |
| Macaroni & Cheese | 500 | 25 | 49 |
| Mashed Potatoes | 470 | 28 | 50 |
| Meatballs in a Cup | 320 | 21 | 17 |
| New England Clam Chowder | 330 | 21 | 24 |
| Seafood Chowder | 210 | 9 | 20 |

**Bakery:**

| | | | |
|---|---|---|---|
| **Croissant,** Plain | 280 | 14 | 35 |
| **Muffins:** Banana Walnut | 670 | 34 | 83 |
| Blueberry | 610 | 30 | 78 |
| Chocolate Chip | 680 | 34 | 86 |
| Corn | 640 | 29 | 87 |

**Hot Beverages:** *Per 16 oz, without Extras*

| | | | |
|---|---|---|---|
| **Hot Cappuccino,** with 2% milk | 130 | 5 | 13 |
| **Mocha Latte,** with 2% milk | 330 | 7 | 59 |

**Smoothie,** Strawberry Banana,

| | | | |
|---|---|---|---|
| without whipped cream, 24 oz | 690 | 0 | 180 |

## Wendy's® (Aug '15)

| Cheeseburgers: | C | F | Cb |
|---|---|---|---|
| *With Standard Toppings* | | | |
| Dave's ¼ lb Single | 580 | 31 | 42 |
| Dave's ½ lb Double | 820 | 47 | 42 |
| Dave's ¾ lb Triple | 1090 | 66 | 43 |
| Baconator | 940 | 57 | 41 |
| Son of Baconator | 630 | 36 | 41 |
| Double Stack | 430 | 23 | 27 |
| Jr. Bacon Cheeseburger | 370 | 21 | 26 |
| Jr. Cheeseburger | 280 | 12 | 26 |
| Jr. Cheeseburger Deluxe | 340 | 18 | 28 |

**Sandwiches:** *With Standard Toppings*

| | | | |
|---|---|---|---|
| Asiago Ranch Club, with Homestyle Chicken | 670 | 32 | 57 |
| Crispy Chicken | 350 | 19 | 34 |
| Homestyle Chicken | 510 | 20 | 54 |
| Spicy Chicken | 510 | 20 | 55 |
| Ultimate Chicken Grill | 370 | 7 | 42 |
| **Go Wraps:** Grilled Chicken | 260 | 10 | 25 |
| Spicy Chicken | 340 | 16 | 30 |

**Chicken Nuggets:**

| | | | |
|---|---|---|---|
| Regular: 6 pieces | 270 | 18 | 14 |
| 10 pieces | 450 | 30 | 24 |
| Spicy: 6 pieces | 260 | 17 | 14 |
| 10 piece | 430 | 28 | 23 |

**Dipping Sauce:** *Per 1 oz*

| | | | |
|---|---|---|---|
| Barbecue | 45 | 0 | 11 |
| Buttermilk Ranch | 120 | 12 | 2 |
| Honey Mustard | 80 | 6 | 7 |
| Sweet & Sour | 45 | 0 | 12 |

**Garden Sensations Salads:** *Full Size With Dressing*

| | | | |
|---|---|---|---|
| Apple Pecan Grilled Chicken | 590 | 26 | 54 |
| Asian Cashew Grilled Chicken | 380 | 13 | 33 |
| BBQ Ranch Grilled Chicken | 580 | 29 | 43 |
| Spicy Grilled Chicken Caesar | 780 | 51 | 41 |

**Sides:**

| | | | |
|---|---|---|---|
| **Baconator Fries** | 490 | 28 | 45 |
| **Baked Potatoes:** | | | |
| Bacon & Cheddar | 520 | 20 | 67 |
| Sour Cream & Chives | 320 | 3.5 | 63 |
| **Ghost Pepper Fries,** 10 oz | 500 | 33 | 44 |
| **Natural Cut Fries:** Value | 220 | 11 | 28 |
| Small, 4 oz | 310 | 15 | 40 |
| Medium, 5 oz | 410 | 20 | 52 |
| Large, 6.5 oz | 500 | 24 | 65 |
| **Rich Meaty Chili:** Small | 170 | 5 | 16 |
| Large | 250 | 7 | 23 |

**Frosty:** *Per Small*

| | | | |
|---|---|---|---|
| Chocolate | 340 | 9 | 56 |
| Vanilla | 330 | 8 | 55 |

## Whataburger® (Aug '15)

### Burgers & Sandwiches:

| | C | F | Cb |
|---|---|---|---|
| A.1. Thick & Hearty Burger | 1040 | 61 | 67 |
| Chop House Cheddar Burger | 1130 | 73 | 63 |
| Green Chili Double | 1000 | 60 | 71 |
| Honey BBQ Chicken Strip S'wich | 1040 | 54 | 89 |
| Sweet & Spicy Bacon Burger | 1070 | 61 | 69 |

### Whataburger:

| | C | F | Cb |
|---|---|---|---|
| Original | 640 | 30 | 63 |
| Double Meat | 880 | 49 | 63 |
| Jalapeno & Cheese | 730 | 37 | 65 |
| Jr. | 340 | 14 | 38 |
| Triple Meat | 1120 | 68 | 63 |

### Chicken:

| | C | F | Cb |
|---|---|---|---|
| **Grilled:** Chicken Sandwich | 490 | 19 | 52 |
| Chicken Melt | 460 | 20 | 39 |

### Whatachick'n:

| | C | F | Cb |
|---|---|---|---|
| Bites: 6 pieces, without sauce | 410 | 18 | 30 |
| 9 pieces, without sauce | 590 | 25 | 42 |
| Sandwiches: Honey Mustard Club | 760 | 31 | 84 |
| Regular | 580 | 24 | 69 |
| Strips, 3 pieces, without sauce | 590 | 33 | 39 |

### French Fries: Small, 3 oz

| | C | F | Cb |
|---|---|---|---|
| Small, 3 oz | 270 | 15 | 36 |
| Medium, 4.5 oz | 410 | 23 | 54 |
| Large, 6 oz | 540 | 30 | 72 |

### Onion Rings:

| | C | F | Cb |
|---|---|---|---|
| Medium, 4.3 oz | 400 | 25 | 37 |
| Large, 6.5 oz | 590 | 38 | 56 |

### Salad: Without Dressing

| | C | F | Cb |
|---|---|---|---|
| **Garden:** With Grilled Chicken | 350 | 17 | 18 |
| With Whatachick'n | 490 | 24 | 40 |
| Without Chicken | 180 | 9 | 16 |

### Breakfast:

| | C | F | Cb |
|---|---|---|---|
| Cinnamon Roll | 390 | 9 | 71 |
| **Biscuits:** Plain | 300 | 17 | 33 |
| With Gravy | 470 | 29 | 45 |
| Honey Butter Chicken | 590 | 36 | 51 |

### Biscuit Sandwiches:

| | C | F | Cb |
|---|---|---|---|
| With Bacon | 490 | 31 | 33 |
| With Sausage | 640 | 45 | 33 |
| **On A Bun:** With Bacon | 390 | 19 | 34 |
| With Sausage | 540 | 33 | 34 |

### Platters:

| | C | F | Cb |
|---|---|---|---|
| With Bacon | 630 | 41 | 37 |
| With Sausage | 780 | 55 | 37 |

### Taquitos:

| | C | F | Cb |
|---|---|---|---|
| With Bacon, Egg & Cheese | 410 | 25 | 28 |
| With Cheese | 360 | 21 | 28 |
| With Potato, Egg & Cheese | 460 | 27 | 40 |

## Whataburger® cont... (Aug '15)

### Desserts:

| | C | F | Cb |
|---|---|---|---|
| Chocolate Chunk Cookie | 230 | 11 | 31 |
| Hot Apple Pie, 3 oz | 270 | 14 | 34 |

### Beverages:

| | C | F | Cb |
|---|---|---|---|
| **Malts:** Chocolate, 20 oz | 600 | 15 | 110 |
| Vanilla, 20 oz | 570 | 16 | 95 |
| **Shake,** Chocolate, 20 oz | 570 | 16 | 98 |

## White Castle® (Aug '15)

*Note:* Nutritional Information varies from state to state. Please check instore

### Sliders:

| | C | F | Cb |
|---|---|---|---|
| Original | 140 | 6 | 13 |
| Bacon, Chedd. Gr. Chkn | 240 | 12 | 15 |
| Cheese | 160 | 9 | 14 |
| Chicken Breast with Cheese | 390 | 28 | 20 |
| Fish, with Cheese | 340 | 24 | 18 |
| Savory Grilled Chicken | 180 | 7 | 13 |
| Wstn BBQ Grilled Chkn | 320 | 16 | 28 |

### Sides:

| | C | F | Cb |
|---|---|---|---|
| **Chicken Rings,** average: | | | |
| 6 rings, 5 oz | 530 | 47 | 12 |
| 9 rings , 7.5 oz | 790 | 71 | 18 |
| French Fries: | | | |
| Small, 5.6 oz | 330 | 21 | 32 |
| Medium | 600 | 39 | 57 |
| Sack | 770 | 49 | 76 |
| Cheese Fries, small | 400 | 27 | 35 |
| Fully Loaded Fries, small | 460 | 38 | 20 |
| Mozzarella Cheese Sticks, 3 sticks | 440 | 33 | 22 |

### Condiments: Per Packet

| | C | F | Cb |
|---|---|---|---|
| Ketchup | 10 | 0 | 2 |
| Mayonnaise | 60 | 7 | 0 |

### Sauces: Per Packet

| | C | F | Cb |
|---|---|---|---|
| BBQ | 10 | 0 | 3 |
| Tartar Sauce | 25 | 1.5 | 1 |

### Breakfast:

| | C | F | Cb |
|---|---|---|---|
| French Toast Sticks, 4 pieces | 460 | 31 | 39 |
| Maple Brown Sugar Oatmeal | 160 | 2 | 32 |
| **Sliders:** Bacon, Egg & Cheese | 210 | 12 | 13 |
| Egg & Cheese | 160 | 7 | 13 |
| Sausage, Egg & Cheese | 310 | 22 | 13 |
| **Toasted Sandwiches:** Egg & Chse | 230 | 9 | 29 |
| Bacon, Egg & Cheese | 340 | 19 | 29 |
| Sausage, Egg & Cheese | 310 | 22 | 13 |

### Sides:

| | C | F | Cb |
|---|---|---|---|
| Hash Brown Nibblers: | | | |
| Small | 360 | 28 | 25 |
| Medium | 600 | 46 | 42 |
| Sack | 1440 | 10 | 101 |

### Dessert:

| | C | F | Cb |
|---|---|---|---|
| **On A Stick:** Fudge Dipped Brownie | 250 | 12 | 33 |
| Fudge Dipped Cheesecake | 180 | 10 | 21 |

Updated Nutrition Data ~ www.CalorieKing.com
Persons with Diabetes ~ See Disclaimer (Page 22)

## Wienerschnitzel® (Aug '15)

*Hot Dogs:*

| | C | F | Cb |
|---|---|---|---|
| **Original:** *On Standard Bun* | | | |
| Chili | 270 | 12 | 32 |
| Chili Cheese | 320 | 16 | 32 |
| Deluxe; Kraut, Plain, average | 245 | 10 | 31 |
| Pastrami | 350 | 18 | 30 |
| **Original:** *On Pretzel Bun* | | | |
| Chili | 400 | 14 | 55 |
| Kraut; Mustard; Plain | 370 | 13 | 53 |
| Relish | 380 | 13 | 55 |
| **Angus All Beef:** *On Pretzel Bun* | | | |
| Chicago | 560 | 26 | 61 |
| Chili Cheese | 590 | 32 | 55 |
| Mustard | 510 | 26 | 52 |
| Relish | 520 | 26 | 55 |
| Junkyard Dog, on Seeded Bun | 600 | 36 | 49 |
| *Specialties:* | | | |
| **Corn Dogs:** Regular | 230 | 13 | 31 |
| Mini (6 pack) | 290 | 16 | 28 |
| **Jalapeno Poppers,** (6 pack) | 300 | 16 | 31 |
| *Sides:* | | | |
| Chili Cheese Fries | 570 | 32 | 59 |
| Fries: Medium | 440 | 23 | 54 |
| Large | 750 | 39 | 92 |
| *Breakfast:* | | | |
| **Biscuits:** Egg, Bacon, Cheese | 450 | 25 | 36 |
| Egg, Sausage, Cheese | 540 | 34 | 40 |
| **Burritos:** Egg, Bacon, Cheese | 370 | 19 | 29 |
| Egg, Sausage, Cheese | 460 | 28 | 33 |
| French Toast Sticks | 530 | 28 | 61 |
| Syrup, 1 oz | 120 | 0 | 31 |
| *Desserts:* | | | |
| **Banana Split** | 820 | 24 | 148 |
| **Cones,** regular | | | |
| Plain, 5 oz | 250 | 9 | 41 |
| Chocolate Dipped, 5 oz | 450 | 27 | 50 |
| **Freezees:** | | | |
| Chocolate Caramel Crunch | 880 | 39 | 133 |
| Chocolate Covered Strawberry | 980 | 56 | 120 |
| Oreo; M&M | 630 | 25 | 99 |
| Reese's Pnut Butter Cup | 630 | 26 | 97 |
| **Shakes,** average all flavors | 650 | 23 | 110 |
| **Sundaes:** | | | |
| Caramel; Hot Fudge, average | 400 | 15 | 64 |
| Chocolate | 390 | 14 | 64 |
| Strawberry | 370 | 14 | 59 |

## Winchell's® (Aug '15)

*Donuts:* Per Donut

| | C | F | Cb |
|---|---|---|---|
| Buttermillk Bars, Choc Iced/Glazed | 420 | 19 | 61 |
| Jelly Filled: | | | |
| Apple with Cinnamon Crumb | 370 | 15 | 53 |
| Raspberry with Glaze | 390 | 13 | 61 |
| Strawberry with Sugar | 380 | 13 | 60 |
| Old Fashioned, Glazed; Maple Iced | 410 | 17 | 60 |
| Raised Ring: Chocolate Iced | 270 | 10 | 41 |
| Sugared | 230 | 9 | 34 |

## WingStreet (Aug '15)

*Chicken:*

| | C | F | Cb |
|---|---|---|---|
| **Breaded Bone In Wings:** *Per 2 Pieces* | | | |
| Buffalo, Mild/Med./Hot, 2.6 oz | 220 | 12 | 19 |
| Garlic Parmesan, 2.5 oz | 290 | 23 | 12 |
| Honey BBQ, 3 oz | 250 | 12 | 28 |
| Honey Sriracha, 2.5 oz | 200 | 10 | 20 |
| Spicy BBQ, 3 oz | 230 | 12 | 24 |
| **Bone Out Wings:** *Per 2 Pieces* | | | |
| Buffalo, Mild/Medium, 2.5 oz | 200 | 9 | 18 |
| Garlic Parmesan, 2.5 oz | 260 | 20 | 11 |
| Honey BBQ, 3 oz | 230 | 9 | 27 |
| Naked | 160 | 9 | 11 |
| **Traditional Wings:** *Per 2 Pieces* | | | |
| Buffalo, Medium/Hot, 2 oz | 130 | 7 | 8 |
| Garlic Parmesan, 2 oz | 200 | 17 | 1 |
| Spicy BBQ, 2.3 oz | 140 | 6 | 12 |
| Sweet Chili, 2.3 oz | 150 | 6 | 13 |

## Woody's Bar-B-Q® (Aug '15)

*Starters:*

| | C | F | Cb |
|---|---|---|---|
| Breaded Wings (10) | 700 | 47 | 13 |
| Beef Chili Cheese Fries | 805 | 38 | 63 |
| *Dinner Entrees:* *Without Sides* | | | |
| ½ Chicken | 840 | 56 | 0 |
| Baby Back Ribs | 520 | 40 | 2 |
| Pork Sampler | 1010 | 62 | 4 |
| *Sandwiches:* *Per Regular, Without Sides* | | | |
| Beef | 390 | 14 | 28 |
| Pork | 490 | 26 | 29 |
| *Wraps:* *Without Sides* | | | |
| Beef BBQ | 380 | 13 | 31 |
| Pork | 440 | 21 | 31 |
| *Extras:* BBQ Beans | 170 | 8 | 20 |
| Cobettes | 80 | 1 | 18 |
| French Fries | 185 | 7 | 28 |
| Garlic Toast | 120 | 6 | 14 |
| Green Beans | 50 | 2.5 | 6 |
| Okra | 95 | 1 | 21 |
| Squash | 140 | 1 | 28 |

*For Complete Nutritional Data ~ see CalorieKing.com*

## Yoshinoya® (Aug '15)

*Appetizers: As Served*

| | C | F | Cb |
|---|---|---|---|
| **Asian BBQ Wings:** 4 pieces | 410 | 25 | 21 |
| 6 peces | 620 | 37 | 32 |

*Entrees: As Served*

| | C | F | Cb |
|---|---|---|---|
| **Angus Steak Bowl:** Regular | 570 | 11 | 97 |
| Large | 850 | 17 | 144 |
| **Beef Bowl:** *With Sauce* | | | |
| Regular | 730 | 27 | 91 |
| Large | 1040 | 38 | 131 |
| With Vegetables: Regular | 650 | 20 | 95 |
| Large | 960 | 29 | 141 |
| **Beef & Teriyaki Chicken Combo:** | | | |
| Large, with skin | 1190 | 36 | 151 |
| Large, without skin | 1150 | 33 | 151 |
| **Teriyaki Chicken Bowl:** | | | |
| Regular, with skin | 790 | 18 | 110 |
| Large, with skin | 1140 | 25 | 165 |
| **Grilled Tilapia:** With Rice & Slaw | 570 | 13 | 91 |
| With Rice & Veggies | 540 | 12 | 88 |
| With Rice, Slaw & Teriyaki Sauce | 620 | 13 | 103 |
| With Rice, Veggies & Teriyaki Sce | 590 | 12 | 100 |
| **Sides,** Clam chowder Soup | 210 | 7 | 34 |
| *Kid's Meals:* Beef | 350 | 11 | 48 |
| Teriyaki Chicken with skin | 360 | 7 | 53 |
| Teriyaki Chicken with skin | 340 | 6 | 53 |

*Please note: Relates only to Northern California Menu*

## Z Pizza® (Aug '15)

*Pizzas: Small, Per Slice*

| | C | F | Cb |
|---|---|---|---|
| **Creations:** Berkeley Vegan | 150 | 5 | 21 |
| California | 140 | 4.5 | 18 |
| Casablanca | 180 | 8 | 17 |
| Greek | 140 | 5 | 17 |
| Italian; Mexican, average | 165 | 7 | 17 |
| Provence; Santa Fe | 150 | 6 | 17 |
| Thai; ZBQ, average | 165 | 5 | 19 |
| **Rusticas:** *Per Slice* | | | |
| Chicken Sausage | 100 | 3.5 | 12 |
| Curry Chicken & Yam | 130 | 3.5 | 16 |
| Mediterranean; Moroccan, av. | 140 | 8 | 13 |
| Pear & Gorgonzola | 130 | 6 | 14 |
| *Calzones:* Meat Calzone | 790 | 36 | 82 |
| Veggie Calzone | 630 | 22 | 86 |
| *Salads:* Small | | | |
| Arugula, with Balsamic Vinaigrette | 450 | 36 | 24 |
| Caesar Side, with Caesar Dressing | 200 | 16 | 8 |
| California, with Chipotle Ranch | 180 | 13 | 16 |

## Zaxby's® (Aug '15)

*Zappetizers: With Sauce*

| | C | F | Cb |
|---|---|---|---|
| Fried White Cheddar Bites w/ sce | 820 | 51 | 62 |
| Onion Rings, 5 oz | 780 | 58 | 59 |
| Spicy Fried Mushroom, 5.7 oz | 620 | 48 | 43 |
| Tater Chips, 5.2 oz | 940 | 69 | 72 |
| *Meal Dealz:* Without Drink | | | |
| Big Zax Snak, with Sauce | 950 | 53 | 82 |
| Buffalo Wings, without sauce | 900 | 57 | 51 |
| Chicken Finger Nibbler, w/ sauce | 1330 | 72 | 137 |
| *Most Popular:* As Served | | | |
| Chicken Finger Plate: Regular | 1260 | 72 | 99 |
| Large | 1990 | 114 | 158 |
| Wings & Things, regular | 1490 | 94 | 85 |
| *Sandwich Baskets: Includes Fries* | | | |
| Cajun Club | 1020 | 50 | 90 |
| Club | 1250 | 74 | 99 |
| *Wings & Fingerz: With Sauce* | | | |
| Buffalo Fingerz: | | | |
| 5 pieces | 630 | 43 | 15 |
| 10 pieces | 1270 | 87 | 30 |
| Buffalo Wings: | | | |
| 5 pieces | 540 | 41 | 3 |
| 10 pieces | 880 | 61 | 4 |
| Chicken Fingerz: | | | |
| 5 pieces | 610 | 39 | 19 |
| 10 pieces | 1230 | 79 | 36 |
| *Zax Kidz: Without Drink* | | | |
| Kiddie Cheese | 800 | 51 | 69 |
| Kiddie Finger | 570 | 36 | 40 |
| Kiddie Nibbler | 550 | 29 | 59 |
| *Zalads: With Texas Toast, Without Dressing* | | | |
| **Blue,** with Blackened Chicken | 580 | 28 | 36 |
| **Caesar:** | | | |
| With Fried Chicken | 730 | 39 | 39 |
| With Grilled Chicken | 540 | 25 | 31 |
| **House Zalad:** With Fried Chicken | 760 | 42 | 44 |
| With Grilled Chicken | 570 | 28 | 36 |
| *Salad Dressings:* | | | |
| Blue Cheese, 1 packet, 1.3 oz | 180 | 19 | 2 |
| Honey French, 1.3 oz | 150 | 12 | 9 |
| Honey Mustard, 1.3 oz | 150 | 13 | 6 |
| Lite Ranch, 1.3 oz | 90 | 8 | 3 |
| Mediterranean, 1.3 oz | 140 | 14 | 4 |
| Ranch, 1.3 oz | 160 | 16 | 2 |
| Thousand Island | 230 | 24 | 3 |
| *Sides:* Celery Basket, | | | |
| with 2 cups Ranch Sauce | 420 | 42 | 10 |
| Cole Slaw, 2.2 oz | 140 | 11 | 12 |
| Crinkle Fries, regular, 5 oz | 360 | 16 | 48 |
| Texas Toast, basket, 3 wedges, 4.3 oz | 440 | 20 | 60 |

## Zero Sub's® ~ *see CalorieKing.com*

## Notes on Cholesterol

- **Cholesterol** is a white waxy substance produced mainly by our liver. It is also found in animal food products. Plant foods have no cholesterol.

- **Cholesterol is essential to life.** It is a structural part of every body cell wall and is the building block for vitamin D, sex hormones, and bile acids which help in the digestion of dietary fats.

- **The body makes sufficient cholesterol** for its needs and does not rely on cholesterol in the diet. Dietary fats have a major influence on blood cholesterol levels - more so than dietary cholesterol.

- **A high blood cholesterol level increases** the risk of atherosclerosis - the thickening of arteries that can reduce or block blood flow to the heart, brain, eyes, kidneys, sex organs and other body parts.

  **This in turn increases the risk of heart attack,** stroke, blindness, kidney failure, impotence and other blood circulatory problems.

  **Other risk factors which increase the risk of atherosclerosis include high blood pressure, smoking, obesity and uncontrolled diabetes.**

### *BLOOD CHOLESTEROL*

### *CHECK YOUR RISK!*

| Total Cholesterol Level (mg/dl) ▼ | | Risk of Heart Attack ▼ |
|---|---|---|
| 240 and above | ~ | **High Risk** |
| 200 - 239 | ~ | **Borderline/High** |
| Below 200 | ~ | **Desirable** |

- 💜 **Know your cholesterol level, particularly if there is a family history of heart disease or stroke. If level is high, see your doctor.**

- 💜 **All adults should have their cholesterol, HDL and triglycerides tested at least every 5 years.**

### *HEART ATTACK WARNING SIGNALS*

Many victims die before reaching the hospital by ignoring warning signals and delaying medical help.
**Symptoms vary and commonly include:**

- **Chest pain,** vice-like squeezing or burning sensation in center of the chest or between the shoulder blades, or in the mid-back. Pain may even feel like severe indigestion.
- **Pain** may be felt in the arms, shoulders, neck or jaw.
- **Shortness of breath** often occurs with or before chest discomfort.
- **Other signs,** with or without pain, include a cold sweat, nausea or light-headedness.

*If you experience any of the above symptoms call IMMEDIATELY for medical help. Every minute counts.*

***Call 9-1-1*** *or your emergency number*

▲ **Atherosclerosis can clog arteries and impede blood flow to the heart or other body organs.**

▼ **A thrombus (blood clot) can form on unstable, festering athero-sclerotic plaque and rapidly block blood flow. A heart attack or stroke can result.**

# Fats & Cholesterol Guide

The amount and type of dietary fat has the greatest influence on blood cholesterol levels.

**Fats in food are a mixture of 3 basic types:** saturated, monounsaturated, and polyunsaturated. Animal fats are mainly saturated while plant oils and fish oils are mainly mono- and polyunsaturated.

**Saturated fats** have subgroups known as long-chain, medium-chain, and short-chain fats. Most of the long chain fats raise blood cholesterol, and increase the risk of blood clots and thrombosis leading to artery blockage.

Long-chain saturated fats are found mainly in full-cream milk, cheese, butter, cream, fatty meats and sausages, and processed foods.

**Monounsaturated fats** tend to more selectively lower 'bad' LDL cholesterol and maintain the protective 'good' HDL cholesterol in the bloodstream – but only if they replace saturated fats in the diet.

Foods rich in monounsaturates include canola and olive oils, canola margarine, peanuts, and avocados.

**Polyunsaturated fats** consist of two main classes. **Omega-6** polyunsaturates tend to lower blood cholesterol. Rich sources include safflower, sunflower and corn oils.

**Omega-3** polyunsaturated fats can lower blood cholesterol; significantly lower blood triglycerides; and reduce the rise of thrombosis, heart arrythmmia, and artery spasm.

**Best practical omega-3 sources** include canola oil and margarine, soybean oil and fish.

**A balanced intake** of the two omega classes is important for optimal health. For most Americans, slightly increasing omega-3 intake would help attain a more ideal balance.

**Trans fats** from hydrogenated vegetable oils and shortenings should also be avoided. They are common in commercial baked and fried food products such as cakes, muffins, pastries, doughnuts, fried snacks and french fries.

Note: All fats are high in calories and need to be limited for weight control.

## DIETARY FATS COMPARISON

■ Saturated Fat ■ Monounsaturated Fat
Polyunsaturated Fats:
□ Linoleic (Omega-6) ■ Alpha-Linolenic (Omega-3)

| OILS | PERCENTAGE CONTENT |
|---|---|
| CANOLA OIL | 7 / 63 / 20 / 10 |
| LINSEED/FLAX OIL | 9 / 19 / 17 / 55 |
| SAFFLOWER OIL | 9 / 14 / 77 |
| GRAPESEED OIL | 10 / 22 / 68 |
| SUNFLOWER OIL | 11 / 23 / 66 |
| CORN OIL | 14 / 32 / 52 / 2 |
| OLIVE OIL | 14 / 76 / 10 |
| SOYBEAN OIL | 15 / 23 / 54 / 8 |
| PEANUT OIL | 19 / 45 / 34 / 2 |
| COTTONSEED OIL | 26 / 16 / 58 |
| PALM OIL | 51 / 39 / 10 |

### SPREADS & FATS
Saturated Fat includes 'Trans Fats'  □ WATER CONTENT

| | |
|---|---|
| LIGHT MARGARINE | 14 / 14 / 21 / 51 |
| CANOLA MARGARINE | 18 / 45 / 12 / 6 / 19 |
| POLYUNSATURATED MARG | 24 / 20 / 36 / 20 |
| BUTTER | 57 / 18 / 2 / 24 |
| LARD | 41 / 47 / 12 |
| BEEF FAT | 44 / 37 / 4 / 15 |

## GOOD SOURCES OF OMEGA-3 FATS

| Plant Sources | Omega-3 Fats (Grams) |
|---|---|
| Canola Oil, 1 Tbsp, ½ fl.oz | 1.5g |
| Flaxseed Oil, 1 Tbsp | 8g |
| Soybean Oil, 1 Tbsp | 1.2g |
| Canola Margarine, 1 Tbsp, ½ oz | 1g |
| Soybeans, cooked, ½ cup, 4 oz | 0.5g |
| Walnuts, ½ oz | 0.5g |

**FISH** - Per 4 oz Serving
**High Content:** Salmon (Chinook), Tuna, Trout (Lake), Sardines, Herring, Mackerel — 3g, 3g
**Medium Content:** Salmon, (Pink/Red/Coho), 4 oz — 2g
**Fair Content:** Per 4 oz Serving
Bass, Catfish, Cod, Grouper, Hake, Halibut, Kingfish, Perch, Pollock, Shark, Trout (Rainbow), Tuna, Crab, Oysters, Blue Mussels, Shrimp, Squid } 0.5-1g

### How Much Is Needed?
**As little as 1-2 grams daily of omega-3 fats** may benefit general health. High doses of fish-oil supplements should only be taken as directed by your doctor.

## Dietary Cholesterol

Cholesterol in food varies in its effect on blood cholesterol level (BCL) from person to person. Much depends on the amount and type of fat and fiber eaten at the same meal.

Any elevating effect of dietary cholesterol on BCL is more likely to occur when the diet is high in saturated fat. Little elevation, if any, generally occurs when dietary fats are balanced in favor of monounsaturated and polyunsaturated fats (including omega-3 fats).

For example, while fish does contain cholesterol, the omega-3 fats can prevent any increase in BCL. Conversely, a meal containing no cholesterol but rich in saturated fat may result in a significant increase in BCL.

**Consequently, the need to be overly concerned about dietary cholesterol is being de-emphasized in favor of the approach of limiting total fat, saturated fat, and trans fat in particular – and substituting unsaturated fats.**

The liver usually cuts back its own cholesterol production in response to cholesterol in the diet. Many people can consume normal amounts of high-cholesterol foods without concern.

However, it is difficult to identify just who is at risk - the so-called 'hyper-responders'. Because over 50% of Americans have a BCL above ideal levels, the **American Heart Association** advises all Americans to be prudent and limit their cholesterol intake to less than 300mg daily, as well as to adopt a heart-healthy diet.

This limitation still allows the inclusion of most foods that are regularly eaten – even the overly maligned egg.

**Eggs contain a modest 5 grams of fat per large egg. Barely 2 grams is saturated, the rest being monounsaturated or polyunsaturated.**

**By comparison, a cup of whole milk has 8g fat of which almost 5g is saturated.**

---

### CHOLESTEROL COUNTER

**Cholesterol is found only in foods of animal origin. Plant foods contain no cholesterol.**

| | Cholesterol mg |
|---|---|
| **Meat** - Average all types: | |
| Lean Meat, cooked, 120g | 100 |
| Fatty Meat, cooked, 120g | 100 |
| Fat, thick strip, 60g | 40 |

*Note: While lean meat and fat have similar amounts of cholesterol, choose lean meat to limit fat intake.*

| | |
|---|---|
| **Chicken/Turkey,** average, 120g | 100 |
| **Organ Meats:** Liver, fried, 4 oz | 500 |
| Brains, beef, pan fried, 3 oz | 1700 |
| **Sausages:** Frankfurter, 40g | 25 |
| Salami, 2 slices, 55g | 40 |
| **Bacon:** 3 slices, cooked, 30g | 20 |
| **Fish:** Fish fillets, average, ckd, 120g | 70 |
| Tuna/Salmon, canned, 100g | 50 |
| Scallops, 9 medium, 3 oz | 30 |
| Prawns, raw, 100g | 110 |
| Oysters, raw, 6 medium, 85g | 45 |
| Crayfish, Crab, cooked, 100g | 70 |
| **Eggs** (Chicken), 1 large | 210 |
| 1 medium | 180 |
| Egg White, *Scramblers* | 0 |
| **Milk/Yoghurt:** Whole, 1 cup, 250ml | 30 |
| Light/low-fat Milk (1%), 1 cup | 10 |
| Skim/Non-fat, 1 cup | 10 |
| **Soy Milk, Tofu, Tempeh** | 0 |
| **Cheese:** Natural/Hard/Cream, 30g | 30 |
| Cottage, low-fat, 2 Tbsp, 40g | 5 |
| Cream Cheese, 30g | 25 |
| **Fats:** Butter, 1 Tbsp, 20g | 45 |
| Margarine, Oils (vegetable) | 0 |
| Mayonnaise, 1 Tbsp | 10 |
| **Cream:** Heavy, whipping, 2 Tbsp, 40g | 40 |
| Light/Sour, 2 Tbsp | 10 |
| **Ice Cream:** Full-fat (10-11%), 100ml/50g | 20 |
| Low-fat (less than 4%), 50g | 5 |
| **Fruit, Vegetables,** Avocados | 0 |
| **Nuts, Seeds, Grains** | 0 |
| **Coffee, Tea, Beer, Wine** | 0 |

*For Comprehensive Food Listings ~ see CalorieKing.com*

# Blood Cholesterol ~ Diet Hints

## DIETARY HINTS TO LOWER BLOOD CHOLESTEROL

1. **Maintain a healthy weight.**
   If overweight, lose weight with a sensible, low-fat meal plan and daily exercise.

2. **Reduce saturated fat intake by:**
   **(a) eating less dairy fat.** Choose low-fat or fat-reduced varieties of milk, yogurt, soy drinks, cheese, and ice cream.

   **(b) replacing saturated fats** with fats and oils rich in monounsaturated and polyunsaturated fats. Choose vegetable oils such as canola, olive, sunflower and soybean. Avoid solid frying fats.

   Note: *Promise Active* and *Benecol* spreads contain plant stanol esters which can lower total and LDL cholesterol.

   **(c) eating less fat from meat and poultry**. Choose lean cuts of meat and skinless chicken. Go easy on lunch meats, salami and fatty sausages. Enjoy fish.

   **(d) eating less saturated and trans fats** from baked and fried fast-foods. Avoid deep-fried foods. Avoid donuts, cakes, pastries and cookies unless made with healthier fats and oils.

3. **Increase your soluble fiber intake.**
   Foods rich in soluble fiber include beans, lentils, chick peas, hummus, nuts, seeds, psyllium-seed husks and psyllium-fiber supplements. Oat bran, rice bran and barley are also good sources, as are fruit, vegetables and avocados.
   (*See Fiber Guide - Page 264-269*).

4. **Eat more soy bean products** such as: soy drinks, tofu, tempeh (cultured soy beans), soy flour, soy vegetarian foods and edamame (fresh green soybeans).

   Soy protein in place of animal protein can significantly decrease high blood cholesterol levels as well as 'bad' LDL cholesterol and blood triglycerides while 'good' HDL cholesterol is maintained. For best results, eat at least 25g of soy protein per day (from 3-4 servings).

5. **Eat more fruit, vegetables, and whole grains** in place of high-fat foods. Aim for 2 fruits and 5 servings of vegetables per day. They also contain valuable antioxidants. The fat of avocados (and most nuts) is mainly unsaturated and can lower blood cholesterol levels.

6. **Limit cholesterol to 300mg per day.**
   (Extra Notes ~ See Previous Page)

7. **Avoid brewed unfiltered coffee** (espresso; plunger-style). Several cups per day may raise blood cholesterol. Filtered coffee is fine.

8. **Spread your food intake over the day.**
   Have 5-6 small meals per day rather than just 2-3 large meals. Nibbling, versus gorging, favors lower blood cholesterol.

## ALCOHOL – WINE

Alcohol is a mixed bag. Moderate amounts of 1-2 drinks daily appear to reduce the risk of heart attack and ischemic stroke in older persons.

However, larger amounts increase the risk of high blood pressure, obesity, heart failure and hemorrhagic stroke, and can aggravate hypertriglyceridemia: as well as many other health hazards. (*See Alcohol Guide – Page 23*)

The speculative benefits of moderate alcohol intake have been overstated in the media. The overriding harmful effects of excess alcohol do not allow its recommendation for any aspects of health promotion.

*Fruit, Vegetables & Tea Also Protect:*
**Red wine and red grapes (more so than white) contain antioxidants which may help protect cholesterol in the blood from becoming oxidized.**

**Many fruits, vegetables, grains, nuts and tea also contain protective antioxidants.**

Fats in the diet affect more than blood cholesterol levels. They can also strongly influence blood clot formation and thrombosis, as well as blood flow and ultimate oxygen delivery to body parts and organs.

While advanced atherosclerosis can impede blood flow to the heart and other organs, it is thrombosis (complete blockage by blood clots) or arterial spasm which commonly results in a heart attack or stroke.

**Plant and fish oils rich in omega-3 fats** lessen the risk of blood clots, thrombus formation, and artery spasm by reducing platelet stickiness and adhesion to artery walls. This reduces the risk of atherosclerotic plaque becoming unstable and reactive.

**Omega-3 fats also improve blood flow** by reducing blood viscosity and increasing the flexibility of red blood cells (RBC) that need to flex and twist on themselves in order to squeeze through tiny narrow capillaries often half their diameter.

**A diet high in saturated fats** has the opposite effect by stiffening RBC membranes and increasing blood viscosity, thereby hindering blood flow. The stiffening of the RBC membrane also reduces its ability to release vital oxygen to body cells and take up carbon dioxide.

Stiff red blood cells may also form aggregates that resemble coin stacks. In narrow blood vessels, this further impedes blood flow and impairs oxygen release through the much-lessened surface area of red blood cell membranes exposed to blood. (Smoking, lack of exercise, and stress can have similar adverse effects on thrombosis, red blood cell flexibility, and blood flow.).

▲ **Picture of Healthy Blood Flow**

*Flexible red blood cells twist and slide through tiny capillaries - often half the diameter of red blood cells.*

▲ **A Not-So-Healthy Picture!**

*Red blood cells have lost their flexibility and ability to twist and slip through capillaries. They are stacked up, thereby impeding blood flow.*

*A diet high in saturated fats can contribute to this picture - as can smoking, lack of exercise, and stress.*

Stay Fit Don't Quit!

Eat Light Eat Right!

Be Smart Don't Start!

# Fiber Guide

## Introduction

Fiber is the general term for those parts of plant food that we cannot digest (although bacteria in the large bowel partly digests fiber through fermentation). It is not found in foods of animal origin (meats, dairy products).

Fiber promotes intestinal health, bowel regularity, can benefit diabetes and blood cholesterol levels, and may help prevent colon cancer. High-fiber foods also assist weight control.

Most Americans don't eat enough fiber – less than 20 grams/day - instead of a healthier 25 to 35 grams/day.

*Fiber promotes good health, and better control of diabetes and cholesterol.*

*'An apple a day keeps the doctor away.'* ... it just might!

## Types of Fiber

Plant foods contain a mixture of different fibers in varying proportions. Insoluble and soluble fiber categories are based on their solubility in water. All types of fiber are beneficial to the body.

◆ Insoluble fibers (cellulose, hemi-celluloses, lignin) make up the structural parts of plant cell walls.

Best food sources are wheat bran, corn bran, rice bran, wholegrain cereals and breads, beans and peas, nuts, seeds, and the skins of fruits and vegetables.

These fibers absorb many times their own weight in water. They create a soft bulk and hasten the passage of waste products through the intestines.

**They promote bowel regularity,** and aid in the prevention and treatment of uncomplicated forms of **constipation, diverticulosis and hemorrhoids.**

**The risk of colon cancer** may also be reduced by fiber's diluting effect on potentially harmful substances.

◆ Soluble fibers (pectin, gums, mucilages) are found mainly within plant cells, soy milk (whole bean) and products.

## Types of Fiber (Cont)

**Best Sources of Soluble Fiber:** Fruits and vegetables, oat bran, barley, beans and peas, prunes, psyllium and flax seed.

These fibers form a gel which slows both stomach emptying and the absorption of sugars from the intestines. **This helps to control blood sugar levels.**

**Weight control** is also aided by the slower emptying of the stomach and the feeling of **fullness provided by soluble fiber.**

Some soluble fibers can lower **blood cholesterol** by binding bile acids and excreting them. More body cholesterol must then be broken down to supply bile acids for emulsification of dietary fats. **Rice bran, while not high in soluble fiber, can also lower blood cholesterol.**

◆ **Resistant starch** is that part of starchy foods (approx. 10%) which is tightly bound by fiber and resists normal digestion. Friendly bacteria in the large bowel ferment and change the resistant starch into short-chain fatty acids, which are important to bowel health and may protect against colon cancer.

Starchy foods include bread, cereals, rice, pasta, potatoes and legumes.

## Fiber & Weight Control

**Fiber can assist weight control** in several ways. Fiber-rich foods such as fresh fruit and vegetables, potatoes and wholegrain bread contain few calories for their large volume (due to their low-fat, high-water content).

**Their bulk fills the stomach** and satisfies the appetite much sooner than fiber-depleted foods. The extra chewing time also contributes to satiety, and gives the stomach time to register a feeling of fullness. Excessive calories are less likely to be consumed.

**Fiber-depleted foods and drinks** are more concentrated in calories; e.g. fats, sugar, candy, soft drinks, fruit juices, alcohol. They require little or no chewing. Large amounts with excessive calories can be consumed before the appetite is satisfied.

**Example:** Whereas one fresh apple might satisfy the appetite, an apple juice drink with the equivalent sugars and calories of 2-3 apples only minimally satisfies the appetite. (See illustration below.)

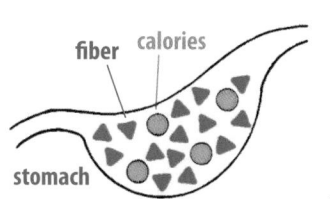

High-fiber foods fill the stomach. Fewer calories are consumed.

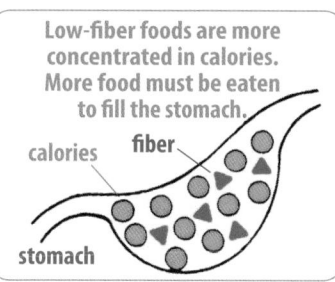

Low-fiber foods are more concentrated in calories. More food must be eaten to fill the stomach.

## EFFECTS OF REMOVING FIBER FROM FOOD

**2-3 pieces of fresh fruit produces 1 glass of fruit juice. The removal of fiber concentrates the sugar and calories.**

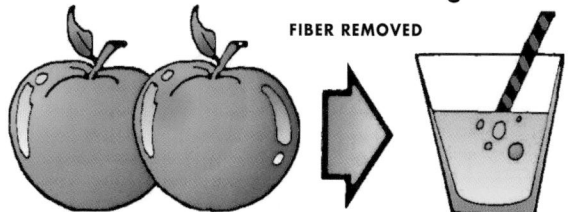

FIBER REMOVED

| Fresh Fruit | | Fruit Juice |
|---|---|---|
| High Fiber | ✦ | Negligible Fiber |
| Low Calorie Density | ✦ | High Calorie Density |
| Long Eating Time | ✦ | No Eating Time (Drink) |
| Satisfies Hunger | ✦ | Does Not Satisfy Hunger |
| Sugar Slowly Absorbed | ✦ | Sugar More Quickly Absorbed |
| Less Insulin Required | ✦ | More Insulin Required |

# Fiber Guide ~ Constipation

## Constipation

**Constipation** can reasonably be defined as a failure to have a bowel movement at least every second day – and just as importantly, without straining or pain.

Typically, constipated stools are too hard, too narrow and too small.

The **main cause** is simply a lack of dietary fiber. Other contributing factors include insufficient fluids, too little exercise, emotional stress, gastrointestinal disease, lack of proper dentition to chew high-fiber foods, and some medications (e.g. some antacids, antidepressants, pain medications).

**Note:** Check with your doctor to rule out any underlying medical problem – especially if you have a change in bowel habits in middle-age or later years.

### DESIRABLE FIBER INTAKE

Adults:  25-35gm per day
Children (under 18):  Age + 5gm
Example: 6-year old (6 + 5)= 11gm

### SAMPLE FOOD QUANTITIES
For 35 Grams of Fiber/Day

| | Fiber |
|---|---|
| Breakfast Cereal (higher-fiber) | 5g |
| **plus**  4 slices wholegrain Bread | 6g |
| **plus**  3 servings fresh Fruit | 9g |
| **plus**  1 medium Potato (w. skin) ⎫ | |
| **or**  1 cup Brown Rice ⎬ 4g | |
| **or**  ½ cup wholegrain Pasta ⎭ | |
| **plus**  3-4 servings Veggies/Salad | 6g |
| **plus**  1 cup Bean Soup ⎫ | |
| **or**  ¼ cup Baked/Soy Beans ⎪ | |
| **or**  ½ cup Corn/Peas/Lentils ⎬ 5g | |
| **or**  1¼ oz Almonds (natural) ⎪ | |
| **or**  3 medium Figs ⎭ | |

## HINTS TO INCREASE FIBER AND AVOID CONSTIPATION

**❶ Breakfast is an important** contributor to daily fiber intake. Eat high-fiber breakfast cereals (bran-based cereals, oatmeal etc.). Add 1-2 tablespoons of unprocessed bran.

Dried fruits, chopped nuts, soy grits, and seeds are also excellent additions to cereals.

*Note:* A gradual increase in fiber will prevent bloating, gas or pain. People intolerant to bran may benefit from psyllium-based fiber supplements and cereals.

**❷ Drink adequate water daily.** Fiber works by absorbing many times its own weight in water.

**❸ Eat wholegrain breads,** or fiber-enriched breads. They have over double the fiber of regular white bread.

**❹ Enjoy fruit as fresh fruit** with skin rather than as fruit juice. Enjoy wholegrain pasta, barley, brown rice, nuts and seeds.

**❺ Eat more vegetables,** salads and legumes – especially cooked beans, lentils, potatoes with skins, avocado, broccoli, brussels sprouts, cabbage, carrots, celery, and peas.

**❻ Add bran** (barley/rice/wheat) or soy grits to soups, casseroles, yogurt, desserts, cookies, cakes. Also use whole-meal flour or soy flour in place of white flour. Use nuts, seeds, and ground linseed.

**❼ Snack** on fresh or dried fruits, carrot or celery sticks, popcorn, nuts or seeds, wholegrain crackers, high-fiber bars (low-fat). Limit amounts if overweight.

**❽ Exercise regularly** to strengthen abdominal muscles and stimulate the gut. Keep up water intake, especially in warm weather.

**❾ Avoid** indiscriminate and regular use of harsh laxatives. They can overstimulate the intestinal muscles and may make normal bowel activity impossible. It may take several weeks to restore normal bowel function.

## FOODS WITH ZERO FIBER

- **Dairy Products (Milk, Cheese, etc)**
- **Meats, Poultry, Fish, Eggs**
- **Fats/Oils, Sugar/Syrups**
  (Only foods of plant origin contain fiber.)

## Breakfast Cereals `Fiber`

**General Mills:**

| | |
|---|---|
| Basic 4, 1 cup, 2 oz | 3 |
| Cheerios (Honey Nut; Multigrain), 1 c., 1 oz | 2 |
| Fiber One, ½ cup, 1.1 oz | 14 |
| Multi-Bran Chex, 1 cup, 2 oz | 7 |
| Oatmeal Crisp Almond, 1 cup, 2 oz | 4 |
| Raisin Nut Bran, 1¼ cup, 2 oz | 6 |
| Total, average all types, ¾ cup, 1 oz | 3 |
| Wheat Chex, 1 cup, 2 oz | 6 |
| Wheaties ¾ cup, 1 oz | 3 |

**Health Valley:**

| | |
|---|---|
| Amaranth Flakes, ¾ cup, 1 oz | 3 |
| Crunches & Flakes, ¾ cup, 1.9 oz | 4 |
| Fiber 7 Flakes, ¾ cup, 1 oz | 7 |
| Golden Flax, ¾ cup, 1.9 oz | 6 |
| Granola (Low-Fat), ⅔ cup, 2 oz | 6 |
| Healthy Fiber Flakes, ¾ cup, 1.1 oz | 4 |
| Oat Bran Flakes, all types, ¾ cup, 1 oz | 2 |
| Oat Bran O's, ¾ cup, 1 oz | 3 |
| Real Oat Bran, ½ cup, 1.7 oz | 5 |

**Kellogg's:**

| | |
|---|---|
| All-Bran, ½ cup, 1.1 oz | 10 |
| All-Bran w. Extra Fiber, ½ cup, 1 oz | 13 |
| All-Bran Bran Buds, ⅓ cup, 1.1 oz | 13 |
| Corn Flakes, Fruit Loops, Smacks 1 cup, 1 oz | 1 |
| Cocoa/Rice Krispies Treats, 1¼ cup, 1 oz | 0 |
| Complete: Wheat Flakes, ¾ c., 1 oz | 5 |
| Oat Bran Flakes, ¾ cup, 1.1 oz | 4 |
| Corn Pops, 1 cup, 1.1 oz | 0 |
| Cracklin' Oat Bran, ¾ cup, 1.7oz | 6 |
| FiberPlus Antioxidants: | |
| Berry Yogurt Crunch, 1 c., 1.9 oz | 10 |
| Cinnamon Oat Crunch ¾ c., 1.1 oz | 9 |
| Frosted Mini Wheats, 24 bisc., 2 oz | 5 |
| Granola w. Raisins, ⅔ cup, 2.1 oz | 3 |
| Raisin Bran, 1 cup, 2.1 oz | 7 |
| Smart Start, Strong Heart, | |
| Cinnamon Raisin, 1 cup, 1.8 oz | 4 |
| Special K, 1 cup, 1.1 oz | 0.5 |

`Fiber` **~ Fiber (grams)**

### Breakfast Cereals (Cont) `Fiber`

**Kashi:**

| | |
|---|---|
| GoLEAN Cereal, 1 cup, 1.8 oz | 10 |
| GoLEAN Crunch!, 1 cup, 1.9 oz | 8 |
| GoLEAN Bars, avg. (1) | 6 |
| Good Friends: Original, 1 cup, 1.9 oz | 12 |
| Cinna-Raisin Crunch, 1 cup, 1.8 oz | 8 |
| Heart to Heart, ¾ cup, 1.2 oz | 5 |
| 7 Whole Grain Pilaf, ½ cup, cooked, 5 oz | 7 |
| 7 Whole Grain Puffs, 1 cup, 0.7 oz | 1 |

**Quaker:**

| | |
|---|---|
| Cap'n Crunch, ¾ cup, 1 oz | 1 |
| 100% Natural Granola, | |
| avg., ½ cup, 1.8 oz | 3 |
| Crunchy Corn Bran, 1 cup, 1 oz | 5 |
| Life Cereal, ¾ cup, 1.1 oz | 2 |
| Oat Bran, ½ cup, 1.4 oz | 6 |
| Oatmeal, average, 1 packet | 3 |

**Post:**

| | |
|---|---|
| 100% Bran, ⅓ cup, 1 oz | 9 |
| Alpha Bits, 1 cup, 1 oz | 2 |
| Blueberry Morning, 1 cup, 1.9 oz | 5 |
| Cranberry Almond Crunch, 1 cup, 1.8 oz | 3 |
| Fruit & Bran, 1 cup, 1.9 oz | 6 |
| Grape-Nuts, ½ cup, 2 oz | 7 |
| Great Grains, ⅔ cup, 1.9 oz | 5 |
| Honey Bunches of Oats, ¾ cup, 1.1 oz | 2 |
| Shredded Wheat & Bran, ½ cup, 2 oz | 8 |

### Brans & Supplements, Metamucil

| | |
|---|---|
| **Oat Bran:** 1 Tbsp (level) | 1 |
| ⅓ cup, (5⅓ Tbsp), 1 oz | 5 |
| **Rice Bran,** raw. ¼ cup, 1 oz | 6 |
| **Wheat Bran,** Unprocessed: | |
| Raw, 1 Tbsp | 1.5 |
| 2 Tbsp (level), ¼ oz | 3 |
| ¼ cup, (4 Tbsp), ½ oz | 6 |
| **Wheat Germ,** Raw, ¼ cup, 1 oz | 4 |
| **Psyllium Seed Husks,** 2 Tbsp | 8 |
| **Fibersure,** 1 heaping tsp | 5 |
| **Metamucil:** Orange, 1 rnd Tbsp, 11g | 3 |
| Fiber Wafers (2) | 6 |

### Hot Cereals, Oatmeal

| | |
|---|---|
| Bulgur (cracked Wheat), ckd, 1 cup | 8 |
| Corn/Hominy Grits, dry, 3 Tbsp, 1 oz | 0.5 |
| Cream of Wheat, cooked, ¾ cup | 1 |
| Oatmeal (uncooked ⅓ cup), ckd, ⅔ cup | 3 |

# Fiber Counter

## Breads & Crackers | Fiber

**Bread:** White, 1 slice, 1 oz — 0.6
Whole-wheat, 1 slice, 1 oz — 1.5
Wholegrain, 1 slice, 1 oz — 2
Rye, Pumpernickel, 1 oz — 1.5
Bagel/Roll/Bun, 1 medium, 2 oz — 1.5
Pita, whole wheat, 6.5″ pocket — 4.5
**Crackers:** Graham, average, 2 — 0.4
Saltine, 4 crackers — 0.4
**Crispbreads,** average, 2 — 4
**Matzo,** 1 board, 1 oz — 1
**Rice Cakes,** average, 1 cake — 0.3
**Tortilla:** Regular, 6″ — 0.5
Whole-wheat, 6″ — 1.3

## Barley, Pasta, Rice & Flours

**Barley,** pearled, raw, ¼ cup, 1.7 oz — 8
**Rice:**
White, cooked, 1 cup — 0.6
Brown, cooked, 1 cup — 3.5
*Rice-A-Roni,* average, 1 cup, prepared — 1.5
**Spaghetti/Noodles:** Cooked, 1 cup — 2
Whole-Wheat, cooked, 1 cup — 4
**Flour:** Wheat, All-purpose, 1 cup, 4.5 oz — 3.5
Whole-Wheat, 1 cup, 4.5 oz — 15
Cornmeal, stone ground, 1 cup, 4.5 oz — 13
Carob Flour, 1 cup, 3.5 oz — 41
Rye Flour, 1 cup, 3.5 oz — 15
Soy Flour: Defatted, 1 cup, 3.5 oz — 17
Full-fat, raw, 1 cup, 3 oz — 8
Soy Meal, defatted, 1 cup, 4.5 oz — 14

## Frozen Entrees & Dinners

*Average All Brands: Per Serving*
Beans/Chili base, average — 6-10
Potato/Pasta base, average — 4-6
Vegetable base, average — 3
Meat/Chicken base, average — 2-3
**Pizzas,** ¼ large, average — 3
**Vegetarian Soy Burgers,** 1 pattie — 4

## Soups

Chicken Noodle, 1 cup — 0.5
Tomato Soup, average, 1 cup — 0.5
Vegetable Soup, average, 1 cup — 3
*Health Valley: Per 1 Cup*
Black Bean; Minestrone — 8
Tomato — 1
5 Bean Vegetable; Lentil & Carrots — 10
Mushroom Barley; Vegetable — 4
Split Pea — 8
*Progresso,* High Fiber, all flavors, 1 cup — 7

## Fast Foods & Restaurants | Fiber

**Hamburgers:** Small, average — 1.5
Large/Whopper, average — 2.5
**Hot Dog,** Regular — 1.5
**French Fries:** Small serving, 2.5 oz — 2.5
Regular/Medium, 3.5 oz — 3.5
**Chicken Nuggets,** 6 pack — 0.5
**Chicken Sandwich,** average — 2
**Taco,** average — 4
**Sundaes,** Shakes, Soft Drinks — 0
*Arby's,* Classic Roast Beef Sandwich — 1
*Denny's:* Grilled Chicken Salad, no bread — 4
Classic Burger, no fries — 4
Club Sandwich, no fries — 2
Grilled Chicken Sandwich, no fries — 4
*Domino's:* 12″, Classic/Thin, 1 slice — 1
Deep Dish, 1 slice — 3
Feast Pizza, Classic/Thin, 1 slice — 2
*McDonald's:* Big Mac — 3
Hamburger; Quarter Pounder — 3
Egg McMuffin — 2
Grilled Chicken Caesar Salad — 4
*Pizza Hut: Per 1 Slice, Medium*
Pan Pizza: Cheese, Pepperoni — 1
Supreme — 2
Thin 'n Crispy, Supreme — 2
Hand-Tossed, average all varieties — 2
*Subway:* Sandwich, white roll, av. — 4
With Honey Wheat Roll, average — 3
Salads, average — 4

## Cakes, Cookies, Snack Bars

**Apple/Fruit Pie,** 1 serving, 4 oz — 2
**Cake:** With plain flour, 1 serving, 3.4 oz — 1.5
With whole-wheat flour, 1 serving — 3
**Carrot Cake,** 4 oz — 4
**Cookies,** oatmeal, (3 small/1 large) — 1
**Donuts,** medium, 1.7 oz — 0.7
**Fruit Cake,** 1 serving, 1.5 oz — 2
**Fig Bars,** 1 cookie, 0.5 oz — 0.7
**Muffins,** Oat Bran (2 small, 1 large), 4 oz — 5
**Granola Bars,** average, 1 bar — 2
*Atkins Advantage Bars,* average — 7
*Clif Bars,* 2.5 oz — 5
*Curves,* Chocolate Peanut Bar, 1 oz — 5
*Fi-Bar Chewy & Nutty,* 1 bar — 1
*Fiber One (Gen. Mills),* 1.4 oz bar — 9
*FiberPlus,* all bars, 1.2 oz — 9
*Health Valley:* Fruit/Granola Bars — 3
Cereal Bars — 1
*Luna Bars,* avg., 1.7 oz — 3
*Special K,* Protein Meal Bar, 1.6 oz — 5

## Chocolate, Chips, Popcorn | Fiber

| | |
|---|---|
| **Cheese Balls/Curls/Twists** | 1 |
| **Chocolate,** Hard Candy, 1 oz | 0 |
| **Chocolate with nuts/fruit,** 2 oz bar | 1.5 |
| *Mars Bar,* 1.8 oz | 1 |
| **Potato Chips; corn chips,** 1 oz | 1 |
| **Popcorn,** 3 cups | 3 |
| **Pretzels,** Twists (6) | 1 |

## Nuts, Seeds

| | |
|---|---|
| **Almonds:** Natural, 25 nuts, 1 oz | 3.5 |
| Blanched (skins removed), 1 oz | 3 |
| **Cashews,** Filberts, Pecans, 1 oz | 1.7 |
| **Peanuts,** Mixed Nuts, Coconut, 1 oz | 2.5 |
| **Peanut Butter,** 2 Tbsp, 1 oz | 2 |
| **Pistachio Nuts,** dried, shelled, 1 oz | 3 |
| **Walnuts,** Black/English, dried, 1 oz | 2 |
| **Seeds:** Amaranth, 2½ Tbsp, 1 oz | 3.5 |
| Flax Seeds, 3 Tbsp, 1 oz | 7 |
| Psyllium Seed Husks, 5 Tbsp, 1 oz | 20 |
| Quinoa Seeds, 3 Tbsp, 1 oz | 1.7 |
| Sesame Seeds, whole, 1 oz | 3.4 |
| Sesame Butter/Tahini, 2 Tbsp, 1.1 oz | 1.4 |
| Sunflower kernels, ¼ cup, 1 oz | 3.8 |
| Teff Seeds, 1 oz | 3.8 |

## Fruit – Fresh

| | |
|---|---|
| **Apples:** 1 medium, 5½ oz (whole) | |
| with skin + core | 3.7 |
| with skin, no core | 3.2 |
| without skin, no core | 1.7 |
| **Apricots,** 2 medium, 4 oz | 1.5 |
| **Avocado,** average, ½ medium | 6 |
| **Banana,** 1 medium, 6 oz (w. skin) | 3 |
| **Blueberries,** raw, ½ cup, 2.5 oz | 1.7 |
| **Cherries,** sweet, raw, 8 fruits, 1.6 oz | 1 |
| **Grapefruit,** average, ½ fruit, 10 oz | 1.4 |
| **Grapes,** 1 medium bunch, seedless, 7 oz | 2 |
| **Kiwifruit,** 1 medium, 2.7 oz | 2.3 |
| **Mango,** 1 medium, 11 oz (whole) | 1.6 |
| **Melons,** Cantaloupe, 4 oz (edible) | 1 |
| **Nectarine,** 1 medium, 4 oz | 1.9 |
| **Olives,** average all types, 7 jumbo, 2 oz | 1.5 |
| **Oranges,** 1 medium (7-8 oz w. skin) | |
| 5½ oz (peeled) | 3.8 |
| **Passionfruit,** 2 medium, 2.5 oz | 5 |
| **Peaches,** 1 large, 6 oz | 2 |
| **Pears,** raw, 1 medium, 6 oz | 4.5 |
| **Pineapple,** 1 slice, 3 oz | 1.2 |
| **Plums,** 2 medium, 6 oz | 1.8 |
| **Strawberries,** 6 medium/3 large, 2 oz | 1 |
| **Watermelon,** 4 oz (edible) | 0.5 |

## Fruit – Dried, Juice | Fiber

| | |
|---|---|
| **Dried** Fruit: Apricots, 8 halves, 1 oz | 2.2 |
| Dates (3 med); Raisins (2 Tbsp), 1 oz | 1.5 |
| Figs, 3 medium,1½ oz | 5 |
| Prunes, 4 medium, 1 oz | 2 |
| **Fruit Juice:** Orange/Apple etc, 1 glass | <0.5 |
| Prune Juice, 5 oz | 1.4 |
| Carrot Juice, 8 oz | 1.8 |

## Vegetables

| | |
|---|---|
| **Asparagus,** 4 medium spears | 1.3 |
| **Bean Sprouts,** ½ cup, 2 oz | 1 |
| **Beans:** Snap/Green, ½ cup, 2 oz | 2 |
| Baked Beans in Tom Sce, ½ c., 4.5 oz | 5 |
| Dried Beans, ckd, average, ½ cup | 7 |
| **Beets,** ckd, slices, ½ cup, 3 oz | 1.7 |
| **Broccoli,** cooked, ½ cup, 3 oz | 2.4 |
| **Brussels Sprouts,** ckd, ½ cup, 3 oz | 3.5 |
| **Cabbage:** White, ckd, ½ cup, 2.5 oz | 1 |
| Red, ckd, ½ cup,2.5 oz | 2 |
| **Carrots,** 1 medium (7½"), ½ cup, 3 oz | 2.5 |
| **Cauliflower,** cooked, 3 flowerets, 2 oz | 1.5 |
| **Celery,** raw, diced, 1 cup, 3.5 oz | 1.6 |
| **Chickpeas (Garbanzos),** ckd, ½ c., 3 oz | 6.5 |
| **Corn:** Kernels, cooked, ½ cup, 2½ oz | 2.5 |
| Corn on the Cob, 1 ear, 5 oz | 4 |
| **Cucumber/Lettuce/Mushrooms,** 2 oz | 0.5 |
| **Eggplant,** raw, sliced, ½ cup , 1.5 oz | 2 |
| **Lentils,** cooked, ½ cup, 3.5 oz | 8 |
| **Mixed Vegetables,** frozen, cooked, ½ cup | 3 |
| **Onions:** Raw, 1 medium, 4 oz | 1.5 |
| Spring Onions, chop., ¼ cup, 1 oz | 0.7 |
| **Peas:** Green, raw, ½ cup, 2.5 oz | 3.7 |
| Cowpeas (Black-eyed), ckd, ½ cup | 10 |
| Split Peas, cooked, ½ cup, 3.5 oz | 8 |
| **Peppers,** sweet, raw, 1 large, 6 oz | 3 |
| **Potatoes:** 1 medium, with skin, 5 oz | 4 |
| 1 medium, without skin | 2.5 |
| ½ cup mashed, 3.5 oz | 1.5 |
| French Fries, small, 2.6 oz | 3 |
| **Spinach,** cooked, ½ cup, 3 oz | 2.2 |
| **Squash:** Summer, cooked, ½ cup, 3 oz | 2.5 |
| Winter, cooked, ½ cup, 3.5 oz | 2.4 |
| **Tomatoes:** 1 medium, 4.5 oz | 1.5 |
| Tomato Sauce, 1 cup | 0.3 |
| **Soybean Products:** Miso, ½ c., 5 oz | 7.4 |
| Tempeh, cooked, 1 piece, 3 oz | 2 |
| Tofu, ½ cup, 4.4 oz | 0.4 |

## Salads:

| | |
|---|---|
| **Side Salad,** average | 1 |
| **Bean Salad,** ½ cup | 5 |
| **Coleslaw,** ½ cup | 1 |
| **Potato Salad,** ½ cup | 2 |

# Protein Guide

## General Notes

- **Protein has many important body functions.** It builds and repairs muscle, and is the basis of our body's organs, hormones, enzymes, and antibodies to fight infection.

- **Protein is also an emergency fuel** in the absence of sufficient carbohydrate and fats. For this reason, weight loss should be gradual so as to preserve protein levels in muscle, the heart and other body organs.

- **It is easy to obtain sufficient protein,** even if vegetarian. **Plant proteins are not inferior to animal proteins.** In fact, eating more soy and other plant proteins, and less animal protein, may help to build stronger bones and prevent osteoporosis, and may help to control blood cholesterol levels.

- **When changing to a vegetarian diet,** include soybeans, and other beans, soy milk drinks (calcium-enriched), lentils, tofu, tempeh, nuts and wholegrain breads and cereals. Milk, yogurt, cheese and eggs can enhance nutrient intake.

## Protein & Muscle

- Although muscles are built of protein, protein is not a special fuel for working muscle cells – carbohydrates and fats are.

- In fact, a diet high in protein (and fat) and low in carbohydrate can significantly reduce the performance of endurance sports athletes. **Carbohydrates** are the best fuel for muscles exercised for long periods.

- Any **extra protein** required by athletes and body-builders can easily be obtained from the extra food eaten to satisfy hunger and energy needs.

- Remember, **excessive protein** intake will not build bigger muscles. Any excess is converted and stored as fat. Excess protein can also strain the kidneys, which excrete the waste products of protein metabolism.

Elderly people (and dieters) must eat sufficient food to ensure adequate protein intake.

Inadequate protein leads to a drop in immune response with greater susceptibility to illness and infections. Muscle strength and muscle mass also drop.

Protein needs are easily met with sensible eating. Athletes who eat enough food for their energy needs can obtain sufficient protein.

### RECOMMENDED DAILY PROTEIN INTAKE
### ~ HEALTHY RANGE ~
(Lower figure is RDA)

| | | PROTEIN |
|---|---|---|
| Children: | 1-3 yrs | 13g-26g |
| | 4-8 yrs | 19g-38g |
| | 9-13 yrs | 34g-64g |
| Males: | 14-18 yrs | 52g-120g |
| | 19+ | 56g-120g |
| Females: | 14+ | 46g-110g |
| Pregnancy: | | 71g-120g |
| Breastfeeding: | | 71g-120g |

**Note:** On lower-calorie diets, aim for higher amounts of protein within the Healthy Range.

**Pro** ~ Protein (grams)

## Meat **Pro**

**Steak:** Average all cuts, lean (no fat)
| | |
|---|---|
| Small (4 oz raw/3 oz cooked) | 23 |
| Medium (6 oz raw/4¼ oz cooked) | 34 |
| Large (10 oz raw/7¼ oz cooked) | 57 |

| | |
|---|---|
| **Roast Beef,** lean, 2 slices, 3 oz | 24 |
| **Ground Beef patty,** lean, cooked, 3 oz | 21 |
| **Lamb chop,** broiled, 3 oz | 22 |
| **Liver,** cooked, 3 oz | 23 |
| **Veal cutlet,** 1 medium | 23 |
| **Pork,** cooked, lean, 3 oz | 24 |
| **Bacon,** 3 medium slices | 6 |
| **Ham,** roasted, 2 pieces, 3 oz | 18 |
| **Ham,** luncheon, 2 slices, 1½ oz | 7 |
| **Pastrami,** 3 sl., 1¾ oz | 10 |
| **Sausages:** Bologna, 2 sl., 2 oz | 7 |
| Braunschweiger, 2 sl., 2 oz | 8 |
| Pork link, thick, 2 oz | 6 |
| Frankfurter, 1⅓ oz | 5 |
| Salami, hard, 3 slices, 1 oz | 7 |
| **Vegetarian,** 1 pattie | 13 |

**Chicken/Turkey:** *Without Skin*
| | |
|---|---|
| **Chicken,** cooked: Breast, Roasted, 4 oz | 36 |
| Leg/Thigh,Roasted, 2 oz | 14 |
| ½ Whole Chicken | 60 |
| Drumstick, Rstd, 1 med., 3 oz | 13 |
| **Turkey:** Light meat, cooked, 3 oz | 28 |
| Dark meat, lean, 3 oz | 24 |

## Fish

**Fresh Fish:** *Per 4 oz, cooked*
| | |
|---|---|
| Cod, Flounder/Sole, Pollock | 28 |
| Catfish, Haddock, Halibut, M/Mahi | 28 |
| Ocean Perch, Swordf., Orange Roughy | 28 |
| **Canned Fish:** Tuna, Light, 3 oz | 25 |
| White, 3 oz | 23 |
| Salmon, pink, 3 oz | 17 |
| Salmon, red, 3 oz | 17 |
| Sardines, 3 whole (3″), 1¼ oz | 9 |
| Anchovies, 1 can, 1½ oz | 13 |
| **Shellfish:** Crabmeat, 3 oz | 17.5 |
| Clams, raw, 4 large/9 sml, 3 oz | 11 |
| Crayfish, cooked, 3 oz | 20 |
| Lobster, cooked, 3 oz | 17 |
| Oysters, raw, 6 medium, 3 oz | 7 |
| Scallops, 2 lge/5 small, 1 oz | 5 |
| Shrimp, raw, 6 large, 1½ oz | 8.5 |
| **Fish Products:** Fish Sticks, 4 sticks | 10 |
| Fish Portions, in batter, 4 oz | 13 |
| Gefilte Fish, 1 medium ball, 2 oz | 8 |

## Eggs **Pro**

| | |
|---|---|
| **1 Large Egg,** whole | 6 |
| Egg Yolk | 3 |
| Egg White | 3 |
| **Omelet:** Plain, 2 eggs | 13 |
| Ham & cheese | 17 |

**Egg Substitutes**, (liquid):
| | |
|---|---|
| *Egg Beaters,* ¼ cup, 2 oz | 4.5 |
| *Better 'n Eggs/Scramblers,* ¼ cup, 2 oz | 6 |

## Milk, Yogurt, Ice Cream

| | |
|---|---|
| **Milk:** Whole: 2%, 1 cup | 8 |
| Low-Fat (1%); Fat-Free, 1 cup | 8.5 |
| **Chocolate Milk,** 1 cup | 8 |
| **Thick Shake:** Chocolate, 10 oz | 9 |
| Vanilla, 10 oz | 11 |
| **Soymilk,** (fortified), average, 1 cup | 7 |
| *Soy Dream,* Enriched, shelf-stable, 1 cup | 7 |

**Yogurt**, average all brands:
| | |
|---|---|
| Plain, 6 oz | 8 |
| Fruit flavors, 6 oz | 7 |
| *Chobani,* Greek, Plain, 6 oz | 14 |
| Soy, fruit flavors, 6 oz | 7 |
| **Ice Cream:** Rich, ½ cup | 2 |
| Regular, Vanilla, ½ cup | 2.5 |
| **Sherbet,** ½ cup | 1 |
| **Custard,** baked, ½ cup | 7 |

## Cheese

| | |
|---|---|
| **Hard Cheeses,** average, 1 oz | 7 |
| **Cottage Cheese,** ½ cup | 13 |
| **Cream Cheese,** avg., 1 oz | 2 |
| **Ricotta,** part skim, ½ cup | 14 |

## Bread, Bagels, Biscuits

**Bread:** *With enriched flour*
| | |
|---|---|
| 1 slice, 1 oz | 2 |
| 4 thin slices, 4 oz | 8 |
| 4 thick slices, 6 oz | 1.2 |
| **Bagel,** plain 2 oz | 6 |
| **Biscuits,** 1 oz | 2 |
| **Pita Bread,** 1 pita, 1½ oz | 4 |
| **Pumpernickel,** 1 slice, 1 oz | 3 |

## Infant/Baby Foods **Pro**

**Infant Formula Milk:**
| | |
|---|---|
| *Enfamil/Gerber/Similac,* | |
| Regular/Low Iron , 5 fl.oz | 2.2 |
| *Isomil/Nursoy/ProSobee,* | 3 |

**Baby Cereals:** *Average all brands*
| | |
|---|---|
| Dry, 4 Tbsp, ½ oz | 1 |
| Jars, with fruit, 4½ oz | 1 |

# Protein Counter

## Breakfast Cereals — Pro

**Hot Cereals** ~ *Cooked:*

| | |
|---|---|
| **Bulgur,** cooked, 1 cup, 5 oz | 9 |
| **Oatmeal:** Reg., non-fortified, 1 cup | 6 |
| Instant, fortified, avg., 1 pkt | 4 |
| *Quaker,* all flavors, ½ cup | 5 |
| **Corn/Hominy Grits:** 1 cup | 3 |
| *Quaker:* Reg., 3 Tbsp, 1 oz | 2 |
| Instant White, 1 packet | 2 |
| **Cream of Wheat,** 1 cup | 4 |

**Brands** ~ *Ready-To-Eat*

*General Mills*:

| | |
|---|---|
| Cheerios, Original, 1 cup, 1 oz | 3 |
| Chex, Corn, 1 cup, 1.1 oz | 2 |
| Kix, Original, 1¼ cups, 1 oz | 2 |
| Lucky Charms, Original, ¾ cup, 1 oz | 2 |
| Total, Raisin Bran, 1 cup, 1.8 oz | 3 |
| Wheaties, ¾ cup, 1 oz | 2 |

*Health Valley:*

| | |
|---|---|
| Amaranth Flakes, 1¼ cups, 2 oz | 6 |
| Bran Flakes, with Raisins, 1 cup, 1.8 oz | 5 |
| Corn Crunch-Ems, 1 cup, 1 oz | 2 |
| Oat Bran Flakes, with Raisins, 1 cup, 1.9 oz | 5 |
| Rice Crunch-Ems, 1¼ cups, 1 oz | 2 |

*Kashi:*

| | |
|---|---|
| Good Friends, 1 cup, 1.9 oz | 5 |
| GoLean Crunch!, 1 cup, 1.9 oz | 9 |
| 7 Whole Grain Flakes, 1 cup, 1.75 oz | 6 |

*Kellogg's:*

| | |
|---|---|
| All-Bran, Original, ½ cup, 1 oz | 4 |
| Apple Jacks, 1 cup, 1 oz | 1 |
| Corn Flakes, 1 cup, 1 oz | 2 |
| Low-fat Granola with Raisins ⅔ cup, 2.1 oz | 5 |
| Product 19, 1 cup, 1 oz | 3 |
| Rice Krispies, 1¼ cup, 1.2 oz | 2 |
| Smart-Start Strong Heart, 1 c., 1.75 oz | 4 |
| Special K: All flavors, 1 c., 1.1 oz | 2 |
| Protein, ¾ cup, 1.1 oz | 10 |

*Post*:

| | |
|---|---|
| Grape Nuts, Original, ½ cup, 2 oz | 8 |
| Raisin Bran, 1 cup, 2 oz | 5 |

*Quaker*:

| | |
|---|---|
| Corn Bran Crunch, ¾ cup, 1 oz | 2 |
| Granola, ½ cup, 1.7 oz | 5 |
| Honey Graham Oh's, ¾ cup, 1 oz | 1 |
| Life, Original, ¾ cup, 1.1 oz | 3 |

## Brans & Wheatgerm — Pro

| | |
|---|---|
| **Oat Bran,** raw, 1 Tbsp | 2 |
| **Rice Bran,** raw, 2 Tbsp | 1 |
| **Wheat Bran,** unprocessed, 2 T. | 1 |
| **Wheat Germ,** 2 Tbsp, ½ oz | 4 |

## Grains & Flours, Yeast

| | |
|---|---|
| **Amaranth,** ½ cup, 3.4 oz | 14 |
| **Barley,** ½ cup, 3.2 oz | 12 |
| **Buckwheat Flour,** Whole-groat, 1 cup | 15 |
| **Carob Flour,** 1 cup, 3.6 oz | 5 |
| **Corn Flour,** 1 cup, 4 oz | 11 |
| **Corn Meal,** 1 cup, 4½ oz | 8 |
| **Flour:** White, 1 cup, 5.6 oz | 9 |
| Wholegrain, 1 cup, 4¼ oz | 16 |
| **Millet,** wholegrain, 1 cup, 3½ oz | 12 |
| **Rye Flour:** Dark, 1 cup, 4½ oz | 18 |
| Light, 1 cup, 3½ oz | 9 |
| **Soy Flour,** full fat, 1 cup, 3 oz | 29 |
| **Yeast:** Brewers, 2 Tbsp, ½ oz | 8 |
| Nutritional Yeast Flakes *(Red Star),* 1 heaping Tbsp, ½ oz | 8 |

## Rice, Spaghetti, Macaroni

| | |
|---|---|
| **Rice:** Brown/White, average 1 cup cooked, 6½ oz | 5 |
| **Spaghetti/Macaroni/Noodles (enriched):** | |
| Cooked, 1 cup, 4½ oz | 7 |
| Canned: in Tomato Sce, ½ cup | 2 |
| with Meatballs, 1 cup, 8 oz | 10 |
| Macaroni & Cheese, 1 cup, 9 oz | 8 |

## Soups

| | |
|---|---|
| With Noodles/Vegetables, 1 cup | 3 |
| With Meat/Beans/Peas, 1 cup | 8 |

## Fruit

**Fresh/Canned:**

| | |
|---|---|
| Average, all types, 1 medium/2 small fruit | 1 |
| **Avocado,** ½ medium | 2 |
| **Dried Fruit:** Apricots, 8 halves, 1 oz | 1 |
| Dates, 6 dates, 2 oz | 1.5 |
| Figs, 4 medium figs, 2 oz | 2 |
| Prunes, 5 medium, 1½ oz | 1 |
| Raisins, 1 oz | 1 |
| **Fruit Juice:** Average, 1 cup | 0.5 |
| Prune Juice, 6 fl.oz | 1 |
| Tomato Juice, 1 cup, 8 fl.oz | 1.5 |

## Vegetables | Pro

| | |
|---|---|
| **Beans:** Snap/green, ½ cup, 2 oz | 1 |
| Dried: Average all types, cooked, ½ cup | 7 |
| Baked Beans, ½ cup 4½ oz | 5 |
| **Bean Sprouts,** mung, 1 c., 4 oz | 3 |
| **Broccoli,** 3 raw, ½ cup, 1½ oz | 1.5 |
| **Cabbage; Cauliflower,** raw, 1 c. 3 oz | 1.5 |
| **Corn:** Raw, ½ cup kernels, 3 oz | 2.5 |
| 1 ear trimmed to 3½" | 2 |
| **Lentils**, cooked, ½ cup, 3½ oz | 9 |
| **Mushrooms,** raw, ½ c., sliced | 1 |
| **Peas:** Green, raw, ½ c., 2½ oz | 4 |
| Split Peas, cooked, 1 cup, 7 oz | 16 |
| **Potatoes:** *Cooked:* | |
| 1 medium, with skin, 5 oz | 3.3 |
| without skin, 4 oz | 2.3 |
| French Fries, small, 2.6 oz | 2 |
| **Potato Salad,** ½ cup, 4 oz | 3.5 |
| **Pumpkin,** ½ cup mashed, 4.3 oz | 1 |
| **Seaweed,** kelp, 1 oz | <1 |
| **Spinach,** cooked, ½ cup, 3 oz | 2.7 |
| **Squash,** ckd, all types, ½ cup | 1 |
| **Tomatoes,** 1 medium, 4½ oz | 1 |
| **Vegetables,** mixed, ckd, 1 cup | 2.5 |
| **Soybeans,** cooked, ½ cup, 3 oz | 14 |

## Tofu, Tempeh, Miso

| | |
|---|---|
| Tofu, raw, firm, ½ cup, 4½ oz | 10 |
| Tempeh, ½ cup, 3 oz | 16 |
| Miso, ½ cup, 5 oz | 16 |
| Miso Soup, 1 cup | 3 |
| **Soybean Protein** *(TVP),* 1 oz | 18 |

## Cakes, Pastries, Pies

| | |
|---|---|
| (Made with enriched flour) | |
| Carrot w. cream cheese frosting, 4 oz | 4 |
| Cheesecake, 1 piece, 4 oz | 6 |
| Chocolate, 1 piece, 2 oz | 2 |
| Fruitcake, 1 piece, 3 oz | 4 |
| Plain, 1 piece, 3 oz | 4 |
| **Croissant,** plain, 2 oz | 4 |
| **Danish Pastry,** 1 pastry, 2¼ oz | 5 |
| **Donuts,** average, 2 oz | 4 |
| **Muffins,** average, 1 med., 1½ oz | 3 |
| **Pancakes,** 4" diam., two, 2 oz | 4 |
| **Pies:** Fruit, 1 piece, 5½ oz | 4 |
| Pecan, 1 piece, 5 oz | 7 |
| **Puddings,** average, ½ cup, 4½ oz | 4 |
| **Waffles,** 1 large, 2½ oz | 7 |

## Peanut Butter | Pro

| | |
|---|---|
| **Regular:** 2 Tbsp, 1.1 oz | 8 |
| *Peter Pan Plus,* 2 Tbsp, 1.1 oz | 8 |

## Sugar, Honey, Jam

| | |
|---|---|
| **Sugar:** White | 0 |
| Brown, 1 Tbsp | 0 |
| **Molasses:** Light/Med., 1 Tbsp | 0 |
| Blackstrap, 1 Tbsp, ¾ oz | 0 |
| **Corn Syrup,** 1 Tbsp, ¾ oz | 0 |
| **Honey, Jams, Jelly** | 0 |

## Candy, Chocolate, Carob

| | |
|---|---|
| **Candy,** sugar-based | 0 |
| **Chocolate:** Plain, 2 oz bar | 4 |
| with nuts, 2 oz bar | 6 |
| **Carob**, plain, 2 oz | 6 |

## Cookies, Crackers, Chips

| | |
|---|---|
| **Cookies**, average, 4 cookies | 2 |
| **Crackers**, Graham, 2½" sq., (2) | 1 |
| **Rice Cakes**, average, one | 1 |
| **Corn/Potato Chips**, 1 oz | 2 |

## Nuts:

| | |
|---|---|
| Almonds, shelled, 20-25 nuts | 6 |
| Brazil Nuts, 7-8 medium nuts, 1 oz | 4 |
| Cashews, 12-16 nuts, 1 oz | 5 |
| Macadamias, 1 oz | 2 |
| Peanuts, dry rsted, 40 nuts, 1 oz | 6 |
| Pecans, 24 halves, 1 oz | 2 |
| Walnuts, 15 halves, 1 oz | 4 |

## Seeds:

| | |
|---|---|
| Sesame Seeds, dry, 1 Tbsp | 2 |
| Pumpkin Kernels, dry, hulled, 1 oz | 7 |
| Sunflower Seeds, dried, hulled, 1 oz | 6 |
| Tahini, 1 Tbsp, ½ oz | 2.5 |

## Granola & Food/Protein Bars

| | |
|---|---|
| **Granola Bars**, average, 1 bar, 2 oz | 2 |
| *Anytime Health,* | |
| Meal Repl. Bars, 80g | 20 |
| Snack Bars, 50g | 12 |
| *Balance* Bars, Original, average all, 1.76 oz | 14 |
| *Bariatrix,* Proti-Bars (1), 1.4 oz | 15 |
| *Dr Soy,* Protein Bars, 1.76 oz | 10 |
| *GeniSoy,* Protein Bar, 1.6 oz | 15 |
| *Jenny Craig,* Bars, av., 1.8 oz | 5 |
| *Met-Rx,* "Big 100", av., 3.5 oz | 27 |
| *Myoplex 30,* all flavors, 3 oz | 30 |
| *Optifast 800,* all flavors, 2 oz | 14 |
| *PowerBar,* Energize, 2 oz | 6 |
| *Slim-Fast,* Protein Meal Bars, 1.7 oz | 10 |
| *Special K:* Protein Meal, 1.6 oz | 10 |
| Protein Snack, 0.9 oz | 4 |

# Protein Counter

## High Protein Drinks **Pro**

| | |
|---|---|
| *Anytime,* Health, Whey Prot. Isolate, all flav., 1 oz | 25 |
| *Atkins,* Shakes, 11 fl.oz | 18 |
| *Boost,* High Protein, 8 fl.oz bottle | 15 |
| *Carnation,* B'fast Essentials, 11 fl.oz | 10 |
| *Curves,* Protein Drink, 2 scoops, dry | 15 |
| *dotFIT,* First String, Choc., 2 scps, 2.65 oz | 21 |
| *Ensure,* Plus, 8 fl.oz bottle | 13 |
| *Gatorade,* Protein Recovery Shake, 11 oz | 20 |
| *GeniSoy,* Protein Shake, 1 scoop, 1.2 oz | 14 |
| *Met-Rx,* Meal Replacement, RTD | 40 |
| *Myoplex,* Original Nutrition Shake, 1 pkt | 42 |
| *Optifast 800,* prepared, 8 fl oz | 14 |
| *Slim-Fast Shakes:* Meal, 10 oz can | 10 |
| High Protein Meal, 10 fl.oz bottle | 20 |
| *Special K$_2$0,* Protein Water, 16 fl.oz | 5 |
| *Weider,* Mass 1000, 4 scoops, 7 oz | 34 |

## Coffee, Tea, Soda

| | |
|---|---|
| Coffee, Coffee Substitutes, 1 cup, 8 fl.oz | 0 |
| Coffee, with 2 oz milk, 1 cup, 8 fl.oz | 2 |
| Caffe latte, large, 16 fl.oz | 12 |
| Cappuccino, large, 16 fl.oz | 8 |
| Frappuccino, average, 16 fl.oz | 6 |
| Hot Chocolate, with milk, 1 cup, 8 fl.oz | 8 |
| Soft Drinks/Soda | 0 |
| Tea, all types | 0 |

## Beer, Wine, Spirits

| | |
|---|---|
| Beer, 12 fl.oz | 1 |
| Wines, red/white, 1 glass | 0 |
| Spirits/Liquor | 0 |

## Fast-Foods/Burgers

| | |
|---|---|
| **Pancakes,** average all outlets, 3 | 8 |
| **Shakes,** Chocolate, 16 fl.oz | 12 |
| **Sundaes,** Average all outlets | 7 |
| *Arby's:* | |
| Chopped Farmhouse Salad, Crispy Chicken | 30 |
| Roast Beef Sandwich: Classic | 23 |
| Max | 45 |
| *Burger King:* Big Fish Sandwich | 18 |
| Double Bacon Cheeseburger | 17 |
| Whopper Sandwich | 22 |

## Fast Foods/Burgers (Cont) **Pro**

| | |
|---|---|
| *Carl's Jr:* | |
| Charbroiled Chicken Club Sandwich | 36 |
| Famous Star Hamburger with Cheese | 28 |
| Super Star Hamburger with Cheese | 48 |
| *Domino's Pizza:* Hand Tossed (12") | |
| Feast, Ultimate Pepperoni, 1 slice | 11 |
| Legend: Buffalo Chicken, 1 slice | 13 |
| Honolulu Hawaiian, 1 slice | 8 |
| *KFC:* Original, Breast | 36 |
| Extra Crispy Tenders, 3 strips | 33 |
| Grilled, Breast | 40 |
| *McDonald's:* Big Mac | 25 |
| Cheeseburger | 15 |
| Chicken McNuggets (6) | 13 |
| Crispy Chicken Classic Sandwich | 24 |
| Filet-O-Fish | 15 |
| Hamburger | 12 |
| Quarter Pounder with Cheese | 30 |
| French Fries: Small, 2.5 oz | 3 |
| Large, 5.4 oz | 6 |
| Salad, with Chicken, average | 26 |
| Shake, McCafe, average, 12 fl.oz | 12 |
| Breakfast: Egg McMuffin | 18 |
| Bacon, Egg & Cheese McGriddles | 19 |
| Sausage Burrito | 12 |
| Sausage McMuffin with Egg | 21 |
| *Pizza Hut:* Per Medium, 1 slice, ⅛ Pizza | |
| Thin 'n Crispy, Supreme | 10 |
| Pan Pizzas, average | 11 |
| Hand Tossed: Pepperoni Lover's | 12 |
| Ultimate Cheese Lover's | 10 |
| *Subway :* 6" Subs with standard toppings, no oil | |
| Applewood Pulled Pork | 25 |
| Meatball Marinara | 21 |
| Spicy Italian | 20 |
| Subway Melt | 23 |
| Turkey Jalapeno Melt | 21 |
| *Taco Bell:* Bean Burrito | 15 |
| Cheesy Gordita Crunch | 20 |
| Chicken Quesadilla | 27 |
| Chicken/Steak Chalupas | 16 |
| Steak Burrito Supreme | 20 |
| Taco Supreme | 9 |
| *Wendy's:* | |
| Asiago Ranch Chicken Club | 38 |
| Dave's ¼lb Single Burger | 30 |
| Jr Hamburger | 14 |

## High Blood Pressure

**Many American adults** have hypertension (high blood pressure), and are unaware of it. It is generally symptomless, so **have your blood pressure checked annually** – particularly if it runs in the family.

**Untreated hypertension** overworks the heart, damages arteries and promotes atherosclerosis. This in turn greatly increases the risk of heart disease, stroke, blindness, kidney disease and impotence. The earlier hypertension is detected, the sooner it can be brought under control.

### BLOOD PRESSURE CLASSIFICATION

*For Adults Age 18 & Older ~ Not Acutely ill or on Medication (American Heart Association)*

|  | DIASTOLIC |  | SYSTOLIC |
|---|---|---|---|
| Normal ➤ | Below 80 | and | Below 120 |
| Prehypertension ➤ | 80-89 | or | 120-139 |
| **Hypertension:** | | | |
| Stage 1 ➤ | 90-99 | or | 140-159 |
| Stage 2 ➤ | 100 or more | or | 160 or more |

### Treating Hypertension

**Prehypertension** (in the chart above) means you don't have high blood pressure now but are likely to develop it in the future.

**You can take steps to lessen the risk by adopting healthy lifestyle habits such as:**
- reducing sodium intake
- eating adequate fruit and vegetables
- losing weight if overweight
- limiting alcohol to 2 drinks or less daily
- quitting smoking
- exercising regularly, managing stress.

**Stage 1 hypertension** can often be treated with the above lifestyle changes.

**Stage 2 hypertension** usually requires drug therapy. However, salt restriction, abstaining from alcohol, and the above lifestyle changes will improve the success of drug therapy, and enable smaller drug doses to be prescribed.

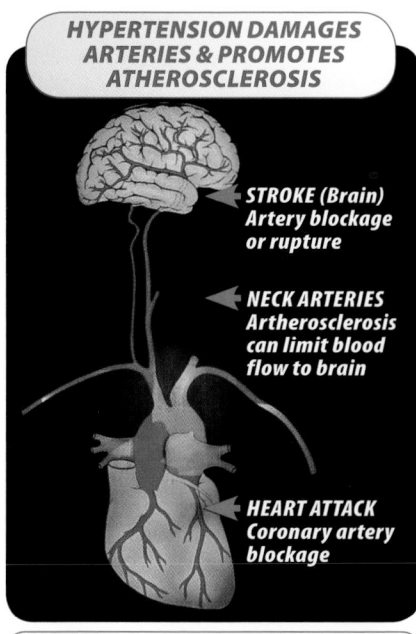

### HYPERTENSION DAMAGES ARTERIES & PROMOTES ATHEROSCLEROSIS

**STROKE (Brain)**
Artery blockage or rupture

**NECK ARTERIES**
Artherosclerosis can limit blood flow to brain

**HEART ATTACK**
Coronary artery blockage

### STROKE
#### KNOW THE WARNING SIGNS

**Stroke is a medical emergency!**
**If you notice one or more of these signs, call 9-1-1 or your doctor immediately.**

These signs may be signalling a possible stroke or transient ischemic attack:

- **Sudden weakness** or numbness in your face, arm, or leg on one side of your body.
- **Sudden confusion,** trouble speaking or understanding. Slurred speech.
- **Sudden trouble seeing,** in one or both eyes
- **Sudden trouble walking,** dizziness, loss of balance or coordination.
- **Sudden severe headache** - 'a bolt out of the blue' – with no apparent cause.

*Extra Info: www.stroke.org*

# Salt & Sodium Guide

## Salt & Sodium

- **Sodium is a mineral element** most commonly found in salt (sodium chloride). It also occurs naturally in much smaller amounts in animal and plant foods, and water – normally sufficient for our needs without having to add salt to our diet.

- **Sodium is required** for nerve and muscle function, as well as to balance the amount of fluid in our tissues and blood. Sodium acts like a sponge to attract and hold fluids in body tissues.

- **Excess sodium** can cause water retention, and increase the risk of developing hyper-tension. Very high salt intake may also increase the risk of stomach cancer.

- **Too little sodium** may cause low blood pressure (hypotension), and decrease blood flow to the heart, brain and kidneys – especially during exercise. (A certain blood volume is required to sustain the blood pressure needed for adequate blood flow in the capillaries).

## Salt-Sensitive Persons

- **Normally, our kidneys** excrete excess dietary sodium. The thirst we feel after a salty meal is the body calling for water to dilute the sodium, and enable the kidneys to flush out excess sodium.

- However, 'salt - sensitive' persons (up to 70% of adults) tend to retain excess sodium (above approximately 3000mg daily) instead of excreting it. Such persons are more likely to develop hypertension and would benefit most from sodium restriction. Assume you are susceptible if there is a family history of hypertension.

- Although not everyone will benefit, all Americans are being asked to moderate their salt and sodium intake as a public health measure – particularly because so many do not know whether or not they have hypertension, and also because we do not know just who is salt-sensitive.

On average, **less than one third of our sodium intake comes from the salt shaker.**
The rest is hidden in processed foods that have salt added during manufacture.

Sodium compounds added to food or medicinals can also contribute significant sodium.

**Sodium bicarbonate** in particular is widely used in antacid tablets (such as *Alka Seltzer*) and powders. Sodium bicarbonate contains 27% sodium by weight. Each gram contributes 270mg sodium. Large amounts of sodium can be unwittingly consumed – up to 600mg per tablet. (See Antacids ~ Page 280)

**Example:** 2 *Alka-Seltzer* Tablets = 1000mg sodium

**Other sodium compounds** include monosodium glutamate (MSG), sodium ascorbate, sodium nitrite, and sodium citrate.

### POTASSIUM BALANCES SODIUM

Potassium helps to balance sodium by helping the kidneys to excrete excess sodium. Fruit and vegetables are rich sources of potassium - another reason to ensure you have your 5-7 servings every day.

Nuts also provide potassium as well as magnesium and other heart-healthy nutrients and anti-oxidants. Eat them unsalted.

*Note: This info is only for people with normal kidney function. Also not for persons on potassium-sparing diuretics.*

### ALCOHOL DANGER

*Excessive alcohol intake contributes to hypertension. Susceptible persons should limit alcohol intake to 1-2 drinks per day.*

Sodium accounts for only 40% of the weight of salt (sodium chloride). Examples:
1 gram (1000mg) Salt has 400mg Sodium
1 teaspoon (5g) Salt has 2000mg Sodium

## HINTS TO REDUCE SODIUM

- **Cut down use of the salt shaker.** Start with an easy 50% cut in sodium by using Lite Salt (*Morton*) or *Cardia* Salt. Then gradually cut back until you can leave the salt shaker off the table. Sea salt is still high in sodium.

- **Use fresh herbs,** and salt-free seasonings to add flavor to food.

- **Choose low-sodium,** sodium-free, and reduced-sodium products in place of regular, salted products.

- **Check food labels for sodium levels.** FDA Guidelines for sodium descriptors are:
  - **Reduced Sodium:** At least 25% less sodium than the original product
  - **Low Sodium:** 140 mg or less/serving
  - **Very Low Sodium:** 35mg or less/serving
  - **Sodium Free:** Less than 5mg/serving
  - **No Salt Added:** Made without the salt normally added, but still contains the sodium that is a natural part of the food

- **Use reduced-sodium breads,** butter and margarine. Regular varieties are considered high in sodium in view of their significant contribution to our diet.

- **Go easy on salty condiments and sauces** such as ketchup, mustard, soy sauce, spaghetti sauces, and salad dressings. Use low-sodium varieties.

- **Limit pizzas and salty fast-foods.** Check the *CalorieKing.com* food database.

- **Avoid salty snack foods** such as potato chips, corn chips, salted nuts, pretzels and cheesy-flavored snacks. **Choose unsalted** popcorn, nuts or seeds. Eat more fruit.

- **Don't salt children's food** to your taste.

- **Avoid antacids with** sodium bicarbonate (such as *Alka-Seltzer*). They are high in sodium. Look for low-sodium alternatives.

- Cheese, Butter, Margarine
- Pickles, Sauerkraut, Olives
- Condiments, Sauces
- Salad Dressings
- Canned vegetables/salads/beans
- Deli Salads (with dressing)
- Frozen/Packaged Meals/Entrees
- Soups: Canned/dry; bouillon cubes
- Meats: Ham, bacon, sausage, luncheon meats, smoked meats
- Canned Fish (in brine/salt)
- Sea Salt, Garlic/Celery Salt
- Snack Foods (potato chips, pretzels)
- Tomato Juice (Canned), V8 Vegetable Juice
- Fast Foods: Pizza, Burgers, Chicken
- *Alka-Seltzer* Antacid
- Bread (regular)

### MODERATE SODIUM

- Meat, Fish, Poultry - Unprocessed
- Milk, Yogurt, Soy Drinks, Eggs
- Peanut Butter
- Breakfast Cereals (less than 200mg/serving)
- Chocolate Candy, Fruit/Nut Bars
- *Reduced Sodium & Low Sodium Products*

### FOODS LOW IN SODIUM

- Products labelled *Very Low Sodium,* or *Sodium Free*
- Bread (No Salt Added)
- Fresh fruits and vegetables
- Canned and Dried Fruits
- Potatoes, Rice, Pasta
- Dried Beans & Lentils, Tofu
- Nuts & Seeds (unsalted)
- Corn & Popcorn (unsalted)
- Pepper, Spices, Herbs
- Jam, Honey, Syrup
- Candy, Gum
- Hard & Jelly Candy
- Coffee, Tea, Alcohol
- Fresh Fruit Juices, Water

# Sodium Counter

**Sodium ~ Sodium (mg)**

## Milk & Dairy Products

| | Sodium |
|---|---|
| **Milk:** Whole/lowfat/skim, average 1 glass, 8 fl.oz | 120 |
| Whole, low sodium, 1 cup | 5 |
| **Choc Milk,** 1 cup | 130 |
| **Soy Milk,** 8 fl.oz | 30 |
| **Buttermilk,** cultured, 8 fl.oz | 250 |
| **Dry/Powder,** skim, ¼ cup, 1 oz | 110 |
| **Yogurt,** with fruit average, 8 oz | 130 |
| **Cheese:** Bleu, 1 oz | 330 |
| Cottage Cheese, Creamed, ½ cup, 4 oz | 450 |
| *Kraft:* Cheddar Singles, 2% milk, 0.7 oz | 290 |
| Philadelphia Cream Cheese Brick, Orig.,1 oz | 105 |
| Parmesan, 1 oz | 450 |
| Process Cheese., average,1 oz | 430 |
| Ricotta Cheese, ½ cup, 4 oz | 150 |
| Swiss, Deli Style, 1 oz | 60 |

## Ice Cream, Frozen Yogurt

| | |
|---|---|
| Icecream, average, ½ cup | 50 |
| Frozen Yogurt, ½ cup | 50 |

## Fats/Oils

| | |
|---|---|
| **Butter/Margarine:** Regular, 2 Tbsp, 1 oz | 230 |
| Unsalted, reg., 2 Tbsp, 1 oz | 5 |
| **Mayonnaise,** avg., 2 Tbsp, 1 oz | 160 |
| **Oils/Lard/Drippings** | 0 |
| **Cream,** average, 1 Tbsp | 5 |
| *Coffee-Mate:* Powdered, 1 tsp | 2 |
| Liquid, 1 Tbsp | 5 |

## Eggs

| | |
|---|---|
| **Whole,** 1 large | 70 |
| **Omelet: 2 egg,** plain | 220 |
| With 1 oz Cheddar Cheese | 400 |
| *Egg Beaters:* Original, ¼ cup | 115 |
| Flavors, average, ¼ cup | 230 |

## Meats

| | |
|---|---|
| **Meat,** average all types, cooked Beef/Lamb/Veal/Pork, 4 oz | 80 |
| **Corned Beef,** cooked, 3 oz | 800 |
| **Bacon,** cooked, 2 slices, 0.5 oz | 270 |
| **Ham,** 3 oz | 1100 |

## Chicken & Turkey

| | |
|---|---|
| **Chicken/Turkey,** cooked, unsalted, 4 oz | 80 |
| **Stuffing Mixes,** average., ½ cup | 500 |

## Sausages & Meats

| | Sodium |
|---|---|
| Bologna, 1 oz | 280 |
| Frankfurter, 2 oz | 640 |
| Ham, chopped, 0.8 oz slice | 290 |
| Liverwurst (Braunschweiger), 1 oz | 320 |
| Pepperoni, 5 slices, 1 oz | 570 |
| Salami: Cooked, 1 oz | 350 |
| dry/hard, 1 oz | 600 |
| Sausage, 1 oz link | 220 |
| Pork, 2 oz patty | 260 |
| **Spam:** Classic, 2 oz | 790 |
| 25% Less Sodium, 2 oz | 580 |
| Turkey Roll, 1 oz | 160 |

## Fish:

| | |
|---|---|
| **Fresh Fish:** average, plain Cooked, 4 oz, without bone | 60 |
| Broiled w. butter, 4 oz | 150 |
| Breaded & fried, 4 oz | 320 |
| Fish fillets, batter-dipped 3 oz | 350 |
| Fish sticks, 1 oz stick | 160 |
| Gefilte Fish, with broth, 1 pce, 1.5 oz | 220 |
| Herring, pickled, 2 pces, 1 oz | 260 |
| Lobster, meat only, 4 oz | 180 |
| Oysters, fresh, 6 med., 3 oz | 95 |
| **Salmon:** Canned, 3 oz | 460 |
| No Salt Added, 3 oz | 65 |
| **Smoked fish,** average, 3 oz | 650 |
| **Tuna:** Canned, drained, 3 oz | 160 |
| Light, drained, 3 oz | 200 |
| No Added Salt, 3 oz | 40 |
| Spicy Flavored, 5 oz | 260 |

## Entrees & Meals

| | |
|---|---|
| **Frozen Meals,** average | 600-900 |
| *Lean Cuisine,* average | 700 |
| *Stouffer's,* average | 580 |
| **Dinners,** average | 900-1200 |
| **Side Dishes,** average | 400-600 |
| **Pizza,** frozen, ¼ large, 6 oz | 800-1200 |
| **Microwave,** Cup Meals | 900-1200 |
| **Cup O'Noodles,** average | 1500 |

**More Sodium Counts: www.CalorieKing.com**

# Sodium Counter

## Soups

| | Sodium |
|---|---|
| **Condensed:** Average, 1 cup, 8 oz | 800-1000 |
| Low Sodium, average | 70 |
| **Chicken Noodle,** average, 1 cup | 900 |
| **Bouillon Cube,** average | 950 |
| **Ramen Noodle Soup,** av., 3 oz pkg | 1500 |
| **Soup Cups,** average | 850 |
| **Soup Mixes,** average, 1 cup | 900 |

## Condiments, Sauces, Dressings

| | |
|---|---|
| **A-1 Sauce,** 1 Tbsp | 280 |
| **Barbecue Sauce,** 1 Tbsp | 130 |
| **Bragg's Liquid Aminos,** 1 tsp | 220 |
| **Chili Sauce,** 1 Tbsp | 230 |
| **Ketchup:** Tomato, 1 Tbsp | 180 |
| Low Sodium, 1 Tbsp | 20 |
| **Mayonnaise,** 1 Tbsp | 80 |
| **Mustard,** 1 tsp | 70 |
| **Pizza Sauce,** ½ cup | 700 |
| **Salad Dressings,** 2 Tbsp, 1 oz | 160-400 |
| **Spaghetti Sauce,** ½ cup | 500 |
| **Soy Sauce:** 1 Tbsp | 900 |
| Lite, 1 Tbsp | 600 |
| **Sweet & Sour,** ½ cup | 250 |
| **Tabasco,** 1 tsp | 25 |
| **Vinegar,** Lemon Juice | 0 |
| **Worcestershire,** 1 Tbsp | 65 |
| **Tomato:** Sauce, 1 cup | 1200 |
| Paste/Puree (salted), ½ cup | 1000 |
| No Salt Added, ½ cup | 75 |

## Salt & Salt Substitutes

| | |
|---|---|
| **Table Salt:** 1 teaspoon, 6g | 2400 |
| Single Serve package, 1 g | 400 |
| *Cardia Salt,* 1 teaspoon | 1080 |
| **Lite Salt,** 1 teaspoon, 6g | 1200 |
| *Morton,* No Salt Substitute, 1 tsp | 5 |
| **Garlic/Onion/Seasoned Salt,** 1 tsp, 4g | 1350 |
| **Garlic/Seasoned Salt** 1 teaspoon, 4g | 1300 |
| **Sea Salt,** 1 teaspoon, 5g | 2250 |

## Seasonings, Herbs & Spices

| | |
|---|---|
| Baking Powder, 1 tsp, 3g | 340 |
| Baking Soda (Sodium bicarb), 1 tsp, 3g | 810 |
| *Accent,* Flavor Enhancer, 1 tsp | 600 |
| Chili Powder, 1 tsp, 3g | 25 |
| Curry Powder | 0 |
| Lemon Pepper 1 tsp | 340 |
| Meat Tenderizer, 1 tsp, 5g | 1750 |
| MSG (Monosodium Glutamate), 5g | 500 |
| *Mrs Dash,* Blends/Marinades | 0 |
| *Old Bay,* Seasoning (Less Sodium), 1 teaspoon, 2.4g | 380 |
| Pepper, Mustard (dry), 1 tsp | 1 |
| Yeast, Nutritional, 1 Tbsp | 10 |

## Breakfast Cereals

| | Sodium |
|---|---|
| **Kellogg's:** | |
| All-Bran, Original, ½ cup, 1 oz | 80 |
| Special K, Original, 1 cup, 1.1 oz | 220 |
| Corn Flakes, 1 cup, 1 oz | 200 |
| Frosted Mini Wheats, Blueb./Strawb., (25) | 0 |
| Raisin Bran, 1 cup | 210 |
| *Quaker:* | |
| Corn Bran Crunch, ¾ cup, 1 oz | 210 |
| Natural Granola, average, ½ cup, 1 oz | 30 |
| Oh's, ¾ cup, 1 oz | 170 |
| Puffed Rice/Wheat, 2 cups, 1 oz | 1 |
| *General Mills,* Total, ¾ cup, 1 oz | 140 |
| **Oatmeal:** Regular, ¾ cup | 1 |
| *Quaker,* Instant, ⅔ cup (1 pkt) | 260 |

## Breads, Bagels, Crackers

| | |
|---|---|
| **Bread:** Thin Slice, average 1 oz | 140 |
| Thick Slice, 1.5 oz | 210 |
| Low Sodium, 1 oz | 10 |
| **Bagels:** Plain, medium, 2 oz | 200 |
| Large, take-out, average, 4 oz | 550 |
| *Panera Bread,* 3.8 oz | 460 |
| **Biscuits,** average, 1 oz | 180 |
| **Bun/Roll:** 1 medium, 1.5 oz | 200 |
| Large, 4 oz | 560 |
| **Crackers:** Saltine, 2 crackers | 70 |
| Low Salt, 2 | 25 |
| Graham, 2 regular | 50 |
| **Croissant,** Plain, average, 2 oz | 280 |
| **Rice Cakes,** average | 25 |
| *Ritz Crackers,* Low-Sodium, 1 oz | 60 |
| *Ry-Krisp,* Crispbread, Sesame, 2 | 90 |

## Cookies, Cakes, Desserts

| | |
|---|---|
| **Cookies:** Average, 2-3 cookies, 1 oz | 100 |
| Average, 1 cookie, 2.5 oz | 180 |
| **Baked Custard,** ½ cup | 100 |
| **Brownie,** 1.5 oz | 130 |
| **Carrot Cake,** 8 oz | 650 |
| **Cheesecake,** 7 oz | 350 |
| **Cinnamon Sweet Roll,** 2 oz | 250 |
| **Danish,** Apple/Fruit | 250 |
| **Donut,** average | 150 |
| **Muffins:** 1 medium, 2 oz | 150 |
| 1 extra large, 4 oz | 300 |
| **Pancakes,** (4"), x 3 | 360 |
| **Fruit Pies,** average, 7 oz | 600 |
| **Pudding:** Average, ½ cup | 160 |
| *Jell-O* (Mix), Instant, 0.9 oz | 350 |
| **Waffles:** Home-made, 7", 2.5 oz | 350 |
| Frozen: Average, 1.2 oz | 260 |
| *Aunt Jemima,* av., 2.5 oz | 336 |

# Sodium Counter

## Fruit & Juices
| | Sodium |
|---|---|
| **Fresh Fruit,** average all types, 1 serving | 1 |
| **Dried/Canned Fruit,** ½ cup | 1 |
| **Fruit Juice:** Fresh, sqz'd, 6 fl.oz | 1 |
| Commercial, aver., 6 fl.oz | 20 |
| **Tomato Juice** *(Campbell's)*, 6 fl.oz | 570 |
| Low Sodium (No Salt Added) | 20 |
| **V8 Vegetable** *(Campbell's)*: 5.5 fl.oz can | 290 |
| 12 fl.oz bottle | 630 |
| Low Sodium, 5.5 fl.oz can | 95 |

## Vegetables
**Fresh/Frozen (No Salt Added):** Per ½ Cup
| | |
|---|---|
| Asparagus, Bean Sprouts, Corn | 3 |
| Beets, Carrots, Celery, ½ cup | 40 |
| Broccoli, Cabbage, Cauliflower | 10 |
| Cucumber, Green Beans, Mushroom, Okra | 3 |
| Onions, Peas, Potato, Pumpkin, Squash | 3 |
| Peppers, Hot Chili, raw, each | 3 |
| Spinach, Turnips, ½ cup, cooked | 40 |
| Tomato, 1 medium, 5 oz | 10 |
| **Canned:** Asparagus, 4 spears | 300 |
| Beans, baked in tomato sauce | 450 |
| Beets, ½ cup, 3 oz | 240 |
| Corn Kernels, ½ cup, 3 oz | 190 |
| Creamed, ½ cup, 4.5 oz | 330 |
| Mushrooms w. butter sce, 2oz | 550 |
| Peas, ½ cup, 3 oz | 250 |
| Sauerkraut, ½ cup, 4 oz | 750 |

## Pickles, Olives
| | |
|---|---|
| **Olives:** pickled: Green, 1 large | 90 |
| Ripe/black, 1 large | 40 |
| **Pickles:** Bread & Butter, 4 slices, 1 oz | 200 |
| Dill, 1 pickle, 2.5oz | 900 |
| Sweet, 1 gherkin, 0.5 oz | 130 |

## Soybean Products
| | |
|---|---|
| **Miso (Soy Paste),** ¼ c., 2.5 oz | 2500 |
| Soybean Protein Isolate, 1 oz | 280 |
| **Tempeh,** Natural, ½ cup, 3 oz | 5 |
| **Tofu,** average, ½ cup, 4 oz | 5 |

## Jam, Honey, Syrups
| | |
|---|---|
| **Jam/Jelly,** 1 Tbsp | 2 |
| **Honey/Maple Syrup,** 1 Tbsp | 1 |
| *Log Cabin,* Syrup, 1 fl.oz | 35 |
| Lite, 1 fl.oz | 90 |

## Peanut Butter
| | |
|---|---|
| **Peanut Butter:** Regular, 2 Tbsp, 0.5 oz | 190 |
| *Jif,* Low Sodium, 2 Tbsp | 65 |
| *Trader Joe's,* Unsalted, 2 Tbsp | 5 |

## Snacks, Nuts
| | Sodium |
|---|---|
| **Cheese Balls/Curls,** 1 oz | 280 |
| **Cheetos,** 1 oz | 290 |
| **Corn/Tortilla Chips:** average, 1 oz | 220 |
| *Fritos,* Lightly Salted, 1 oz | 80 |
| **Granola bars,** average, 1 bar | 80 |
| **Nuts:** Plain, unsalted, 1 oz | 1 |
| Lightly salted, 1 oz | 80 |
| Salted or Honey Roasted, 1 oz | 160 |
| **Popcorn:** Plain (unsalted), 1 cup | 1 |
| Flavored, average, 1 cup | 60 |
| Salt added, 1 cup | 180 |
| **Potato Chips:** Plain, 1 oz | 160 |
| *Lay's,* Lightly Salted, 1 oz | 90 |
| Flavored, average, 1 oz | 250 |
| **Pretzels:** Regular, 3, 1 oz | 450 |
| Soft, salted, large | 1000 |

## Candy, Chocolate
| | |
|---|---|
| **Chocolate,** milk, 1 oz | 30 |
| **Fudge,** chocolate, 1 oz | 55 |
| **Candy Bars,** average, 1.5 oz | 60 |
| **Hard Candy,** 1 oz | 10 |
| **Licorice,** 1 oz | 30 |

## Beverages, Alcohol
| | |
|---|---|
| **Coffee or Tea,** 1 cup | 1 |
| **Cocoa:** Dry, plain, 1 Tbsp | 0 |
| Mix, average, 1 envelope | 120 |
| **Quik,** 2 tsp | 35 |
| **Soft Drinks:** average, 8 fl.oz | 20 |
| **Mineral Water:** Perrier, 8 fl.oz | 5 |
| *Gatorade,* Thirst Quencher, 8 fl.oz | 110 |
| *Red Bull,* 8½ fl.oz can | 200 |
| **Water,** Average, 1 cup, 8 fl.oz | 5 |
| **Alcohol:** Beer, average, 12 fl.oz | 15 |
| Wines, average, 4 fl.oz | 10 |
| Spirits (distilled), 1.5 fl.oz | 1 |

## Antacids ~ Alka-Seltzer
| | Sodium |
|---|---|
| Alka-Seltzer: *Per Tablet* | |
| Original; Heartburn | 570 |
| Extra Strength | 590 |
| Lemon Lime | 500 |
| Gold | 310 |
| *Alka-Mints,* chewable | 0 |
| *Bromo Seltzer,* ¾ capful | 760 |
| *Picot,* 1 packet, 5g | 670 |
| *Rolaids,* All types | 0 |
| *Tums,* Regular/Extra Strength | 0 |

## Cold & Flu ~ Alka-Seltzer Plus
| | |
|---|---|
| Effervescents, average, 1 tablet | 480 |
| Fast Crystal Packs; Liquid Gels | 0 |

## Fast-Foods & Restaurants | Sodium

**Burger King:**

| | |
|---|---|
| **Burgers:** Cheeseburger | 690 |
| **Double Bacon Cheeseburger** | 940 |
| **Hamburger** | 460 |
| **Whoppers:** Original | 980 |
| With Cheese | 1380 |
| Whopper Jr. with Cheese | 730 |
| **Chicken Sandwich,** Original | 1390 |
| **Sides:** French Fries, medium, salted | 570 |
| Onion Rings, medium | 1080 |
| **Breakfast,** Ham, Egg & Cheese Croissan'wich | 1030 |

**Denny's:**

| | |
|---|---|
| **Burgers:** Bacon Avocado Cheeseburger | 1830 |
| Macho Nacho Burger | 1980 |
| **Sandwiches:** Club | 1850 |
| Prime Rib Philly Melt | 2000 |
| **Dinner:** Brooklyn Spaghetti & Meatballs | 2460 |
| Sirloin Steak with bread | 1590 |
| Sides: Broccoli | 20 |
| French Fries, salted, 6 oz | 110 |
| Red-Skinned Potatoes | 627 |
| **Soup:** Chicken Noodle, 12 oz bowl | 1130 |
| Clam Chowder, 12 oz bowl | 1870 |
| **Breakfast:** Buttermilk Pancakes (2) | 1170 |
| Moons Over My Hammy Omelette, w/ Hash | 2530 |
| Hearty Breakfast Skillet | 2130 |
| Sides: Hash Browns, 1 serving | 650 |
| Hearty Breakfast Sausage | 830 |
| **Desserts:** Apple Pie, 7 oz | 580 |
| Hot Fudge Brownie al la Mode, 9 oz | 520 |

**Jack In The Box:**

| | |
|---|---|
| **Burgers:** Bacon Untimate Cheeseburger | 2190 |
| Hamburger | 680 |
| Jumbo Jack with Cheese | 1310 |
| Sandwiches: Homestyle Ranch Chicken Club | 2010 |
| Sourdough Grilled Chiken Club | 1490 |

**KFC:**

| | |
|---|---|
| **Chicken Breast:** Original | 1130 |
| Extra Crispy | 1140 |
| Grilled | 730 |
| **Popcorn Chicken,** | |
| Value Box | 2160 |
| **Sandwich,** Crispy Twister | 1260 |
| **Strips,** Extra Crispy Tenders, 3 pieces | 940 |
| **Sides:** Macaroni & Cheese | 830 |
| Mashed Potatoes with Gravy | 530 |
| Potato Wedges | 810 |
| **Wings,** HBBQ Hot (1) | 160 |

## Fast-Foods & Restaurants | Sodium

**McDonalds:**

| | |
|---|---|
| **Burgers:** Big Mac | 970 |
| Cheeseburger | 680 |
| Double | 1050 |
| Hamburger | 480 |
| Quarter Pounder with Cheese | 1100 |
| **Chicken McNuggets:** 6 pieces | 540 |
| Chipotle BBQ Sauce, 1 package, 1 oz | 190 |
| **Sandwich,** Prem. Grilled Chicken Ranch BLT | 1210 |
| **French Fries:** Small, 2.5 oz | 160 |
| Medium, 4 oz | 270 |
| Large, 5.4 oz | 350 |
| Ketchup, 1 package, 10g | 100 |
| **Breakfast:** Egg McMuffin | 780 |
| Big Breakfast, reg. size Biscuit | 1560 |
| Hash Browns, 2 oz | 310 |
| Hotcakes, with Syrup & Whipped Margarine | 665 |
| Sausage Burrito | 790 |
| Southern Style Chicken Biscuit, regular bisc. | 1180 |
| **Desserts/Shakes:** Hot Fudge Sundae | 170 |
| Strawberry McCafe Shake, 12 fl.oz | 240 |

**Pizza Hut:**

**Pan Pizza:** *12", Per ½ Pizza, 4 Slices*

| | |
|---|---|
| Meat Lovers | 3280 |
| Cheese; Chicken Supreme; average | 2110 |
| Pepperoni; Supreme, average | 2560 |
| Pepperoni Lover's: Super Supreme, av. | 3120 |

**Subway:**

**6" Lowfat Sandwich:** *W/ Set Menu Board Toppings, no oil*

| | |
|---|---|
| Chicken, oven roasted | 610 |
| Roast Beef | 660 |
| Subway Club | 850 |
| Sweet Onion Chicken Teriyaki | 840 |

**6" Sandwiches:** *With Set Menu Board Toppings, no Oil*

| | |
|---|---|
| BLT; Tuna, average | 625 |
| Meatball Marinara | 920 |
| Spicy Italian | 1490 |
| **12" Footlong** ~ Double above figures | |

**Taco Bell:**

| | |
|---|---|
| **Burritos:** Combo, 8.2 oz | 1380 |
| Supreme, Chicken; Steak, average | 1065 |
| **Chapulas,** Chicken; Steak, average | 515 |
| **Gorditas,** Cheesy Crunch | 830 |
| **Nachos:** Regular | 420 |
| BellGrande | 1270 |
| **Specialties,** Cheese Quesadillas | 990 |
| **Tacos:** Chicken, Soft | 480 |
| Crunchy Supreme | 340 |

# Index A - C

# Index C - E

## e-BOOK EDITIONS

### NOW AVAILABLE FOR
### KINDLE • 0 iPAD • iPHONE
### Fully Searchable & Enhanced

# Index E - J

**FAST-FOODS INDEX**
**~ PAGE 175 ~**

# Index O - S

**FAST-FOODS INDEX**
**~ PAGE 175 ~**